Social and Interpersonal Dynamics in Pain

Tine Vervoort • Kai Karos
Zina Trost • Kenneth M. Prkachin
Editors

Social and Interpersonal Dynamics in Pain

We Don't Suffer Alone

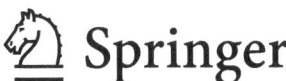 Springer

Editors
Tine Vervoort
Department of Experimental-Clinical and
Health Psychology
Ghent University
Ghent, Belgium

Zina Trost
Department of Psychology
University of Alabama at Birmingham
Birmingham, AL, USA

Kai Karos
Research Group on Health Psychology
KU Leuven
Leuven, Belgium

Kenneth M. Prkachin
Department of Psychology
University of Northern British Columbia
Prince George, BC, Canada

ISBN 978-3-030-08680-0   ISBN 978-3-319-78340-6   (eBook)
https://doi.org/10.1007/978-3-319-78340-6

Printed on acid-free paper

This Springer imprint is published by the registered company Springer International Publishing AG part of Springer Nature.
The registered company address is: Gewerbestrasse 11, 6330 Cham, Switzerland

Preface

We have come a long way in understanding and treating pain. Any contemporary model of pain includes both medical and psychosocial factors and acknowledges the reciprocal influences among these factors in understanding pain. Early theories of pain, however, were very different. Descartes' explanation of pain assumed sensory experience of pain resulting directly from stimulation of specific noxious receptors. Building on Descartes' notion of pain, a biomedical approach to pain dominated its conceptualization and treatment for a long time. The traditional biomedical model of pain focuses on structural and biological abnormalities to explain the occurrence and the maintenance of pain. The biomedical perspective assumes linear one-to-one relationships between tissue damage, pain, and disability (Waddell, 1992). Postulation of the "Gate Control Theory," Melzack and Wall (1965) marked a turning point in our understanding of pain in two respects. The first was in terms of the mechanisms of the transmission and modulation of nociceptive signals, the second was in terms of its recognition of pain as a psychophysiological phenomenon resulting from the interaction between physiological and psychological events. In contrast to Descartes' ideas, the transmission of information about painful events in the periphery is not a simple one-way system. The Gate Control Theory suggested that several processes mediated by the central nervous system, including cognition and affect, could directly impact the transmission and perception of nociceptive sensory information from the periphery.

The Gate Control Theory framework conferred legitimacy upon the idea that a complete understanding of pain required appreciation of its regulation by psychological factors. It was, in essence, a biopsychological model. A more precise understanding of what psychological factors are involved in pain and how they work inevitably invited questions embedded in the recognition that pain and its underlying mechanisms occur in living organisms in which its presence has implications not only for the sufferer but also for her or his conspecifics. In humans, the implications of pain play out from the simple level of the interaction between someone who is in pain and a companion to the complex ways in which societies and cultures have organized collective responses to the fact of pain, such as in how health care is delivered. Observations, empirical studies, conceptual frameworks, and theoretical models implicating social influences in the explanation of pain phenomena emerged with increasing frequency toward the latter half of the twentieth century and an even more accelerated pace since then. This expansion of the domain of influences affirms that a comprehensive understanding of pain requires the application of a biopsychosocial perspective, which brings insights from the study and conceptualization of social processes to bear on pain phenomena.

Specifically, it has become increasingly clear that although pain is commonly defined as private, highly personal, and subjective, it is, *in essence*, also a social experience; pain, as an archetypal sign of threat, not only demands the attention of the sufferer (Eccleston & Crombez, 1999), it also demands, through behavioral manifestations, the attention and potentially the concern of others in the social environment (Craig, 2004; Hadjistavropoulos & Craig, 2002; Hadjistavropoulos et al., 2011). Others' responses, in turn, might have a tremendous impact upon the sufferer's pain experience. For example, families may influence children's experiences of pain through family members' own experiences of pain and use of coping strategies in dealing with their own pain and their child's pain (Goodman & McGrath, 2003; Schanberg et al., 2001), as well as by a range of diverse caregiving behaviors that differentially impact upon the child's pain responses (Peterson & Palermo, 2004; Vervoort et al., 2011; Walker, Claar & Garber, 2002). A comprehensive understanding of pain as a *social* experience, i.e., the dynamic interplay between a sufferer's pain experience and the social environment in which pain emerges, requires consideration of social or communication features of the pain as these are important determinants of pain experience, pain expression, and related disability and suffering (Craig, 2004; Hajistavropolous & Craig, 2002; Hadjistavropoulos et al., 2011).

It is now generally accepted that the association between physical impairment and pain intensity and pain-related disability is loose and that psychological and social factors play a crucial role in understanding pain and pain-related problems. However, empirical inquiry has focused largely upon the biological and psychological dimensions of pain; the social dimension has long been neglected. Yet, it has become increasingly clear that pain affects others in a myriad of ways. Observer' responses, in turn, impact sufferers' pain experience and expression. Indeed, we rarely suffer alone. Pain almost always occurs in the context of a dynamic and influential social network with others. This book is devoted to this idea, and the realization that we can only fully understand and treat pain, when we also acknowledge the interpersonal or social context in which pain occurs.

This book originated in the spring of 2015, when we were invited to present a symposium entitled "We do not suffer alone: recent insights into interpersonal dynamics of pain" at the 28th convention for the Association for Psychological Science in New York City. The symposium was intended to give an overview of recent advances in the research on interpersonal factors in pain. It covered a wide area of topics including injustice perceptions in pain sufferers, the effect of threatening social environments on fear learning, the role of emotion regulation in parents of children in pain, and the empathic reaction of others to someone else's pain. In the course of preparing the symposium and in subsequent discussions among us and

Springer representative Morgan Ryan, it became apparent that the specific topics addressed were a mere sampling of work from a much larger domain that had, since the turn of the twenty-first century, acquired sufficient breadth and sophistication to warrant the term "field," and that, despite this, a comprehensive treatment of the field in the form of a book did not exist. It did not take much convincing before we all realized the promise and potential of such a project. We felt that this endeavor was both timely and potentially rewarding and would appeal to a diverse audience of researchers, clinicians, and patients who deal with pain in their daily lives and all those who are interested in pain.

Leading authorities in the field of interpersonal dynamics of pain were invited to provide a compelling overview of where the field is coming from, where it currently stands, and which promising avenues lay ahead of us. The first part of this book is devoted to *Theoretical foundations* upon which most of the research in this area has been based. The second part is devoted to *Pain expression*, the vehicle through which pain essentially becomes an interpersonal phenomenon. The third part is devoted to underlying *Neuroscience* of interpersonal pain dynamics. With recent advances in neuroscience and fundamental research in nonhuman species, we now understand much more about the biological and evolutionary mechanisms that underlie interpersonal dynamics in pain. Part IV is devoted to the effect of *Facing pain in others* and explores the myriad of influences that contextual factors can have on observers' cognitive, affective, and behavioral responses to someone else's pain. This part is closely linked to Part V, which describes *Observer responses* to other's pain, with a special focus on caregivers. The focus of this part is on the effect that observer responses have on the person in pain. Part VI, *Across the lifespan*, provides a developmental perspective on interpersonal pain dynamics and highlights crucial changes across infancy, childhood, adulthood, and elderly. Part VII explores the effect of the larger *Societal context* on pain, with a focus on gender and race. Part VIII, *towards change,* takes on a clinical focus and demonstrates how insights from interpersonal pain dynamics can be translated to assessment and treatment of pain.

All in all, the aim of this book is to highlight the crucial importance of interpersonal dynamics in the understanding and treatment of acute and chronic pain by summarizing the significant advances that have been made in this field in the past, and by formulating specific goals for the future which we discuss within the concluding chapter "Where we have been, where we need to go."

Ghent, Belgium   Tine Vervoort
Leuven, Belgium   Kai Karos
Birmingham, AL, USA   Zina Trost
Prince George, BC, Canada   Kenneth M. Prkachin

References

Craig, K. D. (2004). Social communication of pain enhances protective functions: A comment on Deyo, Prkachin and Mercer. *Pain, 107*, 5–6.

Eccleston, C., & Crombez, G. (1999). Pain demands attention: A cognitive-affective model of the interruptive function of pain. *Psychological Bulletin, 125*, 356–366.

Goodman, J. E., & McGrath, P. J. (2003). Mothers' modelling influences children's pain during a cold pressor task. *Pain, 104*, 559–565.

Hadjistavropoulos, T., & Craig, K. D. (2002). A theoretical framework for understanding self-report and observational measures of pain: A communications model. *Behaviour Research and Therapy, 40*, 551–570.

Hadjistavropoulos, T., Craig, K. D., Duck, S., Cano, A., Goubert, L., Jackson, P. L., …, Fitzgerald, T. D. (2011). A biopsychosocial formulation of pain communication. *Psychological Bulletin, 137*, 910–939.

Melzack, R., & Wall, P. D. (1965). Pain mechanisms. *Science*, 150, 971–979.

Peterson, C. C., & Palermo, T. M. (2004). Parental reinforcement of recurrent pain: The moderating impact of child depression and anxiety on functional disability. *Pain, 131*, 132–141.

Schanberg, L. E., Anthony, K. K., Gil, K. M., Lefebvre, J. C., Kredich, D. W., & Macharoni, L. M. (2001). Family pain history predicts child health status in children with chronic rheumatic disease. *Pediatrics, 108*, 247–254.

Vervoort, T., Caes, L, Trost, Z., Sullivan, M. J. L., Vangronsveld, K., & Goubert, L. (2011). Social modulation of facial pain display in high catastrophizing children: An observational study in schoolchildren and their parents. *Pain, 152*, 1591–1599.

Waddell, G. (1992). Biopsychosocial analysis of low back pain. *Baillieres Clinical Rheumatology, 6*, 523–557.

Walker, L. S., Claar, R. L., & Garber, J. (2002). Social consequences of children's pain: When do they encourage symptom maintenance? *Journal of Pediatric Psychology, 27*, 689–698.

Contents

Contributors

Erinn L. Acland Department of Psychology, University of Toronto Mississauga, Mississauga, ON, Canada

Line Caes Faculty of Natural Sciences, Division of Psychology, University of Stirling, Stirling, UK

Annmarie Cano Wayne State University, Detroit, MI, USA

Shannon M. Clark Wayne State University, Detroit, MI, USA

Jeffrey F. Cohn University of Pittsburgh, Pittsburgh, PA, USA

Kaytlin Constantin Department of Psychology, University of Guelph, Guelph, ON, Canada

Kenneth D. Craig University of British Columbia, Vancouver, BC, Canada

Julie K. Cremeans-Smith Department of Psychological Sciences, Kent State University at Stark, North Canton, OH, USA

Lies De Ruddere Department of Experimental-Clinical and Health Psychology, Ghent University, Ghent, Belgium

Rocio de la Vega Department of Rehabilitation Medicine, University of Washington, Seattle, WA, USA

Center for Child Health, Behavior, and Development, Seattle Children's Research Institute, Seattle, WA, USA

Brian Blake Drwecki Regis University, Denver, CO, USA

M. Erin Browne University of Regina, Regina, SK, Canada

Emma Fisher Center for Child Health, Behavior, and Development, Seattle Children's Research Institute, Seattle, WA, USA

Natasha L. Gallant Department of Psychology and Centre on Aging and Health, University of Regina, Regina, SK, Canada

Hannah Gennis Department of Psychology, York University, Toronto, ON, Canada

Liesbet Goubert Department of Experimental-Clinical and Health Psychology, Ghent University, Ghent, Belgium

Thomas Hadjistavropoulos Department of Psychology and Centre on Aging and Health, University of Regina, Regina, SK, Canada

Zakia Hammal The Robotics Institute, Carnegie Mellon University, Pittsburgh, PA, USA

Lauren C. Heathcote Stanford University, Stanford, CA, USA

Philip L. Jackson École de Psychologie, Université Laval, Québec, QC, Canada

Centre interdisciplinaire de recherche en réadaptation et intégration sociale, Québec, QC, Canada

Centre de recherche de l'Institut universitaire en santé mental de Québec, Québec, QC, Canada

Judith Kappesser Department of Clinical Psychology, Justus-Liebig-University Giessen, Giessen, Germany

Kai Karos Research Group on Health Psychology, KU Leuven, Leuven, Belgium

Kimberley A. Kaseweter University of British Columbia, Okanagan Campus, Kelowna, BC, Canada

Edmund Keogh Department of Psychology, University of Bath, Bath, UK

Miriam Kunz Department of General Practice and Elderly Care Medicine, University of Groningen, University Medical Center Groningen, Groningen, The Netherlands

Michelle T. Leonard University of Michigan–Dearborn, Dearborn, MI, USA

Navdeep K. Lidhar Department of Psychology, University of Toronto Mississauga, Mississauga, ON, Canada

Marc O. Martel Faculties of Dentistry and Medicine, McGill University, Montreal, QC, Canada

Loren J. Martin Department of Psychology, University of Toronto Mississauga, Mississauga, ON, Canada

Department of Cell Systems and Biology, University of Toronto Mississauga, Mississauga, ON, Canada

C. Meghan McMurtry Department of Psychology, University of Guelph, Guelph, ON, Canada

Pediatric Chronic Pain Program, McMaster Children's Hospital, Hamilton, ON, Canada

Children's Health Research Institute, London, ON, Canada

Department of Paediatrics, Schulich School of Medicine & Dentistry, Western University, London, ON, Canada

Aurore Meugnot Centre interdisciplinaire de recherche en réadaptation et intégration sociale, Québec, QC, Canada

Centre de recherche de l'Institut universitaire en santé mental de Québec, Québec, QC, Canada

Rachel L. Moline Department of Psychology, University of Guelph, Guelph, ON, Canada

Melanie Noel University of Calgary, Calgary, AB, Canada

Tonya M. Palermo Center for Child Health, Behavior, and Development, Seattle Children's Research Institute, Seattle, WA, USA

Department of Anesthesiology and Pain Medicine, University of Washington, Seattle, WA, USA

Bethany Pester Wayne State University, Detroit, MI, USA

Rebecca Pillai Riddell Department of Psychology, York University, Toronto, ON, Canada

Department of Psychiatry, Hospital for Sick Children, Toronto, ON, Canada

Department of Psychiatry, University of Toronto, Toronto, ON, Canada

Kenneth M. Prkachin Department of Psychology, University of Northern British Columbia, Prince George, BC, Canada

Laura Simons Department of Anesthesiology, Perioperative and Pain Medicine, Stanford University School of Medicine, Stanford, CA, USA

Michael J. L. Sullivan Department of Psychology, McGill University, Montreal, QC, Canada

Raymond Tait Department of Psychiatry and Behavioral Neuroscience, Saint Louis University School of Medicine, St. Louis, MO, USA

Marie-Pier B. Tremblay École de Psychologie, Université Laval, Québec, QC, Canada

Centre interdisciplinaire de recherche en réadaptation et intégration sociale, Québec, QC, Canada

Centre de recherche de l'Institut universitaire en santé mental de Québec, Québec, QC, Canada

Zina Trost Department of Psychology, University of Alabama at Birmingham, Birmingham, AL, USA

Tine Vervoort Department of Experimental-Clinical and Health Psychology, Ghent University, Ghent, Belgium

Amanda C de C Williams Clinical. Educational & Health Psychology, University College London, London, UK

About the Editors

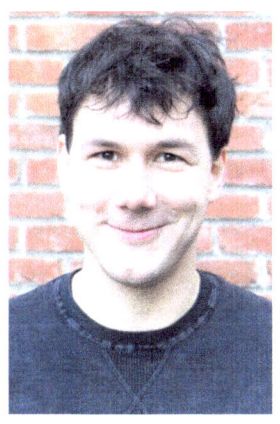

Kai Karos is a PhD student at the Research Group for Health Psychology at the KU Leuven, Belgium. He received his bachelor's in psychology from Maastricht University in 2009 and finished the research master in psychopathology at Maastricht University in 2012. His research concerns the effects of threatening interpersonal environments on the experience and expression of pain. Drawing from social, evolutionary, learning and health psychology, he is interested in how interpersonal threat affects facial expression of pain, self-reported pain ratings, learning of pain-related fear, and interpersonal processes such as aggression and empathy. Moreover, he developed a theoretical, motivational framework which outlines how acute and chronic pain challenge several interpersonal human needs such as the need to belong, the need for autonomy, and the need for justice. His work has been presented at several international congresses and published in internationally peer-reviewed papers.

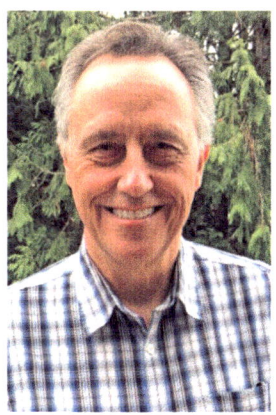

Kenneth M. Prkachin is Professor Emeritus of Psychology at the University of Northern British Columbia. He trained in clinical psychology at the University of British Columbia where he developed an abiding interest in the communication of emotion and its role in interpersonal relationships and health. This, combined with his early experience as a clinician working with patients suffering from pain, led him to embark on a clinician-scientist's journey to understand the process of pain communication and the insights that this can provide toward understanding their lives. His published work has examined various components of the pain process articulated in the earliest communication model of pain, including studies of the nature of pain expression, the ways in which others respond to people in pain, and the clinical implications of pain expression. He was a central contributor to the first studies examining brain systems involved in interpreting pain in others and the development of automated systems for detecting pain. Retired from teaching, he maintains a clinical practice and active involvement in programs of research on empathy and clinical applications of knowledge about pain expression when he is not watching the sailboats and cruise ships plying the waters of the Salish Sea from his deck.

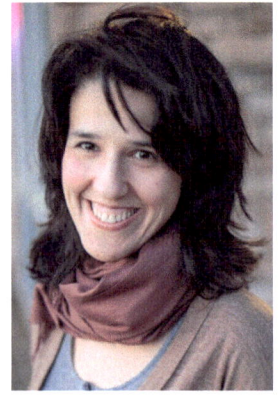

Zina Trost received her Bachelor's in Psychology in 2003 from Fordham University in New York City, where she grew up after her family immigrated from St. Petersburg, Russia, in 1991. She received her doctorate in clinical health psychology from Ohio University where she first began to explore her interests in chronic pain and illness, subsequently completing an internship at the University of Washington Medical Center, and postdoctoral fellowship at McGill University in Montreal, Canada. Dr. Trost's research addresses how individuals cope with pain and physical trauma—specifically cognitive, emotional, and behavioral responses to pain that can contribute to disability or facilitate positive adjustment, as well as the potential modulating influence of social, cultural, and contextual factors. Her work uses both clinical and laboratory paradigms to examine the mechanisms and impact of psychological constructs such as pain-related fear, catastrophizing, and perceptions of injustice among individuals with pain, injury, and illness. Dr. Trost's recent work has adapted virtual reality and gaming technologies (including augmented reality and simulation) to aid in pain coping and rehabilitation among individuals with chronic pain and physical trauma, in particular spinal cord injury. She is working on harnessing these technologies to examine interpersonal processes in the context of pain and illness. Dr. Trost has received national and international recognition for her work and is grateful for wonderful colleagues worldwide.

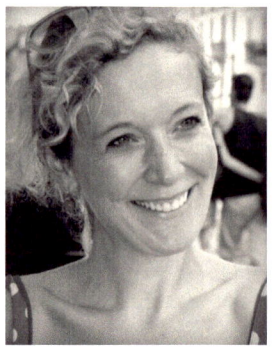

Tine Vervoort is a Research Professor at the Department of Experimental-Clinical and Health Psychology, Ghent University, Belgium. Dr. Vervoort came to her career as a research psychologist interested in pediatric psychology with a background in psychiatric (child/adolescent) nursing and clinical psychology. Having completed her PhD in clinical psychology on social determinants of child pain expression she has systematically conceptualized the dynamic interaction between children in pain and caregivers in terms that facilitate empirical study of family socialization and social context as determinants of child pain experience. Drawing upon an affective-motivational account of pain, she has developed a theoretically integrative and clinically informative program of research addressing (1) the nature and (social) determinants of child (facial) pain expression/pain experience; (2) emotion regulatory function of child pain-related attention and behavioral impact; (3) the nature and role of observer emotion regulation in understanding observers' emotional and behavioral responses; and, most recently, (4) the nature and role of parental injustice appraisals in the context of their child's pain. Her work has been presented at numerous international congresses and published in internationally peer-reviewed papers. She is likewise the recipient of a number of prestigious national and international awards/grants. She is also the proud mother of four boys.

Part I
Theoretical Foundations

Chapter 1
Why Do We Care? Evolutionary Mechanisms in the Social Dimension of Pain

Amanda C de C Williams and Judith Kappesser

Abstract Human expression of pain and others' responses to it are explored using an evolutionary framework. Pain itself functions to promote recovery, and both the capacity to react to damaging stimuli and many behaviors showing the aversive nature of the event are widespread in animals. One of the behaviors, facial expression of pain, is described in detail, as it is a direct communication of pain to those close by, and is understood across ages, ethnicities, roles, and relationships. Those who observe another's pain may respond in various ways, from empathy to exploitation. Evolutionary mechanisms help us understand the biases in how we perceive and judge behavior that indicates pain, and how this informs social responses to pain, particularly in clinical and caregiving settings.

Keywords Evolutionary psychology · Facial expression · Social interaction · Empathy · Help-giving

We care because we are wired to care: to attend to other people's expression of pain and to understand its meaning; to feel distress in relation to their distress; and to be motivated to reduce their distress, and ours, if we are able to do so. All those processes are the results of evolution, evident not only in humans but also in other mammals, and extensively described in rodents. In this chapter, we give a brief introduction to evolution and pain in humans and other animals and then attempt to show how considering an evolutionary psychology perspective in pain research could broaden our understanding. Few studies have been designed to investigate evolutionary hypotheses, so we also draw on results of a wider set of studies that can be reinterpreted within an evolutionary psychology framework. With regard to this literature, we first explore the evolved expression of pain and its recognition and

A C de C Williams (✉)
Clinical. Educational & Health Psychology, University College London, London, UK
e-mail: amanda.williams@ucl.ac.uk

J. Kappesser
Department of Clinical Psychology, Justus-Liebig-University Giessen, Giessen, Germany

© Springer International Publishing AG, part of Springer Nature 2018
T. Vervoort et al. (eds.), *Social and Interpersonal Dynamics in Pain*,
https://doi.org/10.1007/978-3-319-78340-6_1

3

interpretation by those around the person in pain and then describe the evolutionary background of empathic and helpful responses. We close with questions and unexplored areas that need attention.

Evolution and Pain

Despite wide acceptance, evolutionary theory is surprisingly often misunderstood or misapplied. Genes are passed to the next generations when they confer survival and/or reproductive advantage, or did so in our ancestral environment, not because they determine physical and mental superiority or well-being. The concept of the "selfish gene" (Dawkins, 1976/1989) was intended to show how different alleles of genes compete by improving the reproductive success of individuals carrying those alleles. Far from making the individual "selfish," in pursuing his or her survival and reproductive success, as often misinterpreted, these alleles can encourage altruistic behavior towards kin who may also carry those alleles, even if such behavior seems disadvantageous to the altruist.

There is little disagreement that acute pain is an essential survival mechanism, with striking conservation of physiological processes and cellular substrates across vertebrates and invertebrates (St. John Smith & Lewin, 2009; Walters, 1994, 2016). People with congenital insensitivity to pain (Nagasako, Oaklander, & Dworkin, 2003) have their lives drastically shortened by this dysfunction. There is less certainty about chronic pain, often asserted to have no purpose but being the inevitable cost of the efficient acute pain alarm system (Nesse & Stearns, 2008). There are alternative theories, not so widely adopted: one concerns the failure of reregulation of a dysregulated (i.e., sensitized) nervous system because of prolonged protective behavior (Williams, 2016); another concerns pain as a signal to elicit help (Finlay & Syal, 2014). However, data on chronic pain in nonhuman animals are scarce, so many of the studies on which we draw in this chapter do not, unfortunately, concern chronic pain.

Pain and Behavior

In relation to pain, we know almost nothing about the behavior of our remote ancestors when injured or affected by painful disease, except that there is sufficient evidence from healed major fractures (Mithen, 1996; Redfern, 2010) to recognize that injured members of hominid groups were not necessarily abandoned to die, but supported through healing and, presumably, recovery of function. We know a little about pain-related behavior in situations where health-care is scarce or inaccessible, but studies framing observed behavior in Western norms tell us little (Encandela, 1993) since they use the implicit norm of the white Western male as the ideal both of sensitivity to pain and of correct expression of pain (Bourke, 2014).

The similarities in behavioral effects of pain across only very distantly related animals demonstrate its powerful motivational effects. Here, though, we need to appreciate that we have virtually no accounts of chronic pain in wild animals, only in animals that are captive in zoos, in farming, as companion animals or in research laboratories (Williams, 2016). As with early hominids, skeletal remains and observations of injured animals in the wild indicate that they do not necessarily fall victim to predators or lethal infection, but may heal, recover, and function remarkably well despite enduring such disabilities as missing digits or limbs, or dysfunctional joints including jaws (Beamish & O'Riain, 2014; Byrne & Stokes, 2002; Chapman & Chapman, 1969; Forsman, Otto, & Muths, 2006; Jurmain, 1997; Malgorzata, Carey, & Molleman, 2009).

Are skeletons with healed injuries those of lone injured individuals who somehow survived, or might conspecifics have helped, actively or passively? Pain from injury maintains attention on the wound and on priorities for recovery (Wall, 1979); the acutely injured animal behaves in very consistent ways across many species, reducing nonessential activity, often eating and socializing less and resting and sleeping more (Wall, 1979; Walters, 1994). These behaviors reduce strain on the injured site/s that might exacerbate injury or prolong healing, and allow energy resources to be committed to mobilizing an effective, but energy-demanding, immune response (Shakhar & Shakhar, 2015), given the serious threat of infection to survival. Sensitization is central to the state of acute pain (Walters, 1994), fostering wound care and sparing of the affected part, and heightening vigilance to potential threats. Again, it is shared not only by vertebrates but also invertebrates (Elwood, 2011; St. John Smith & Lewin, 2009; Tobin & Bargmann, 2004; Walters, 2016), from mollusks (Walters & Moroz, 2009) and flatworms (St. John Smith & Lewin, 2009; Tobin & Bargmann, 2004) to insects (Adamo, 2016; St. John Smith & Lewin, 2009).

Function is gradually recovered, possibly with limping or guarding of the injured area or limb, observed not just in mammals or (terrestrial) vertebrates but also in some crustaceans (Dyuizen, Kotsyuba, & Lamash, 2012) and cephalopods (Alupay, Hadjisolomou, & Crook, 2014). Although there are excellent accounts of the withdrawn state in undomesticated deer and dogs (Wall, 1979), and in literature on the welfare of laboratory and farm animals (e.g., Anil, Anil, & Deen, 2005; Whittaker & Howarth, 2014), they are surprisingly few, and there is almost no observation of behavior during recovery. In the wild, the need to conserve resources conflicts with needs to obtain food and ensure safety (which usually require mobility, whether to forage or hunt, to evade predators or to stay within the social group, such as family or herd). It is not clear how this conflict is resolved.

Animal behaviors associated with pain and injury promote survival and return to function. Interestingly, they also share features with an evolutionary model of depression as a way to survive defeat and entrapment (Gilbert & Allan, 1998). In humans, however, pain behaviors have mainly been studied in clinical settings, using the framework of a particular psychological theory, operant learning. This in turn arose from a radical behaviorist stance in which evolution was acknowledged as having shaped the human body but was rarely referred to in descriptions of human behavior or psychological capacities. Reinforcers available in the environment of the person with pain, often social behaviors of family members but also relief from feared activities (avoidance), and analgesic and psychotropic effects of prescribed or self-selected drugs, were identified as important contingencies for behavior expressing pain. While not doubting that behaviors associated with pain, including facial expression (Kunz, Rainville, & Lautenbacher, 2011), can come under operant reinforcement, the concern is that reinforcement is assumed rather than demonstrated in many clinical settings. The operant behavior paradigm was applied to chronic pain, on the basis of careful observation and discussion with the person in pain, with considerable benefits (Fordyce, 1982; Main, Keefe, Jensen, Vlaeyen, & Vowles, 2014) and still informs much of current cognitive behavior therapy practice in the field of pain treatment (Morley, 2011).

The varied behaviors expressing pain, for which Fordyce (1976) established the term "pain behaviors," are commonly classified as verbal and nonverbal (e.g., Hadjistavropoulos & Craig, 2002): verbal behaviors include crying out, exclaiming, and pain self-reports and description; nonverbal behaviors range from paralinguistic features of vocalization, other nonverbal qualities of speech, physiological and bodily activity to facial expressions. Pain behaviors also include such complex behaviors as seeking medical help or the help or support of nonprofessional others: these are further explored below. Of all the behaviors associated with pain, facial expression dominates observers' estimates of pain and other impressions of the person in pain (Hadjistavropoulos, Breau, & Craig, 2011; Poole & Craig, 1992).

Facial Expression of Pain

Evolutionary psychologists assume that facial expressions of emotions in general have two functions: (1) to communicate information about internal state (e.g., "I am in pain"), and (2) to identify the (evolutionarily recurrent) situation facing the person (e.g., "Something/somebody hurt me."). Others emphasize that facial expressions communicate intention (Fridlund, 1994). All such information is potentially of value to observers, and humans have a coevolved ability to decode facial expressions of others into knowledge about their states, discussed below under *Others' responses to facial expression of pain* (see also Cosmides & Tooby, 2000).

Facial expressions of emotion, with a focus on the "core" emotions of happiness, fear, anger, surprise, disgust, and sadness (but not pain), have been studied in humans for several decades (Ekman, 1992, 1993). Studies of facial expression mainly use the Facial Action Coding System (FACS: Ekman & Friesen, 1978; Ekman, Friesen, & Hager, 2002) that identifies over 40 distinct muscular movements in the face: in various combinations, these constitute expressions of the core emotions. The expressions appear to be produced in a consistent way across ages and cultures, and are universally recognized at a level better than chance (Calvo & Nummenmaa, 2016; Ekman, 1989) (although with an in-group advantage: Elfenbein & Ambady, 2002; Xu, Zuo, Wang, & Han, 2009). They appear to be processed categorically and rapidly, even under suboptimal visual conditions (Calvo & Nummenmaa, 2016).

The same is, as far as can be ascertained, also true of facial expression of pain (Williams, 2002). The facial actions that characterize human pain expression are distinguishable from those of other emotions (Kappesser & Williams, 2002; Prkachin & Solomon, 2008; Williams, 2002). There may be ways to analyze facial expression of pain other than by separate facial actions, such as by clustering groups (Kunz & Lautenbacher, 2014). Facial expression of pain has not only been identified in humans but also in mammals, notably rodents (Chambers & Mogil, 2015; Langford et al., 2010), in which grimace scales are now used as the most sensitive indicator of pain in analgesic research (NC3), rabbits (Keating, Thomas, Flecknell, & Leach, 2012), cats (Holden et al., 2014), and horses (Dalla Costa et al., 2014), the latter despite the assumption that prey animals would suppress all expression of pain (Underwood, 2002), and others.

To date, findings on facial expression of emotions come mainly from studies that use posed expressions of single emotions in still photographs. In everyday life, expressions are dynamic, often blended with other emotional expression or communicative messages in the face (e.g., Kunz, Prkachin, & Lautenbacher, 2013), spontaneous rather than posed, and may be amplified or suppressed deliberately. Under these conditions, recognition may be more (Krumhuber, Kappas, & Manstead, 2013) or less accurate (Calvo & Nummenmaa, 2016) but still better than chance; cultural differences emerge although strong similarities remain (Sneddon, 2011); perceptual processing takes precedence, with affective processing relatively independent; context is used much more to assign meaning to the expression (Calvo & Nummenmaa, 2016), and the categories of basic emotions themselves may differ from those described above (Jack, Garrod, & Schyns, 2014). This means that exposure to a particular facial expression is expected to improve identification of that expression (Calvo & Nummenmaa, 2016; Elfenbein & Ambady, 2003), an issue discussed later in relation to clinician estimation of patients' pain. Unfortunately, much of the focus of automatic (i.e., performed by technology not humans) detection of facial expression of pain has been on faked pain or deception (e.g., Bartlett, Littlewort, Frank, & Lee, 2014), easy to produce in experimental situations but of little clinical use in detecting subtle or suppressed pain expression.

Facial Expression of Pain in Social Settings

Of major importance is the recognition that facial expression of pain is communicative, and has no direct protective function (Salomons, Coan, Hunt, Backonja, & Davidson, 2008) in the way that limping, for instance, directly spares the injured limb; there may, of course, be indirect benefit by mobilizing others' help. There is evidence on rapid processing as an alerting signal for others (Khatibi et al., 2015; Reicherts et al., 2012), with facial expression of pain recognized even before gender (Czekala, Maguière, Mazza, Jackson, & Frot, 2015) or other emotions (Reicherts et al., 2012). Facial expression of pain is understood across differences in age and culture (Prkachin, 2011; Williams, 2002), although issues of cultural differences and similarity in all facial expression of emotion are complex and await a better generation of studies (Jack, 2013). The social communication model of pain (Craig, 2015; Hadjistavropoulos & Craig, 2002) details the encoding and decoding processes and internal and external influences on them. These include such factors as sex differences in both encoding and decoding pain expression (Keogh, 2014); and differences between facial expression of pain and other communication, particularly verbal pain ratings (Kunz, Mylius, Schepelmann, & Lautenbacher, 2004; Labus, Keefe, & Jensen, 2003).

Evolutionary psychologists propose that all communication systems require rules on whether to transmit information or not. When over evolutionary time it was, on average, beneficial to share emotional state and risk assessment with conspecifics nearby, species-typical facial and other expressions of emotion were selected (Cosmides & Tooby, 2000). In such a framework, expressing pain in the face provides information to those close by (e.g., kin and cooperators) on a possible proximate danger to them, and might elicit their help. Averaged across individuals over evolutionary time, not all emotional states are advantageous for an organism to share in every setting. Among the factors governing whether a particular emotion should be expressed are the relationship between displayer and observer, as well as the information that the particular expression would reveal (Cosmides & Tooby, 2000). For pain information, it is likely more beneficial to share information with closer cooperators than with potential competitors or adversaries.

These effects can be simulated using artificial life experiments, and predictions about evolutionary processes can be tested by experiments in silico (Niazi & Hussain, 2011). Such experiments can simulate complex behaviors in combination with environmental pressures over evolutionary time. Eventual simulation outcomes, therefore, can demonstrate which behaviors are more or less adaptive in certain environments. For pain (Williams, Gallagher, Fidalgo, & Bentley, 2016), agents were programed to show certain behavioral strategies: (1) to express pain or not, and (2) when encountering others who showed pain to help (altruistic strategy), ignore (non-altruistic strategy) or exploit them (selfish strategy). Agents then interacted randomly while foraging, i.e., gaining energy. Random injury interrupted energy gain for a fixed time unless help from an altruistic agent speeded recovery. Showing altruistic behavior, however, was associated with a loss of energy. The initial proportions of each behavior were varied, as were injury severity and interaction rates. Each model was run for 10,000 iterations. Results showed that over evolutionary time, helpful behaviors were more robust to variation in environmental and behavioral conditions than was expression of pain. Expression of pain was particularly disadvantageous for agents when they were exploited or when injury was frequent. Results were meaningful since the behavioral interactions found in this simulation study resembled those evident from mammalian pain research which covers only a few interactions rather than an evolutionarily relevant time span.

The evolutionary theories described above relate well to experimental results, where the presence of a stranger, although intended as a neutral observer, inhibits facial expression of pain; it is only if the observer is known to be friendly that this inhibition is released (Krahé, Springer, Weinman, & Fotopoulou, 2013). The same effect holds for an observer of different ethnicity (Hsieh, Tripp, & Ji, 2011). In one experimental study, social threat resulted in people with high catastrophizing scores suppressing facial pain expression, while verbal report increased (Peeters & Vlaeyen, 2011). It is quite possible that the expression of pain to a clinician, but not to strangers in a waiting room, represents the same phenomenon (i.e., a release of suppression) rather than the "exaggeration" often assumed (Williams, 2002). Understanding of children's expression of pain, and its modulation in front of their caregivers, would benefit from similar analysis (Zeltzer & Tsao, 2006). Such encounters are also modulated by characteristics such as sex of person in pain and observer, with boys and men subject to more pervasive cultural expectations to suppress expression of pain (Keogh, 2014).

Others' Responses to Facial Expression of Pain

Facial expression of emotion necessarily coevolves with attention to it and comprehension of its meaning (Fridlund, 1994), providing relevant information for the observer without disadvantaging the sender. Observers' recognition of emotional facial displays including pain are found to be above chance (Calvo & Nummenmaa, 2016; Kappesser & Williams, 2002; Simon, Craig, Gosselin, Belin, & Rainville, 2008), although influenced by characteristics of the person observed and by beliefs and role of the observer (Tait, Chibnall, & Jovel, 2014; Tait, Chibnall, & Kalauokalani, 2009), as well as the social context (Schiavenato & Craig, 2010). In particular, ethnicity and sex of the person in pain affect pain ratings: clinicians (predominantly white and male) are far more likely to rate the pain of black African-Americans (Staton et al., 2007) and of women (Pronina & Rule, 2014; Schäfer, Prkachin, Kaseweter, & Williams, 2016) lower than they rate their own pain.

In an application of signaling theory, an evolutionary mechanism whereby a signal of need has a cost to the signaler that thereby indicates its honesty, Steinkopf (2016) has proposed that given observers' less than perfect accuracy distinguishing genuine from faked pain facial expression (Hill & Craig, 2004), and the potential waste of resources of the individual who responds to the faked expression, observers refer to the context to help them to judge credibility of the pain/need signal. This explains the weight put on medical validation (Chibnall & Tait, 2009) by laypeople and health care personnel; on opportunity costs by laypeople (Kappesser & Williams, 2008); and perhaps the weight given to beliefs about people in the particular category of the person in need (such as sex or ethnicity). Some studies suggest that these contextual variables are particularly important where pain is perceived by the observer as high intensity (De Ruddere, Goubert, Stevens, Williams, & Crombez, 2013; Tait, 2013).

Since the facial expression of pain is communicative in function and communication gains the attention of those sufficiently close, it is not surprising that it is processed in the brain in many (Jackson, Rainville, & Decety, 2006) of the same areas as those that are active in emotional processing of (the observer's) experienced pain (Hari & Kujala, 2009). Further, seeing another person in pain directs attention to pain and facilitates processing of nociceptive stimuli subsequently delivered to the observer (Khatibi, Vachon-Presseau, Schrooten, Vlaeyen, & Rainville, 2014).

In the context of judging pain, decoding of the facial expression often includes not only a judgment of the presence or absence of pain but also of intensity (Saarela et al., 2007). Particularly when made by clinicians, that judgment is substantially lower than the target person's self-rating, whether in experimental or clinical studies (Pronina & Rule, 2014; Schäfer et al., 2016; Tait et al., 2009). While underestimation of pain is a matter of clinical concern, the expectation that the two judgments be identical has no basis given that the person in pain and the observer have different data available to them (Kappesser & Williams, 2010).

As described above, the facial expression of pain may elicit help from others, behavior which is also important to understand in an evolutionary context. Despite widespread misunderstanding, the selfish gene concept (Dawkins, 1976/1989) was hugely important in generating new understandings of Darwinian theory. It led to studies of cooperation and altruism that explained why they were advantageous, rather than disadvantageous, in terms of selection. From a gene's viewpoint, the gene-bearer, who by his or her behavior fosters the survival of others who share some of those genes (depending on the degree of relatedness), makes it more likely that those genes will be passed to the next generation. This is kin altruism, for which evidence is plentiful across species (Hamilton, 1971/1996; Tooby & Cosmides, 1996). However, social species show extensive cooperation and sharing between unrelated individuals, reciprocal altruism, with punishment or exclusion of those who fail to fulfil their part of the exchange (Tooby & Cosmides, 1996; Trivers, 1971). This is discussed further below. Beyond this, altruism is also extended to those who are unlikely to be encountered again (Krasnow, Delton, Tooby, & Cosmides, 2013), or to be able to reciprocate, and the predominant explanation for this concerns reputation, of considerable value in sexual selection and in indirect reciprocation towards those known to be generous and fair (Kelly & Dunbar, 2001; Tooby & Cosmides, 1996).

It is therefore entirely consistent that, within a fairly stable social group such as characterized humans' ancestral past, kin and reciprocal altruism in particular led us to expect help-giving to those who are temporarily unable to look after themselves through painful injury or disease. Help is not the only possibility, however: conspecifics can take advantage of the injured or diseased member of their group, taking food, status, mates, and other resources, and observations of chimpanzees in the wild provide examples of such behaviors (Drews, 1996; Fabrega, 1997; Goodall, 1986). Curiously, almost all research on humans and on other primates focuses on empathy and altruism with little or no mention of the possibilities of exploitation and even cruelty to those who are temporarily or permanently in pain or disabled. That exploitation and cruelty have largely been neglected with regard to pain (with a few notable exceptions such as the Milgram experiment) may be due to the challenges of meeting ethical requirements in experimental investigations, and the barriers to careful observation and recording when exploitation and cruelty occur spontaneously. Beyond anecdotal evidence, one way to better understand the conditions that foster exploitation, and the variables affecting the relevant behaviors, is the use of simulation studies such as the one referred to in *Facial expression of pain in social settings*, and their comparison with real-world observations.

Further Pain Behaviors

Given how commonly the term "pain behavior" is used, we know surprisingly little about the behaviors: it is not even clear whether these descriptions of behavior are distinct and can be reliably applied. One reason might be that the operant approach which dominated the study of pain behaviors paid no attention to the morphology or function of the particular behavior, since, consistent with Skinnerian principles, the focus was far more on cues, reinforcers, and contingencies. This position was later modified as principles of operant learning were better understood. Another reason might be that empirical evidence regarding pain behaviors other than facial expressions, such as paravocalizations or body movements, is scarce, possibly because these categories cover a variety of behaviors of multiple levels of complexity (e.g., body movement behaviors range from reflexive withdrawal to changes in activity patterns associated with anticipated pain). With regard to vocalizations, a few studies on cries of neonates focus on cry characteristics such as pitch or frequency, and their deviation from typical cries, using automatic analysis by software programs. Parents as potential caregivers were found to be responsive to deviation in cry characteristics, although context and mood had moderating effects (LaGasse, Neal, & Lester, 2005).

Posture and body movement may also convey that emotion is positive or negative (Aviezer, Trope, & Todorov, 2012) or may specifically communicate pain (Walsh, Eccleston, & Keogh, 2014), but this area of work is in its infancy. It also appears that facial expression is used exclusively or predominantly, rather than movement abnormalities, by clinicians even when viewing pain-relevant movements (Courbalay et al., 2016), so it is not clear what importance posture and movement characteristics have in observer judgments.

From an evolutionary point of view, it is likely that behaviors indicative of pain are not a unitary group of equivalent behaviors and different behaviors may serve different functions (Prkachin, 1986). Whereas a cry of a neonate, for example, could serve as a call for closer attention from a caregiver who may be out of sight but not of hearing, facial expression would convey information about the infant's need-state (Hadjistavropoulos, Craig, Grunau, & Johnston, 1994). Further, pain behaviors differ considerably in morphology, visibility, occurrence, and interrelationships with other behaviors and characteristics (Prkachin, 1986), so it is likely that they are diverse in their functions, and possibly even in their association with particular pains. For instance, visceral pains provoke writhing and stretching in rodents (Langford et al., 2006; Roughan & Flecknell, 2004; Whittaker & Howarth, 2014) and in human infants, in whom the movements possibly have the purpose of untrapping wind that is painfully distending some part of the gut. Writhing and stretching are not described in relation to headache or musculoskeletal pains in general. When explored for association with disability, only guarding (from the list rubbing, bracing, limping, supporting, and guarding) shows a consistent relationship (Jensen, Turner, & Romano, 2007).

This evolutionarily functional diversity of pain behaviors contrasts strongly with the realization of pain behaviors in currently available observational pain assessment tools (see Cook et al., 2013; Keefe & Block, 1982; Revicki et al., 2009) that consist of lists of behaviors that are equally weighted in a single total score whose meaning and clinical implications are obscure. More recently, there have been some notable attempts at distinctions. One of the most widely adopted is that of protective (often escape-related) versus communicative behaviors (Sullivan, 2008). Often described as if mutually exclusive, although not originally represented as such (Sullivan, 2008), this is far from the case, since any visible behavior (including immobility and silence) is potentially communicative, whatever the intentions of the agent producing the behavior. And if communication successfully elicits help from others, then communicative behavior also has a protective function. Another distinction is based in spontaneous classifications of pain behavior observed in others, and describes behavior as automatic or controlled (Craig, Versloot, Goubert, Vervoort, & Crombez, 2010; McCrystal, Craig, Versloot, Fashler, & Jones, 2011). Automatic behaviors are immediate, reflexive, and consist mainly of facial expression and paralinguistic behavior, while controlled behaviors aim to exercise control over pain or distress or instrumentally over the social environment. While these classifications address function of the behaviors, both are derived from impressions of function rather than from direct testing.

Evolution, Social Exchange and Pain Judgments

One area in which evolutionary psychology has successfully informed experimental pain research is that of social exchange, a particular form of social interaction. Social exchange, also known as reciprocal altruism, reciprocity, or tit-for-tat, occurs in situations in which two or more individuals cooperate for mutual benefit by exchanging goods or services. Technically speaking, in this exchange an "individual is required to pay a cost (or meet a requirement) to an individual (or group) in order to be eligible to receive a benefit from that individual" or group (Cosmides, 1989, p. 197); for example, "I will help you if you are in reasonable need."

However, "always cooperate" would not be an evolutionarily stable strategy since then cheaters (individuals who take benefits without reciprocating) could invade the group of cooperators, exploit their help, and out-reproduce them. On the other hand, "always cheat" would not be evolutionarily stable either since a group of cheats could be invaded by people who cooperate selectively with non-cheats (rather than indiscriminately). The vital point that was demonstrated by evolutionary game theory is that selective cooperation cannot work without a cognitive heuristic for detecting cheats—or, more precisely, a heuristic for directing an individual's attention to information that could reveal that s/he is being cheated (Cosmides & Tooby, 1992; Gigerenzer, 2000).

Interestingly, not only humans but also some animals (e.g., chimpanzees, baboons, and vampire bats) are able to recognize and expel cheats from their buddy systems (e.g., Wilkinson, 1990). The fact that not all animals are able to do so supports the assertion that it is a specific cognitive mechanism evolved to detect cheaters rather than a general learning mechanism (e.g., classical or operant conditioning) applied to the situation. Thus only animals with this cognitive capacity can successfully engage in social exchange. Moreover, there is neurological evidence for humans indicating that social exchange reasoning can be selectively impaired while reasoning about other domains is left intact (Stone, Cosmides, Tooby, Kroll, & Knight, 2002).

Empirical studies of reasoning about social exchange mostly use the Wason selection task. This is a test of conditional reasoning in which participants are shown four cards, given a conditional rule ("If P, then Q") and asked to identify possible violations of this rule. Cosmides (1989) showed that participants were successful in solving the Wason selection task when the conditional rule expressed a *social* contract, i.e., when violations corresponded to detecting cheats, at a much greater rate than detecting violations of conditional rules concerning nonsocial exchange or abstract problems (Cosmides, 1989), or when conditional rules lacked a single key defining feature of social exchange (Fiddick, Cosmides, & Tooby, 2000; Gigerenzer & Hug, 1992; Platt & Griggs, 1993). Further support comes from similar results in an Ecuadorian Amazon hunter-horticulturalist tribe (Sugiyama, Tooby, & Cosmides, 2002).

Situations in which patients' pain has to be estimated could be regarded as social exchange situations since judges (e.g., health care professionals, relatives) are potential sources of help or resources ("provide a benefit") so long as patients are genuinely in pain ("meet a requirement"). Correspondingly, if judges suspect that patients in pain do not satisfy the requirements—for instance, are exaggerating or even faking their pain in order to receive a benefit—the cheater detection mechanism is alerted, prompting skepticism and more conservative judgments of patients' pain intensity and needs. Accordingly, deliberate exaggeration of pain is usually met with anger and alarm by health care professionals (Craig, Hill, & McMurtry, 1999).

In a review of scientific evidence for behavior or conditions suggestive of cheating in chronic pain patients, Fishbain and colleagues (Fishbain, Rosomoff, Cutler, & Rosomoff, 1995) found that studies can be divided into two areas of inquiry. The first concerns marital reinforcement (often termed spouse solicitousness: see Fordyce, 1976; Main et al., 2014), which purportedly motivates the patient to maintain the sick role. The second represents compensation receipt as a maintaining factor in disability. Other potential benefits of pain could be analgesic medication for patients with acute pain (particularly opioids, given concern about addiction; Main et al., 2014) or medication producing desirable psychoactive effects such as sedation or euphoria. Another cue that might raise suspicion in judges (and be associated with pain underestimation) is the absence of medical findings to support patients' pain complaints; a common interpretation is that pain is psychogenic (e.g., De Ruddere et al., 2014).

To summarize, the cheater detection device may be activated by the presence of certain context cues (such as the absence of supporting medical evidence), and possibly associated with secondary gains (such as marital reinforcement or compensation status). As a result, these factors lead to more conservative judgments of pain, effectively pain underestimation (Kappesser & Williams, 2010). Kappesser, Williams, and Prkachin (2006) studied this concept experimentally, asking health care professionals to watch facial expressions of shoulder pain patients undergoing painful movements and to rate the patients' pain on the same scale as used by the patients. Participants were randomly assigned to one of three conditions: the first group saw only facial pain expressions; the second group saw the facial pain expressions and were told the patients' self-report of pain intensity; and the third group were given the same information as the second with the additional information that some patients had faked their pain in order to obtain opioid medication, thereby alerting the cheater detection mechanism. Those health care professionals who based their estimation solely on the facial pain expression (first group) showed significant and substantial underestimation of pain compared with the patients' self-report. When health care professionals were given the patients' self-report (second group), underestimation was almost removed. For the third group, the cue priming health care professionals to expect cheating was enough to reinstate underestimation, eliminating the effect obtained by providing patients' self-reports. In answer to a further question, health care professionals quantified their expectations about exaggeration of pain: across the three groups, the higher their expectation of exaggeration, the greater their underestimation of pain. These results strongly support the model of a cheater detection mechanism that, when activated, contributes significantly to pain underestimation.

Since the cheater detection mechanism can operate in any social exchange situation, it should be expected also to influence judgments by nonclinical observers who hold potential benefits; the content of social exchange, and therefore the cues to possible cheating, are likely to differ somewhat from those identified in clinical contexts. Family members and close friends of people with persistent pain provide substantial amounts of care, making demands on their limited resources of time and energy (Newton-John & Williams, 2006), but there is little research on cues affecting an observer's pain estimation when that observer is a family carer. In an experimental study, Kappesser and Williams (2008) asked relatives and friends of chronic pain patients to read vignettes of fictitious people with chronic pain. Within the vignettes, four cues were systematically varied: self-reported pain intensity was high or low, medical evidence was absent or present, and liked and disliked activities were reported to be continued or abandoned by the fictitious person with pain. The latter two behavioral cues were designed using the hypothesis that "continuing a pleasant activity despite the pain but stopping an unpleasant duty because of the pain" would (unlike the other three combinations) be regarded as unfair, thereby alerting the cheater detection mechanism and resulting in lower pain estimates. Results showed that high pain self-reports and discontinuing all tasks (liked and disliked) led to highest pain estimates, while the lowest estimates of pain were given to people who stopped tasks they disliked while they continued with tasks they liked. Interestingly, this combination of behavioral cues was also rated as the least fair way to behave. From these results, it seems reasonable to deduce that behaviors judged as unfair by taking advantage of the pain can activate the cheater detection mechanism, which in turn leads to lower pain intensity estimates.

A more implicit method of alerting the cheater detection mechanism was used in an experimental study by de Ruddere et al. (2013). Using the cover story of a delayed memory task that took place before the actual experiment, participants read either a neutral text on the Belgian health care system or a text on its misuse by undeserving people. In the "real" experiment, participants then watched videos of chronic pain patients performing activities that exacerbated pain, and estimated patients' pain as well as their own sympathy for the patient. Next, participants reestimated patients' pain after being provided with patients' pain self-report. Last, photos of patients' faces were presented and participants indicated how positively or negatively they perceived each. Results show that, while priming for cheating had no direct effect on pain estimation, primed participants perceived patients more negatively, which in turn led to lower pain estimates and more pain underestimation compared with patients' own ratings.

Conclusion and Outlook

In this chapter we consider the social dimension of pain from an evolutionary psychology perspective, focusing on facial display of the pain experience as well as on its decoding by onlookers. We review consistent evidence of facial expression of pain, modulated according to context; of how the expression is understood by observers; and of responses characterized by the evolutionary mechanism of social exchange supported by cheater detection.

We hope that describing and discussing pain expression and others' responses within an evolutionary framework would encourage readers to consider more closely the functions of behaviors associated with pain, behaviors with which we are all familiar. To suggest that these ways of behaving owe much to evolution is not to suggest that they are automatic or without conscious control, that they are unchangeable, or that factors such as learning and contingencies do not have an impact, but that they are tendencies and tools with which humans approach problems, particularly those where they need to influence others' behavior in order to improve their own situation or to mitigate risk. This is of particular relevance in the clinical context where patients and clinicians interact.

Given the resources available in clinical settings, from permission to be absent from work to prescribed opioids, and clinicians' role as gatekeepers of these resources, it is unsurprising that some of the most marked underestimation effects are evident in these settings. While the assertion that pain was the "fifth vital sign," to be assessed in patients alongside temperature, respiration rate, pulse, and blood pressure, was intended to raise awareness of pain and ensure proper assessment, it ignored the obviously subjective nature of the pain self-rating compared to the other four signs (Schiavenato & Craig, 2010), and clinicians' uncertainty about how to interpret it (Backonja & Farrar, 2015). We care about others in pain because it is in our interest to care, since we in our turn may require it from others, but the power imbalance in the clinician–patient relationship, the pressures on clinicians not to dispense limited resources too freely, and the unverifiable nature of pain complaint produce a situation where skepticism and beliefs about patients' tendency to exaggerate and fake pain far outweigh what is justified. Because patients often anticipate this, they may make strenuous efforts to establish their honesty and the extent of their need, efforts that may only increase clinicians' suspicions.

Another area with many open questions, the further development of which could benefit from considering an evolutionary psychology perspective, is pain assessment. Taking into account the different agendas patients and clinicians bring to the assessment situation, unidimensional scales seem inadequate to represent clinical pain experience. Most such scales depend on self-report as the only source of information, neglecting assessment of patients unable temporarily or permanently to communicate their pain experience verbally. From an evolutionary perspective, we need to further examine the different functions of pain behaviors, since this would help clinicians to better understand and evaluate behaviors occurring in situations in which they assess pain. Clarity on the functions of behaviors might also help to produce better tools for pain assessment using observable behaviors, recognizing that clinical expertise is no protection against bias from evolved systems such as that of cheater detection, and that judgments about pain are made in a social and societal context.

References

Adamo, S. A. (2016). Do insects feel pain? A question at the intersection of animal behavior, philosophy and robotics. *Animal Behaviour, 118*, 75–79.

Alupay, J. S., Hadjisolomou, S. P., & Crook, R. J. (2014). Arm injury produces long-term behavioral and neural hypersensitivity in octopus. *Neuroscience Letters, 558*, 137–142.

Anil, L., Anil, S. S., & Deen, J. (2005). Pain detection and amelioration in animals on the farm: Issues and options. *Journal of Applied Animal Welfare Science, 8*(4), 261–278.

Aviezer, H., Trope, Y., & Todorov, A. (2012). Body cues, not facial expressions, discriminate between intense positive and negative emotions. *Science, 338*, 1225.

Backonja, M., & Farrar, J. T. (2015). Are pain ratings irrelevant? *Pain Medicine, 16*, 1247–1250.

Bartlett, M. S., Littlewort, G. C., Frank, M. G., & Lee, K. (2014). Automatic decoding of facial movements reveals deceptive facial expressions. *Current Biology, 24*, 738–743.

Beamish, E. K., & O'Riain, M. J. (2014). The effects of permanent injury on the behavior and diet of commensal Chacma baboons (*Papio ursinus*) in the Cape Peninsula, South Africa. *International Journal of Primatology, 35*, 1004–1020.

Bourke, J. (2014, June 19). This won't hurt a bit: the cultural history of pain. *New Statesman*. Retrieved from http://www.newstatesman.com/culture/2014/06/wont-hurt-bit-cultural-history-pain

Byrne, R. W., & Stokes, E. J. (2002). Effects of manual disability on feeding skills in gorillas and chimpanzees. *International Journal of Primatology, 23*(3), 539–554.

Calvo, M. G., & Nummenmaa, L. (2016). Perceptual and affective mechanisms in facial expression recognition: An integrative review. *Cognition & Emotion, 30*(6), 1081–1106.

Chambers, C. T., & Mogil, J. S. (2015). Ontogeny and phylogeny of facial expression of pain. *Pain, 156*(5), 798–799.

Chapman, D. I., & Chapman, N. (1969). Observations on the biology of fallow deer (*Dama dama*) in Epping Forest, Essex, England. *Biological Conservation, 2*(1), 55–62.

Chibnall, J. T., & Tait, R. C. (2009). Long term adjustment to work related low back pain: Associations with sociodemographics, claim processes, and post settlement adjustment. *Pain Medicine, 10*(8), 1378–1388.

Cook, K. F., Keefe, F., Jensen, M. P., Roddey, T. S., Callahan, L. F., Revicki, D., … Amtmann, D. (2013). Development and validation of a new self-report measure of pain behaviors. *Pain, 154*(12), 2867–2876.

Cosmides, L. (1989). The logic of social exchange: Has natural selection shaped how humans reason? Studies with the Wason selection task. *Cognition, 31*(3), 187–276.

Cosmides, L., & Tooby, J. (1992). Cognitive adaptations for social exchange. In J. H. Barkow, L. Cosmides, & J. Tooby (Eds.), *The adapted mind. Evolutionary psychology and the generation of culture* (pp. 163–228). New York, NY and Oxford, England: Oxford University Press.

Cosmides, L., & Tooby, J. (2000). Evolutionary psychology and the emotions. In M. Lewis & J. M. Haviland-Jones (Eds.), *Handbook of emotions* (pp. 91–115). New York, NY: Guilford Press.

Courbalay, A., Deroche, T., Descarreaux, M., Prigent, E., O'Shaughnessy, J., & Amorim, M.-A. (2016). Facial expression overrides lumbopelvic kinematics for clinical judgement about low back pain intensity. *Pain Research & Management, 9*. https://doi.org/10.1155/2016/7134825

Craig, K. D. (2015). Social communication model of pain. *Pain, 156*(7), 1198–1199.

Craig, K. D., Hill, M. L., & McMurtry, B. W. (1999). Detecting deception and malingering. In E. F. Kremer (Ed.), *Handbook of pain syndromes: Biopsychosocial perspectives* (pp. 41–58). Mahwah, NJ: Lawrence Erlbaum.

Craig, K. D., Versloot, J., Goubert, L., Vervoort, T., & Crombez, G. (2010). Perceiving pain in others: Automatic and controlled mechanisms. *Journal of Pain, 11*(2), 101–108.

Czekala, C., Maguière, F., Mazza, S., Jackson, P. L., & Frot, M. (2015). My brain reads pain in your face, before knowing your gender. *Journal of Pain, 16*(12), 1342–1352.

Dalla Costa, E., Minero, M., Lebelt, D., Stucke, D., Canali, E., & Leach, M. C. (2014). Development of the Horse Grimace Scale (HGS) as a pain assessment tool in horses undergoing routine castration. *PLoS One, 9*(3), e92281.

Dawkins, R. (1976/1989). *The selfish gene*. Oxford, England: Oxford University Press.

De Ruddere, L., Goubert, L., Stevens, M., Williams, A. C. d. C., & Crombez, G. (2013). Discounting pain in the absence of medical evidence is explained by negative evaluation of the patient. *Pain, 154*, 669–676.

De Ruddere, L., Goubert, L., Stevens, M. A. L., Deveugele, M., Craig, K. D., & Crombez, G. (2014). Health care professionals' reactions to patient pain: Impact of knowledge about medical evidence and psychosocial influences. *The Journal of Pain, 15*(3), 262–270.

Drews, C. (1996). Contexts and patterns of injuries in free-ranging male baboons (Papio cynocephalus). *Behaviour, 133*, 443–474.

Dyuizen, I. V., Kotsyuba, E. P., & Lamash, N. E. (2012). Changes in the nitric oxide system in the shore crab *Hemigrapsus sanguineus* (Crustacea, decapoda) CNS induced by a nociceptive stimulus. *Journal of Experimental Biology, 215*, 1668–1676.

Ekman, P. (1989). The argument and evidence about universals in facial expressions of emotion. In H. Wagner & A. Manstead (Eds.), *Handbook of social psychophysiology* (pp. 143–164). Oxford, England: John Wiley & Sons.

Ekman, P. (1992). An argument for basic emotions. *Cognition & Emotion, 6*, 169–200.

Ekman, P. (1993). Facial expression and emotion. *American Psychologist, 48*, 384–392.

Ekman, P., & Friesen, W. V. (1978). *Facial action coding system*. Palo Alto, CA: Consulting Psychologists Press.

Ekman, P., Friesen, W. V., & Hager, J. C. (2002). *Facial action coding system (FACS): Manual*. Salt Lake City, UT: A Human Face.

Elfenbein, H. A., & Ambady, N. (2002). On the universality and cultural specificity of emotion recognition: A meta-analysis. *Psychological Bulletin, 128*, 203–235.

Elfenbein, H. A., & Ambady, N. (2003). When familiarity breeds accuracy: Cultural exposure and facial expression recognition. *Journal of Personality and Social Psychology, 85*, 276–290.

Elwood, R. W. (2011). Pain and suffering in invertebrates? *ILAR Journal, 52*(2), 175–184.

Encandela, J. A. (1993). Social science and the study of pain since Zborowski: A need for a new agenda. *Social Science & Medicine, 36*(6), 783–791.

Fabrega, H. (1997). *Evolution of sickness and healing*. Berkeley, CA: University of California Press.

Fiddick, L., Cosmides, L., & Tooby, J. (2000). No interpretation without representation: The role of domain-specific representations and inferences in the Wason selection task. *Cognition, 77*(1), 1–79.

Finlay, B. L., & Syal, S. (2014). The pain of altruism. *Trends in Cognitive Science, 18*(12), 615–617.

Fishbain, D. A., Rosomoff, H. L., Cutler, R. B., & Rosomoff, R. S. (1995). Secondary gain concept: A review of the scientific evidence. *Clinical Journal of Pain, 11*(1), 6–21.

Fordyce, W. E. (1976). *Behavioral methods for chronic pain and illness*. St. Louis, MO: C.V. Mosby Company.

Fordyce, W. E. (1982). A behavioural perspective on chronic pain. *British Journal of Clinical Psychology, 21*, 313–320.

Forsman, E. D., Otto, I. A., & Muths, E. (2006). Healed fractures and other abnormalities in bones of small mammals. *Northwestern Naturalist, 87*(2), 143–146.

Fridlund, A. J. (1994). *Human facial expression: An evolutionary view*. San Diego, CA: Academic Press.

Gigerenzer, G. (2000). *Adaptive thinking: Rationality in the real world*. Oxford, England: Oxford University Press.

Gigerenzer, G., & Hug, K. (1992). Domain-specific reasoning: Social contracts, cheating, and perspective change. *Cognition, 43*(2), 127–171.

Gilbert, P., & Allan, S. (1998). The role of defeat and entrapment (arrested flight) in depression: An exploration of an evolutionary view. *Psychological Medicine, 28*, 585–598.

Goodall, J. (1986). *The chimpanzees of Gombe: Patterns of behaviour*. Cambridge, MA: Harvard University Press.

Hadjistavropoulos, H. D., Craig, K. D., Grunau, R. V. E., & Johnston, C. C. (1994). Judging pain in newborns: Facial and cry determinants. *Journal of Pediatric Psychology, 19*(4), 485–491.

Hadjistavropoulos, T., Breau, L. M., & Craig, K. D. (2011). Assessment of pain in adults and children with limited ability to communicate. In D. C. Turk & R. Melzack (Eds.), *Handbook of pain assessment* (pp. 260–280). New York, NY: Guilford Press.

Hadjistavropoulos, T., & Craig, K. D. (2002). A theoretical model for understanding self-report and observational measures of pain: A communications model. *Behaviour Research & Therapy, 40*, 551–570.

Hamilton, W. D. (1971/1996). Selection of selfish and altruistic behaviour in some extreme models. In W. D. Hamilton (Ed.), *Narrow roads to gene land: Vol. 1*. Oxford, England: Macmillan Press.

Hari, R., & Kujala, M. V. (2009). Brain basis of human social interaction: From concepts to brain imaging. *Physiological Reviews, 89*, 453–479.

Hill, M. L., & Craig, K. D. (2004). Detecting deception in facial expressions of pain. *Clinical Journal of Pain, 20*(6), 415–422.

Holden, E., Calvo, G., Collins, M., Bell, A., Reid, J., Scott, E. M., & Nolan, A. M. (2014). Evaluation of facial expression of acute pain in cats. *Journal of Small Animal Practice, 55*, 615–621.

Hsieh, A. Y., Tripp, D. A., & Ji, L.-J. (2011). The influence of ethnic concordance and discordance on verbal reports and nonverbal behaviours of pain. *Pain, 152*, 2016–2022.

Jack, R. E. (2013). Culture and facial expressions of emotion. *Visual Cognition, 21*(9–10), 1248–1286.

Jack, R. E., Garrod, O. G. B., & Schyns, P. G. (2014). Dynamic facial expressions of emotion transmit an evolving hierarchy of signals over time. *Current Biology, 24*, 187–192.

Jackson, P. L., Rainville, P., & Decety, J. (2006). To what extent do we share the pain of others? Insight from the neural bases of pain empathy. *Pain, 125*, 5–9.

Jensen, M. P., Turner, J. A., & Romano, J. M. (2007). Changes after multidisciplinary pain treatment in patient beliefs and coping are associated with concurrent changes in patient functioning. *Pain, 131*(1–2), 38–47.

Jurmain, R. (1997). Skeletal evidence of trauma in African apes, with special reference to Gombe chimpanzees. *Primates, 38*(1), 1–14.

Kappesser, J., & Williams, A. C. d. C. (2002). Pain and negative emotions in the face: Judgements by health professionals. *Pain, 99*, 197–206.

Kappesser, J., & Williams, A. C. d. C. (2008). Pain judgements of patients' relatives: Examining the use of social contract theory as theoretical framework. *Journal of Behavioral Medicine, 31*(4), 309–317. https://doi.org/10.1007/s10865-008-9157-4

Kappesser, J., & Williams, A. C. d. C. (2010). Pain estimation: Asking the right questions. *Pain, 148*, 184–187.

Kappesser, J., Williams, A. C. d. C., & Prkachin, K. M. (2006). Testing two accounts of pain underestimation. *Pain, 124*(1), 109–116. https://doi.org/10.1016/j.pain.2006.04.003

Keating, S. C., Thomas, A. A., Flecknell, P. A., & Leach, M. C. (2012). Evaluation of EMLA cream for preventing pain during tattooing of rabbits: Changes in physiological, behavioural and facial expression responses. *PLoS One, 7*(9), e44437.

Keefe, F. J., & Block, A. R. (1982). Development of an observation method for assessing pain behavior in chronic low back pain patients. *Behavior Therapy, 13*, 363–375.

Kelly, S., & Dunbar, R. (2001). Who dares wins: Heroism versus altruism in female mate choice. *Human Nature, 12*, 89–105.

Keogh, E. (2014). Gender differences in the nonverbal communication of pain: A new direction for sex, gender and pain research? *Pain, 155*, 1927–1931.

Khatibi, A., Schrooten, M., Bosmans, K., Volders, S., Vlaeyen, J. W. S., & Van den Bussche, E. (2015). Sub-optimal presentation of painful facial expressions enhances readiness for action and pain perception following electrocutaneous stimulation. *Frontiers in Psychology, 6*, 913. https://doi.org/10.3389/fpsyg.2015.00913

Khatibi, A., Vachon-Presseau, E., Schrooten, M., Vlaeyen, J., & Rainville, P. (2014). Attention effects on vicarious modulation of nociception and pain. *Pain, 155*(10), 2033–2039.

Krahé, C., Springer, A., Weinman, J. A., & Fotopoulou, A. (2013). The social modulation of pain: Others as predictive signals of salience—a systematic review. *Frontiers in Human Neuroscience, 7*, 386. https://doi.org/10.3389/fnhum.2013.00386

Krasnow, M. M., Delton, A. W., Tooby, J., & Cosmides, L. (2013). Meeting now suggests we will meet again: Implications for debates on the evolution of cooperation. *Scientific Reports, 3*, 1747. https://doi.org/10.1038/srep01747

Krumhuber, E. G., Kappas, A., & Manstead, A. S. R. (2013). Effects of dynamic aspects of facial expressions: A review. *Emotion Review, 5*(1), 41–46.

Kunz, M., & Lautenbacher, S. (2014). The faces of pain: A cluster analysis of individual differences in facial activity patterns of pain. *European Journal of Pain, 18*(6), 813–823.

Kunz, M., Mylius, V., Schepelmann, K., & Lautenbacher, S. (2004). On the relationship between self-report and facial expression of pain. *Journal of Pain, 5*(7), 368–376.

Kunz, M., Prkachin, K., & Lautenbacher, S. (2013). Smiling in pain: Exploration of its social motives. *Pain Research & Treatment* 8, 128093. https://doi.org/10.1155/2013/128093

Kunz, M., Rainville, P., & Lautenbacher, S. (2011). Operant conditioning of facial displays of pain. *Psychosomatic Medicine, 73*, 422–431.

Labus, J. S., Keefe, F. J., & Jensen, M. P. (2003). Self-reports of pain intensity and direct observations of pain behavior: When are they correlated? *Pain, 102*, 109–124.

LaGasse, L. L., Neal, A. R., & Lester, B. M. (2005). Assessment of infant cry: Acoustic cry analysis and parental perception. *Mental Retardation and Developmental Disabilities Research Reviews, 11*(1), 83–93.

Langford, D. J., Bailey, A. L., Chanda, M. L., Clarke, S. E., Drummond, T. E., Echols, S., … Mogil, J. S. (2010). Coding of facial expressions of pain in the laboratory mouse. *Nature Methods, 7*, 447–449.

Langford, D. J., Crager, S. E., Shehzad, Z., Smith, S. B., Sotocinal, S. G., Levenstadt, J. S., … Mogil, J. S. (2006). Social modulation of pain as evidence for empathy in mice. *Science, 312*, 1967–1970.

Main, C. J., Keefe, F. J., Jensen, M. P., Vlaeyen, J. W. S., & Vowles, K. E. (Eds.). (2014). *Fordyce's behavioral methods for chronic pain and illness.*, republished with invited commentaries. Philadelphia, PA: IASP Press/Wolters Kluwer.

Malgorzata, E. A., Carey, J. R., & Molleman, F. (2009). Species, age and sex differences in type and frequency of injuries and impairments among four arboreal primate species in Kibale National Park, Uganda. *Primates, 50*, 65–73.

McCrystal, K., Craig, K. D., Versloot, J., Fashler, S. R., & Jones, D. N. (2011). Perceiving pain in others: Validation of a dual processing model. *Journal of Pain, 152*, 1083–1089.

Mithen, S. (1996). *The prehistory of the mind*. London, England: Thames & Hudson.

Morley, S. (2011). Efficacy and effectiveness of cognitive behaviour therapy for chronic pain: Progress and some challenges. *Pain, 152*(3), S99–S106.

Nagasako, E. M., Oaklander, A. L., & Dworkin, R. H. (2003). Congenital insensitivity to pain: An update. *Pain, 101*, 213–219.

Nesse, R. M., & Stearns, S. C. (2008). The great opportunity: Evolutionary applications to medicine and public health. *Evolutionary Applications, 1*, 28–48.

Newton-John, T. R., & Williams, A. C. d. C. (2006). Chronic pain couples: Perceived marital interactions and pain behaviours. *Pain, 123*(1), 53–63.

Niazi, M., & Hussain, A. (2011). Agent-based computing from multi-agent systems to agent-based models: A visual survey. *Scientometrics, 89*(2), 479–499.

Peeters, P. A., & Vlaeyen, J. W. (2011). Feeling more pain, yet showing less: The influence of social threat on pain. *Journal of Pain, 12*(12), 1255–1261.

Platt, R. D., & Griggs, R. A. (1993). Darwinian algorithms and the Wason selection task: A factorial analysis of social contract selection task problems. *Cognition, 48*(2), 163–192. https://doi.org/10.1016/0010-0277(93)90029-U

Poole, G. D., & Craig, K. D. (1992). Judgments of genuine, suppressed, and faked facial expressions of pain. *Journal of Personality and Social Psychology, 63*(5), 797–805.

Prkachin, K. M. (1986). Pain behavior is not unitary. *Behavioral & Brain Sciences, 9*(4), 754–755.

Prkachin, K. M. (2011). Facial pain expression. *Pain Management, 1*, 367–376.

Prkachin, K. M., & Solomon, P. E. (2008). The structure, reliability and validity of pain expression: Evidence from patients with shoulder pain. *Pain, 139*(2), 267–274.

Pronina, I., & Rule, N. O. (2014). Inducing bias modulates sensitivity to nonverbal cues of others' pain. *European Journal of Pain, 18*, 1452–1457.

Redfern, R. (2010). A regional examination of surgery and fracture treatment in Iron Age and Roman Britain. *International Journal of Osteoarchaeology, 20*, 443–471.

Reicherts, P., Wieser, M. J., Gerdes, A. B., Likowski, K. U., Weyers, P., Mühlberger, A., & Pauli, P. (2012). Electrocortical evidence for preferential processing of dynamic pain expressions compared to other emotional expressions. *Pain, 153*(9), 1959–1964.

Revicki, D. A., Chen, W. H., Harnam, N., Cook, K. F., Amtmann, D., Callahan, L. F., … Keefe, F. J. (2009). Development and psychometric analysis of the PROMIS pain behavior item bank. *Pain, 146*(1), 158–169.

Roughan, J. V., & Flecknell, P. A. (2004). Behaviour-based assessment of the duration of laparotomy-induced abdominal pain and the analgesic effects of carprofen and buprenorphine in rats. *Behavioural Pharmacology, 15*, 461–472.

Saarela, M. V., Hlushchuk, Y., Williams, A. C. d. C., Schürmann, M., Kalso, E., & Hari, R. (2007). The compassionate brain: Humans detect intensity of pain from another's face. *Cerebral Cortex, 17*, 230–237.

Salomons, T. V., Coan, J. A., Hunt, S. M., Backonja, M.-M., & Davidson, R. J. (2008). Voluntary facial displays of pain increase suffering in response to nociceptive stimulation. *Journal of Pain, 9*(5), 443–448.

Schäfer, G., Prkachin, K. M., Kaseweter, K. A., & Williams, A. C. d. C. (2016). Health care providers' judgments in chronic pain: The influence of gender and trustworthiness. *Pain, 157*, 1618–1625. https://doi.org/10.1097/j.pain.0000000000000536

Schiavenato, M., & Craig, K. D. (2010). Pain assessment as a social transaction: Beyond the "gold standard". *Clinical Journal of Pain, 26*, 667–676.

Shakhar, K., & Shakhar, G. (2015). Why do we feel sick when infected—can altruism play a role. *PLoS Biology, 13*(10), e1002276.

Simon, D., Craig, K. D., Gosselin, F., Belin, P., & Rainville, P. (2008). Recognition and discrimination of prototypical dynamic expressions of pain and emotions. *Pain, 135*, 55–64.

Sneddon, L. (2011). Pain perception in fish. *Journal of Consciousness Studies, 18*(9–10), 209–229.

St. John Smith, E., & Lewin, G. R. (2009). Nociceptors: A phylogenetic view. *Journal of Comparative Physiology A, 195*, 1089–1106.

Staton, L. J., Panda, M., Chen, I., Genao, I., Kurz, J., Pasanen, M., … Cykert, S. (2007). When race matters: Disagreement in pain perception between patients and their physicians in primary care. *Journal of the National Medical Association, 99*(5), 532–538.

Steinkopf, L. (2016). An evolutionary perspective on pain communication. *Evolutionary Psychology, 14*(2), 1474704916653964.

Stone, V. E., Cosmides, L., Tooby, J., Kroll, N., & Knight, R. T. (2002). Selective impairment of reasoning about social exchange in a patient with bilateral limbic system damage. *Proceedings of the National Academy of Sciences, 99*(17), 11531–11536.

Sugiyama, L. S., Tooby, J., & Cosmides, L. (2002). Cross-cultural evidence of cognitive adaptations for social exchange among the Shiwiar of Ecuadorian Amazonia. *Proceedings of the National Academy of Sciences, 99*(17), 11537–11542.

Sullivan, M. J. L. (2008). Toward a biopsychomotor conceptualization of pain. *Clinical Journal of Pain, 24*(4), 281–290.

Tait, R. C. (2013). Pain assessment—an exercise in social judgment? *Pain, 154*, 625–626.

Tait, R. C., Chibnall, J. T., & Jovel, A. (2014). Accountability and empathy effects on medical students' clinical judgments in a disability determination context for low back pain. *Journal of Pain, 15*(9), 915–924.

Tait, R. C., Chibnall, J. T., & Kalauokalani, D. (2009). Provider judgments of patients in pain: Seeking symptom certainty. *Pain Medicine, 10*, 11–34.

Tobin, D. M., & Bargmann, C. I. (2004). Invertebrate nociception: Behaviors, neurons and molecules. *Journal of Neurobiology, 61*, 161–174.

Tooby, J., & Cosmides, L. (1996). Friendship and the banker's paradox: Other pathways to the evolution of adaptations for altruism. *Proceedings of the British Academy, 88*, 119–143.

Trivers, R. L. (1971). The evolution of reciprocal altruism. *Quarterly Review of Biology, 46*, 35–57.

Underwood, W. J. (2002). Pain and distress in agricultural animals. *Journal of the American Veterinary Medical Association, 221*(2), 208–211.

Wall, P. D. (1979). On the relation of injury to pain. *Pain, 6*, 253–264.

Walsh, J., Eccleston, C., & Keogh, E. (2014). Pain communication through body posture: The development and validation of a stimulus set. *Pain, 155*(11), 2282–2290.

Walters, E. T. (1994). Injury-related behavior and neuronal plasticity: An evolutionary perspective on sensitization, hyperalgesia and analgesia. *International Review of Neurobiology, 36,* 325–427.

Walters, E. T. (2016). Pain-capable neural substrates may be widely available in the animal kingdom. *Animal Sentience (electronic resource),* 063.

Walters, E. T., & Moroz, L. L. (2009). Molluscan memory of injury: Evolutionary insights into chronic pain and neurological disorders. *Brain Behaviour & Evolution, 74,* 206–218.

Whittaker, A. L., & Howarth, G. S. (2014). Use of spontaneous behaviour measures to assess pain in laboratory rats and mice: How are we progressing? *Applied Animal Behaviour Science, 151,* 1–12.

Wilkinson, G. S. (1990). Food sharing in vampire bats. *Scientific American, 262,* 76–82.

Williams, A. C. d. C. (2002). Facial expression of pain: An evolutionary account. *Behaviour & Brain Sciences, 25,* 439–488.

Williams, A. C. d. C. (2016). What can evolutionary theory tell us about chronic pain? *Pain, 157*(4), 788–790.

Williams, A. C. d. C., Gallagher, E., Fidalgo, A. R., & Bentley, P. J. (2016). Pain expressiveness and altruistic behavior: An exploration using agent-based modeling. *Pain, 157*(3), 759–768.

Xu, X., Zuo, X., Wang, X., & Han, S. (2009). Do you feel my pain? Racial group membership modulates empathic neural responses. *Journal of Neuroscience, 29*(26), 8525–8529.

Zeltzer, L. K., & Tsao, J. C. I. (2006). What's in a face? Can parents "read pain" in their children's faces? *Pain, 126,* 1–2.

Chapter 2
Toward the Social Communication Model of Pain

Kenneth D. Craig

Abstract Understanding the impact of the social environment on human pain is essential to development of pain prevention and intervention strategies. Social factors determine whether there is exposure to pain, how it is experienced and expressed, and whether adequate treatment is provided. Inadequate prevention, assessment, and treatment are common, leading to high levels of needless pain. The importance of social factors as determinants of pain appears particularly the case for humans. The evolved human brain permitted adaptations to complex social environments and considerable sensitivity to social contexts with an impact on how pain is experienced. Cognitive and social processes assume more important roles in experiencing and responding to pain with humans than is the case with less complex species. The social communications model of pain integrates an understanding of social determinants of pain with psychological and biological systems. The biological systems evolved to support healthy behavioral adaptations to the challenges of living in complex environments.

Keywords Social communication · Social learning · Evolution · Human brain · Social contexts · Prevention · Assessment · Treatment

Introduction

Ronald Melzack (1990) described the tragedy of needless pain several decades ago. This classic, inspiring, change-provoking paper reported on effective treatments not made available to patients who would benefit from them. More than 25 years later the observation that "patients worldwide continue to be undertreated and to suffer unnecessary agony" (p. 27) remains current. The case can be stated for acute pain arising from injury, disease, surgery, and other medical procedures as well as persistent and recurring chronic pain. Large numbers of people are implicated, with

K. D. Craig (✉)
University of British Columbia, Vancouver, BC, Canada
e-mail: kcraig@psych.ubc.ca

© Springer International Publishing AG, part of Springer Nature 2018   23
T. Vervoort et al. (eds.), *Social and Interpersonal Dynamics in Pain*,
https://doi.org/10.1007/978-3-319-78340-6_2

vulnerable populations, including infants and children, people with developmental disabilities and seniors with dementia, even less likely to receive adequate care (Hadjistavropoulos, Breau, & Craig, 2011; Hadjistavropoulos et al., 2011). The suffering that was the focus of Professor Melzack's paper arose "because physicians are often reluctant to prescribe morphine" (p. 27). While prescription practices remain a serious issue, currently accentuated by deaths resulting from overprescription, misuse and illicit use of opioids (Lynch, 2016), we now appreciate that failures in the treatment of pain also are a consequence of failures to recognize pain, inadequate or inappropriate assessment, underestimation of people's pain and suffering, inadequate or inappropriate treatment, social biases and failures to adequately educate health-care professionals to understand pain and its management (Craig & Fashler, 2014).

It is noteworthy that the tragedies Melzack so powerfully evoked arise not so much from a misunderstanding of the biology of pain or lack of efficacy of the withheld care, but from social pressures on physicians and their inability and reluctance to deliver appropriate care. For example, at the time of writing, there is much tumult in the public health community relating to concerns about underprescribing and overprescribing opioids, as well as concerns about imposition of guidelines and mandatory regulations concerning their prescription (Lynch & Katz, 2017). Diverse social factors determine whether people will be exposed to pain, how it is experienced, how it is communicated to others and the adequacies of care they will receive. These social dimensions of pain experience and pain care delivery are complex and deserving of careful study if optimal care is to be provided.

A Sociobehavioral Evolutionary Perspective

The evolutionary perspective informs our understanding of pain as it relates to the behavioral capabilities and social nature of the human animal. Biological systems became organized to support actions needed to protect organisms from environmental insult long ago—even the tropisms of unicellular organisms demonstrate this to be the case. All creatures are vulnerable to physical harm from disease, predators and environmental risks. Survival and procreation depend upon adaptive behaviors and biological systems that were conserved in ancient species and perpetuated through to the human lineage. A basis for human pain emerged in far simpler organisms, although it is unknown just when in the long course of phylogenetic change resulting from adaptations to different ecological niches pain emerged to function as an adaptive strategy. Our current understanding of the neural substrates needed to support simple forms of pain and pain behavior suggests the possibility that "raw experiences" or "primitive feelings" were present even in invertebrates, e.g., the large, slug-like marine snails, *Aplysia*, squid and fish (Crook & Walters, 2011), but transformations in the nervous system would be associated with greater complexity in pain experiences and behavior.

At present, pain is accepted as a feature of life in all mammals. Hence, the considerable use of rodents in preclinical research on pain. While rodent brains are dramatically smaller than those of humans (the mouse brain weighs about 0.4 g, whereas the human brain weighs about 1400 g), the presence of a cerebral cortex in mice appears to support feelings and behaviors humans recognize as pain (Mogil, 2015), albeit the experiences must differ from those of humans.

The legacy of pain-related functional behavior and its biological substrates dating back to simpler organisms is most evident in human automatic/reflexive reactions to threat of physical harm, including "hard-wired" nociceptive escape reflexes and protective body movements (Craig, Versloot, Goubert, Vervoort, & Crombez, 2010). Defensive actions have some species-specificity, reflecting adaptations to unique ecological niches, but some features of the functional systems persisted across species to the extent they remained adaptive. At early stages of evolutionary development, the actions would largely be self-directed; for example, facilitating escape from dangerous settings or adopting protective postures. Demanding environments and continuing evolution led to more efficient and often more complex adaptive mechanisms. Addressing imminent or actual threat would be supported by increasingly robust capacities to recognize, learn about and remember dangers that signal potential harm; hence, cognition became a part of the adaptive pain systems. Increasingly complex nervous systems evolved, culminating in the human brain capable of goal-directed behavior, benefiting from learning about the experiences of others (Craig, 1986; Goubert, Vlaeyen, Crombez, & Craig, 2011) and discovering how to care for others and to enlist their care (Craig, 2004), as epitomized by human use of problem-solving, language, other forms of communication, and cooperation in complex social environments, rather than the fixed reactions to immediate environmental demands observed in less complex organisms.

Evolution of the nervous system needed to support complex pain behavior is evident in changes to the human brain over extended spans of time. Gross anatomical comparisons indicate that the human brain became capable of responding to the demands of increasingly complex multifaceted human environments. During evolution from ancient *hominins* 2–3 million years ago, brains grew from about 600 cm^3 to a current size of 1300–1400 cm^3 in *Homo sapiens*. A look at the size of the newborn human brain relative to the adult brain also is instructive of the emergent behavioral capabilities of the mature adult. The brain grows from about 350–400 g at birth to 1300–1400 in the adult. Of great importance in phylogenetic development of species (Zhang & Sejnowski, 2000) and ontogenetic development of human children are changes in the ratio of cortical gray and white matter (Lenroot & Giedd, 2006). Myelinization of human neurons means human brains are composed of ~80% fat tissue, whereas rodent brains have ~30% fat tissue. This supports the structures and functions that permit truly extraordinary complex processes in the adult at biological, psychological, and sociocultural levels of analysis (Melchert, 2016). Evolution provided organisms with increasingly complex biological capabilities needed to adapt to increasingly complex ecological systems. Mammalian carnivore species with larger brains, relative to their body size, are better problem-solvers (Benson-Amram, Dantzer, Stricker, Swanson, & Holekamp,

2016). This would support more complex reactions in humans to the challenges posed by pain.

These differences in brain size and cerebral maturation have been associated with increases in social intelligence. It now seems evident that the unusually large brains of primates, relative to their body size and compared to all other vertebrates, evolved to manage particularly complex social systems (Dunbar, 2009). While brain size cannot be equated with intelligence, the larger, more sophisticated brain of humans supports substantially more complex behavior (Roth & Dicke, 2005) and this has been associated with sociality (Schultz, Dunbar, & Lovejoy, 2010). While nonhuman primates often display considerable social intelligence (de Waal, 2009), comparatively this is unusually enhanced in humans, as displayed by human capacities for theory of mind, imitation and language (Roth & Dicke, 2005). The human brain perhaps evolved in size and complexity to support the demands of human cooperation and competition, or evolution of the human brain for other reasons permitted and supported these complexities of human social living.

Appreciating the importance of social interaction is key to understanding human brain function. "People are embedded in social interaction that shapes their brains throughout their lifetime." (Hari, Henriksson, Malinen, & Parkkonen, 2015). The nature of human pain experience, its social expression and the care systems designed to minimize exposure to pain need to be understood accordingly. The social complexities are evident at the simplest level in expressive and receptive communication among individuals using both language and nonverbal expression and at more complex levels in the social institutions humans have invented to minimize pain and distress, including health care professionals specialized in providing care for pain and underlying conditions, hospitals and the bureaucratic systems that support them and public health consciousness and willingness to provide resources.

Continuities Across Species

Certain systems that protected ancestral species and earlier hominins appear to have been well-conserved over evolutionary time. Protopathic sensory and emotional qualities would have been the most ancient features of pain, manifested through bodily actions in the form of spontaneous limb and torso movements and postures. These reflexive, automatic protective reactions serve homeostatic functions and would be associated with the more primitive feelings of pain that emerge in consciousness. Touching a hot element on a stove illustrates experiential and expressive features of pain of this type. There is a quick apprehension of pain and reflexive withdrawal of the hand. This pattern appears typical in virtually all species given its capacity to protect from physical danger and threats to safety. There also would be only a limited capacity to inhibit escape from the source of pain in species capable of this, albeit, purposeful action might inhibit the reaction.

Discontinuities Across Species

While human pain reactions display many of the ancient features that would have emerged and been conserved in progenitor species, one would expect unique features of pain to be associated with species discontinuities in structure and function. These are likely to reflect the adaptations of different species to ecological niches. For example, young pigs, dogs and humans typically make considerable noise when hurt, but young sheep do not (Broom, 1998). Humans and other large primates, as well as pigs and dogs, who live socially, likely benefit from receiving and helping conspecifics when attacked by predators or conspecifics (Broom & Fraser, 2007). Vocalization is likely to be advantageous for social species helped by conspecifics, but disadvantageous (i.e., attracting predators) for prey species that do not help injured conspecifics, such as sheep and antelope (Cantor & Craig, 2017). As a further example, the facial expression of pain displays consistencies across mammals, with variations reflecting evolved structural and functional differences among species (Chambers & Mogil, 2015; Langford et al., 2010). As well, the apparently hard-wired, automatic reactions described above appear to have acquired greater flexibility as the human brain evolved, permitting purposive and controlled actions designed to protect the individual. In their fullest expression, these features of human pain reflect enhanced cognitive and social features of the experience. Other species display evidence of sociality, including insects (e.g., bees, termites and ants), fish, birds and mammals, including nonhuman primates, but none approach the complexity to be observed in the social arrangements in which human life is embedded.

Evolution of course added enormous complexity to brains, as emotional systems emerged to provide sustained action adaptations to sensory processing and the mantle of cortex emerged in mammals to support problem-solving adaptations. The capacity to engage in purposeful control of pain perhaps is most evident in development of the cortical mantle in humans through the first 15–20 years of life. Notably late to reach adult levels of cortical thickness is the dorsolateral prefrontal cortex, involved in circuitry subserving control of impulses, judgment, and decision-making. The human brain can be characterized as comprising modules suited to social demands and capable of the calculations and information processing associated with life in human society. These capabilities are enlisted in human pain experience and expression. Table 2.1 contrasts a popular intrapersonal conception of the function of pain with an extended perspective which incorporates social functions.

Appreciation of developmental changes in pain experience and expression requires recognition of the interactions between biological maturation and life experience (see Chap. 3). The hardwired biological features of pain appear best captured in study of the genetics and epigenetics of pain and the neurophysiological systems needed for nociception and central processing. Genetic variations reflect ancient histories of primordial ancestors, with further variation contributed through epigenetic mechanisms and the consequences of nutrition, disease, stress, and life experience. Nonhuman pain would appear to be more reflexive than human pain. Human

Table 2.1 Pain serves both intrapersonal and interpersonal functions

Intrapersonal functions of pain
• Warns the individual of real or potential biological threat in the form of tissue damage and motivates escape

Interpersonal functions of pain
• Behavioral reactions alarm conspecifics; warn of risk of personal danger (self-interested responses)
• Informs others of situational factors capable of harm or care, how they might respond and the success of these efforts (observational learning)
• Instigates empathetic reactions and perhaps sympathy and care (altruistic responses) or sadistic satisfaction in observers
• Instructs concerning the behavioral capabilities of the person; people in pain are vulnerable and perhaps less capable of contributing to the social fabric

pain incorporates the primal features, but also reflects biological systems that permit flexible adaptations to complex environments because of experience. Humans appear particularly predisposed to change or benefit from personal and social histories of experiences with pain, even during earliest stages of life. This includes biological dispositions transformed by familial and cultural socialization and the acquisition of skills that determine how one should anticipate and experience pain and how to respond before, during, and following painful events. Both variability in the biological systems manifest during pain and variability in histories of life experience are responsible for the considerable individual differences observed when people experience pain.

Characterizations of pain experience typically focus upon sensory and emotional processes, for example, the International Association for the Study of Pain definition of pain describes it as "an unpleasant sensory and emotional experience associated with actual or potential tissue damage, or described in terms of such tissue damage" (1979). This characterization of the subjective experience of pain serves research with nonhuman species reasonably well, but neglects cognitive and social features that exist in both nonhuman and human organisms, a problem particularly in the case of humans where cognitive mechanisms associated with attention, expectations, thinking, and problem-solving and the social contexts of people's lives are of great importance. An alternative definition has been proposed that explicitly acknowledges these features of life in social environments, "Pain is a distressing experience associated with actual or potential tissue damage with sensory, emotional, cognitive and social components" (Williams & Craig, 2016).

Integration of Automatic and Controlled Features of Human Pain Experience and Expression

Relatively independent, dual neuroregulatory systems (Craig et al., 2010; Hadjistavropoulos & Craig, 2002) are responsible for (a) automatic/reflexive pain behavior in both humans and other animals, reflecting the long line of human progenitor species, and (b) controlled/purposive behaviors, evident in mammals and other nonhuman animals, but never in such substantial and complex forms as in humans; for example, in the use of verbal report, self-directed coping, including use of pharmaceuticals, and seeking care from others. Humans are born with tremendous potential to exercise cognitive control, but they are born helpless and require nurturing environments that support physical and psychological development for an extended period of time if they are to survive and thrive as adults. They depend upon parents and others to care for their physical well-being as well as to help them acquire adaptive psychological, behavioral and social skills. Learning to anticipate danger, understanding the meaning and emotional significance of painful events and behaving in a proactive manner, including recognizing how to effectively access care from others, are challenging tasks. The capacity to engage in voluntary behavior leading to self-management of pain emerges slowly during infancy and childhood and may decline toward the end of life, leading one to anticipate life span changes in the experience and expression of pain.

Thus, continuity with nonhuman species is evident in the various automatic/reflexive behaviors and discontinuity is manifest primarily in controlled/purposive behaviors. The former stimulus driven features of pain largely address intrapersonal functional benefits; this component of the pain system warns of tissue damage or stress, motivates escape or avoidance and facilitates learning about dangerous situations. Emergence of the latter more proactive system greatly extended adaptive benefits by facilitating interpersonal adaptive behavior, including benefiting from the experiences of others, altruistic actions, and development of social systems accommodating the needs of people in pain. While conscious planning of actions able to minimize exposure to pain need not be social, humans can be distinguished from other species by the complexity of social actions and related institutions engaged to prevent exposure to pain and to ameliorate distress. Health care systems and the specialized knowledge and skills of health care professionals are but one example of complex human cultures that are characterized by high levels of social cooperation and competition giving rise to economic, political, cultural, commercial, transportation, educational, and health care systems.

Slow Emergence of Recognition of Social Determinants of Pain

The burgeoning strengths of scientific medicine in the nineteenth century supported an early biomedical focus on pain as a sensory process (Foster & Sherrington, 1897). Most people continue to see pain as a basic bodily sensation induced by a noxious stimulus. In an effort to rectify this narrow perspective, Melzack and Casey (1968) noted: "To consider only the sensory features of pain, and ignore its motivational and affective properties, is to look at only part of the problem, and not even the most important part at that" (p. 423). Over time, complexity of the experience has been acknowledged. Debates over a 100 years ago led to a focus on negative affect as the central feature (Marshall, 1894). The major twentieth century definition of pain, quoted above, came to dominate the fields of research and pain management. This biomedical approach emphasizes a close relationship between tissue pathology and painful experience, peripheral afferent systems, which transmit sensory information concerning damage caused by injury or disease to the brain, and use of medical interventions, including pharmaceuticals, surgery, nerve blocks, and peripheral or central nervous system stimulators designed to modulate nociception.

The approach harmonizes with most people's everyday experiences of pain, including cuts, bruises, sprains, and burns, and acute clinically significant pain requiring medical care. These relatively short-term painful experiences are often associated with diagnosable tissue pathology, but not invariably, satisfactorily resolve with time, and are responsive to analgesic drugs and other medical interventions during tissue healing. Most of us would hope that both our personal and others' experiences of pain would conform to these characteristics, but the reality is that not all episodes of pain have these characteristics.

The biomedical model has severe limitations. There is only a moderate relationship between the experience of pain and demonstrable tissue pathology. In fact, tissue pathology can often be demonstrated in the absence of pain, and very often considerable clinical pain can be found to have no specific diagnosable tissue pathology associated with it. Chronic pain, which persists beyond the expected healing time, usually specified as 3 or 6 months, defies the common expectation that pain will resolve after a period of time, minutes or hours in the case of everyday pain, and days and weeks, or maybe months, in the case of clinically important acute pain. Chronic persistent or recurrent pain often does not resolve. Indeed, it has been suggested that the majority of patients suffering from chronic pain do not have a medically diagnosable condition associated with their pain. For them, the best medical diagnostic and treatment procedures will have proven inadequate to patients' needs, leaving them suffering debilitating pain that does not benefit from traditional medical care, whether pharmaceuticals, surgery, or other medical interventions. The health care system, a human social institution, is in many ways not designed to care for people with chronic pain; it is heavily structured to care for people suffering medically diagnosable injuries and diseases. The dogma of the biomedical model, the inertia of established medical institutions and the vested financial and professional interests of health care practitioners and those supporting this establishment have led to resistance to advances. From this perspective, social factors are typically ignored, understated, or conceptualized as important only to the extent that pain creates havoc with people's working, family, and recreational lives. Fortunately, alternatives have been proposed and are slowly becoming established because they are supported by scientific knowledge and unmet needs of large numbers of people.

More than 50 years ago, Gate Control Theory (GCT) was proposed as an alternative model of pain to address the limitations of biomedical formulations that focused upon pain as a nociceptive sensation specific to tissue pathology (Melzack & Wall,

1965). The evidence-based GCT model described physiological mechanisms capable of modulating electrochemical activity associated with pain and recognized the spinal cord and brain as dynamic systems that facilitate or inhibit transmission of information in the nervous system. Melzack and Wall state that "the theory proposes that the dorsal horn of the spinal cord acts like a gate which modulates the flow of nerve impulses from the peripheral fibers to the central nervous system. The gate is influenced by peripheral fiber activity and by descending influences from the brain" (Melzack & Wall, 1982). As Katz and Rosenbloom (2015) observed, the theory helped understand "previously inexplicable, 'bizarre' symptoms (e.g., phantom limb pain) believed to arise from psychopathology" (Gagliese & Katz, 2000), discouraged the use of surgery as a tool for interrupting sensory input, encouraged development of neuromodulation stimulation interventions and established an important role for such psychological factors as depression and anxiety in modulating pain. As Melzack and Wall (1965) put it, "Thus, it is possible for central nervous system activities subserving attention, emotion, and memories of prior experience to exert control over the sensory input." (p. 976). While not directly addressing social influences on pain, it is clear they contemplated their role, as they referred to classic work by Beecher (1956) who described soldiers wounded in battle who denied pain and declined analgesics because they were "overjoyed" at having escaped with their lives. Social contexts can begin to explain why there is not a relationship between wounds and pain.

Environmental and contextual input to the experience of pain was also acknowledged in Melzack's neuromatrix theory of pain (Melzack, 2001) which proposed that pain is a multidimensional experience produced by a "neurosignature" or patterns of widely distributed neural activity in the brain. A major source of input to the neuromatrix is described as "cognitive-evaluative," or tonic input from cultural learning, past experience and personality variables. This explicit recognition of social factors, through referencing cultural learning, supports the enormous range of research elaborating social determinants of pain, the thrust of this volume. Of course, these interact with other determinants, including the evolved biological systems that permit intentional/voluntary behavior.

At present, it is not unusual for clinicians and researchers to acknowledge the importance of the "biopsychosocial model of pain," but then to attend primarily to "biopsycho" parameters. Thus, the major emphasis remains on intrapersonal factors (biological and psychological). The broad acknowledgment of a role for social determinants is encouraging, but there remains resistance to detailing the importance of social factors or to seriously focus on social dimensions of pain to improve health care (Craig & Fashler, 2014; Hadjistavropoulos et al., 2011). Williams and Craig (2016) noted that the current IASP definition of pain, quoted above, dates back 50 years and deserves revision in light of a flood of advances in our understanding and management of pain since then. An updated definition was proposed: "Pain is a distressing experience associated with actual or potential tissue damage with sensory, emotional, cognitive and social components" (p. 2423). Among other changes proposed leading to the revised definition, cognitive and social factors are to be recognized explicitly as much the essence of the experience as sensory and emotional factors. Both research and clinical practice now incorporate consideration of these features to a considerable extent. But a request to the International Association for the Study of Pain to reconsider the long-lasting definition quoted above was met with the observation that the leadership of the IASP ICD-11 Task Force and the Pain Terminology Task Force did not consider revising the definition of pain a priority at this time.

The Social Communication Model of Pain

A considerable evidence-base now supports social factors as potent determinants of (a) exposure to risks or prevention of pain, (b) how pain is experienced, including vulnerability and resilience, (c) its debilitating impact and how pain becomes disclosed to others, and (d) the social consequences of painful events, in particular whether and how care is provided (Craig & Fashler, 2014). The impact of prior and current social factors is perhaps most evident on inspection of single episodes of acute pain which unfold over a relatively brief span of time, characteristically ranging between seconds and weeks. But social factors also are evident as determinants of pain when very different time scales are examined. Chronic pain typically is defined as enduring at least 3–6 months and could encompass a substantial portion of any person's life span. As well, the social events delineated can be seen as influencing pain over the long spans of time represented by the bioevolutionary process, as described earlier, perhaps best represented by geological time spans. Thus, what is experienced during any painful event is determined by cumulative ancestral as well as personal histories with current social factors playing important roles.

What has been needed is a conceptual framework which would direct attention in our understanding of pain to a fine-grained appreciation of social factors integrated with biological and psychological factors (Craig, 2009; Hadjistavropoulos et al., 2011). The social communication model of pain attempts to provide a comprehensive perspective on determinants of pain by including the three sets of determinants in the temporal sequence of events associated with any experience of pain, including antecedents, impact on the individual, and consequences in the social behavior of others. Figure 2.1 depicts this cycle. The model proposes reducing the complexities by nesting within this framework mini-models of component processes whose fine-grained analysis would address specific issues at stages of the temporal dynamics. Biological, psychological, and social features at different stages can be examined as they reflect various processes engaged, thereby encouraging different levels of analysis. Figure 2.1 focuses on social and psychological processes rather than biological processes that are subservient. The perspective does not specify the hypotheses to be tested, as would a theory. It serves to integrate and attract attention to the numerous "sociopsychobio" features of pain that must be considered in efforts to either understand or to provide care for people in pain. Other interpersonal models of chronic pain (e.g., operant (Fordyce, 1984; Main, Keefe, Vlaeyen, & Vowles, 2014); intimacy (Cano & Williams, 2010) or communal coping

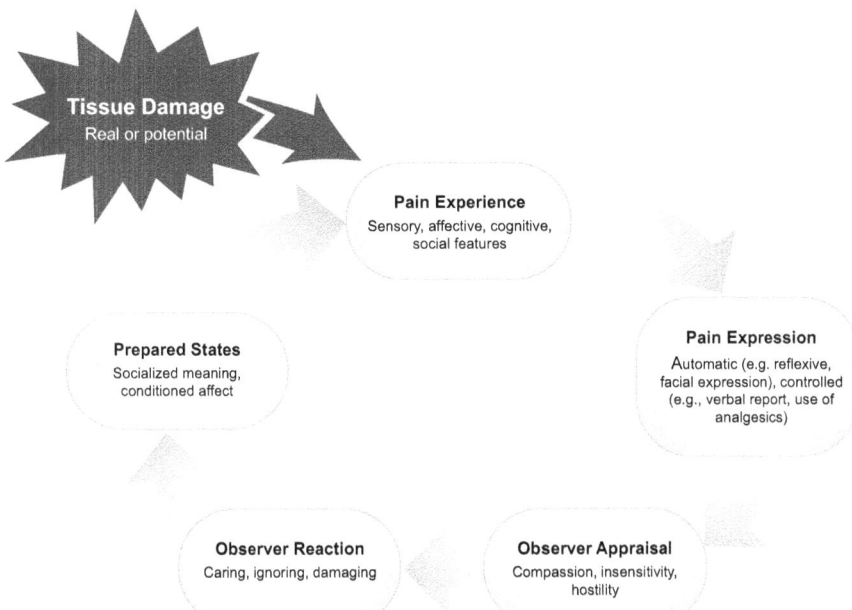

Fig. 2.1 The pain social communications cycle. All stages (1) operate within causal, social, and ecological contexts, (2) have biological substrates, (3) are amenable to change through social and biological interventions. The process is recursive, reciprocal, and dynamic

models (Sullivan, 2012)) appear to select and attach importance to particular features of the dynamic social interactions related to pain.

Social influences vary between those that can be characterized as operating at macro-levels (e.g., cultural, ethnic, economic, health care system, and political) and micro-levels (e.g., linguistic, facial expression, and social neuroscience). Our attempt to provide a conceptual structure has focused upon the intermediate level characteristics of dyadic transactions; how individuals communicate with and influence other individuals (Hadjistavropoulos et al., 2011), but the broader social ecosystem cannot be ignored as social norms, public standards, regulations, and laws set limits on the nature of dyadic communications. For example, consider the challenges of pain management in resource limited economies that are restricted in their capacity to provide medical care (Cleary, Husain, & Maurer, 2016). The study of dyadic transactions represents a level of analysis that directly addresses how people influence each other, with more detailed analyses nested within stages of the temporal sequence and the dyadic transaction recognized as nested within broader contexts. Key features of a social communications analysis concern how pain is encoded behaviorally by the suffering person and how observing others decode this expression. One can examine what is expressed, on the one hand, and what is received on the other. This also lends itself to study of communications as interactions; the correspondence between the message as intended and the message as interpreted, leaving room for accuracy and errors in communication. In turn, communications can be examined as transactions. In patient–physician transactions, accurate communication fulfills both in their roles and a likelihood of effective care; in contrast, errors can lead to both patients and doctors feeling dissatisfied and aggrieved (Hadjistavropoulos et al., 2011).

The typical temporal sequence described above lends itself to isolating factors associated with (a) predispositions to experiencing pain, (b) the pain experience itself, (c) how pain is expressed, and (d) the reactions of parties attendant to the pain (Prkachin & Craig, 1995). The process is recognized as dynamic and recursive with substantial reciprocal influences. A further logical and heuristic distinction can be made between environmental events impacting at biological, psychological, and social levels of analysis that are historical, or in the past for the person, and those that are contemporary and immediately present. The former cannot be changed, while the latter are amenable to change as a feature of protecting or caring for the individual.

Predispositions and Antecedents People are biologically, psychologically, and behaviorally predisposed or prepared to experience and express pain instigated by threshold level internal or external noxious events. The individual's past, very broadly conceived, and the present context, complex in its own right, must interact to determine whether there indeed is exposure and the experience of pain. Evolutionary processes responsible for phylogenetic variation in how pain is experienced have already been described. The unique genetic inheritance of any given individual must be recognized as responsible for ontogenetic emergence of life span changes, in interaction with epigenetic processes that represent interactions between the individual and her/his unique environments, ultimately responsible for the individual's phenotype. The individual's current situation would then determine whether there was exposure to pain and whether vulnerability or resilience was displayed. Moderate to severe pains tend to be traumatic and to have a traumatic enduring impact—witness the large numbers of people who appear to have acquired needle, dental, or medical phobias by virtue of routine painful vaccination needle injections (Taddio et al., 2010) and the benefits derived from current programs designed to minimize pain during immunization injections (Taddio et al., 2013). Screening for psychological vulnerability and resilience can be undertaken with success (Esteve, Bendayan, Lopez-Martinez, & Ramirez-Maestre, 2017). The socially constructed physical environment is important in determining protection or exposure to pain. Numerous environmental factors can be identified, both physical and social, including workplace features that place employees at risk, recreational and sport settings that similarly pose or minimize threats, whether inoculation programs designed to prevent contagious diseases minimize the pain infants and children experience, and availability and access to medical care.

The Experience of Pain: Sensory, Affective, Cognitive, and Social Features Accepting pain as an integrated whole experience with cognitive, emotional, and social as well as sensory features implicates a very broad range of psychosocial determinants. Processing pain must entail at least attention to it, comprehending its meaning, evaluating it favorably or unfavorably, deciding how to react and acting, with both conscious and unconscious mechanisms engaged. Personal experiences with pain have a feed forward impact as they determine subsequent reactions. Both implicit and explicit learning can be involved. Fear conditioning as a result of painful injury is an obvious illustration. For example, medical prophylaxis, diagnosis, and treatment all can have long lasting impact, perhaps in the form of phobias, but also as leading to dispositions toward tolerance during inevitable exposure to pain. The human capacity for knowing the pain of others (Goubert, Craig, & Buysse, 2009) and vicarious learning processes (Boerner, Chambers, McGrath, LoLordo, & Uher, 2017; Goubert et al., 2011) multiply the potential for social learning about pain through acquisition of understanding about risks and protection from pain, what one is likely to experience, and how various actions diminish or potentiate the painful experience. Human use of language further expands the potential for observational learning, as written texts and oral communications can effectively transmit the experiences of others, promoting the types of learning just articulated. These different forms of social learning provide the opportunities for families, and the ethnic contexts within which they are embedded, to transmit beliefs, expectations, values, social norms, and social standards across generations. A growing body of research suggests that it is not the intensity of the pain itself, but rather the extent to which pain interferes with valued, daily activities that is the primary motivation for seeking treatment, and may be the key trigger for subsequent coping (Crombez, Eccleston, Van Damme, Vlaeyen, & Karoly, 2012). Such findings underscore the importance of targeting psychosocial aspects of the pain experience. Psychological states prognostic of adverse reactions to noxious events (e.g., negative schemas, anxiety sensitivity or catastrophizing) can be identified, assessed and potentially changed through social interventions. But this perhaps places too much emphasis on the individual's past and fails to adequately recognize the immediate effect of the setting and the social audience on both pain experience and the behavioral reaction. Cues signaling safety or danger, availability of relief or further threat, or the presence of friends or adversaries trigger less or more severe reactions (e.g., Leknes et al., 2013; Van Damme et al., 2003).

Expressive Actions   Pain may be a private, subjective experience, but that does not preclude almost inevitable public manifestations that permit others to infer painful experience. Surprisingly, there has been little detailed description of how people react when in pain, with most attention devoted to the presumed important manifestations, self-report and nonverbal expression. Melzack and Wall (1965) described how people react to sudden unexpected damage to the skin, including a startle response, a flexion reflex, postural readjustment, vocalization, orientation of the head and eyes to examine the damaged area, autonomic responses, evocation of past experience in similar situations and prediction of the consequences of the stimulation, and many other patterns of behavior aimed at diminishing the sensory and affective components of the whole experience, such as rubbing the damaged area and avoidance behavior. But there have been few systematic descriptive studies. These immediate largely involuntary reactions carry considerable credibility as expressive of pain for observers. In a systematic review of observational scales designed to assess children's pain, Sekhon, Fashler, Versloot, Lee, and Craig (2017) noted fully 66 different behavioral items to be observed in 21 different scales. A study using factor analyses to characterize observer ratings of these behavioral items on the automatic/controlled distinction noted above indicated that "Automatic" items included facial expression, paralinguistic qualities of the use of language and consolability of the child, "Controlled" items included intentional movements, verbalizations and social actions, and items that were ambiguous on these dimensions included voluntary facial expressions, supporting the dual-processing, neuroregulatory model of pain expression (Craig et al., 2010).

While biological and personal histories constrain how pain may be expressed, current setting and social events determine personal modulation of the expression. Self-report of pain is highly modulated to be appropriate to the situation, whereas nonverbal expression, including facial expression, tends to be more spontaneous and less ambiguous with respect to whether these manifestations are caused by pain rather than other factors, including purposeful efforts to control the situation. Schiavenato and Craig (2010) have argued that considering pain assessment to be a social transaction would permit a greater understanding of the process. Variations in pain during intimate sexual relationships are instructive. For example, in vulvodynia, the pain interferes with both sexuality and romantic relationships, two highly valued aspects of life. Rosen, Muise, Bergeron, Delisle, and Baxter (2015) and Rosen, Sadikaj, and Bergeron (2015) summarize a substantial literature indicating that facilitative partner responses were associated with women's lower intercourse pain and better sexual functioning, as well as couples' greater relationship and sexual satisfaction. Conversely, greater negative and solicitous partner responses were associated with more pain and depressive symptoms in women, as well as lower sexual functioning and relationship and sexual satisfaction in couples. The functional significance of pain communications is considerable and deserving of greater attention (Steinkopf, 2016).

The focus on pain experience can lead to less attention to the debilitating effects of pain and the ability to work, benefit from school, fulfill domestic responsibilities, or maintain social relationships. Increasing attention is being paid to the impact of pain upon interpersonal functioning. For example, one of the more common measures of pain disability, the Pain Disability Index (Chibnall & Tait, 1994) examines the impact of pain on seven domains of an individual's life: family, recreation, social activities, occupation, sexual behavior, self-care, and life support activities. All are social in different ways.

Others' Judgments and Decision-Making When Pain Is Expressed Attention and care provided to the person experiencing clinical pain will depend upon the sensitivity, disposition, and skills of others. Their relationship (family member, health care practitioner, stranger, enemy, etc.), training, and commitment to the person in pain will be crucial. Reactions to witnessing pain in others can be characterized using the dual automatic/controlled neuroregulatory systems already described (Braver, 2012). Seeing others in pain can instigate automatic empathetic reactions (for example, gut level reactions) as well as reflective effort to understand what is happening to the person. Observers readily distinguish these two categories of protective behavior in adults (McCrystal et al., 2011) and children (Sekhon et al., 2017). Automatic, spontaneous reactions provide a relatively unambiguous readout of painful experience. Controlled, self-directed behavior may have determinants other than painful experience, including conscious efforts to control both the experience and its behavioral impact on others, either by inhibiting or facilitating the display, or, at an extreme, feigning painful distress when pain is not present (Hill & Craig, 2002).

Both self-interest and other-interest may be engaged (Goubert et al., 2009). There is considerable potential for suspicion and distrust concerning the credibility of people's complaints of pain (De Ruddere & Craig, 2016). People who perceive injustice as associated with their pain are more likely to become depressed (Scott & Sullivan, 2012).

A greater understanding of social factors governing whether observers are indifferent, compassionate or perpetrators of further distress is needed. Partner responses can be solicitous (attention and sympathy), negative (hostility and frustration), and facilitative (encourage adaptive coping) (Rosen, Muise, et al., 2015; Rosen, Sadikaj, et al., 2015). The distinction between historical and current determinants of pain also applies to observer reactions. Personal backgrounds, including dispositions to be sensitive to others, medical histories, and perhaps formal training as health care professionals would affect judgments about a person's pain and how it should be managed. Perhaps specialized training in pain research and management will dictate sensitivity and decision-making for the person in pain, within the scope of the individual's capabilities.

All interventions administered by other people could be reconceptualized as social interventions, regardless of whether they arise from the biomedical model (e.g., pharmaceuticals, surgery, or stimulators), or from a broader biopsychosocial perspective (for example, cognitive-behavioral or self-management therapies). The placebo phenomenon is increasingly conceptualized as a social intervention rather than the application of an inert substance. Expectancies acquired through socialization now are recognized as the active ingredient.

The Broad Socio-ecological Contexts of Environments in Which Pain Is Experienced Access to care for both acute and chronic pain depends upon the nature and quality of the health system. This varies substantially by geographic location. Public demand, willingness of politicians to create and fund programs, and scientific research creating knowledge and interventions are some of the determinants of willingness to commit resources to care for people in pain. Access to care is presently a major issue. Whether the focus of available care is upon biomedical or biopsychosocial care is important. There are big differences in care provided to vulnerable populations, including infants and young children, people with intellectual disabilities or brain damage, and seniors, including those with dementias. Care invariably relates to the broad differences represented by demographic characteristics, e.g., age, sex, ethnicity, race, or socioeconomic status? Also important is whether caregivers are educated in up-to-date evidence-based intervention strategies.

Concluding Remarks

The social communications perspective emerged from recognition of the all-embracing and powerful role of social determinants of pain and pain-related disabilities. The intent here was to demonstrate that social determinants and the social context are particularly important for humans. A heavy clinical and research focus on sensory features of pain has led to a neglect of interpersonal and contextual factors that could be controlled, thereby reducing the likelihood of exposure to painful distress, appraising the experience in dark and distressing ways, inappropriate or ineffective demands for help, and inadequate or iatrogenic clinical care. Ignoring social factors does not mean that they are unimportant—their impact will remain substantial, only unintentional and unappreciated. Clinical management of painful conditions needs to go beyond medical interventions to include use of social interventions, psychological and contextual in ongoing care to reduce pain and suffering.

References

Beecher, H. K. (1956). Relationship of significance of wound to pain experienced. *JAMA, 161*, 1609–1613.

Benson-Amram, S., Dantzer, B., Stricker, G., Swanson, E., & Holekamp, K. (2016). Brain size predicts problem solving ability in mammalian carnivores. *PNAS, 113*, 2532–2537.

Boerner, K. E., Chambers, C. T., McGrath, P. J., LoLordo, V., & Uher, R. (2017). The effect of parental modeling on child pain responses: The role of parent and child sex. *Journal of Pain, 18*, 702–715.

Braver, T. S. (2012). The variable nature of cognitive control: A dual-mechanisms framework. *Trends in Cognitive Sciences, 16*, 106–113.

Broom, D. M. (1998). Welfare, stress, and the evolution of feelings. *Advances in the Study of Behavior, 27*, 371–404.

Broom, D. M., & Fraser, A. F. (2007). Behavior towards predators and social attackers. In D. M. Broom & A. F. Fraser (Eds.), *Domestic animal behavior and welfare* (4th ed., pp. 73–76). Wallingford, England: CAB International.

Cano, A., & Williams, A. C. d. C. (2010). Social interaction in pain: Reinforcing pain behaviors or building intimacy? *Pain, 149*, 9–11.

Cantor & Craig (2017). Chronic pain, recuperation and cooperation: Evolution and signaling theory perspectives. unpublished.

Chambers, C. T., & Mogil, J. S. (2015). The ontogeny and phylogeny of facial expression of pain. *Pain, 156*, 798–799.

Chibnall, J. T., & Tait, R. C. (1994). The pain disability index: Factor structure and normative data. *Archives of Physical Medicine and Rehabilitation, 75*, 1082–1086.

Cleary, J. F., Husain, A., & Maurer, M. (2016). Increasing worldwide access to medical opioids. *Lancet, 387*(10028), 1597–1599.

Craig, K. D. (1986). Social modeling influences: Pain in context. In R. A. Sternbach (Ed.), *The psychology of pain* (2nd ed., pp. 67–96). New York, NY: Raven Press.

Craig, K. D. (2004). Editorial—social communication of pain enhances protective functions: A comment on Deyo, Prkachin and Mercer (2003). *Pain, 107*, 5–6.

Craig, K. D. (2009). The social communication model of pain. *Canadian Psychology, 50*, 22–32.

Craig, K. D., & Fashler, S. (2014). Social determinants of pain. In J. Strong, A. Unruh, & H. van Griensven (Eds.), *A textbook for healthcare practitioners*. London, England: Elsevier.

Craig, K. D., Versloot, J., Goubert, L., Vervoort, T., & Crombez, G. (2010). Perceiving others in pain: Automatic and controlled mechanisms. *Journal of Pain, 11*, 101–108.

Crombez, G., Eccleston, C., Van Damme, S., Vlaeyen, J. W. S., & Karoly, P. (2012). Fear-avoidance model of chronic pain: The next generation. *Clinical Journal of Pain, 28*, 475–483.

Crook, R. J., & Walters, E. T. (2011). Nociceptive behavior and physiology of molluscs: Animal welfare implications. *ILAR Journal, 52*, 185–195.

De Ruddere, L., & Craig, K. D. (2016). Understanding stigma and chronic pain: A state of the art review. *Pain, 157*, 1607–1610.

De Waal, F. (2009). *The age of empathy: Nature's lessons for a kinder society*. New York, NY: Harmony Books.

Dunbar, R. I. (2009). The social brain hypothesis and its implications for human evolution. *Annals of Human Biology, 36*, 562–572.

Esteve, R., Bendayan, R., Lopez-Martinez, A. E., & Ramirez-Maestre, C. (2017). Resilience and vulnerability factors when pain is acute as predictors of disability: Findings from a two-year longitudinal study. *Pain Medicine, 18*, 2116–2125.

Fordyce, W. E. (1984). Behavioral science and chronic pain. *Postgraduate Medical Journal, 60*, 865–868.

Foster, M., & Sherrington, C. S. (1897). *A textbook of physiology* (7th ed.). New York, NY: Macmillan.

Gagliese, L., & Katz, J. (2000). Medically unexplained pain is not caused by psychopathology. *Pain Research & Management, 5*, 251–257.

Goubert, L., Craig, K. D., & Buysse, A. (2009). Perceiving others in pain: Experimental and clinical evidence on the role of empathy. In W. Ickes & J. Decety (Eds.), *The social neuroscience of empathy* (pp. 153–166). Cambridge, MA: MIT Press.

Goubert, L., Vlaeyen, J. W. S., Crombez, G., & Craig, K. D. (2011). Learning about pain from others: An observational learning account. *Journal of Pain, 12*, 167–174.

Hadjistavropoulos, T., Breau, L., & Craig, K. D. (2011). Pain assessment in adults and children with limited ability to communicate. In D. C. Turk & R. Melzack (Eds.), *Handbook of pain assessment* (3rd ed., pp. 260–282). New York, NY: Guilford Press.

Hadjistavropoulos, T., & Craig, K. D. (2002). A theoretical framework for understanding self-report and observational measures of pain: A communications model. *Behaviour Research and Therapy, 40*(5), 551–570.

Hadjistavropoulos, T., Craig, K. D., Duck, S., Cano, A. M., Goubert, L., Jackson, P., … Dever Fitzgerald, T. (2011). A biopsychosocial formulation of pain communication. *Psychological Bulletin, 137*(6), 910–939.

Hari, R., Henriksson, L., Malinen, S., & Parkkonen, L. (2015). Centrality of social interaction in human brain function. *Neuron, 88*, 181–193.

Hill, M. L., & Craig, K. D. (2002). Detecting deception in pain expressions: The structure of genuine and deceptive facial displays. *Pain, 98*, 135–144.

Katz, J., & Rosenbloom, B. (2015). The golden anniversary of Melzack and Wall's gate control theory of pain: Celebrating fifty years of pain research and management. *Pain Research & Management, 20*, 285–286.

Langford, D. J., Bailey, A. L., Chanda, M. L., Clarke, S. E., Drummond, T. E., Echols, S., … Mogil, J. S. (2010). Coding of facial expressions of pain in the laboratory mouse. *Nature Methods, 7*(6), 447–449.

Leknes, S., Berna, C., Lee, M. C., Snyder, G. D., Biele, G., & Tracey, I. (2013). The importance of context: When relative relief renders pain pleasant. *Pain, 154*, 402–410.

Lenroot, R. K., & Giedd, J. N. (2006). Brain development in children and adolescents: Insights from anatomical magnetic resonance imaging. *Neuroscience and Biobehavioral Reviews, 30*, 718–729.

Lynch, M. (2016). The opioid pendulum and the need for better pain care. *Pain Medicine, 17*, 1215–1219.

Lynch, M., & Katz, J. (2017). "One size fits all" doesn't fit when it comes to long-term opioid use for people with chronic pain. *Journal of the Canadian Pain Society, 1*, 2–7.

Main, C. J., Keefe, F. J., Vlaeyen, J. W. S., & Vowles, K. E. (2014). *Fordyce's behavioral methods for chronic pain and illness*. Seattle, WA: IASP Books.

Marshall, H. R. (1894). *Pain, pleasure, and aesthetics*. London: Macmillan.

McCrystal, K. N., Craig, K. D., Versloot, J., Fashler, S. R., & Jones, D. M. (2011). Perceiving pain in others: Validation of a dual processing model. *Pain, 152*, 1083–1089.

Melchert, T. P. (2016). Leaving behind our preparadigmatic past: Professional psychology as a unified clinical science. *American Psychologist, 71*, 486–496.

Melzack, R. (1990). The tragedy of needless pain. *Scientific American, 262*, 27–33.

Melzack, R. (2001). Pain and the neuromatrix in the brain. *Journal of Dental Education, 65*, 1378–1382.

Melzack, R., & Casey, K. L. (1968). Sensory, motivational, and central control determinants of pain: A new conceptual model. In D. R. Kenshalo (Ed.), *The skin senses* (pp. 423–439). Springfield, IL: Charles C. Thomas.

Melzack, R., & Wall, P. D. (1965). Pain mechanisms: A new theory. *Science, 150*, 971–979.

Melzack, R., & Wall, P. D. (1982). Citation classic—pain mechanisms: A new theory. *Current Contents, 22*.

Mogil, J. S. (2015). Social modulation of and by pain in humans and rodents. *Pain, 156*(Suppl. 1), S35–S41.

Prkachin, K. M., & Craig, K. D. (1995). Expressing pain: The communication and interpretation of facial pain signals. *Journal of Nonverbal Behavior, 19*, 191–205.

Rosen, N. O., Muise, A., Bergeron, S., Delisle, I., & Baxter, M. L. (2015). Daily associations between partner responses and sexual relationship in couples coping with provoked vistibulodynia. *Journal of Sexual Medicine, 12*, 1028–1039.

Rosen, N. O., Sadikaj, G., & Bergeron, S. (2015). Within-person variability in relationship satisfaction moderates pain estimation among couples with vulvodynia. *Pain*. https://doi.org/10.1097/j.pain.0000000000001015678

Roth, G., & Dicke, U. (2005). Evolution of the brain and intelligence. *Trends in Cognitive Science, 9*, 250–257.

Schiavenato, M., & Craig, K. D. (2010). Pain assessment as a social transaction: Beyond the "gold standard". *Clinical Journal of Pain, 26*, 667–676.

Schultz, S., Dunbar, R., & Lovejoy, C. O. (2010). Encephalization is not a universal macroevolutionary phenomenon in mammals but is associated with sociality. *Proceedings of the National Academy of Sciences, 107*(50), 21582–21586.

Scott, W., & Sullivan, M. J. L. (2012). Perceived injustice moderates the relationship between pain and depressive symptoms among individuals with persistent musculoskeletal pain. *Pain Research & Management, 17*, 335–340.

Sekhon, K. K., Fashler, S. R., Versloot, J., Lee, S., & Craig, K. D. (2017). Children's behavioral pain cues: Implicit automaticity and control dimensions in observational measures. *Pain Research & Management, 2017*, 3017837. Published online February 21, 2017. https://doi.org/10.1155/2017/3017837

Steinkopf, L. (2016). An evolutionary perspective on pain communication. *Evolutionary Psychology*. https://doi.org/10.1177/1474704916653964

Sullivan, M. J. L. (2012). The communal coping model of pain catastrophizing: Clinical and research implications. *Canadian Psychology, 53*, 32–41.

Taddio, A., Appleton, M., Bortolussi, R., Chambers, C., Dubey, V., Halperin, S., … Shah, M. (2010). Reducing the pain of childhood vaccination: An evidence-based clinical practice guideline (summary). *CMAJ, 182*, 1989–1995.

Taddio, A., Shah, V., Leung, E., Wang, J., Parikh, C., Smart, S., … Franck, L. (2013). Knowledge translation of the HELPinKIDS clinical practice guideline for managing childhood vaccination pain: Usability and knowledge uptake of educational materials directed to new parents. *BMC Pediatrics, 13*, 13–23. https://doi.org/10.1186/1471-2431-13-23

Van Damme, S., Lorenz, J., Eccleston, C., Koster, E. H. W., Clercq, A. D., & Crombez, G. (2003). Fear-conditioned cues of impending pain facilitate attentional engagement. *Clinical Neurophysiology, 34,* 33–39.

Williams, A. C. d. C., & Craig, K. D. (2016). Updating the definition of pain. *Pain, 157,* 2420–2423.

Zhang, K., & Sejnowski, T. J. (2000). A universal scaling law between gray matter and white matter of cerebral cortex. *PNAS, 97,* 5621–5626.

Chapter 3
Developmental Dimensions in Understanding Interpersonal Features of Pain

Rebecca Pillai Riddell and Kenneth D. Craig

Abstract Lifespan stage must be considered among the innumerable biological, cognitive, emotional, behavioral, and social determinants of individual variations in pain. Pain experience and expression are dynamic products of interactions among biological inheritance and daily living within diverse physical and social environments that vary substantially over the course of a lifetime. This chapter presents an overview of basic concepts needed to understand developmental changes in both intrapersonal and interpersonal features of pain in complex human environments. While one's physiology, genetics, maturational stage, nutritional history, disease and injury exposure, and other features of biological well-being are important determinants of pain experience and expression, at all stages of life the social environment has powerful impacts on whether there is exposure to pain, how pain is experienced and expressed, how others react and deliver care to the person and, frequently, whether pain is controlled. Consideration is given to the relevance of these concepts for developmentally appropriate care and to addressing their relevance for pain assessment and management.

Keywords Lifespan · Intrapersonal factors · Interpersonal factors · Psychosocial mechanisms · Developmental

R. Pillai Riddell (✉)
Department of Psychology, York University, Toronto, ON, Canada

Department of Psychiatry, Hospital for Sick Children, Toronto, ON, Canada

Department of Psychiatry, University of Toronto, Toronto, ON, Canada
e-mail: rpr@yorku.ca

K. D. Craig
University of British Columbia, Vancouver, BC, Canada

© Springer International Publishing AG, part of Springer Nature 2018
T. Vervoort et al. (eds.), *Social and Interpersonal Dynamics in Pain*,
https://doi.org/10.1007/978-3-319-78340-6_3

Introduction

Pain is known to be a complex, highly personal, subjective experience. Its multiple dimensions were traditionally characterized as sensory and affective (Merskey et al., 1979), but decades of research have compelled recognition of cognitive and social parameters of the experience (Williams & Craig, 2016). Efforts to understand this complexity have focused upon physiological, psychological, and social-environmental determinants. Pain experience is not only a product of evolved biological mechanisms, but also is determined by psychological and social processes. Pain is a synthesis—a sum that is greater than its parts.

The brain has a remarkable capacity to modulate perception of sensory input through the biological substrates of emotion, cognition, and social processes. While innate systems provide the initial biological architecture for the experience of pain, this framework is remarkably plastic, particularly in humans, with transformations throughout the lifespan shaped by biological changes and personal experiences. The changes to the nociceptive system can be described by biological scientists at the level of epigenetic, anatomical, and physiological systems, but the role of psychological and social-environmental determinants of pain requires description in terms of how the organism acts, thinks, and feels. Memory, attention, expectations, and appraisals are intimately involved in cognitive and emotional modulation of pain, with appraisals of its meaning and associative emotion determined by social contexts. These sensitivities and capabilities exist because they have functional value— they facilitate adaptation to physical and social environmental demands and challenges.

Social communication models of pain (in text ref) distinguish (Craig, 2009; Hadjistavropoulos et al., 2011; Pillai Riddell, Racine, Craig & Campbell, 2014) distinguishes stages of painful events that occur in the context of social influences (see Craig, Chap. 2). Individuals of all ages bring predispositions to react to painful events with varying sensitivities and patterns of experience and expression. Tissue damage associated with injury or disease instigates the sensory, emotional, cognitive, and social features of the experience of pain. Tissue damage triggers automatic, reflexive features of homeostatic systems as well as behaviors designed to protect the individual that can be classified as either involuntary or controlled, including more complex controlled behavior that permits escape from noxious events or engagement of the care of others (Hadjistavropoulos et al., 2011). These allow caregivers to determine the nature of care to be provided. In adolescents and adults, the majority of painful events are managed through personal care interventions or through self-regulation of distress/stress. However, intellectually disabled individuals and younger children may not have the personal skills accessible; thus, the interventions of others may be necessary. Hence, the model incorporates consideration not only of the person who is in pain but also the appraisals and behavior of others responding to the person in distress and the interplay between the two. The influence and importance of individuals who respond to a person in distress varies greatly according to the developmental stage of the individual in pain.

For example, mothers involved in infant care monitor them intensely and are highly protective, whereas older children typically can be presumed to have some of the cognitive, emotional, behavioral, and social skills needed to care for themselves. Of course, in the case of clinically significant pain, these skills may be insufficient, at any age, requiring the intercessions of professionals, including physicians who may deliver medical care or other health care professionals able to address more complex psychological and social issues. Successful delivery of care for pain, either a reduction or a resolution, depends upon the capacities of caregivers to recognize pain, evaluate its nature within the context of the person and the setting, and their decisions and actions designed to deliver care. To accomplish this successfully requires sensitivity to developmental stage.

This chapter examines developmental changes in the phenomenon of pain, particularly how the interpersonal environment shapes the nature of pain experience and its expression in the course of lifespan development. The focus is upon humans.

Infants, children, adolescents, and adults (early, midlife, and older) suffering from pain vary considerably in physical, cognitive, emotional, behavioral, and social characteristics. Pain is a major feature of life across the lifespan, but developmental differences necessitate consideration of what the commonalities are at different stages of life and how differences over the lifespan and among people will influence pain experience and expression. Before examining mechanisms of how the social context influences pain experience and expression, the different domains of pain experience will be discussed through a developmental lens.

Developmental Domains of Pain Experience and the Influence of the Social Context

Transformations in biological development, cognitive capabilities, emotional processes, behavioral competence, and patterns of social interaction are conspicuous during different phases of the lifespan. All are affected by and influence in turn interpersonal features of pain. Each cannot be addressed in isolation as they interact with each other through reciprocal influence processes. For example, physical growth is optimized by healthy environments which provide adequate nutrition, exercise, and social stimulation. Physical growth constrains maturation of cognitive and affective systems that underlie the experience and behavioral expression of pain.

Pain is usually thought of as a unitary state—people talk about their pain experiences and are asked about their pain as if it were one construct. Nevertheless, the experience is recognized as comprising an amalgam of differentiable thoughts, feelings, and sensory features, with older children and adults able to talk about separately when asked to do so. It is useful to separately conceptualize different components of the experience from the lifespan perspective and examine how each feature interacts with the social context. In the following we briefly examine features of pain, the intersection with social processes, and how they may vary over developmental life stage.

Sensory/Discriminative Features

Fundamental to the experience of pain are sensations associated with real or potential tissue damage. In competent children and adults, these can be described in terms of a location on the body, different sensory qualities (Melzack, 1975; Melzack & Casey, 1968), and perceived intensity. Even the most premature newborn typically displays reactions to tissue damage or stress, and these patterns remain obvious throughout the lifespan (Vinall & Grunau, 2014). These painful responses become more differentiated, specific to pain, and reliable with age, as cognitive sophistication increases for humans to be better able to differentiate pain physiologically (e.g., intensity levels, visceral versus musculoskeletal) and pain psychologically (e.g., physical pain from loneliness, fear, and social rejection).

Unlike other sensory phenomenon represented in the brain, pain is distinct. Rather than have brain architecture that is specific to pain, neuroscientists have posited that networks of cortical and subcortical connections are orchestrated to result in the sensations, cognitions, emotions and social perceptions that synergize to form pain experience (Verriotis, Chang, Fitzgerald, & Fabrizi, 2016). Thus, development of the sensory/discriminative features across the lifespan is dependent not only on the maturation of individual brain structures, but also on the maturity of the connective relationships between brain structures that form the adult nociceptive network. Adding to the complexity of understanding the development of cortical underpinnings of the sensory/discriminative aspects of pain development is that, in the adult brain, similar networks are activated when social pain is experienced. For example, using a repeated-measures design on emerging adulthood participants, a lab-based social exclusion task was shown to involve the same somatosensory components of the lab-based physical pain paradigm (electrical pain stimuli), namely the posterior insular cortex and secondary somatosensory cortex (November, Zanon, & Silani, 2015).

The sensory/discriminative features of painful experience come closest to representing "bottom-up" determinants of the experience, i.e., the sensory input, but they are subject to facilitative and inhibitory modulation by emotional and cognitive states, the "top-down" determinants of the experience.

Affective/Motivational Features

Painful experience is also defined by the powerful motivational and emotional features that drive defensive escape or avoidance of further tissue stress. These are intrinsic aversive and noxious features of noxious experience that are influenced by dispositions and the situational context. They are capable of driving other emotions including fear, anger, or disgust. Evidence of the aversive impact of painful experience is as evident in preterm newborns as it is later in life, including when capacities for cognizant awareness may have diminished through dementias or developmental stage. Emotional distress is roughly correlated with the magnitude of the painful experience (Craig, Best, & Best, 1978).

The raw negative emotions observed in infant facial expressions after painful procedures have been shown to be relatively undifferentiated over the first year of life (Ahola Kohut, Pillai Riddell, Flora, & Oster, 2012). However, consistent with the child's attachment capabilities (i.e., how an infant uses the caregiver to regulate distress) after the first year of life, social emotions such as shame and guilt, appear. The presence of these emotional displays suggests emerging cognizance of the social environment. Most infants learn on a rudimentary level, through repeated interactions with their caregivers during painful and distressing events (i.e., social-ization), to modify distress signaling, based on what strategies are successful in achieving soothing from a parent (Horton, Pillai Riddell, Flora, Moran, & Pederson, 2015). Negative emotional expression through toddlerhood and preschooler age has also been shown to be multidetermined. To illustrate, a large genotype by environ-ment interaction study recently demonstrated that challenges with the expression of negative emotionality were a product not only of adoptive parents who had diffi-culty regulating their own emotion but also of a genetic predisposition for negative emotionality in the birth mother (Lipscombe, Leve, Shaw, & Neiderhiser, 2012). In late childhood and adolescence, affective capabilities are more advanced and a more introspective perspective of one's pain experience becomes possible. The child's or teen's pain experience gradually gains an increasingly private dimension and they are more able to control affective displays in response to pain. This increased self-regulatory ability comes in tandem with greater control of the pain signaling they want to send to other people (Larochette, Chambers, & Craig, 2006).

Cognitive Features

Cognitive features of the pain experience appear subject to the greatest progressive differentiation and change from infancy through to the mature adult years. These intrinsically represent an amalgam of life experiences structured through mecha-nisms of attention, memory, language, thought, and decision making. Infants and people with limited cognitive capabilities are dependent upon others to assess and manage their pain. For young children, emergence of self-management capabilities over development allows for gradual independence in assessing and managing mun-dane painful experiences. While infants initially display sensory and diffuse negative emotional reactions as prominent features of their primal painful experience, capaci-ties for the more refined characteristics of cognitive processing become manifest early in life. Over the first year of life, individual differences in how infants behav-iorally respond to tissue damage increasingly display greater variability, in signifi-cant part reflecting how the infant was socialized in pain contexts by their parents (Pillai Riddell et al., 2013). It is argued elsewhere in this book that at no other stage in the lifespan does the social context play such a large part in the construction of an individual's pain experience (See Gennis and Pillai Riddell, Chap. 17).

Through infancy into the early years of life there is an increased capacity to modu-late reactions during painful events and shape those reactions based on interactions with primary caregivers and other members of the family. Using the perspectives of attachment theory and research, Bowlby (1969/1982) described as "internal working models" (IWMs) the early social cognitions of infants relating to distress and beliefs about caregiving they anticipate receiving. Generally speaking, IWMs represent cognitive schema that emerge in early life but continue to be activated over the lifespan when appropriate to life events, for example when in pain. IWMs are critical determinants of the emotions experienced and social behaviors enacted to elicit support. The sophistication of IWMs would be impacted by developing cortical capacities, including the capacity for long-term memory storage and retrieval, emerging language abilities, and the ability to use abstract reasoning. Their emergence is associated with capacities for descending inhibitory control over pain during early childhood. The fully developed capacity to assess and cope with pain largely appears to come on board around the transition into adolescence. While a family's social influences on pain cognitive processing (directly or indirectly) are ubiquitous, at any stage in the lifespan another major influence on a person's cognitive schemas would be substantial exposure to clinical and hospital environments or chronic pain. Medical challenges would lead individuals coming to understand pain differently than those without such exposure based on different needs for their caregiver. For example, research has shown that individuation from parents may be delayed with adolescents who experience a chronic pain condition (Logan & Scharff, 2005).

As a function of increasing cognitive complexity over the lifespan, pain reactions become less reflexive and people become more deliberate in their pain behavior, coordinating pain expression with situational social demands in their perceived best interests. In this manner, self-management skills supplant reflexive homeostatic regulatory systems and children come to exercise skill in coping with painful events, including through active engagement with other people. It should be recognized that this only describes typical development. People with intellectual disabilities or loss of these cognitive capabilities through injury or disease may not have these facilities in the first instance or may lose the capacities. The inability to understand or report pain should never preclude appropriate pain assessment and management.

Social Features of Pain

Humans are social animals. Adapting to the broad range of natural and social ecological niches that modern humans inhabit has been accomplished primarily through innovative social institutions. Social environments largely provide the contexts in which the perception of pain emerges. The primacy of the social context in the development of pain and distress responses appears codified in human genes. By virtue of first cries at birth, humans are born capable of signaling others and socialization of distress immediately begins. They do not learn to cry or mount a distress expression, yet these instinctual behaviors over time become deliberate behaviors. Infants are strikingly sensitive to their mother's emotional states when they are in pain. Their ability to regulate from the pain and distress of painful procedures has been shown to be contingent upon their primary caregiver's reactions during the first year of life (Din Osmun, Pillai Riddell, & Flora, 2014; Racine et al., 2016).

As children grow older, social experiences in family, school and peer contexts teach about settings associated with pain, what types of pain expressions are appropriate in what contexts, and how they might avoid or manage pain (Goubert, Vlaeyen, Crombez, & Craig, 2011). The meaning of pain is learned through experiences of pain in social contexts. The importance of social cueing becomes recognizable when problematic issues that confront clinicians are considered. For example, the salience of the social context can be recognized when one appreciates that a hospitalized infant mounts a distress response when they hear a nurse opening an alcohol swab or an adult claims they would rather face illness or disease than receive a routine vaccination. How the social context becomes internalized into one's pain experience and expression will be the subject of the following section.

Understanding Mechanisms for the Interpersonal Factors in Pain

Ontogenetic Transformations

Developmental changes in pain experience and expression have a basis in biological maturation. The invariant sequence of progression through infancy, childhood, adolescence, adulthood and older life and the substantial variations in pain expression at any age can be conceptualized as having their origins in (1) the biological legacy inherited by the individual and its maturational unfolding over the lifespan, (2) prenatal and postnatal environmental factors influencing unfolding of these systems, including those described by epigenetics and the impact of disease and injury, (3) environmental factors such as nutrition or toxic environmental exposures, and (4) the impact of the unique social environments to which people are exposed through the course of life from birth to death. The substantial sex and gender differences in pain experience and expression are the consequence of interactions between biological inheritance and social experience with the latter recognized as of considerable importance (Greenspan et al., 2007).

Brain and nervous system development are substantial during infancy and childhood, paralleling the more obvious physical maturity as children grow older. Advances in understanding epigenetics have made it clear that genetic unfolding is responsive to experience, with early life medical, nutritional, and social histories having an impact on genetic outcomes. Thus, we increasingly appreciate of the role of early life experiences with pain as they lead to changes in neurobiological development and the experience and expression of pain. Early and/or severe events are able to change the brain and nervous system (Fitzgerald & Walker, 2009; Grunau, 2013). Biological processes are often conceptualized as reflexive and automatic, but in more evolved species, humans in particular, the biological capabilities provide for capacities to learn and problem-solve. The large human cerebrum provides for intergenerational transmission of knowledge, learning through personal and social experience, and the ability to problem-solve when confronted with life challenges, including the dilemmas associated with pain.

Social and Environmental Influences

Social and environmental influences have an impact on the children's emotional experiences, their thoughts and the skills they exercise to influence their environment. From earliest infancy, maternal care and other adult care are essential if the child is to thrive. Working in tandem with the attachment behavioral control system postulated by Bowlby (1969/1982), is a caregiving behavioral control system. This is believed to be a hardwired system, seen in early childhood and changing over development. It draws humans to attend to the distress of others and to engage in sympathetic and altruistic behaviors (Goubert et al., 2005). How parents and other caregiving adults respond to the child in pain influences the child's perception of pain in the moment and how they learn to express pain with others, both verbally and nonverbally. The following describes mechanisms whereby humans learn about the nature of pain, how to express it, and how others react when people are in pain.

Direct Experience Early in the evolution of protohuman species, the biological systems needed to escape from physical harm would have been present, thereby improving chances of survival (Crook & Walters, 2011) (see also Craig, Chap. 2, this volume). Nociceptive reflexes leading to escape from physical harm illustrate these systems. These were conserved through the long continuity of human precursors and ancestors and provided the basis for human pain, with modification as brains evolved, culminating in the capacities afforded by the complex brains of *Homo sapiens*. Early in development, young human children have the capacity to withdraw from painful stimuli and to benefit from painful experiences. Through age and direct experience, humans learn personalized strategies to minimize painful experiences such as the self-administration of medication.

Conditioning and Associative Learning A capacity to associate the potential for harm with specific environmental cues or settings represents an evolved, more sophisticated strategy for harm avoidance. The capacity for classical conditioning or respondent learning of fear in environments that have provoked pain is evident in early mammals and has been demonstrated in newborn human infants (Taddio, Shah, Gilbert-MacLeod, & Katz, 2002). Fear conditioning is conspicuous in infants as a result of painful vaccinations. Needle fears/phobias have long been recognized as a primary source of aversions to dental and medical care with 63% of children and about 24% of parents reporting some degree of needle fear (Taddio et al., 2012). While the fears may appear asocial, they have major social parameters: the content of the fear experience typically has social components as people (e.g., parents, physicians, peers, etc.)

typically are responsible for inflicting pain upon children. Associative learning would account for generalization of the fears to other people and settings involved, and consequent avoidant behavior would include reluctance to access health care provided by social institutions (health care providers and settings). Vicarious classical conditioning of emotional states can also ensue. This type of social learning provides a basis not only for learning about pain and illness behavior, but it supports most patterns of socialization in family and culture sanctioned roles.

Observational Learning Humans, and some other social species, benefit from observation of others experiencing pain (Goubert et al., 2011; Helsen, Goubert, Peters, & Vlaeyen, 2011). Observers may recognize that (a) conspecifics are experiencing pain, (b) certain events and situations pose threats of danger and can instigate pain, (c) specific actions lead to escape from pain or further harm avoidance, (d) and the efforts of other people can be engaged to deliver comfort and care by certain actions. Infants display considerable empathy towards the emotional reactions of their mothers and other children very early in life (Liddle, Bradley, & McGrath, 2015). Newborns in hospital nurseries cry when others cry—the synchronization can be striking (Provasi, Anderson, & Barbu-Roth, 2014).

In older children and adults, acquisition of skills in managing pain is greatly enhanced through observational learning. Humans in particular benefit from observing what others consider to be dangerous situations, how to avoid or control pain in those settings, and how others are likely to react to various ways of coping with pain. Observational learning is a particularly important modality of human learning (Bandura, 1986; Craig, 1986). Social skills determine the child's capacity to communicate pain and to influence others. Children learn by watching others, with children then reacting both spontaneously and using other's behavior as models for how to behave in the most efficient manner possible. Feedback from age peers, parents and others would shape conformity to familial and cultural expectations. Children with chronic pain may not have the same opportunities to learn and practice social skills in day-to-day interactions. Thus, pain can interfere with a child's ability to observe adaptive responses to pain and distress from peers. Moreover, even what an adult or a child selectively attends to when observing others in pain can be influenced by cognitive schemas that are shaped by earlier observations of other in pain (Goubert et al., 2011).

Social Influences on Cognitive Processing of Pain

The concept that how we think about pain is shaped by our social context is an intriguing one. Humans, perhaps more so than other species, are capable of cognizing the nature or their experience, a facility that enables memory, attention, problem-solving, language skills, and judgmental processes to assist in managing the challenges pain provokes. The full complement of cognitive processes becomes engaged in the various modalities of learning already described, vis-à-vis expectations, attention, appraisal, and beliefs. Cognitive factors influence a child's ability to learn and understand the nature of pain, as well as how to cope with pain (see also Chap. 18). As children grow up, their capacity to use cognitive skills transforms, with the mature child or adolescent frequently capable of moderating pain and its expression using self-management control strategies. Cognitive features of pain include basic features such as whether a child interprets bodily distress as indicative of pain but also includes more complex schemas such as the meaning of the pain, the long-term threat of the pain, and different courses of action related to reacting and recovering from pain that impact not only themselves but also other individuals in their social network. The capacity to exercise cognitive skills when attempting to cope with pain is developmentally acquired. Language becomes available to understand and interpret personal reactions, including pain, and to describe these reactions to others as a means of seeking help. The importance of language is evident when one considers the limitations of children with developmental disabilities who cannot clearly articulate the nature and nuances of their pain and the pain relief, if any, that has resulted from caregiver intervention (Craig, Stanford, Fairbairn, & Chambers, 2006).

The end product of learning about the natural and social environment by any given person through a massive number of interactions should be a capacity to realistically and effectively respond to challenges. Acquiring a capacity to understand and cope with pain resembles other life skills in this respect. The family is of considerable importance in providing instruction and supporting these skills (Lewandowski, Palermo, Stinson, Handley, & Chambers, 2010; Palermo & Holley, 2013). This is the primary source of observational learning. Parental support (e.g., special attention, relief from responsibilities or attending school) may strengthen pain behavior leading to greater functional handicaps (Peterson & Palermo, 2004). Learning is not always efficient or effective—children can learn not only effective social skills, but they may learn maladaptive habits of avoidance, catastrophizing, maladaptive thinking and helplessness in this manner.

Ethnocultural factors are also important to how individuals create cognitive frameworks around pain, but are not well documented. Cultures appear to vary in the acceptability of pain expression, although the overall norm for Western cultures would appear to be towards conservative expression, encouraging self-control and use of interpersonal resources only when the need is substantial. There are similar restraints in how others react when they see people in pain, again with the tendency towards committing resources only when the need is deemed substantial. Judgments as to whether care should be provided no doubt vary with the age of the child. Differences exist in how people interact with the health care system, whether they seek treatment, and whether they adhere to care. Bolstering the impact of family, the impact of ethnic and cultural variations on pain schemas would seem to first take root through the family when an individual is learning other social norms and practices. Family members generally model normative standards for their culture, although the nature of the influence of early familial learning later in life would depend greatly on the individual. Zeman and Garber (1996) described how even children as young as 9 years old can demonstrate a sophisticated understanding of how emotional display rules would vary according to who is watching them.

The complexity of the socialization process is now evident through a variety of studies. For example, caregivers who identified with a heritage culture that was more highly individualistic tended to show greater attention to the infant's pain-related distress during immunization injections, which in turn predicted decreased infant pain expression at 1 and 2 min post-needle (O'Neill, Pillai Riddell, Garfield, & Greenberg, 2016). With older children, self-reported pain was significantly lower when they were observed by a parent in contrast to when they are alone (Vervoort et al., 2011). As well, girls' self-reported pain was influenced by whether their mothers engaged in pain-promoting (e.g., reassurance, apologies, criticism) or pain-reducing (e.g., distraction, humor, and task orientation) behavior, though no such effect was observed in mother–son interactions (Chambers, Craig, & Bennett, 2002).

Concluding Observations

The sensations, feelings, and thoughts associated with painful experiences are communicated to others through both verbal and nonverbal expression. The communication of pain reflects a complex interplay of biological, cognitive, and emotional modalities that always occur in a social context. However, this context may be present in the moment of pain or codified in multimodal schemas from long ago socializations. Success in securing the care of others is intimately locked to the ability to attract their attention and the ability of observers to interpret what is happening.

A developmental sequence in the cues available to others is readily observed, with the painful experiences of infants and younger children largely made manifest by automatic, reflexive displays (e.g., nociceptive reflexes, facial expression, and cry), with these complemented by more readily controlled expressions of pain (asking for help, intentional movements, taking medication) as humans progress through the lifespan.

The ever-present social context surrounds both signaling from the pained individual and empathy or caregiving responses from those who witness the pain signals. Ultimately, while no one can truly know another's pain experience, the very nature of having an experience with multiple features that are each influenced by behaviors in another strongly supports the premise that both pain experience and pain expression are a socially constructed psychobiological phenomenon.

References

Ahola Kohut, S., Pillai Riddell, R. R., Flora, D., & Oster, H. (2012). A longitudinal analysis of the development of infant facial expressions in responses to acute pain: Immediate and regulatory expressions. *Pain, 153*(12), 2458–2465.

Bandura, A. (1986). *Social foundations of thought and action: A social cognitive theory.* Englewood Cliffs, NJ: Prentice-Hall.

Bowlby, J. (1969/1982). *Attachment and loss, Vol. 1: Attachment*. New York, NY: Basic Books.

Chambers, C. T., Craig, K. D., & Bennett, S. M. (2002). The impact of maternal behavior on children's pain experiences: An experimental analysis. *Journal of Pediatric Psychology, 27*, 293–301.

Craig, K. D. (1986). Social modeling influences: Pain in context. In R. A. Sternbach (Ed.), *The psychology of pain* (2nd ed., pp. 67–96). New York, NY: Raven Press.

Craig, K. D. (2009). The social communication model of pain. *Canadian Psychology, 50*, 22–32.

Craig, K. D., Best, H., & Best, J. A. (1978). Self-regulatory effects of monitoring sensory and affective dimensions of pain. *Journal of Consulting and Clinical Psychology, 46*, 573–574.

Craig, K. D., Stanford, E. A., Fairbairn, N. S., & Chambers, C. T. (2006). Emergent pain language communication competence in infants and children. *Enfance, 1*, 52–71.

Crook, R. J., & Walters, E. T. (2011). Nociceptive behavior and physiology of molluscs: Animal welfare implications. *ILAR Journal, 52*, 185–195.

Din Osmun, L., Pillai Riddell, R. R., & Flora, D. (2014). Infant negative affect at 12 months of age: Caregiver and infant predictors. *Journal of Pediatric Psychology, 39*(1), 23–34.

Fitzgerald, M., & Walker, S. M. (2009). Infant pain management: A developmental neurobiological approach. *Nature Clinical Practice. Neurology, 5*, 35–50.

Goubert, L., Craig, K. D., Vervoort, T., Morley, S., Sullivan, M. J. L., Williams, A., … Crombez, G. (2005). Facing others in pain: The effects of empathy. *Pain, 118*, 286–288.

Goubert, L., Vlaeyen, J. W. S., Crombez, G., & Craig, K. D. (2011). Learning about pain from others: An observational learning account. *Journal of Pain, 12*, 167–174.

Greenspan, D., Craft, R. M., LeResche, L., Arendt-Nielsen, L., Berkley, K. J., Fillingim, R. B., … Traub, R. J. (2007). Studying sex and gender differences in pain and analgesia: A consensus report. *Pain, 132*(Supplement 1), S26–S45.

Grunau, R. E. (2013). Neonatal pain in very preterm infants: Long-term effects on brain, neurodevelopment and pain reactivity. *Rambam Maimonides Medical Journal, 4*, e0025. https://doi.org/10.5041/RMMJ.10132

Hadjistavropoulos, T., Craig, K. D., Duck, S., Cano, A. M., Goubert, L., Jackson, P., … Dever Fitzgerald, T. (2011). A biopsychosocial formulation of pain communication. *Psychological Bulletin, 137*, 910–939.

Helsen, K., Goubert, L., Peters, M. L., & Vlaeyen, J. W. S. (2011). Observational learning and pain-related fear: An experimental study with colored cold pressor tasks. *Journal of Pain, 12*, 1230–1239.

Horton, R., Pillai Riddell, R. R., Flora, D., Moran, G., & Pederson, D. (2015). Distress regulation in infancy: Attachment and temperament in the context of acute pain. *Journal of Developmental and Behavioral Pediatrics, 36*(1), 35–44.

Larochette, A. C., Chambers, C. T., & Craig, K. D. (2006). Genuine, suppressed and faked facial expressions of pain in children. *Pain, 126*, 64–71.

Lewandowski, A. S., Palermo, T. M., Stinson, J., Handley, S., & Chambers, C. T. (2010). Systematic review of family functioning in families of children and adolescents with chronic pain. *Journal of Pain, 11*, 1027–1038.

Liddle, M. J. E., Bradley, B. S., & McGrath, A. (2015). Baby empathy: Infant distress and peer prosocial responses. *Infant Mental Health Journal, 36*, 446–458.

Lipscombe, S., Leve, L., Shaw, D., & Neiderhiser, J. (2012). Negative emotionality and externalizing problems in toddlerhood: Overreactive parenting as a moderator of genetic influences. *Development and Psychopathology, 24*, 167–179.

Logan, D., & Scharff, L. (2005). Relationships between family and parent characteristics and functional abilities in children with recurrent pain syndromes: An investigation of moderating effects on the pathway from pain to disability. *Journal of Pediatric Psychology, 30*(8), 698–707.

Melzack, R. (1975). The McGill Pain Questionnaire: Major properties and scoring methods. *Pain, 1*, 277–299.

Melzack, R., & Casey, K. L. (1968). Sensory, motivational and central control determinants of pain: A new conceptual model. In D. L. Kenshalo (Ed.), *The skin senses* (pp. 423–443). Springfield, IL: Charles C Thomas.

Merskey, H., Albe-Fessard, D., Bonica, J. J., Carmon, A., Dubner, R., Kerr, F. W. L., … Sunderland, S. (1979). Pain terms: A list with definitions and notes on usage. Recommended by the IASP Subcommittee on Taxonomy. *Pain, 6*, 249–252.

November, G., Zanon, M., & Silani, G. (2015). Empathy for social exclusion involves the sensory-discriminative component of pain: A within-subject fMRI study. *SCAN, 10*, 153–164. https://doi.org/10.1093/scan/nsu038

O'Neill, M., Pillai Riddell, R., Garfield, H., & Greenberg, S. (2016). Does caregiver behavior mediate the relationship between cultural individualism and infant pain at 12 months of age? *Journal of Pain, 197*(12), 1273–1280.

Palermo, T. M., & Holley, A. L. (2013). The importance of the family environment in pediatric chronic pain. *JAMA Pediatrics, 167*, 93–94.

Peterson, C. C., & Palermo, T. (2004). Parental reinforcement of recurrent pain: The moderating impact of child depression and anxiety on functional disability. *Journal of Pediatric Psychology, 29*, 331–341.

Pillai Riddell, R., Racine, N., Craig, K. D., & Campbell, L. (2014). Biopsychosocial models of pediatric pain. In P. J. McGrath, B. Stevens, S. Walker, & W. Zempsky (Eds.), *Oxford textbook of pediatric pain* (pp. 85–94). Oxford: Oxford University Press.

Pillai Riddell, R. R., Flora, D. B., Stevens, S. A., Stevens, B. J., Cohen, L. L., Greenberg, S., & Garfield, H. (2013). Variability in infant acute pain responding meaningfully obscured by averaging pain responses. *Pain, 154*(5), 714–721.

Provasi, J., Anderson, D. I., & Barbu-Roth, M. (2014). Rhythm perception, production, and synchronization during the perinatal period. *Frontiers in Psychology, 5*, 1048. https://doi.org/10.3389/fpsyg.2014.01048

Racine, N., Pillai Riddell, R., Flora, D., Taddio, A., Greenberg, S., & Garfield, H. (2016). Preschool anticipatory distress to immunization pain: Understanding development. *Pain, 157*(9), 1918–1932.

Taddio, A., Shah, V., Gilbert-MacLeod, C., & Katz, J. (2002). Conditioning and hyperalgesia in newborns exposed to repeated heel lances. *JAMA, 288*, 857–861.

Verriotis, M., Chang, P., Fitzgerald, M., & Fabrizi, L. (2016). The development of the nociceptive brain. *Neuroscience, 338*, 207–219. https://doi.org/10.1016/j.neuroscience.2016.07.026

Vervoort, T., Caes, L., Trost, Z., Sullivan, M., Vangronsveld, K., & Goubert, L. (2011). Social modulation of facial pain display in high-catastrophizing children: An observational study in school children and their parents. *Pain, 152*, 1591–1599.

Vinall, J., & Grunau, R. (2014). Impact of repeated procedural pain-related stress in infants born very preterm. *Pediatric Research, 75*, 584–587. https://doi.org/10.1038/pr.2014.16

Williams, A. C. d. C., & Craig, K. D. (2016). Updating the definition of pain. *Pain, 157*, 2420–2423.

Zeman, J., & Garber, J. (1996). Display rules for anger, sadness, and pain: It depends on who is watching. *Child Development, 67*, 957–973.

Chapter 4
An Affective-Motivational Account of Interpersonal Dynamics in Pain

Tine Vervoort and Zina Trost

Abstract Pain is a disruptive experience occurring within an interpersonal context of multiple goal pursuit for both the pain sufferer and the pain observer. The observer's affective-motivational response to another's pain and caregiving behavior in turn impact the sufferers' pain experience. Understanding the specific dynamics of interaction between the sufferer and the observer is crucial for theoretical development and clinical intervention within this area. Further, an integrative account that acknowledges emotional, motivational, and interpersonal dimensions as integral to pain experience is critical to capture the complexity and nuance of interpersonal pain dynamics. Drawing on recent advances in interpersonal pain–empathy research and established insights from appraisal theory of emotion, influential behavioral models, and social psychology literature, we present a theoretical framework for interpersonal pain dynamics to guide research in this area. Specifically, we highlight the interpersonal nature of pain and the relationship between motivation and emotion in the context of pain. We discuss the distinction and tension between self- and other-oriented goals to explain the occurrence of differential emotional-motivational responses in pain observers, associated distinctions in the nature and effectiveness of caregiving, and highlight possible underlying mechanisms. We hypothesize that observer emotional responses and emotion regulatory capacities facilitate optimal caregiving behaviors and, by extension, affect the sufferer's pain experience. The merit of adopting emotion regulation theory and paradigms to guide research on observer–sufferer interactions is supported by recent evidence regarding the role of observer emotion regulation in caregiver behavior in the context of pain. We conclude by outlining a foundation for an integrative theoretical account and directions for future research.

Keywords Pain · Interpersonal dynamics · Observer · Behavioral responses · Empathy · Appraisal · Emotion · Emotion regulation · Motivation · Goals

T. Vervoort (✉)
Department of Experimental-Clinical and Health Psychology, Ghent University,
Ghent, Belgium
e-mail: Tine.Vervoort@Ugent.be

Z. Trost
Department of Psychology, University of Alabama at Birmingham, Birmingham, AL, USA

© Springer International Publishing AG, part of Springer Nature 2018
T. Vervoort et al. (eds.), *Social and Interpersonal Dynamics in Pain*,
https://doi.org/10.1007/978-3-319-78340-6_4

57

Imagine this scenario: *Sitting on the kitchen counter, a 5-year old girl accidentally places her hand on the hot electrical stove. Her happy expression immediately turns into a painful grimace as she snatches her hand away, drops her toys, and wails. Seeing the crying girl cradle her hand in pain, the mother drops her cooking and, with her heart pounding, quickly takes action to cool the burn and comfort her child.*

Pain is a multidimensional aversive experience that is undoubtedly adaptive. Pain serves protective functions in the face of physical threat; upon exposure to a hot surface, the sudden experience of pain promptly captures a child's attention, leading to a quick reflexive withdrawal. Behavioral manifestations of pain—such as the child's grimace and crying—also capture her mother's attention, motivating the parent to come to her daughter's aid and, in all likelihood, attempt to soothe the pain. The potential for pain to not only grasp the attention of the person in pain but also others in the environment, as well as the substantial personal and social consequences arising from another's sensitivity to the sufferer's pain expression may have an evolutionary basis (Craig, 2004; Eccleston & Crombez, 1999; Hadjistavropoulos & Craig, 2002; Williams, 2002; Williams & Craig, 2006). Attention to another's expression of pain may trigger an observer's approach and targeted helping behavior, which increases the survival chances of offspring or the group as a whole. The pain reactions of another may also serve as a warning signal of potential threat to the observer, and motivate observer avoidance of personal harm when the cost of helping is too high (Craig, 2004; Hadjistavropoulos et al., 2011; Vervoort & Trost, 2016; Williams, 2002).

We wish to highlight several characteristics of pain that form the basis of the current chapter. First, pain is closely tied to motivation and hence to emotions. As will be discussed below, goal (in)congruence is conceptualized as a key feature of emotional processes. Fundamentally, pain is incongruent with the goal of preserving physical integrity. Once a pain stimulus is appraised as being incongruent with this goal, it leads to action tendencies, somatic responses, expressive behavior, and subjective feelings that constitute an emotional episode. Second, and related to this, pain is likely to be highly disruptive and hence incongruent with the pursuit of goals *other than physical integrity*, such as daily goals (e.g., to work, to play) and broader identity-relevant goals (e.g., to be a good colleague, spouse, friend, or parent). Thus, pain occurs in a motivational context consisting of *multiple* goals. Third, pain occurs in and is shaped by an *interpersonal* context. The experience of pain does not take place in a social vacuum but rather within a rich social environment comprising individuals (both pain sufferers and observers) that each has their own distal and proximal goals or concerns. Accordingly, an observer's optimal response to another's pain experience reflects an ability to regulate emotional responses through appropriate attunement to (and in many cases juggling between) goals central to the self (i.e., self-oriented goals) and to the person in pain (i.e., other-oriented goals). As we will highlight within this chapter, it is ultimately other-oriented goals and associated emotions that facilitate adaptive interpersonal dynamics and caregiving. Because emotional responses are key in shaping behavior, emotion regulation is likely key in this regard.

While each of the above elements is a fundamental moderator of pain experience, research on each aspect has proceeded in a relatively independent fashion, with largely disparate attention allotted to either the emotional, broader motivational, and interpersonal dimensions of pain. In this chapter, we argue that the understanding of one aspect is incomplete without an understanding of the other two aspects and that theory that acknowledges each of these elements is critical to capture the complexity and nuance of interpersonal dynamics. As part of this multidimensional approach, the current chapter focuses on observer emotion and emotion regulation in response to another person's pain experience, examining the role of appraisal processes against the backdrop of changes in goal pursuit or concerns. To begin, we discuss the conceptual relationship between emotion and motivation, noting the centrality of appraisal processes and the multiplicity of goals and emotions. We then discuss how an interpersonal lens on pain experience involves a fundamental tension between two types of goals: *self-oriented goals*, which are directed toward the observer him/herself and *other-oriented goals*, which are directed toward the pain sufferer. We will highlight how different goals facilitate differential emotional and motivational processes that can impact the nature and effectiveness of observer behavioral responses to sufferers' pain. In this context, we describe potential mechanisms of actions that may underlie commonly observed paradoxical effects of ostensibly prosocial behaviors or differential effects of ostensibly similar caregiving responses.

After highlighting the relevance of the three central elements—emotions, goals/concerns, and the interpersonal context—to the pain experience as well as the inherently interdependent relationship among these constructs, we describe the role of emotion regulation and strategies that may facilitate optimal interpersonal pain dynamics and caregiving within a multiple goal context. Finally, we present a foundation for an integrative motivational account of emotion (and, by extension, of emotion regulation) within the interpersonal pain context and provide directions for future research.[1]

Pain Is Closely Intertwined with Emotional Processes Involving Appraisal of the Pain Stimulus

The importance of emotion in understanding pain experience is reflected in the original definition provided by the International Association for the Study of Pain (IASP). IASP reached consensus in defining pain as '*an unpleasant sensory and emotional experience associated with actual or potential tissue damage*' (International Association for the Study of Pain Task Force on Taxonomy, 1994, p. 210). This definition highlighted the central role of emotion in pain, recognizing that without emotion, the sensory perception of pain is insufficient to reflect pain

---

[1]A condensed synthesis of the current chapter is available as a focus article; Vervoort and Trost (2017).

experience as we know it. Critically, this IASP definition also recognizes the lack of absolute correspondence between pain experience and tissue damage. As pain experience can occur in the absence of objective damage, a necessary and sufficient characteristic of pain experience is that it is perceived or *appraised* as harmful or threatening for physical integrity. Accordingly, this definition recognizes that emotions *arising from subjective appraisals* (that in turn feed emotional responses) are at the heart of the response system by which pain is understood and dealt with.

Pain-Related Emotion Occurs Within a Broader Motivational (Goal) Context

The connection between emotion and motivation is articulated by appraisal theories of emotion. Appraisal theories take emotions to be relatively short-lived episodes that unfold over time and that can be deconstructed into components comprising changes in the following organismic subsystems: (a) a *cognitive* component, with changes in stimulus evaluation or appraisal (subserved by perception, memory, and attention), (b) a *motivational* component, with changes in action tendencies, preparing the organism to undertake a behavior, (c) a *somatic* component with changes in (neuro)physiological responses, (d) a *motor* component, with changes in expressive behavior (e.g., facial and vocal expressions and gross motor behavior or actions), and (e) a *subjective* component, with changes in feelings. Together, these components of emotion work toward prioritizing energy and behavior in ways that optimize the individual's adjustment to the demands of the physical and social environment (Frijda, 2007; Keltner & Gross, 1999; Moors, 2009; Oatley & Johnson-Laird, 1987).

The presence of all these components is nonetheless insufficient to classify a given episode as an emotional one. Appraisal theories suggest that emotions occur when a *stimulus is appraised as relevant for and/or (in)congruent with a central goal or concern* (Frijda, 2007; Moors, 2009; Moors & Scherer, 2013). Dropping a glass while washing dishes may be relevant to a goal of minor importance, thereby eliciting no emotion or weak emotion. However, if the glass was a cherished family heirloom, the meaning of the event and the emotional consequences may be quite different. As long as a discrepancy exists between the goal or desired state/situation on the one hand, and the *actual* situation on the other hand, the person strives to reduce the discrepancy. Emotions are thought to "unfold over time", with the appraisal component driving changes in all the other components of emotion. For instance, appraisal that an event mismatches with one's goal activates motive to do something about the situation, together with associated physiological responses that prepare and support actual behavior to change the situation. Ultimately, the subjective "feeling" component is conceptualized as the totality of traces that all other components leave in consciousness. Contemporary appraisal theorists also assume that changes in later components feedback to earlier components (Moors, 2013).

For example, feedback from physiological responses may modify attentional focus and hence bias further reappraisal and adjustment in action tendencies; in the same manner, characterizing experience with emotion labels (e.g., "fear," "anger," "anxiety") may further color the emotional experience (e.g., "If I feel anxious, there must be danger.").

When pain is perceived as a sign of tissue damage it is at odds with the goal of self-preservation; accordingly, negative emotions elicited by pain (primarily fear) can be considered goal-directed in that they facilitate the prompt and efficient pursuit of pain control/avoidance via engagement of cognitive (e.g., narrowed attention), motivational (e.g., increased action readiness), motor (e.g., increased expressive behavior), and somatic processes (e.g., increased sympathetic activation; Eccleston & Crombez, 1999; Hamilton, Karoly, & Kitzman, 2004; Vlaeyen & Linton, 2000). Within the literature on individuals' responses to *personal* pain experience, emotions in response to pain are often subsumed under the umbrella of *pain-related fear,* which has emerged as a central variable in current pain theorizing.

As a case in point, the fear–avoidance model of chronic pain developed by Vlaeyen and Linton (2000) has evolved as a leading account of how some individuals with an acute musculoskeletal injury go on to develop chronic pain and disability whereas others do not. Briefly, the fear–avoidance model posits that pain-related appraisals, associated fear responses, and avoidant motivational tendencies drive the pain–disability cycle. Following acute injury, individuals are differentially susceptible to pain-related fear (also referred to as fear of movement and re/injury) based on catastrophic appraisals of pain stimuli, that is, interpretation of pain as a potential sign of serious tissue damage and hence a threat to physical integrity (Sullivan et al., 2001). In turn, pain-related fear promotes hypervigilance, biased interpretation of pain sensations, and defensive behavior to escape/avoid potentially painful situations. The superordinate goal of highly fearful/catastrophizing individuals is to avoid pain/injury experience. Although the above processes are a natural and adaptive responses to facilitate pain control after acute injury (Eccleston & Crombez, 1999; Suls & Fletcher, 1985), adult and child findings indicate that excessive or prolonged avoidance of daily activities may actually promote disability (Leeuw et al., 2007; Simons & Kacynski, 2012; Zale, Lange, Fields, & Ditre, 2013). Disability is further exacerbated by the negative physical/physiological sequelae of avoidance behavior (Crombez, Vlaeyen, Heuts, & Lysens, 1999; Moseley, Nicholas, & Hodges, 2004; Vlaeyen & Linton, 2000).

In this sense, a clearly adaptive response can become problematic in circumstances where pain relief is not likely—e.g., when pain becomes chronic. Under such circumstances, continuous prioritization of pain control goals—underpinned by negative emotion and characterized by immediate motivation to end pain—can come at the expense of other goals broadly identified as "non-pain related" (Crombez, Eccleston, Van Damme, Vlaeyen, & Karoly, 2012; Karoly & Ruehlman, 1996; Van Damme, Legrain, Vogt, & Crombez, 2010). Such goals can include engagement in daily activities or pursuits that contribute to one's identity as a good partner, worker, or spouse. Both acute and chronic pain experience can present a challenge of integrating immediate motivation to end pain (pain-control goals) with valued non-pain goals. Indeed, in a typically complex social environment, one and the same event inevitably touches on multiple goals simultaneously. It follows that stimuli are appraised as relevant to *a number of goals*. Because people want multiple and often contradictory things, competing goals/concerns likely inform much emotional complexity and conflict. Understanding the role of emotion in pain clearly requires consideration of the broad motivational context (comprised of both proximal and distal goals) in which pain emerges.

Pain-Related Goals and Emotion Within an Interpersonal Context

Pain is often considered a personal experience but is in fact rarely private. A pain sufferer's voluntary and involuntary behaviors communicate distress to others, eliciting others' emotional and caregiving responses that will in turn impact the sufferer's pain experience and expression (Craig, 2004; Goubert et al., 2005; Goubert, Vervoort, & Craig, 2013; Hadjistavropoulos et al., 2011; Vervoort, Caes, et al., 2011; Vervoort, Huguet, Verhoeven, & Goubert, 2011). Further, observation of pain may activate neural representations of the observer's own pain experiences. In this way, observing another's pain automatically references the self (e.g., Decety & Jackson, 2006; Goubert, Vervoort, & Crombez, 2009; Lamm, Decety, & Singer, 2011; Loggia, Mogil, & Bushnell, 2008; Yamada & Decety, 2009) and underscores the intrinsically interpersonal nature of pain, whereby pain not only touches on the goals relevant for the person in pain but also for observers.

The interpersonal nature of pain is likely reflected in a basic motivational distinction that directs an observer's behavior when faced with another in pain. Specifically, we hypothesize that observers are faced with a tension between two types of goals: *self-oriented goals*, which are directed toward the observer himself/herself (and potentially subserved in part by shared neural representations; e.g., protecting oneself) and *other-oriented goals*, which are directed toward the pain sufferer (e.g., protecting the other in pain). This notion is supported by social psychology research indicating that almost all goal pursuit occurs in a relationship context where joint and personal goals exist in tension (Vanderdrift & Agnew, 2015) as well as findings that multiple goal pursuit pulls resources away from individual goal efforts, and may thus be difficult (Fishbach & Ferguson, 2007). As goal incongruence is central to emotion, preferential attunement to self-oriented goals will likely result in self-focused aversive emotional states; these will prioritize avoidance motives and result in behavior directed toward one's own needs (Dix, 1991; Gable & Gosnell, 2013; Martini & Busseri, 2010; Strough, Berg, & Sansone, 1996). In contrast, attunement to other-oriented goals will likely promote an other-oriented emotional state—often denoted as sympathy—prioritizing approach motives and resulting in behaviors directed at and appropriately responsive to another's needs (Batson, Fultz, & Schoenrade, 1987; Eisenberg et al., 1989; Elliot, Eder, & Harmon-Jones, 2013; Lin

& McFatter, 2012). Behavioral traditions, most notably operant behavioral theory (Fordyce, 1976), have long recognized the key role of interpersonal responses in determining pain behavior, yet the likely tension between self- and other-oriented goals, and related observer emotional, motivational, and behavioral responses has yet to be fully explicated.

In response to the pain of another, observer behavioral responses can be broadly categorized as behaviors intended to control pain (pain-control behaviors) and those not focused on pain control (non-pain-control behaviors). Pain-control behaviors, encompassing behaviors such as comforting, reassuring, or restricting pain sufferer activities, are behaviors that direct sufferer attention toward pain and hence, are also referred to as *pain attending behaviors*. Conversely, non-pain-control behaviors, encompassing behaviors such as the use of humor, distraction, or encouraging activity, are behaviors that direct sufferer attention away from pain and are referred to as *non-pain attending behaviors* (Atkinson, Gennis, Racine, & Pillai Riddell, 2015; Hamilton et al., 2004; Jensen, Karoly, & Huger, 1987). Studies have shown that whereas pain-control/attending behaviors contribute to increased sufferer pain and distress, non-pain control/attending behaviors contribute to increased sufferer coping (Atkinson et al., 2015; Hamilton et al., 2004; Jensen et al., 1987). However, evidence is not unequivocal; some studies have failed to find expected associations (see for example Campbell, Jordan, & Dunn, 2012; Flor, Kerns, & Turk, 1987) or have observed evidence counter to expectations (e.g., Vervoort, Huguet, et al., 2011). For example, observer pain control behaviors, such as providing reassurance or taking over household chores (Kerns, Turk, & Rudy, 1985) are expected to increase pain behaviors, yet evidence has shown that this is not always the case; these types of support behaviors do not always reinforce pain expression (Newton-John, 2002). Emerging research suggests that one particular type of behavioral response cannot, in and of itself, be considered adaptive or maladaptive (e.g., Bolger, Foster, Vinokur, & Ng, 1996; Bolger, Zuckerman, & Kessler, 2000). A priori categorizations about beneficial or detrimental qualities of behavioral responses can underrepresent the complexity of the interaction between observers and co-actors and pain sufferers.

Self-Oriented Versus Other-Oriented Goals: Behavioral Implications and Mechanisms of Action

In line with the motivational distinction outlined above, we hypothesize that *ostensibly similar caregiving behavior* may be underpinned by either approach or avoidance motives; this is the case both for pain control and non-pain related behaviors. For instance, the same pain control behavior (e.g., comforting a child, offering medication), may be motivated by the self-oriented goal to avoid another's pain underpinned by an aversive emotional state or by an other-oriented approach motive. A similar distinction between other-oriented approach motives (attuned to the needs of the other) and self-oriented avoidance motives (attuned to the needs of the self) can likewise underlie a non-pain oriented caregiving response, such as encouraging the pain sufferer to engage in daily activities. This notion is in line with findings that approach motivation does not necessarily manifest as behavioral approach; similarly, avoidance motivation does not always manifest as behavioral avoidance (Elliot et al., 2013). For example, a partner reassuring a distressed spouse (an ostensible approach behavior) may be underpinned by approach motivation (reflecting an other-oriented goal of providing comfort); alternatively, the same reassuring behavior may be underpinned by avoidance motivation (reflecting self-oriented goals of wanting to regulate self-oriented emotional distress). It stands to reason that observable approach or avoidant responses cannot be defined as such without understanding of their underlying motivational substrates.

Further, we hypothesize that a seemingly similar behavioral response to another's pain—when underpinned by either approach versus avoidance motives—is likely to exert differential effects (see for example Dix, Gershoff, Meunier, & Miller, 2004; Hastings & Grusec, 1998). Such associations have been noted elsewhere. For instance, social support literature suggests that more favourable outcomes are observed following similar partner actions when they arise from approach motivation rather than from avoidance motivation (Impett, Peplau, & Gable, 2005). To date, potential consequences of motivational tensions in response to another's pain, and explanatory mechanisms of action, have received limited empirical scrutiny. At the same time, emerging research suggests that the effectiveness of caregiver behavior may depend upon the extent to which such behavior matches the specific *needs* of the person in pain. For instance, intimacy process models in the context of pain (see for example Laurenceau, Barrett, & Rovine, 2005) posit that observer caregiving exerts positive effects and empowers individuals in pain when it matches individuals' *needs* for emotional intimacy and closeness. An empathic or validating response following an emotional self-disclosure may thus empower the sufferer to better cope with pain and promote closeness/relationship satisfaction, rather than reinforcing the pain response (Edmond & Keefe, 2015; Laurenceau et al., 2005). To date, it remains unclear *when* caregivers' behavior will be more or less attuned to the needs of the person in pain. We suggest that recognition of differential affective-motivational substrates plays a major role in this regard and that various mechanisms may account for differential effects.

One potential mechanism is *quality of caregiving response* reflected in nonverbal elements such as caregiver tone of voice or facial expression (see also Chap. 14). For instance, parental efforts to distract a child suffering from pain with humor are likely to rely a great deal on what is communicated by the facial expression of the parent (e.g., fearful facial expression vs. neutral facial expression). Another mechanism may be caregivers' *sensitivity to feedback cues* provided by the person in pain. For instance, self-oriented affective states and associated avoidance motives may impede caregiver receptivity to sufferer feedback, potentially contributing to rigid or inflexible caregiving behavior (e.g., persistently trying to control pain at the expense of non-pain goals, or, vice versa, excessive focus on non-pain goals at the expense of adequate pain control). Accordingly, attention to differential affective-motivational substrates of caregiving behavior may provide input regarding the paradoxical findings in pain literature regarding the effect of seemingly prosocial action (McMurthry, Chambers, McGrath, & Asp, 2010; Newton-John, 2002; Newton-John & Williams, 2006).

Drawing upon the above reasoning and empirical evidence, we propose that, for optimal behavioral response to the pain of another, other-oriented goals and other-oriented emotional states (i.e., sympathy, with corresponding approach motives) must to some extent prevail over their counterparts, thus prioritizing the goals/needs of the person in pain. Given the centrality of emotion in response to another's pain, we propose that emotion regulation is key in facilitating this other-oriented perspective.

Caregiver Emotion Regulation Within the Interpersonal Context of Pain

Emotion regulation may be defined as a goal-directed process, functioning to influence the type, intensity, and duration of emotional experience (Gross, 2013; Gross & Thompson, 2007; Koole, 2009: Moors, 2013). Emotion regulation can occur in an automatic or controlled manner (Koole & Rothermund, 2011; Mauss, Bunge, & Gross, 2007) and successful emotion regulation permits flexibility in emotional responding in accordance with current proximal or distal goals. In line with this, emerging research on emotion regulation suggests that people do not seek to regulate emotional responses for strictly hedonistic purposes i.e., to avoid unpleasant feelings and maximize pleasant feelings. Instead, emotion regulatory efforts appear based on instrumental motives—that is, people are willing to forgo immediate pleasure to maximize attainment of valued goals (Tamir, 2009; Tamir, Chiu, & Gross, 2007; Tamir, Mitchell, & Gross, 2008). Within the interpersonal pain context, these may involve both self-oriented goals as well as other-oriented goals and, as noted above, adaptive interpersonal dynamics and pain outcomes likely emerge when the latter prevail.

Any activity that impacts a person's' emotion may serve a regulatory function. Attempts have been undertaken to classify the myriad of potential emotion regulation strategies. According to Gross's process model (Gross, 1998; Gross & Thompson, 2007)—considered one of the most comprehensive models on emotion regulation—emotion regulation strategies can be classified by their targeted component and differentiated along the timeline of the unfolding emotional response. Strategies occurring before appraisals that give rise to full-blown emotions are considered *antecedent-focused* and encompass *situation selection* (i.e., selecting a situation expected to give rise to desired emotions and prevent unwanted emotions), *situation modification* (i.e., directly attempting to change a situation so as to modify its emotional impact), *attentional deployment* (i.e., influencing emotional response by redirecting attention and thus selecting incoming information), and *cognitive change/reappraisal* (i.e., changing the value of appraisal variables such as goal relevance or coping potential). Antecedent-focused strategies can be contrasted with *response-focused* emotion regulation or *response modulation*, which occurs later in the emotional episode and refers to efforts to control ongoing physiological or behavioral responding, and feelings following appraisal. Common forms of response modulation may include drug consumption (serving to decrease the physiological component) or direct suppression of expressive behavior and feeling. Appraisal theory and Gross's process model coincide in identifying appraisal as the central process responsible for emotion generation and regulation and thus driving the changes in other components of emotion. In this way, both theoretical accounts point to reappraisal as a particularly important emotion regulatory strategy. Indeed, a considerable number of findings suggest that reappraisal is an efficacious and adaptive strategy (see for example Ray, McRae, Ochnser, & Gross, 2010; Webb, Miles, & Sheeran, 2012). Antecedent-focused strategies that target the emotion-eliciting stimulus (e.g., attention deployment) should likewise be effective and adaptive as they influence appraisal (Johnson, 2009a, 2009b; Moors, 2013).

Evidence attesting to the critical emotion regulatory role of reappraisal mainly stems from studies examining the role of exposure-based interventions. Exposure relies on the assumption that repeated experiences of being able to perform various feared and avoided activities without accompanying harm/(re)injury facilitate reappraisal of the harm value of pain/avoided activity. Indeed, findings suggest that exposure contributes to reduced appraisals of pain-related harm, lower self-reported fear, and decreased avoidance behavior (Boersma et al., 2004; de Jong, Vlaeyen, Van Eijsden, Loo, & Onghena, 2012; Trost, France, & Thomas, 2008). Such findings are in line with recent studies employing interpretation bias modification paradigms (i.e., whereby participants are trained to make a nonthreatening interpretation of pain) and showing that decreasing negative interpretations of pain contributes to decreased avoidance behavior (Jones & Sharpe, 2014). Research further confirms that modifying attention to pain using distraction or attention modification training leads to diminished pain aversiveness and appraisals of harm as well as increased pain tolerance (Elommaa, Williams, & Kalso, 2009; Malloy & Milling, 2010), decreases in self-reported negative affect and lower pain interference (Schoth, Georgallis, & Liossi, 2013; Sharpe et al., 2012). To our knowledge, only one study has examined emotion regulation within the interpersonal pain context; specifically, Vervoort et al. (Vervoort, Trost, Sutterlin, Caes, & Moors, 2014; described in detail below) offered initial evidence regarding observer attentional deployment as an emotion regulatory strategy with implications for caregiving behavior.

Given the multiplicity of goals, continuous adjustment is necessary for multiple and optimal goal pursuit; it follows that continuous and flexible emotional regulation (*emotion regulatory flexibility*) is likely to be most adaptive (see for example Bonnano & Burton, 2013; Bonnano, Papa, Lalande, Westphal, & Coifman, 2004; Sheppes et al., 2014). Emotion regulatory flexibility is thought to include at least three characteristics: (a) context-sensitive emotional responding, (b) associated utilization of a broad repertoire of regulatory strategies, and (c) the ability to monitor feedback and maintain or readjust regulatory strategies as needed (Bonnano &

Burton, 2013). A flexibly attuned emotion regulation process aims to achieve optimal emotion dynamics in order to facilitate appropriate responding to the ever-changing demands of the environment. For instance, while other-orientation is hypothesized to be fundamental to effective caregiving, flexible attunement to self vs. other-oriented goals is also critical (e.g., engaging in appropriate self-care while caring for a loved one with chronic illness; Manczak, DeLongis, & Chen, 2016). The notion of emotion regulatory flexibility is in line with findings indicating that psychological flexibility—modifying behavior in accordance with situational demands and one's personal goals and values (Hayes, Pistorello, & Levin, 2012; Wicksell, Olsson, & Hayes, 2011)—attenuates the negative impact of pain experience on psychological well-being and is associated with improved emotional functioning (McCracken & Keogh, 2009; McCracken & Vowles, 2014).

Critically, emotion regulatory flexibility implies that, in itself, no emotion regulation strategy can be considered efficacious vs. nonefficacious or adaptive vs. maladaptive. Growing evidence indicates that the efficacy or adaptivity of a strategy depends on *the goal context* in which it emerges (Aldao, 2013). For example, using a reappraisal strategy when your friend once again stands you up for a dinner date ("she's probably in a traffic jam, it's not so bad") would be helpful to reduce feeling of anger/disappointment in the service of an overarching social goal (e.g., maintaining harmony). However, the same anger-diffusing reappraisal would not serve the goal of maintaining personal assertiveness. As goals frequently coexist and are in conflict, it would be in one's best interest to flexibly implement specific emotion regulation strategies in accordance with prioritized goals based on a variety of contextual feedback relevant to a given situation (Bonnano et al., 2004; Bonnano & Burton, 2013).

In the context of pain, literature on catastrophizing about personal pain offers an illustrative example of the context sensitivity of emotion regulation. High catastrophizing individuals appraise their pain as signalling physical danger, leading to the prioritization of pain control goals. Accordingly, such individuals adopt emotion regulation strategies to optimize escape from and avoidance of pain, which is paradoxically manifested in attentional hyper-vigilance toward pain sensations and associated negative emotional states. In line with this, there is evidence that those who catastrophize about imminent pain find less benefit from distraction (Campbell et al., 2010; Goubert, Eccleston, Crombez, & Devulder, 2004; Heyneman, Fremouw, Gano, Kirkland, & Heiden, 1990; Verhoeven et al., 2010) *unless* the salience of competing goals (e.g., working toward a reward in spite of pain) is enhanced (see for example Verhoeven et al., 2010). These findings suggest that differential prioritization of goals (and associated emotional states) may inform the utility of a given emotion regulatory strategy and—as individuals hold multiple goals simultaneously—highlight the possible malleability and utility of modifying goal context. Such findings likewise also underscore the therapeutic value of broadening goal context beyond pain control; indeed, this is a central tenet of treatment approaches such as Acceptance and Commitment Therapy (McCracken & Keogh, 2009; McCracken & Vowles, 2014).

   In their 2014 study Vervoort et al. provided evidence regarding the impact of differential emotional states (and hence, differential goals) on the utility of emotion regulatory strategy. This was the first study to examine attentional deployment (i.e., attention toward child's pain vs. attention away from child's pain) as an emotion regulatory strategy within the interpersonal (child/parent) context. Vervoort et al. found that directing attention away from their child's pain was associated with improved emotional outcomes and caregiving responses among low-anxious but not high-anxious parents, who benefitted more from directing attention toward their child. Findings indicated that whereas *low anxious* parents reported more distress and demonstrated more pain control behavior in the *"Attend to Pain"* condition, *high anxious* parents reported more distress and showed more pain control behavior in the *"Avoid Pain"* condition. This inverse pattern for high versus low anxious parents was also reflected in indices of physiological distress regulation, such as heart rate. Given the early nature of this research, it is premature to draw firm conclusion about what time of person (i.e., which goals or emotional states) benefits most from which emotion regulatory strategy. However, while Vervoort et al. did assess parental experienced anxiety and not parent's goals, their findings highlight the value of exploring the effect of differential goals on various pain outcomes, their potential relation to self- versus other-oriented processes (e.g., does high parental anxiety reflect a self-oriented goal?), and potential mechanisms of action.

   The Affective-Motivational Model of Interpersonal Pain Dynamics that appears in Fig. 4.1 represents a preliminary framework that integrates the concepts outlined in previous sections. We expect this preliminary model to be refined through future research. The Model proposes that an observer's attention to a sufferer's pain expression triggers an inherent tension between appraisals of *self-* versus *other-*oriented goals. Attunement to self-oriented goals is hypothesized to promote *self-focused emotional states* (with corresponding elements of emotion, described above); self-oriented emotional states in turn prioritize *avoidance motives*. On the other hand, we hypothesize that preferential attunement to other-oriented goals will promote *other-oriented emotional states* that in turn prioritize *approach motives*. It is important to point out that these very different affective-motivational substrates may form the foundation of *caregiving behavior* that is ostensibly similar. As noted in the previous section, differential motives may affect caregiving response via subtle mechanisms (e.g., nonverbal features) that impact on the quality of caregiving behavior as well as a caregiver's receptivity to feedback cues and potential (in)flexibility in caregiving strategy. *Emotion regulation* (subserved by such regulatory strategies as attentional deployment and reappraisal) is a central feature of the model, suggested to be key in promoting a balance of self- versus other-oriented goals and emotions to facilitate optimal caregiving and pain outcomes.

   As depicted in the model, these affective-motivational dynamics are likely to be modulated by contextual and individual difference factors. For instance, individual and contextual factors will likely affect the value observers place on various self- vs. other-oriented goals, in turn shaping emotional responses and associated efficacy of regulatory strategies. Research has previously examined such contextual influences as presence versus absence of organic pathology, perceived similarity/familiarity

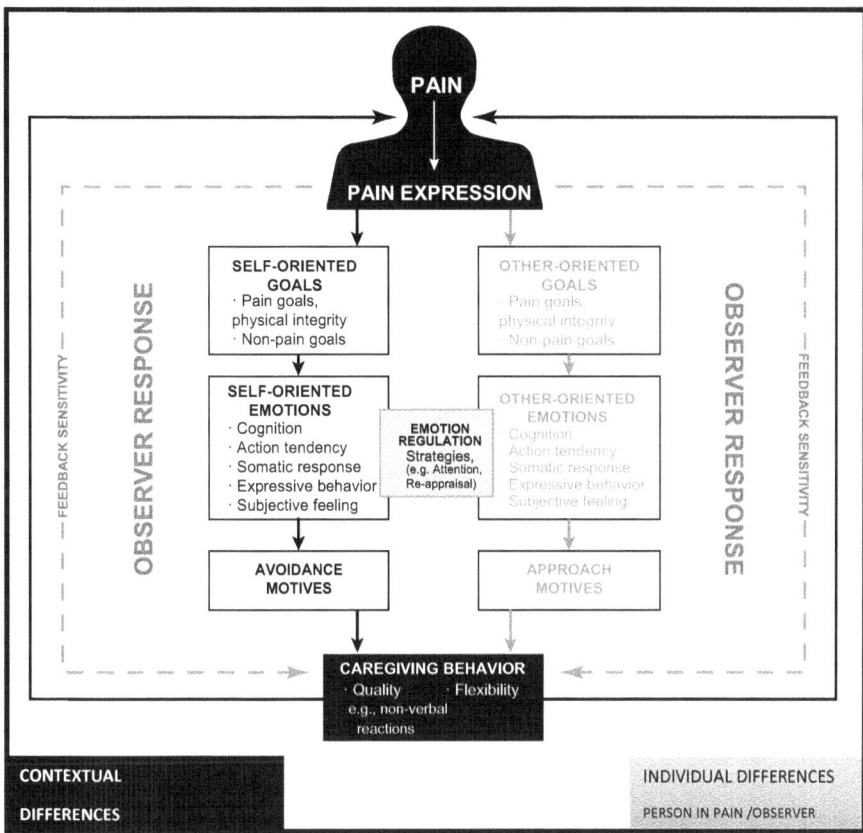

Fig. 4.1 An integrative affective-motivational account of interpersonal dynamics in pain

with the pain sufferer, perceived unfairness of the pain experience, and prejudicial/ discriminatory attitudes (Azevedo, Macaluso, Avenanti, Santangelo, & Aglioti, 2013; De Coster, Verschuere, Goubert, Tsakiris, & Brass, 2013; De Ruddere, Goubert, Vervoort, Kappesser, & Crombez, 2013; De Ruddere, Goubert, Vervoort, Prkachin, & Crombez, 2012; Hein & Singer, 2008; Vervoort, Caes, et al., 2011; Vervoort, Huguet, et al., 2011) The nature of various dyadic relationships in the context of pain is also likely to influence the above processes, modulating prioritization and impact of self vs. other-oriented goals, associated affective-motivational states, and behavioral responses. Such dyadic relationships may include that between parent and child, patient and health provider, strangers, or spouses. For instance, as children are often dependent upon others' care and likely have a more limited coping repertoire than adults, the impact of parental responses may be much more pronounced.

Finally, individual differences characterizing either observers or persons in pain are also likely to modulate interpersonal pain dynamics; such factors may include (but are not limited to) prior (inter)personal pain experience, available coping resources, dispositional empathy, and specific pain beliefs (Caes, Vervoort, Eccleston, & Goubert, 2012; Leonard & Cano, 2006). The role of individual difference factors is supported by recent findings (Vervoort et al., 2014), that observer characteristics (e.g., observer state anxiety) may significant affect the utility/effectiveness of specific emotion regulatory strategy (e.g., attending away vs. toward another's pain) in ways that can be explained by the proposed model.

Conclusions and Future Directions

The current chapter and proposed model are intended to synthesize and foster inquiry regarding affective-motivational dynamics within the interpersonal pain context. The proposed model aims to extend existing frameworks in several ways. Specifically the model (a) addresses goals both related and not related to physical integrity, (b) distinguishes affective-motivational and behavioral processes oriented toward the self vs. the person in pain, (c) proposes mechanisms (e.g., feedback sensitivity and nonverbal features) that may interact with affective-motivational processes to influence the nature and efficacy of caregiving response, and (d) highlights the role of emotion regulation strategies within a multiple goal context. Finally, given the centrality of emotion to pain experience, we hope to highlight a more nuanced conceptualization of emotion in the context of pain, one that recognizes emotions as stemming from goals and consisting of multiple components that may all constitute targets for regulation.

Future research will ideally draw on both clinical and experimental approaches to refine specific hypotheses stemming from this model (e.g., associations between self- vs. other-oriented affective-motivational processes, specific observable behaviors, moderating contextual/individual differences, and pain outcomes). Research on prosocial/caregiving behavior requires attention to potential social desirability bias; it is likely that creative and implicit mythologies (e.g., to assess observer self- vs. other-orientations) will be particularly useful [85]. Manipulations of perspective-taking (e.g., imagining self vs. another in pain; Craig, 1968; Jackson, Brunet, Meltzoff, & Decety, 2006) and goal manipulation (e.g., modifying the value or salience of self- vs. other-oriented goals (Claes, Karos, Meulders, Crombez, & Vlaeyen, 2014; Schrooten et al., 2012) may also be valuable in this line of research. Although discussion of clinical implications is premature, future research may wish to consult treatment modalities (such as dialectical behavioral therapy; Kirby & Baucom, 2007) which explicitly address emotion dysregulation within intrapersonal and interpersonal functioning, as these may offer insights regarding both research and clinical targets. In summary, the current account offers an initial conceptualization of processes increasingly recognized as central to the pain experience. It is hoped and expected that the proposed framework will be further advanced and refined through empirical and clinical efforts.

References

Aldao, A. (2013). The future of emotion regulation research: Capturing context. *Perspectives on Psychological Science, 8,* 155–172.

Atkinson, N. H., Gennis, H., Racine, N. M., & Pillai Riddell, R. (2015). Caregiver emotional availability, caregiver soothing behaviors, and infant pain during immunization. *Journal of Pediatric Psychology, 40,* 1105–1114.

Azevedo, R. T., Macaluso, E., Avenanti, A., Santangelo, V., Cazzato, V., & Aglioti, S. M. (2013). Their pain is not our pain: Brain and autonomic correlates of empathic resonance with the pain of same and different race individuals. *Human Brain Mapping, 34,* 3168–3181.

Batson, C. D., Fultz, J., & Schoenrade, P. A. (1987). Distress and empathy—2 qualitatively distinct vicarious emotions with different motivational consequences. *Journal of Personality, 55,* 19–39.

Boersma, K., Linton, S., Overmeer, T., Jansson, M., Vlaeyen, J., & de Jong, J. (2004). Lowering fear-avoidance and enhancing function through exposure in vivo—a multiple baseline study across six patients with back pain. *Pain, 108,* 8–16.

Bolger, N., Foster, M., Vinokur, A. D., & Ng, R. (1996). Close relationships and adjustment to a life crisis: The case of breast cancer. *Journal of Personality and Social Psychology, 70*(2), 283–294.

Bolger, N., Zuckerman, A., & Kessler, R. C. (2000). Invisible support and adjustment to stress. *Journal of Personality and Social Psychology, 79*(6), 953–961.

Bonnano, G. A., & Burton, C. L. (2013). Regulatory flexibility: An individual differences perspective on coping and emotion regulation. *Psychological Science, 8,* 591–612.

Bonnano, G. A., Papa, A., Lalande, K., Westphal, M., & Coifman, K. (2004). The importance of being flexible: The ability to both enhance and suppress emotional expression predicts long-term adjustment. *Psychological Science, 15,* 482–487.

Caes, L., Vervoort, T., Eccleston, C., & Goubert, L. (2012). Parents who catastrophize about their child's pain prioritize attempts to control pain. *Pain, 153,* 1695–1701.

Campbell, C. M., Witmer, K., Simango, M., Carteret, A., Loggia, M. L., Campbell, J. N., … Edwards, R. R. (2010). Catastrophizing delays the analgesic effect of distraction. *Pain, 149,* 202–207.

Campbell, P., Jordan, K. P., & Dunn, K. M. (2012). The role of relationship quality and perceived partner responses with pain and disability in those with back pain. *Pain Medicine, 13*(2), 204–214.

Claes, N., Karos, K., Meulders, A., Crombez, G., & Vlaeyen, J. W. S. (2014). Competing goals attenuate avoidance behaviour in the context of pain. *Journal of Pain, 15,* 1120–1129.

Craig, K. D. (1968). Physiological arousal as a function of imagined, vicarious, and direct stress experiences. *Journal of Abnormal Psychology, 73,* 513–520.

Craig, K. D. (2004). Social communication of pain enhances protective functions: A comment on Deyo, Prkachin and Mercer. *Pain, 107,* 5–6.

Crombez, G., Eccleston, C., Van Damme, S., Vlaeyen, J. W. S., & Karoly, P. (2012). Fear-avoidance model of chronic pain: The next generation. *Clinical Journal of Pain, 28,* 475–483.

Crombez, G., Vlaeyen, J. W. S., Heuts, P. H. T. G., & Lysens, R. (1999). Pain-related fear is more disabling than pain itself: Evidence on the role of pain-related fear in chronic pain disability. *Pain, 80,* 329–339.

De Coster, L., Verschuere, B., Goubert, L., Tsakiris, M., & Brass, M. (2013). I suffer more from your pain when you act like me: Being imitated enhances affective responses to seeing someone else in pain. *Cognitive, Affective, & Behavioral Neuroscience, 13,* 519–532.

de Jong, J. R., Vlaeyen, J. W. S., van Eijsden, M., Loo, C., & Onghena, P. (2012). Reduction of pain-related fear and increased function and participation in work-related upper extremity pain (WRUEP): Effects of exposure in vivo. *Pain, 153,* 2109–2118.

De Ruddere, L., Goubert, L., Vervoort, T., Kappesser, J., & Crombez, G. (2013). The impact of being primed with social deception upon observer responses to other's pain. *Pain, 154*, 221–226.

De Ruddere, L., Goubert, L., Vervoort, T., Prkachin, K., & Crombez, G. (2012). We discount the pain of others when pain has no medical explanation. *Pain, 13*, 1195–1205.

Decety, J., & Jackson, P. L. (2006). A social-neuroscience perspective on empathy. *Current Directions in Psychological Science, 15*, 54–58.

Dix, T. (1991). The affective organization of parenting: Adaptive and maladaptive processes. *Psychological Bulletin, 110*, 3–25.

Dix, T., Gershoff, E. T., Meunier, L. N., & Miller, P. C. (2004). The affective structure of supportive parenting: Depressive symptoms, immediate emotions, and child-oriented motivation. *Developmental Psychology, 40*, 1212–1227.

Eccleston, C., & Crombez, G. (1999). Pain demands attention: A cognitive-affective model of the interruptive function of pain. *Psychological Bulletin, 125*, 356–366.

Edmond, S. N., & Keefe, F. J. (2015). Validating pain communication. *Pain, 156*(2), 215–219.

Eisenberg, N., Fabes, R. A., Miller, A., Fultz, J., Shell, R., Mathy, R. M., & Reno, R. R. (1989). Relation of sympathy and personal distress to prosocial behaviour: A multimethod study. *Journal of Personality and Social Psychology, 57*, 55–66.

Elliot, A. J., Eder, A. B., & Harmon-Jones, E. (2013). Approach-avoidance motivation and emotion: Convergence and divergence. *Emotion Review, 5*, 308–311.

Elommaa, M. M., Williams, A. C. D., & Kalso, E. A. (2009). Attention management as a treatment for chronic pain. *European Journal of Pain, 13*, 1062–1067.

Fishbach, A., & Ferguson, M. J. (2007). The goal construct in social psychology. In A. W. Kruglanski & E. T. Higgins (Eds.), *Social psychology: Handbook of basic principles* (pp. 490–515). New York, NY: Guilford Press.

Flor, H., Kerns, R. D., & Turk, D. C. (1987). The role of spouse reinforcement, perceived pain, and activity levels of chronic pain patients. *Journal of Psychosomatic Research, 31*(2), 251–259.

Fordyce, W. E. (1976). *Behavioural methods in chronic pain and illness*. St. Louis, MO: Mosby.

Frijda, N. H. (2007). *The laws of emotion*. New York, NY: Routledge.

Gable, S. L., & Gosnell, C. L. (2013). Approach and avoidance behaviour in interpersonal relationships. *Emotion Review, 5*, 269–274.

Goubert, L., Craig, K. D., Vervoort, T., Morley, S., Sullivan, M. J. L., Williams, A. C. d. C., … Crombez, G. (2005). Facing others in pain: The effects of empathy. *Pain, 118*, 285–288.

Goubert, L., Eccleston, C., Crombez, G., & Devulder, J. (2004). Distraction from chronic pain during a pain-inducing activity is associated with greater post-activity pain. *Pain, 110*, 220–227.

Goubert, L., Vervoort, T., & Craig, K. D. (2013). Empathy and pain. In R. F. Schmidt & G. F. Gebhart (Eds.), *Encyclopedia of pain* (2nd ed., pp. 1128–1134). Heidelberg, Germany: Springer-Verlag.

Goubert, L., Vervoort, T., & Crombez, G. (2009). Pain demands attention from others: The approach/avoidance paradox. *Pain, 143*, 5–6.

Gross, J. J. (1998). The emerging field of emotion regulation: An integrative review. *Review of General Psychology, 2*, 271–299.

Gross, J. J. (2013). Emotion regulation: Taking stock and moving forward. *Emotion, 13*, 359–365.

Gross, J. J., & Thompson, R. A. (2007). Emotion regulation: Conceptual foundations. In J. J. Gross (Ed.), *Handbook of emotion regulation* (pp. 3–20). New York, NY: Guilford Press.

Hadjistavropoulos, T., & Craig, K. D. (2002). A theoretical framework for understanding self-report and observational measures of pain: A communications model. *Behaviour Research and Therapy, 40*, 551–570.

Hadjistavropoulos, T., Craig, K. D., Duck, S., Cano, A., Goubert, L., Jackson, P. L., … Fitzgerald, T. D. (2011). A biopsychosocial formulation of pain communication. *Psychological Bulletin, 137*, 910–939.

Hamilton, N., Karoly, P., & Kitzman, H. (2004). Self-regulation and chronic pain: The role of emotion. *Cognitive Therapy and Research, 28*, 559–576.

Hastings, P. D., & Grusec, J. E. (1998). Parenting goals as organizers of responses to parent-child disagreement. *Developmental Psychology, 34*, 465–479.

Hayes, S. C., Pistorello, J., & Levin, M. E. (2012). Acceptance and commitment therapy as a unified model of behavior change. *The Counseling Psychologist, 40*, 976–1002.

Hein, G., & Singer, T. (2008). I feel how you feel but not always: The empathic brain and its modulation. *Current Opinion in Neurobiology, 18*, 153–158.

Heyneman, N., Fremouw, W. J., Gano, D., Kirkland, F., & Heiden, L. (1990). Individual differences and the effectiveness of different coping strategies for pain. *Cognitive Therapy and Research, 14*, 63–77.

Impett, E. A., Peplau, L. A., & Gable, S. L. (2005). Approach and avoidance sexual motivation: Implications for personal and interpersonal well-being. *Personal Relationships, 12*, 465–482.

International Association for the Study of Pain Task Force on Taxonomy. (1994). *Classification of chronic pain: Descriptions of chronic pain syndromes and definitions of pain terms* (2nd ed.). Seattle, WA: IASP Press.

Jackson, P. L., Brunet, E., Meltzoff, A. N., & Decety, J. (2006). Empathy examined through the neural mechanisms involved in imagining how I feel versus how you feel pain. *Neuropsychologia, 44*, 752–761.

Jensen, M. P., Karoly, P., & Huger, R. (1987). The development and preliminary validation of an instrument to assess patients' attitudes toward pain. *Journal of Psychosomatic Research, 31*, 393–400.

Johnson, D. R. (2009a). Emotional attention set shifting and its relationship to anxiety and emotion regulation. *Emotion, 9*, 681–690.

Johnson, D. R. (2009b). Goal-directed attentional deployment to emotional faces and individual differences in emotional regulation. *Journal of Research in Personality, 43*, 8–13.

Jones, E. B., & Sharpe, L. (2014). The effect of cognitive bias modification for interpretation (CBM-I) on avoidance of pain during an acute experimental pain task. *Pain, 155*, 1569–1576.

Karoly, P., & Ruehlman, L. S. (1996). Motivational implications of pain: Chronicity, psychological distress, and work goal construal in a national sample of adults. *Health Psychology, 15*, 383–390.

Keltner, D., & Gross, J. J. (1999). Functional accounts of emotions. *Cognition and Emotion, 13*, 467–480.

Kerns, R. D., Turk, D. C., & Rudy, T. E. (1985). The West Haven-Yale Multidimensional Pain Inventory (WHYMPI). *Pain, 23*, 345–356.

Kirby, J. S., & Baucom, D. H. (2007). Integrating dialectical behavior therapy and cognitive-behavioral couple therapy: A couples skills group for emotion dysregulation. *Cognitive and Behavioral Practice, 14*, 394–405.

Koole, S. L. (2009). The psychology of emotion regulation: An integrative review. *Cognition and Emotion, 23*, 4–41.

Koole, S. L., & Rothermund, K. (2011). "I feel better but I don't know why": The psychology of implicit emotion regulation. *Cognition and Emotion, 25*, 389–399.

Lamm, C., Decety, J., & Singer, T. (2011). Meta-analytic evidence for common and distinct neural networks associated with directly experienced pain and empathy for pain. *NeuroImage, 54*, 2492–2502.

Laurenceau, J.-P., Barrett, L. F., & Rovine, M. J. (2005). The interpersonal process model of intimacy in marriage: A daily-diary and multilevel modeling approach. *Journal of Family Psychology, 19*(2), 314–323.

Leeuw, M., Goossens, M. E. J. B., Linton, S. J., Crombez, G., Boersma, K., & Vlaeyen, J. W. S. (2007). The fear-avoidance model of musculoskeletal pain: Current state of scientific evidence. *Journal of Behavioral Medicine, 30*, 77–94.

Leonard, M. T., & Cano, A. (2006). Pain affects spouses too: Personal experience with pain and catastrophizing as correlates of spouse distress. *Pain, 126*, 139–146.

Lin, H., & McFatter, R. (2012). Empathy and distress: Two distinct but related emotions in response to infant crying. *Infant Behavior and Development, 35*, 887–897.

Loggia, M. L., Mogil, J. S., & Bushnell, M. C. (2008). Empathy hurts: Compassion for another increases both sensory and affective components of pain perception. *Pain, 136*, 168–176.

Malloy, K. M., & Milling, L. S. (2010). The effectiveness of virtual reality distraction for pain reduction: A systematic review. *Clinical Psychology Review, 30*, 1011–1018.

Manczak, E. M., DeLongis, A., & Chen, E. (2016). Does empathy have a cost? Diverging psychological and pshysiological effects within families. *Health Psychology, 35*, 211–218.

Martini, T. S., & Busseri, M. A. (2010). Emotion regulation strategies and goals as predictors of older mothers' and adult daughters' helping-related subjective well-being. *Psychology and Aging, 25*, 48–59.

Mauss, I. B., Bunge, S. A., & Gross, J. J. (2007). Automatic emotion regulation. *Social and Personality Psychology Compass, 1*, 146–167.

McCracken, L. M., & Keogh, E. (2009). Acceptance, mindfulness, and values-based action may counteract fear and avoidance of emotions in chronic pain: An analysis of anxiety sensitivity. *Journal of Pain, 10*, 408–415.

McCracken, L. M., & Vowles, K. E. (2014). Acceptance and commitment therapy and mindfulness for chronic pain model, process, and progress. *American Psychologist, 69*, 178–187.

McMurthry, C. M., Chambers, C. T., McGrath, P. J., & Asp, E. (2010). When "don't worry" communicates fear: Children's perceptions of parental reassurance and distraction during a painful medical procedure. *Pain, 150*, 52–58.

Moors, A. (2009). Theories of emotion causation: A review. *Cognition and Emotion, 23*, 625–662.

Moors, A. (2013). Understanding emotion change requires an understanding of emotion causation. In D. Hermans, B. Mesquita, & B. Rimé (Eds.), *Changing emotions* (pp. 144–150). New York, NY: Psychology Press.

Moors, A., & Scherer, K. R. (2013). The role of appraisal in emotion. In M. Robinson, E. Watkins, & E. Harmon-Jones (Eds.), *Handbook of cognition and emotion* (pp. 135–155). New York, NY: Guilford Press.

Moseley, G. L., Nicholas, M. K., & Hodges, P. W. (2004). Does anticipation of back pain predispose to back pain trouble? *Brain, 127*, 2339–2347.

Newton-John, T. R. (2002). Solicitousness and chronic pain: A critical review. *Pain Reviews, 9*, 7–27.

Newton-John, T. R., & Williams, A. (2006). Chronic pain couples: Perceived marital interactions and pain behaviours. *Pain, 123*, 53–63.

Oatley, K., & Johnson-Laird, P. N. (1987). Towards a cognitive theory of emotions. *Cognition and Emotion, 1*, 29–50.

Ray, R. D., McRae, K., Ochsner, K. N., & Gross, J. J. (2010). Cognitive reappraisal of negative affect: Converging evidence from EMG and self-report. *Emotion, 10*, 587–592.

Schoth, D. E., Georgallis, T., & Liossi, C. (2013). Attentional bias modification in people with chronic pain: A proof of concept study. *Cognitive Behaviour Therapy, 42*, 233–243.

Schrooten, M. G. S., Van Damme, S., Crombez, G., Peters, M. L., Vogt, J., & Vlaeyen, J. W. S. (2012). Nonpain goal pursuit inhibits attentional bias to pain. *Pain, 153*, 1180–1186.

Sharpe, L., Ianiello, M., Dear, B. F., Perry, K. N., Refshauge, K., & Nicholas, M. K. (2012). Is there a potential role for attention bias modification in pain patients? Results of 2 randomised controlled trials. *Pain, 153*, 722–731.

Sheppes, G., Scheibe, S., Sure, G., Radu, P., Blechert, J., & Gross, J. J. (2014). Emotion regulation choice: A conceptual framework and supporting evidence. *Journal of Experimental Psychology: General, 143*, 163–181.

Simons, L. E., & Kacynski, K. J. (2012). The fear avoidance model of chronic pain: Examination for pediatric application. *Journal of Pain, 13*, 827–835.

Strough, J., Berg, C. A., & Sansone, C. (1996). Goals for solving everyday problems across the life span: Age and gender differences in the salience of interpersonal concerns. *Developmental Psychology, 32*, 1106–1115.

Sullivan, M. J. L., Thorn, B., Haythornthwaite, J., Keefe, F., Martin, M., Bradley, L., & Lefebvre, J. C. (2001). Theoretical perspectives on the relation between catastrophizing and pain. *Clinical Journal of Pain, 17*, 52–64.

Suls, J., & Fletcher, B. (1985). The relative efficacy of avoidant and non-avoidant coping strategies: A meta-analysis. *Health Psychology, 4*, 249–288.

Tamir, M. (2009). What do people want to feel and why? Pleasure and utility in emotion regulation. *Current Directions in Psychological Science, 18*, 101–105.

Tamir, M., Chiu, C., & Gross, J. J. (2007). Business or pleasure: Utilitarian versus hedonic considerations in emotion regulation. *Emotion, 7*, 546–554.

Tamir, M., Mitchell, C., & Gross, J. J. (2008). Hedonic and instrumental motives in anger regulation. *Psychological Science, 19*, 324–328.

Trost, Z., France, C. R., & Thomas, J. S. (2008). Exposure to movement in chronic back pain: Evidence of successful generalization across a reaching task. *Pain, 137*, 26–33.

Van Damme, S., Legrain, V., Vogt, J., & Crombez, G. (2010). Keeping pain in mind: A motivational account of attention to pain. *Neuroscience and Biobehavioral Reviews, 34*, 204–213.

Van Ryckeghem DM, De Houwer J, Van Bockstaele B, Van Damme S, De Schryver M, Crombez G. (2013). Implicit assocations between pain and self-schema in patients with chronic pain. Pain, 154, 2700-2706.

VanderDrift, L. E., & Agnew, C. R. (2015). Relational consequences of personal goal pursuits. *Journal of Personality and Social Psychology, 106*, 927–940.

Verhoeven, K., Crombez, G., Eccleston, C., Van Ryckeghem, D. M. L., Morley, S., & Van Damme, S. (2010). The role of motivation in distracting attention away from pain: An experimental study. *Pain, 149*, 229–234.

Vervoort, T., Caes, L., Trost, Z., Sullivan, M. J. L., Vangronsveld, K., & Goubert, L. (2011). Social modulation of facial pain display in high catastrophizing children: An observational study in schoolchildren and their parents. *Pain, 152*, 1591–1599.

Vervoort, T., Huguet, A., Verhoeven, K., & Goubert, L. (2011). Mothers' and fathers' responses to their child's pain moderate the relationship between the child's pain catastrophizing and disability. *Pain, 152*(4), 786–793.

Vervoort, T., & Trost, Z. (2016). The interpersonal function of pain: Conserving multiple resources. *Pain, 157*, 773–774.

Vervoort, T., & Trost, Z. (2017). Examining affective-motivational dynamics and behavioural implications within the interpersonal context. *Journal of Pain, 18*, 1174–1183.

Vervoort, T., Trost, Z., Sutterlin, S., Caes, L., & Moors, A. (2014). The emotion regulatory function of parent attention to child pain and associated implications for parental pain control behaviour. *Pain, 155*, 1453–1463.

Vlaeyen, J. W. S., & Linton, S. J. (2000). Fear-avoidance and its consequences in chronic musculoskeletal pain: A state of the art. *Pain, 85*, 317–332.

Webb, T. L., Miles, E., & Sheeran, P. (2012). Dealing with feeling: A meta-analysis of the effectiveness of strategies derived from the process model of emotion regulation. *Psychological Bulletin, 138*, 775–808.

Wicksell, R. K., Olsson, G. L., & Hayes, S. C. (2011). Mediators of change in acceptance and commitment therapy for pediatric chronic pain. *Pain, 152*, 2792–2801.

Williams, A. C. d. C. (2002). Facial expression of pain: An evolutionary account. *Behavioral and Brain Sciences, 25*, 439–488.

Williams, A. C. d. C., & Craig, K. D. (2006). A science of pain expression? *Pain, 125*, 202–203.

Yamada, M., & Decety, J. (2009). Unconscious affective processing and empathy: An investigation of subliminal priming on the detection of painful facial expressions. *Pain, 143*, 71–75.

Zale, E. L., Lange, K. L., Fields, S. A., & Ditre, J. W. (2013). The relation between pain-related fear and disability: A meta-analysis. *Journal of Pain, 14*, 1019–1030.

Part II
A Science of Pain Expression

Chapter 5
Pain Behavior: Unitary or Multidimensional Phenomenon?

Marc O. Martel and Michael J. L. Sullivan

Abstract The behavioral alterations observed in individuals experiencing pain have been referred to as "pain behavior." This chapter begins with a brief overview of protocols that have been developed for the assessment of pain behaviors, both in clinical and nonclinical settings. We then provide an overview of studies that have been conducted on the functions, determinants, and consequences of pain behaviors. We conclude the chapter by summarizing arguments and evidence in support of a multidimensional conceptualization of pain behavior. The multidimensional view of pain behavior is supported by evidence indicating that different types of pain behaviors are only modestly interrelated, and that different types of pain behaviors have different degrees of temporal stability. The multidimensional view is also supported by research suggesting that different types of pain behaviors likely serve different functions and have different determinants. Importantly, research indicates that different types of pain behaviors have a differential impact on functional and occupational disability outcomes, which provides further support the multidimensional nature of pain behavior. On the basis of research conducted to date, it appears clear that a multidimensional conceptualization of pain behavior will be required to further advance our knowledge on the functions, determinants and consequences of pain behaviors. A multidimensional conceptualization of pain behavior will also be required in order to pave the way for the development of new treatment interventions designed to minimize pain behaviors and their potentially negative impact on pain-related outcomes.

Keywords Pain · Pain behavior · Determinants · Functions · Communication · Protection

M. O. Martel (✉)
Faculties of Dentistry and Medicine, McGill University, Montreal, QC, Canada
e-mail: marc.o.martel@mcgill.ca

M. J. L. Sullivan
Department of Psychology, McGill University, Montreal, QC, Canada

Introduction

Pain does not only affect how people feel, it also affects what people "do." Individuals in pain "behave" differently from individuals without pain. Compared to individuals without pain, individuals with pain will often display facial expressions such as grimaces or frowns, they might emit utterances such as moans or sighs, they might hold, guard, or touch body parts affected by pain, they might exhibit an altered gait, they might move slower, and they might discontinue or avoid activities associated with pain. Collectively, the behavioral alterations observed in individuals experiencing pain have been referred to as "pain behavior."

In the pain literature, there is a long history of viewing pain behavior as a unitary construct. That is, it has often been implicitly invoked that different types of pain behaviors are equivalent, and that different types of pain behaviors simply reflect a common underlying internal experience (i.e., pain) (Loeser & Melzack, 1999; Rachlin, 2010). Research has now accumulated indicating that different types of pain behaviors have different functions, determinants, and consequences. In this chapter, we begin with a brief overview of protocols that have been developed for the assessment of pain behaviors, both in clinical and non-clinical settings. We then provide an overview of studies that have been conducted over the past few decades on the functions, determinants, and consequences of pain behaviors. We conclude the chapter by summarizing arguments and evidence in support of a multidimensional conceptualization of pain behavior.

The Assessment of Pain Behavior

Over the past few decades, procedures have been developed for the assessment of pain behavior among patients with pain. Early approaches to pain behavior assessment relied on semi-structured interviews (Cinciripini & Floreen, 1983), self-recording methods (Follick, Ahern, & Aberger, 1985; Kerns et al., 1991), or direct observation methods (Keefe & Block, 1982; Richards, Nepomuceno, Riles, & Suer, 1982; Romano et al., 1992). To date, the most widely used method is that based on the work of Keefe and his colleagues (Keefe et al., 1987; Keefe & Block, 1982), who developed a direct observation method for assessing pain behaviors while patients engage in a series of functional tasks such as reclining, standing, and walking. During these tasks, patients' pain behaviors are videotaped and then quantified by trained coders, who record the occurrence of pain behaviors based on a variety of predefined pain behavior categories. The Keefe and Block method was initially developed to be carried out as part of physical or medical examination procedures, but is now used in a variety of research laboratory settings. Studies have provided support for the reliability and validity of the Keefe and Block method among patients with a variety of pain conditions, including back pain (Keefe et al., 1987; Keefe & Block, 1982; Sullivan et al., 2006), osteoarthritis (Keefe et al., 1987), and rheumatoid arthritis (Anderson et al., 1987; Anderson, Bradley, Turner, Agudelo, & Pisko, 1994; McDaniel et al., 1986).

In recent years, adaptations and refinements have been made to the Keefe and Block pain behavior observation protocol. For example, Prkachin and his colleagues (Prkachin, Hughes, Schultz, Joy, & Hunt, 2002; Prkachin, Schultz, Berkowitz, Hughes, & Hunt, 2002) incorporated greater focus on facial pain behaviors, and developed a procedure enabling "in vivo" assessment of pain behaviors as a way to reduce resource demands associated with pain behavior coding. More recently, Sullivan, Thibault, et al. (2006) adapted the Keefe and Block method to a simulated occupational lifting task designed to yield indices of pain behavior, along with broader indices of physical performance. Pain behavior observation methods based on the Keefe and Block system are now widely used, and have allowed researchers to investigate the functions, determinants, and consequences of different types of pain behaviors. Although other assessment procedures can be used for the assessment of pain behavior, such as the Facial Action Coding System (FACS; Ekman & Friesen, 1978), the FACS is limited to facial pain expressions, which considerably limits its utility when other types of pain behaviors are also of interest.

Pain behavior assessment protocols modeled after the Keefe and Block system have proven particularly useful for examining the consistency across different types of pain behaviors. For instance, while the FACS has contributed to identifying a core set of facial muscles that are reliably involved in generating facial pain expressions, studies based on the Keefe and Block system revealed only modest interrelationships across different types of pain behaviors (Prkachin, Hughes, et al., 2002; Prkachin, Schultz, et al., 2002). Test-retest studies conducted among patients with pain have also found that different types of pain behaviors have different degrees of temporal stability (Martel, Thibault, & Sullivan, 2010; Prkachin, Hughes, et al., 2002). That is, certain types of pain behaviors are displayed more frequently and consistently over time than others.

Functions of Pain Behavior

To date, evolutionary theories have provided the most powerful theoretical frameworks within which to understand the functions of pain behaviors. From an evolutionary perspective, pain has been discussed as an internal mechanism that increases the probability of survival (Damasio, 1994; Wall, 1999). Pain alerts the individual to the possibility that the integrity of the body has been potentially compromised. Central to the survival value of the pain system is the mobilization of behaviors that will act on the source of the pain, or tend to the consequences of pain. Building upon evolutionary and functional perspectives, Sullivan (Sullivan, 2008) recently argued that the pain system can only be adaptive if pain sensations are accompanied by behavioral programs designed to deal with pain, and further argued that different forms of pain behavior are likely to serve different adaptive functions. In the following sections, two separate functions of pain behavior will be addressed, namely, (1) protective functions and (2) communicative functions.

The Protective Functions of Pain Behavior

Descartes was likely the first theorist to address the protective functions of pain behavior. Descartes proposed that once pain information had been "reflected" by the pineal gland, pain signals activated motor mechanisms that would move the body away from the noxious stimulus (Descartes, 1662). As such, reflexive and protective withdrawal from a painful stimulus was considered as part of the pain system. The Gate Control Theory also addressed an action system that would be elicited to promote withdrawal from the source of pain (Melzack & Wall, 1965). Insofar as reflexive withdrawal minimizes the probability of further injury, it can be construed as a protective pain behavior. For example, the withdrawal of a limb from a hot surface can serve to terminate the action of a noxious stimulus and, in turn, protect the limb from further injury (Wall, 1999). Withdrawal can be reflexive, involving the simple movement of a limb, or it can be more complex, involving the coordinated engagement of a larger repertoire of behavior. Escape behavior (e.g., discontinuation of behavior causing pain) might represent an extension of reflexive withdrawal (Vlaeyen & Linton, 2000). Escape behavior might serve a protective function by allowing individuals to avoid activities that could potentially contribute to increasing pain. Similarly, the use of limping to alter weight distribution during ambulation might minimize pain to an injured limb and reduce the probability of injury exacerbation (Corbeil, Blouin, & Teasdale, 2004; Decchi et al., 1997). Individuals might also alter their gait in order to minimize pain associated with weight bearing on an arthritic joint. Other pain behaviors such as performing actions in a rigid or halting manner, or engaging in behaviors such as holding or guarding might also serve a protective function by minimizing movements that cause pain (Lund, Donga, Widmer, & Stohler, 1991; Moseley, Nicholas, & Hodges, 2004; Waddell, 1998). Protective pain behaviors are thus viewed as any action primarily aimed at minimizing the experience of pain, promoting recovery from injury, or reducing the probability of further injury. Although protective pain behaviors may have some adaptive value shortly after injury and/or in acute pain situations, evidence indicates that the frequent and persistent display of protective pain behaviors may become maladaptive under chronic pain conditions. This will be discussed in subsequent sections of this chapter.

The Communicative Functions of Pain Behavior

There has been considerable discussion on the communicative function of pain behavior. Craig and his colleagues (Craig, 2009; Hadjistavropoulos & Craig, 2002; Prkachin & Craig, 1995) have proposed a model of pain communication that addresses how pain information is communicated to others in the social environment. According to this model, facial responses accompanying pain are "broadcast" into the social world where they may be perceived and interpreted (i.e., decoded) by others. Of all the pain behaviors, facial pain expressions are assumed to exert the greatest impact upon observers by rapidly communicating information about pain, distress, and suffering (Craig, 2009). Other types of communicative pain behaviors include verbal or paraverbal pain expressions such as pain words, grunts, sighs, and moans. These behaviors communicate pain experience to others, but they are not assumed to serve a direct protective function. Unlike protective pain behaviors, they cannot eliminate or terminate the source of pain other than through eliciting the interventions of others (Sullivan, 2008; Williams, 2002). The effective communication of pain through facial, verbal, or paraverbal expressions may be critical to survival, especially when injury is severe and others' assistance is required for protection or care. Facial displays can be an important channel of pain communication when others are in close proximity; vocalizations can be an important channel of pain communication when others are not in view (Craig, 2009; Williams, 2002). From an evolutionary standpoint, facial displays could be considered "safer" than vocalizations when there is a predator/antagonist present because they are silent and would not attract attention from an enemy yet could communicate suffering to an ally (Williams, 2002).

Over the years, considerable studies have been conducted to examine the communicative value of facial pain expressions. Numerous studies, for instance, revealed that greater inferential weight is typically given to the face than to the body when observers make judgments about others' pain (Martel, Thibault, Roy, Catchlove, & Sullivan, 2008; Martel, Thibault, & Sullivan, 2011; Prkachin, Currie, & Craig, 1983; Sullivan, Martel, Tripp, Savard, & Crombez, 2006a). These studies provided support for the communicative value of facial pain expressions, and supported the functional distinctiveness of different types of pain behaviors. In another study (Sullivan, Thibault, et al., 2006), patients with low back pain were asked to lift a series of weights under two communication goal conditions. In one condition, patients were asked to estimate the weight of the object lifted, and in another condition, patients were asked to rate their pain when they lifted the object. Facial displays of pain were more pronounced during the pain rating task than the weight estimation task. Other pain behaviors (e.g., holding, guarding) were not affected by the communication goal manipulation. Findings showing that facial displays, and not other forms of pain behavior, are influenced by the manipulation of communication goals further support the functional distinctiveness of different forms of pain behavior.

In sum, there is both conceptual and empirical support for the functional distinctiveness of different forms of pain behavior. It is likely, however, that the functional distinctiveness of communicative and protective pain behaviors is restricted to their primary function, not their sole function (Hadjistavropoulos & Craig, 2002; Sullivan, 2008; Williams, 2002). For instance, protective pain behaviors (e.g., limping) can be understood in terms of the way they protect individuals from further injury or symptom exacerbation, but they may also serve a communicative function insofar as they are perceived by others. Similarly, facial expressions have been discussed as having a primary communicative function, but they can also serve a protective function by soliciting assistance or caregiving from others in the social environment.

Determinants of Pain Behavior

One of the most consistent findings emerging from studies on pain behavior is the large variability across individuals in the display of pain behaviors. Some patients display high levels of pain behavior, whereas other patients display very few pain behaviors. There is likely an innate and genetic component to pain behaviors, as evidence indicates that newborns have the ability to express pain (Craig, Whitfield, Grunau, Linton, & Hadjistavropoulos, 1993; Grunau & Craig, 1987). Albeit innate, pain behaviors, like any other form of human behavior, are likely to be influenced by a multitude of other biological, psychological, and social factors.

Biomedical Determinants of Pain Behavior

Early biomedical models have led to the widespread assumption that pain perception and pain expression should be proportionate to injury severity and the extent of tissue damage. Research, however, has now accumulated indicating that biomedical variables cannot fully account for the large variability observed across patients in the expression of pain behaviors. For instance, weak-to-modest associations have been found between measures of disease severity (e.g., joint counts, erythrocyte sedimentation rate) and displays of protective pain behaviors such as guarding and rubbing among patients with rheumatoid arthritis (McDaniel et al., 1986; Parker et al., 1993). Weak associations between measures of disease severity and pain behaviors have also been observed among patients with knee osteoarthritis (Keefe et al., 1987, 1991).

Pain Intensity Several studies have examined the association between self-reports of pain and the expression of pain behaviors. Studies have generally revealed significant positive associations between self-reports of pain intensity and pain behaviors (for a review, see Labus, Keefe, & Jensen, 2003). That is, higher levels of pain intensity have been found to be associated with heightened pain behaviors. Research, however, indicates that the relation between self-reports of pain intensity and pain behaviors is generally weak-to-modest, with reports of pain intensity rarely accounting for more than 10–15% of the variance in measures of communicative and protective pain behavior (Labus et al., 2003). This has been observed across a wide range of pain conditions, including musculoskeletal, visceral, orofacial, and neuropathic pain conditions. Based on these findings, it has become clear that the subjective experience of pain and the display of pain behavior are distinct phenomena, and that pain behaviors are not simply a proxy for pain experience (Hadjistavropoulos & Craig, 2002; Sullivan, 2008). The weak overlap between reports of pain and pain behaviors is also consistent with the biopsychomotor model of pain (Sullivan, 2008), which postulates that sensory and behavioral dimensions of pain are independent and only partially overlapping dimensions of the pain system.

Psychological Determinants of Pain Behavior

Considerable research has been conducted to examine the psychological determinants of pain behaviors. Some of the psychological factors that have been found to be most consistently associated with the expression of pain behaviors include depression, catastrophizing, and pain-related fear. Other psychological factors, however, have also been found to be associated with pain behaviors, including self-efficacy (Buckelew et al., 1994; Buescher et al., 1991), anger (Burns, Quartana, & Bruehl, 2011), and perceived injustice (Sullivan, Davidson, Garfinkel, Siriapaipant, & Scott, 2009).

Depression and Anxiety Studies examining the influence of depression and anxiety on the expression of pain behaviors have primarily been conducted among patients with pain. In these studies, it has been found that patients who are depressed display more intense communicative and protective pain behaviors than patients who are not depressed (Keefe, Wilkins, Cook, Crisson, & Muhkbaier, 1986; Kleinke, 1991; Krause, Wiener, & Tait, 1994; Romano et al., 1988). Similarly, several studies have found that patients scoring high on measures of anxiety tend to display more pain behaviors than patients low in anxiety (Burns et al., 2008; Hadjistavropoulos & LaChapelle, 2000; Tang et al., 2007).

Catastrophizing Studies have been consistent in showing that individuals who have a tendency to catastrophize during pain display higher levels of pain behaviors than patients who do not catastrophize. The term "pain catastrophizing" refers to a particular response to pain that includes elements of rumination, magnification, and helplessness (Sullivan et al., 2001). Pain catastrophizing has been associated with the expression of a variety of pain behaviors, both in clinical (Keefe et al., 1987, 2000; Sullivan et al., 2009) and non-clinical (Kunz, Chatelle, Lautenbacher, & Rainville, 2008; Sullivan, Adams, & Sullivan, 2004; Sullivan, Martel, et al., 2006a; Sullivan & Neish, 2000) populations. In a sample of patients with back pain, catastrophizing was found to be associated with the expression of communicative and protective pain behaviors even when controlling for patients' self-reports of pain (Thibault, Loisel, Durand, Catchlove, & Sullivan, 2008). It has been argued that high pain catastrophizers might engage in exaggerated pain expression in order to maximize proximity, or to solicit assistance or empathic responses from others (Sullivan et al., 2001). This notion is supported by studies showing that the expression of pain behaviors among high catatrophizers is sensitive social context. For instance, one experimental study showed that the presence of an observer led to increases in pain behaviors for pain catastrophizers but not for non-catastrophizers (Sullivan et al., 2004). In another study, the association between catastrophizing and self-reports of pain was found to be higher among pain patients living with a supportive spouse or caregiver (Giardino, Jensen, Turner, Ehde, & Cardenas, 2003). These studies provided indirect evidence that overt expressions of pain among high catastrophizers might serve a communal or intepersonal coping function.

There is evidence to suggest that catastrophizing might account, in part, for the observed sex differences in the expression of pain behaviors. Women have been found to display higher levels of pain behaviors than men, both in clinical (Keefe et al., 1987, 2000) and nonclinical (Kunz, Gruber, & Lautenbacher, 2006; Sullivan, Tripp, & Santor, 2000) populations. In one study, Keefe et al. (2000) found that catastrophizing mediated the relationship between sex and pain behaviors in patients with osteoarthritis. Likewise, Sullivan et al. (2000) found that sex differences in pain behaviors during experimentally induced cold pressor pain were no longer significant after controlling for pain catastrophizing. Results of these two mediational studies suggest that catastrophizing might account for the observed sex differences in the expression of pain behaviors.

Pain-Related Fear Pain-related fear is another psychological factor that has been found to be associated with the expression of pain behaviors. Much of the research examining the association between pain-related fear and pain behaviors has been conducted among patients with chronic back pain, and has relied on self-report questionnaires such as the Fear-Avoidance Beliefs Questionnaire (FABQ; Waddell, Newton, Henderson, Somerville, & Main, 1993) and the Tampa Scale for Kinesiophobia (TSK; Kori, Miller, & Todd, 1990). The FABQ was designed to assess pain-related fear from physical activity, and the TSK was designed to assess fear of movement and reinjury. Two studies have revealed significant positive correlations between the FABQ and "objective" measures of guarding using electromyographic (EMG) activity of paraspinal muscles in patients with chronic back pain (Main & Walson, 1996; Watson, Booker, Main, & Chen, 1997). Studies have also revealed significant positive correlations between the TSK and measures of pain behaviors such as facial expressions and guarding (Gauthier, Thibault, & Sullivan, 2011; Koho, Aho, Watson, & Hurri, 2001; Thibault et al., 2008). In one study (Thibault et al., 2008), the TSK was associated with protective pain behaviors such as guarding, holding, or rubbing, but not with communicative pain behaviors (e.g., facial and paraverbal pain expressions).

Unconscious and Automatic Processes There is reason to believe that psychological factors operating outside of conscious awareness might contribute, at least in part, to the expression of pain behaviors. Traditional psychodynamic models of persistent pain conditions proposed that unconscious psychological conflicts may, in some cases, take the form of physical symptoms and expressive behaviors (Engel, 1959; Pilowsky & Spence, 1976). Interestingly, Burns and his colleagues (Burns, 2000) found that emotional repression, a concept with psychodynamic roots, is associated with negative pain-related outcomes among patients with chronic pain. Although it is not readily feasible to reliably assess the influence of unconscious factors on the expression of pain behaviors, the contribution of these factors should not be completely ruled out. In recent years, there has been growing interest in examining the degree of automaticity and cognitive control that might underlie the expression of pain behaviors. For instance, Craig, Versloot, Goubert, Vervoort, and Crombez (2010) argued that pain behaviors are likely to vary along a continuum ranging from fully automatic to fully controlled (i.e., intentional). On the one hand, it is possible that pain behaviors are mainly governed by the operation of automatic processes that are independent of cognitive control. This perspective implies that pain behaviors occur without intention, planning, or awareness (Craig et al., 2010; Hadjistavropoulos et al., 2011; Hadjistavropoulos & Craig, 2002). On the other hand, it is possible that pain behaviors are mainly governed by the operation of cognitive control processes that allow the intentional expression of various forms of pain behavior. One recent study provided preliminary evidence that communicative pain behaviors (e.g., facial pain expressions) are likely to be under greater cognitive control than protective pain behaviors (Martel, Trost, & Sullivan, 2012). Although communicative pain behaviors have been discussed in terms of their automaticity (Hadjistavropoulos & Craig, 2002; Williams, 2002), they are not impervious to cognitive control. Additional research will be needed to further explore the degree of automaticity and cognitive control underlying different types of pain behaviors.

Social Determinants of Pain Behavior

Over the past few decades, considerable efforts have been devoted to examining the social determinants of pain behaviors. Most of the studies examining the social determinants of pain behaviors were grounded in the operant view of pain behaviors (Fordyce, 1976, 1984). Proceeding from principles of operant conditioning, Fordyce suggested that pain behaviors, like any other behaviors, are influenced by their consequences (Fordyce, 1984). He suggested that pain behaviors could be systematically shaped by environmental and interpersonal reinforcers such as increased attention or reduced demands. For instance, a particular behavior (e.g., moaning) that is followed by a positive consequence (e.g., empathic attention) will have a higher probability of being emitted in the future, regardless of pain. In this case, "moaning" becomes instrumental in achieving empathic attention.

A considerable amount of research has supported the operant view of pain behaviors. For instance, it has been found that chronic pain patients who live with solicitous spouses display higher levels of communicative and protective pain behaviors than patients who live with non-solicitous spouses (Block, 1981; Kerns et al., 1991; Romano et al., 1992, 1995). In a study of patient–spouse interactions during a series of household chores (Romano, Jensen, Turner, Good, & Hops, 2000), spouse solicitous behaviors contributed significant variance to the prediction of patients' pain behaviors even after controlling for patients' self-reports of pain. Other studies have found that patients who report high satisfaction with their social support display significantly higher levels of pain behaviors than patients who report low social support satisfaction (Gil, Keefe, Crisson, & Van Dalfsen, 1987). Findings such as these have been interpreted in terms of operant learning, with spouse support and solicitousness reinforcing patients' displays of pain behavior. Alternate explanations, though, should also be considered. For instance, among adults living with pain, the expression of pain behaviors in day-to-day situations is likely to be under some degree of inhibitory control. However, when individuals in pain are in the presence of significant others with whom they are familiar and/or comfortable (e.g., spouses), especially supportive ones, inhibition might be released, which in turn might contribute to the expression of pain behaviors (Cano & Williams, 2010).

Potential Consequences of Pain Behavior

Although pain behaviors are assumed to have adaptive value by serving protective and communicative functions, research has accumulated indicating that the expression of pain behaviors may lead to a number of negative pain-related outcomes.

Impact of Pain Behavior on Physical Performance Studies have examined the association between pain behaviors and patients' performance during the execution of a variety of physical and functional tasks. In three studies, higher levels of communicative and protective pain behaviors were found to be associated with reduced performance on physical tasks such as forward flexion, rotation, and sit-to-stand (Koho et al., 2001; Lindstrom, Ohlund, & Nachemson, 1995; Watson et al., 1997). In another study, displays of protective pain behaviors such as guarding and rubbing have been found to be associated with decreased physical tolerance during the performance of a physically demanding lifting task (Thibault et al., 2008). Finally, in a study of gait biomechanics, Keefe and Hill (1985) found that higher levels of communicative and protective pain behaviors were associated with shorter steps and slower walking during a 15-m walk. On the basis of these studies, it was concluded that the expression of pain behaviors may directly interfere with patients' performance on a variety of physical and functional tasks.

Impact of Pain Behavior on Functional and Occupational Disability Studies have also found associations between pain behaviors and indices of pain-related disability. For example, a number of cross-sectional studies have found that higher levels of pain behaviors are associated with higher levels of self-reported functional disability (Prkachin, Schultz, & Hughes, 2007; Romano et al., 1988; Sullivan, Thibault, et al., 2006). In two studies, higher levels of pain behaviors were associated with higher levels of self-reported functional disability even after controlling for patients' self-reports of pain intensity (Koho et al., 2001; McCahon, Strong, Sharry, & Cramond, 2005). In the majority of these studies, different forms of pain behavior were assessed, and guarding emerged as the strongest predictor of patients' self-reports of functional disability.

A number of studies have also revealed significant prospective associations between pain behaviors and occupational disability outcomes (Crook, Moldofsky, & Shannon, 1998; Ohlund et al., 1994; Prkachin et al., 2007; Schultz et al., 2002). In one study, Schultz et al. (2002) examined the contribution of different forms of pain behavior, measured shortly following work injury, to the prediction of patients' return-to-work (RTW) status 3 months later. Pain behaviors were assessed in the context of a standardized physical examination procedure, and included behaviors such as grimacing, sighing, moaning, and guarding. Of these behaviors, guarding emerged as the only significant prospective predictor of patients' RTW status, with higher levels of guarding associated with a reduced likelihood of returning to work. Importantly, multivariate analyses indicated that guarding was a significant prospective predictor of patients' RTW status over and above the influence of a number of demographic, medical, workplace, and psychosocial variables. Using the same population of patients and the same categories of pain behavior, Prkachin et al. (2007) also found guarding to be a significant prospective predictor of patients' RTW status 3 months following work injury. In this study, guarding emerged as a significant predictor of other occupational disability outcomes, including days lost from work and compensation costs. Verbal pain behaviors (e.g., pain words) were also significantly associated with days lost from work and compensation costs, but not with patients' RTW status. As in Schultz et al.'s study (Schultz et al., 2002), other forms of pain behavior such as grimacing, sighing, or moaning were not related to any of the occupational disability outcomes. The differential impact of protective (i.e., guarding) and communicative (e.g., facial expressions) pain behaviors on disability outcomes supports the multidimensional nature of the pain behavior construct.

Impact of Pain Behaviors on Pain and Disability Judgments Given their overt nature, pain behaviors may exert an impact on how patients with pain are perceived by others in the social environment. In clinic settings, for example, it is well known that clinicians routinely make judgments about the severity of patients' pain conditions (Hadjistavropoulos et al., 2011; Tait & Chibnall, 1997). In making judgments about patients' pain, clinicians may rely on various sources of information, including patients' pain behaviors, self-reports of pain severity (i.e., intensity), and other pain-relevant contextual information (e.g., pain diagnosis). According to the Social Communication Model of Pain (Craig, 2009; Hadjistavropoulos & Craig, 2002; Prkachin & Craig, 1995), the experience of pain is communicated through various behavioral displays (i.e., pain behaviors) that are perceived and interpreted by observers as a function of contextual information. In line with this model, studies have been consistent in showing that pain behaviors account for significant variance in observers' inferences about others' pain (Hadjistavropoulos, Craig, Grunau, & Whitfield, 1997; Prkachin et al., 1983; Sullivan, Martel, et al., 2006a; Sullivan, Martel, Tripp, Savard, & Crombez, 2006b). Behaviors such as facial expressions and bodily movements accompanying pain are generally used by observers to make inferences of pain, with greater inferential weight being given to the face than to the body (Prkachin et al., 1983); (Sullivan, Martel, et al., 2006a). The weight given to pain behaviors in drawing inferences about others' pain, however, has been found to vary as a function of the amount of pain-relevant contextual information available to observers (Kappesser, Williams, & Prkachin, 2006; Martel et al., 2008; Poole & Craig, 1992).

In the treatment of patients with pain conditions, clinicians may also sometimes be called upon to make judgments about patients' levels of disability or readiness to work. These judgments may arise in the context of routine clinical practice, or in the context of disability determination practices (Main, Sullivan, & Walson, 2008; Pransky, Katz, Benjamin, & Himmelstein, 2002; Schultz, Joy, Crook, & Fraser, 2008). Considering that pain behaviors may convey salient information about patients' pain severity and pain-related limitations (Craig, 2009; Hadjistavropoulos & Craig, 2002; Sullivan, 2008), it is possible that patients presenting with high levels of pain behaviors might lead clinicians to infer high levels of pain and, in turn, consider prescribing an extended period of sick leave. The observation of heightened levels of pain behavior might also lead an employer to consider that the employee is unable to meet his or her occupational responsibilities. In a recent study, chronic pain patients who displayed high levels of protective pain behaviors (e.g., guarding) during a physically demanding task were perceived as being less ready to return to work than patients displaying other types of pain behaviors (Martel, Wideman, & Sullivan, 2012). Although speculative, there is reason to believe that specific types of pain behaviors might contribute to occupational disability indirectly by influencing clinicians' judgments about patients' readiness to work.

Impact of Pain Behaviors on Social Impressions Given the overt nature of pain behavior, the "information" conveyed by patients' pain behaviors might not be limited to patients' pain severity or pain-related limitations. For instance, one study found that patients displaying protective pain behaviors (e.g., guarding) were perceived as being significantly less "likable" and "dependable" than patients displaying communicative behaviors (Martel, Wideman, & Sullivan, 2012). Another study showed that individuals displaying pain behaviors were perceived as being less "warm" and "competent" than individuals displaying no pain behavior.[3] Taken together, these findings suggest that pain behaviors may not only convey information about patients' pain and limitations but also about patients' personality traits. Research will be needed to further examine the nature of social judgments that may be formed based on the observations of patients' pain behaviors, especially in the context of clinical practice. One might assume that negative personality trait inferences arising from the observation of patients' pain behaviors might affect pain management decisions as well as the quality of the therapeutic relationship between patients and clinicians (Hall, Epstein, DeCiantis, & McNeil, 1993; Hall, Roter, & Rand, 1981).

In the treatment of patients with pain conditions, clinicians are sometimes invited to participate in discussions concerning the authenticity or the genuineness of patients' symptoms of pain and disability. In patients with pain conditions, the incidence of faking is known to be low (Fishbain, Cutler, Rosomoff, & Rosomoff, 2004). However, when concerns that patients may be exaggerating or faking pain arise, clinicians may be called upon to render opinions or judgments about the genuineness of patients' symptoms of pain. To date, there are no objective measures that allow to determine whether a patient is exaggerating or faking pain. When clinicians are asked to make judgments about the genuineness of patients' pain, they are most often left with their own clinical intuitions, and their judgments tend to be based on ambiguous behavioral signs and symptoms, including patients' pain behaviors

(Craig & Badali, 2004; Main et al., 2008; Sullivan & Main, 2007). These judgments are most often based on clinicians' own intuitions or idiographic interpretations of patients' pain behaviors (Craig & Badali, 2004; Sullivan & Main, 2007), and there is abundant anecdotal evidence indicating that patients who present with high levels of pain behavior encounter the risk of being perceived as exaggerating or faking pain (Craig & Badali, 2004; Keefe & Dunsmore, 1992; Main et al., 2008). Such perceptions or judgments may lead to negative consequences for the patient, including undertreatment, frustration, and reduced quality of life (Craig & Badali, 2004; Main et al., 2008; Schiavenato & Craig, 2010).

Research efforts have been devoted to examining the influence of different forms of pain behavior when observers make judgments about the genuineness of others' pain. One line of research has shown that observers do rely on specific facial actions when making judgments about the genuineness of others' pain (Hadjistavropoulos, Craig, Hadjistavropoulos, & Poole, 1996; Hill & Craig, 2004; Poole & Craig, 1992; Prkachin, 1992), but research has also been conducted to examine the relative weight given to different forms of pain behavior (e.g., communicative vs protective) when observers make judgments about pain genuineness. If suspicion is raised about the genuineness of patients' pain, one study found that communicative pain behaviors (e.g., facial expressions) become the main behavioral cues from which observers make inferences about faking (Martel et al., 2011). Other studies have found that the pain of patients expressing pain behaviors in the absence of medical evidence to support their condition tends to be perceived as less intense and to be taken less seriously by observers (De Ruddere et al., 2014; De Ruddere, Goubert, Stevens, Williams, & Crombez, 2013). Collectively, these findings corroborate clinical anecdotes suggesting that patients who present with high pain behaviors might place themselves at greater risk of being accused of exaggerating or faking pain, particularly if there is no identifiable organic pathology that may account for their pain symptoms.

Pain Behavior and Pain Management

Given the potential deleterious consequences of pain behaviors, there is reason to believe that interventions designed to reduce patients' pain behaviors might contribute to improving pain-related outcomes. Interventions aimed at reducing the expression protective pain behaviors (e.g., guarding, limping) may be particularly important given that these behaviors appear to contribute to functional and occupational disability (Prkachin et al., 2007; Schultz et al., 2002). To date, the majority of pain management programs are still dominated by the view that pain behaviors are secondary to pain, and that effective pain relief will lead to a reduction in patients' pain behaviors. Research, however, suggests that patients' pain behaviors are likely to persist over time if treatment efforts are solely devoted toward the reduction of patients' pain intensity (Martel et al., 2010). Pain behaviors may thus continue to exert deleterious effects on pain-related outcomes unless they are targeted directly and extinguished using specific treatment interventions.

The idea of targeting pain behaviors as part of pain management programs is not new. In the 1970s and 1980s, William Fordyce and his colleagues applied the principles of operant learning theory to chronic pain (Fordyce, 1976, 1984). The focus of Fordyce's approach to treatment was not on reducing the experience of pain, but on reducing the overt display of pain behaviors. The targets selected for treatment were pain behaviors such as distress vocalizations, facial grimacing, limping, guarding, medication intake, activity withdrawal and activity avoidance. These first behavioral approaches to the management of pain and disability were conducted within inpatient settings that permitted systematic observation of pain behaviors, as well as control over environmental contingencies influencing pain behavior. Staff were trained to monitor pain behavior, and to selectively reinforce 'well behaviors' and selectively ignore "pain behaviors." The manipulation of reinforcement contingencies was found to exert a powerful influence on the frequency of pain behaviors (Fordyce, 1984). The manipulation of reinforcement contingencies was then applied to other domains of pain-related behavior and shown to be effective in reducing medication intake, reducing downtime and maximizing participation in goal-directed activity. In recent years, interventions have been specifically developed for chronic pain patients' spouses to educate them on the meaning of pain behaviors, and on the importance of selectively reinforcing patients' pain coping efforts (Keefe et al., 1996, 2004). Interventions have also been put forward to help spouses develop effective communication skills, especially when having to deal with their partners' pain-related distress and pain behaviors (Cano & Leonard, 2006; Cano & Williams, 2010).

Although early behaviorally oriented pain management programs did recognize the importance of using treatment interventions to reduce patients' pain behaviors (e.g., Fordyce, 1976, 1984), these pain management programs have not emphasized the distinction between different forms of pain behavior. As noted by Sullivan (2008), some patients may present with an overrepresentation of communicative pain behaviors, while other patients may present with an overrepresentation of protective pain behaviors. Considering that these two forms of pain behavior might have different functions and determinants, one would assume that they might respond differently to treatment interventions. Moreover, given that these two forms of pain behavior are likely to persist over time independently from each other (Martel et al., 2010; Prkachin, Hughes, et al., 2002), the complete elimination of patients' pain behaviors might require considering communicative and protective pain behaviors as two distinct treatment targets.

One of the challenges in the treatment of patients with pain is that patients may not be aware of their own patterns of pain behaviors. It has been proposed that the use of innovative tools such as video feedback interventions may help patients become more aware of their pain behavior displays (Keefe, Williams, & Smith, 2001; Sullivan, 2008). To our knowledge, however, research has yet to test the effectiveness of these interventions for reducing pain behaviors. Emerging evidence suggests that the degree of automaticity and cognitive control underlying different types of pain behaviors will need to be considered when developing new treatment interventions. To the extent that patients may exert different degrees of cognitive control over the expression of communicative and protective pain behaviors, these two types of pain behaviors might respond differently to treatment interventions. Clinical studies conducted among non-pain populations, for instance, have shown that automatic behaviors tend to be more resistant to treatment interventions than behaviors that are governed by cognitive control processes (Hunt, Matarazzo, Weiss, & Gentry, 1979; Verplanken & Faes, 1999). To the extent that communicative and protective pain behaviors involve different degrees of automaticity and cognitive control, these two forms of pain behavior might thus be differently resistant to treatment interventions. Further research examining the degree of automaticity and cognitive control underlying different forms of pain behavior might point to specific treatment interventions allowing the successful reduction of pain behaviors in patients with pain.

Conclusion

There is a long history in the pain literature of viewing pain behavior as a "unitary" construct. This has led to the widespread assumption that different types of pain behaviors are equivalent, and that pain behaviors are simply the product of nociceptive processes and/or pain perception. There is now a compelling body of evidence suggesting that the unitary view of pain behavior is flawed, and that a multidimensional conceptualization of pain behavior is needed in order to account for the different types of behavioral manifestations that may accompany pain. The multidimensional view of pain behavior is supported by evidence indicating that different types of pain behaviors are only modestly interrelated, and that different types of pain behaviors have different degrees of temporal stability. The multidimensional view is also supported by research suggesting that different types of pain behaviors likely serve different functions and have different determinants. Importantly, research indicates that different types of pain behaviors have a differential impact on functional and occupational disability outcomes, which provides further support the multidimensional nature of pain behavior. Finally, research indicates that different types of pain behaviors convey different information to observers with regard to patients' pain intensity, pain-related limitations, and personality traits, suggesting that different types of pain behaviors are certainly not equivalent to the eyes of observers. On the basis of research conducted to date, it appears clear that a multidimensional conceptualization of pain behavior will be required to further advance our knowledge on the functions, determinants and consequences of pain behaviors. A multidimensional conceptualization of pain behavior will also be required in order to pave the way for the development of new treatment interventions designed to minimize pain behaviors and their potentially negative impact on pain-related outcomes.

References

Anderson, K. O., Bradley, L. A., McDaniel, L. K., Young, L. D., Turner, R. A., Agudelo, C. A., … Semble, E. L. (1987). The assessment of pain in rheumatoid arthritis: Disease differentiation and temporal stability of a behavioral observation method. *The Journal of Rheumatology, 14*(4), 700–704.

Anderson, K. O., Bradley, L. A., Turner, R. A., Agudelo, C. A., & Pisko, E. J. (1994). Pain behavior of rheumatoid arthritis patients enrolled in experimental drug trials. *Arthritis Care and Research, 7*(2), 64–68.

Ashton-James, C. E., Richardson, D. C., de Williams, A. C. C., Bianchi-Berthouze, N., & Dekker, P. H. (2014). Impact of pain behaviors on evaluations of warmth and competence. *Pain, 155*(12), 2656–2661.

Block, A. R. (1981). Investigation of the response of the spouse to chronic pain behavior. *Psychosomatic Medicine, 43*(5), 415–422.

Buckelew, S. P., Parker, J. C., Keefe, F. J., Deuser, W. E., Crews, T. M., Conway, R., … Hewett, J. E. (1994). Self-efficacy and pain behavior among subjects with fibromyalgia. *Pain, 59*(3), 377–384.

Buescher, K. L., Johnston, J. A., Parker, J. C., Smarr, K. L., Buckelew, S. P., Anderson, S. K., & Walker, S. E. (1991). Relationship of self-efficacy to pain behavior. *The Journal of Rheumatology, 18*(7), 968–972.

Burns, J. W. (2000). Repression predicts outcome following multidisciplinary treatment of chronic pain. *Health Psychology, 19*(1), 75–84.

Burns, J. W., Quartana, P., & Bruehl, S. (2011). Anger suppression and subsequent pain behaviors among chronic low back pain patients: Moderating effects of anger regulation style. *Annals of Behavioral Medicine, 42*(1), 42–54. https://doi.org/10.1007/s12160-011-9270-4

Burns, J. W., Quartana, P., Gilliam, W., Gray, E., Matsuura, J., Nappi, C., … Lofland, K. (2008). Effects of anger suppression on pain severity and pain behaviors among chronic pain patients: Evaluation of an ironic process model. *Health Psychology, 27*(5), 645–652. https://doi.org/10.1037/a0013044

Cano, A., & Leonard, M. (2006). Integrative behavioral couple therapy for chronic pain: Promoting behavior change and emotional acceptance. *Journal of Clinical Psychology, 62*(11), 1409–1418. https://doi.org/10.1002/jclp.20320

Cano, A., & Williams, A. C. (2010). Social interaction in pain: Reinforcing pain behaviors or building intimacy? *Pain, 149*(1), 9–11. https://doi.org/10.1016/j.pain.2009.10.010

Cinciripini, P. M., & Floreen, A. (1983). An assessment of chronic pain behavior in a structured interview. *Journal of Psychosomatic Research, 27*(2), 117–123.

Corbeil, P., Blouin, J. S., & Teasdale, N. (2004). Effects of intensity and locus of painful stimulation on postural stability. *Pain, 108*(1–2), 43–50.

Craig, K. D. (2009). The social communication model of pain. *Canadian Psychology-Psychologie Canadienne, 50*(1), 22–32. https://doi.org/10.1037/a0014772

Craig, K. D., & Badali, M. A. (2004). Introduction to the special series on pain deception and malingering. *The Clinical Journal of Pain, 20*(6), 377–382.

Craig, K. D., Versloot, J., Goubert, L., Vervoort, T., & Crombez, G. (2010). Perceiving pain in others: Automatic and controlled mechanisms. *The Journal of Pain, 11*(2), 101–108. https://doi.org/10.1016/j.jpain.2009.08.008

Craig, K. D., Whitfield, M. F., Grunau, R. V., Linton, J., & Hadjistavropoulos, H. D. (1993). Pain in the preterm neonate: Behavioural and physiological indices. *Pain, 52*(3), 287–299.

Crook, J., Moldofsky, H., & Shannon, H. (1998). Determinants of disability after a work related musculetal injury. *The Journal of Rheumatology, 25*(8), 1570–1577.

Damasio, A. (1994). *Descartes' error: Emotion, reason and the human brain.* New York, NY: Macmillan.

De Ruddere, L., Goubert, L., Stevens, M., Williams, A. C. d. C., & Crombez, G. (2013). Discounting pain in the absence of medical evidence is explained by negative evaluation of the patient. *Pain, 154*(5), 669–676. https://doi.org/10.1016/j.pain.2012.12.018

De Ruddere, L., Goubert, L., Stevens, M. A., Deveugele, M., Craig, K. D., & Crombez, G. (2014). Health care professionals' reactions to patient pain: Impact of knowledge about medical evidence and psychosocial influences. *The Journal of Pain, 15*(3), 262–270. https://doi.org/10.1016/j.jpain.2013.11.002

Decchi, B., Zalaffi, A., Spidalieri, R., Arrigucci, U., Di Troia, A. M., & Rossi, A. (1997). Spinal reflex pattern to foot nociceptive stimulation in standing humans. *Electroencephalography and Clinical Neurophysiology, 105*(6), 484–489.

Descartes, R. (1662). *De Homine*. Leyden: Moyardus and Leffen.

Ekman, P., & Friesen, W. V. (1978). *The facial action coding system*. Palo Alto, CA: Consulting Psychologists Press.

Engel, G. L. (1959). Psychogenic pain and pain-prone patient. *The American Journal of Medicine, 26*(6), 899–918.

Fishbain, D. A., Cutler, R. B., Rosomoff, H. L., & Rosomoff, R. S. (2004). Is there a relationship between nonorganic physical findings (Waddell signs) and secondary gain/malingering? *The Clinical Journal of Pain, 20*(6), 399–408.

Follick, M. J., Ahern, D. K., & Aberger, E. W. (1985). Development of an audiovisual taxonomy of pain behavior: Reliability and discriminant validity. *Health Psychology, 4*(6), 555–568.

Fordyce, W. E. (1976). *Behavioral methods in chronic pain and illness*. St. Louis, MO: C.V. Mosby.

Fordyce, W. E. (1984). Behavioral science and chronic pain. *Postgraduate Medical Journal, 60*(710), 865–868.

Gauthier, N., Thibault, P., & Sullivan, M. J. (2011). Catastrophizers with chronic pain display more pain behaviour when in a relationship with a low catastrophizing spouse. *Pain Research & Management, 16*(5), 293–299.

Giardino, N. D., Jensen, M. P., Turner, J. A., Ehde, D. M., & Cardenas, D. D. (2003). Social environment moderates the association between catastrophizing and pain among persons with a spinal cord injury. *Pain, 106*(1–2), 19–25.

Gil, K. M., Keefe, F. J., Crisson, J. E., & Van Dalfsen, P. J. (1987). Social support and pain behavior. *Pain, 29*(2), 209–217.

Grunau, R. V., & Craig, K. D. (1987). Pain expression in neonates: Facial action and cry. *Pain, 28*(3), 395–410.

Hadjistavropoulos, H., Craig, K. D., Grunau, R. V. E., & Whitfield, M. F. (1997). Judging pain in infants: Behavioural, contextual, and developmental determinants. *Pain, 73*, 319–324.

Hadjistavropoulos, H. D., Craig, K. D., Hadjistavropoulos, T., & Poole, G. D. (1996). Subjective judgments of deception in pain expression: Accuracy and errors. *Pain, 65*(2–3), 251–258.

Hadjistavropoulos, H. D., & LaChapelle, D. L. (2000). Extent and nature of anxiety experienced during physical examination of chronic low back pain. *Behaviour Research and Therapy, 38*(1), 13–29. https://doi.org/10.1016/s0005-7967(99)00024-8

Hadjistavropoulos, T., & Craig, K. (2002). A theoretical framework for understanding self-report and observational measures of pain: A communication model. *Behaviour Research and Therapy, 40*, 551–570.

Hadjistavropoulos, T., Craig, K. D., Duck, S., Cano, A., Goubert, L., Jackson, P. L., … Fitzgerald, T. D. (2011). A biopsychosocial formulation of pain communication. *Psychological Bulletin, 137*(6), 910–939. https://doi.org/10.1037/a0023876

Hall, J. A., Epstein, A. M., DeCiantis, M. L., & McNeil, B. J. (1993). Physicians' liking for their patients: More evidence for the role of affect in medical care. *Health Psychology, 12*(2), 140–146.

Hall, J. A., Roter, D. L., & Rand, C. S. (1981). Communication of affect between patient and physician. *Journal of Health and Social Behavior, 22*(1), 18–30.

Hill, M. L., & Craig, K. D. (2004). Detecting deception in facial expressions of pain: Accuracy and training. *The Clinical Journal of Pain, 20*(6), 415–422.

Hunt, W. A., Matarazzo, J. D., Weiss, S. M., & Gentry, W. D. (1979). Associative learning, habit, and health behavior. *Journal of Behavioral Medicine, 2*, 111–124.

Kappesser, J., Williams, A. C., & Prkachin, K. M. (2006). Testing two accounts of pain underestimation. *Pain, 124*(1–2), 109–116. https://doi.org/10.1016/j.pain.2006.04.003

Keefe, F., & Block, A. (1982). Development of an observational method for assessing pain behavior in chronic pain patients. *Behavior Therapy, 13*, 363–375.

Keefe, F., Wilkins, R., Cook, W., Crisson, J., & Muhkbaier, L. (1986). Depression, pain and pain behavior. *Journal of Consulting and Clinical Psychology, 54*, 665–669.

Keefe, F. J., Blumenthal, J., Baucom, D., Affleck, G., Waugh, R., Caldwell, D. S., … Lefebvre, J. (2004). Effects of spouse-assisted coping skills training and exercise training in patients with osteoarthritic knee pain: A randomized controlled study. *Pain, 110*(3), 539–549. https://doi.org/10.1016/j.pain.2004.03.022

Keefe, F. J., Caldwell, D. S., Baucom, D., Salley, A., Robinson, E., Timmons, K., … Helms, M. (1996). Spouse-assisted coping skills training in the management of osteoarthritic knee pain. *Arthritis Care and Research, 9*(4), 279–291.

Keefe, F. J., Caldwell, D. S., Martinez, S., Nunley, J., Beckham, J., & Williams, D. A. (1991). Analyzing pain in rheumatoid arthritis patients. Pain coping strategies in patients who have had knee replacement surgery. *Pain, 46*(2), 153–160.

Keefe, F. J., Caldwell, D. S., Queen, K., Gil, K. M., Martinez, S., Crisson, J. E., … Nunley, J. (1987). Osteoarthritic knee pain: A behavioral analysis. *Pain, 28*(3), 309–321.

Keefe, F. J., & Dunsmore, J. (1992). Pain behavior: Concepts and controversies. *American Pain Society Journal, 1*, 92–100.

Keefe, F. J., & Hill, R. W. (1985). An objective approach to quantifying pain behavior and gait patterns in low back pain patients. *Pain, 21*(2), 153–161.

Keefe, F. J., Lefebvre, J. C., Egert, J. R., Affleck, G., Sullivan, M. J., & Caldwell, D. S. (2000). The relationship of gender to pain, pain behavior, and disability in osteoarthritis patients: The role of catastrophizing. *Pain, 87*(3), 325–334.

Keefe, F. J., Williams, D. A., & Smith, S. (2001). Assessment of pain behaviors. In D. C. Turk & R. Melzack (Eds.), *Handbook of pain assessment* (pp. 170–187). New York, NY: Guilford Press.

Kerns, R. D., Haythornthwaite, J., Rosenberg, R., Southwick, S., Giller, E. L., & Jacob, M. C. (1991). The Pain Behavior Check List (PBCL): Factor structure and psychometric properties. *Journal of Behavioral Medicine, 14*(2), 155–167.

Kerns, R. D., Southwick, S., Giller, E. L., Haythornthwaite, J. A., Jacob, M. C., & Rosenberg, R. (1991). The relationship between reports of pain-related social interactions and expressions of pain and affective distress. *Behavior Therapy, 22*, 101–111.

Kleinke, C. (1991). How chronic pain patients cope with depression: Relation to treatment outcome in a multidisciplinary clinic. *Rehabilitation Psychology, 36*, 207–218.

Koho, P., Aho, S., Watson, P., & Hurri, H. (2001). Assessment of chronic pain behaviour: Reliability of the method and its relationship with perceived disability, physical impairment and function. *Journal of Rehabilitation Medicine, 33*(3), 128–132.

Kori, S., Miller, R., & Todd, D. (1990). Kinesophobia: A new view of chronic pain behavior. *Pain Management Nursing, 3*, 35–43.

Krause, S. J., Wiener, R. L., & Tait, R. C. (1994). Depression and pain behavior in patients with chronic pain. *The Clinical Journal of Pain, 10*(2), 122–127.

Kunz, M., Chatelle, C., Lautenbacher, S., & Rainville, P. (2008). The relation between catastrophizing and facial responsiveness to pain. *Pain, 140*(1), 127–134. https://doi.org/10.1016/j.pain.2008.07.019

Kunz, M., Gruber, A., & Lautenbacher, S. (2006). Sex differences in facial encoding of pain. *The Journal of Pain, 7*(12), 915–928. https://doi.org/10.1016/j.jpain.2006.04.012

Labus, J. S., Keefe, F. J., & Jensen, M. P. (2003). Self-reports of pain intensity and direct observations of pain behavior: When are they correlated? *Pain, 102*(1–2), 109–124.

Lindstrom, I., Ohlund, C., & Nachemson, A. (1995). Physical performance, pain, pain behavior and subjective disability in patients with subacute low back pain. *Scandinavian Journal of Rehabilitation Medicine, 27*(3), 153–160.

Loeser, J. D., & Melzack, R. (1999). Pain: An overview. *Lancet, 353*(9164), 1607–1609. https://doi.org/10.1016/s0140-6736(99)01311-2

Lund, J. P., Donga, R., Widmer, C. G., & Stohler, C. S. (1991). The pain-adaptation model: A discussion of the relationship between chronic musculoskeletal pain and motor activity. *Canadian Journal of Physiology and Pharmacology, 69*, 683–694.

Main, C., Sullivan, M., & Walson, P. J. (2008). *Pain management: Practical applications of the biopsychosocial perspective in clinical and occupational settings.* Edinburgh, England: Churchill Livingstone.

Main, C., & Walson, P. J. (1996). Guarded movements: Development of chronicity. *Journal of Musculoskeletal Pain, 4*, 163–170.

Martel, M. O., Thibault, P., Roy, C., Catchlove, R., & Sullivan, M. J. (2008). Contextual determinants of pain judgments. *Pain, 139*(3), 562–568. https://doi.org/10.1016/j.pain.2008.06.010

Martel, M. O., Thibault, P., & Sullivan, M. J. (2010). The persistence of pain behaviors in patients with chronic back pain is independent of pain and psychological factors. *Pain, 151*(2), 330–336. https://doi.org/10.1016/j.pain.2010.07.004

Martel, M. O., Thibault, P., & Sullivan, M. J. (2011). Judgments about pain intensity and pain genuineness: The role of pain behavior and judgmental heuristics. *The Journal of Pain, 12*(4), 468–475. https://doi.org/10.1016/j.jpain.2010.10.010

Martel, M. O., Trost, Z., & Sullivan, M. J. (2012). The expression of pain behaviors in high catastrophizers: The influence of automatic and controlled processes. *The Journal of Pain, 13*(8), 808–815. https://doi.org/10.1016/j.jpain.2012.05.015

Martel, M. O., Wideman, T. H., & Sullivan, M. J. (2012). Patients who display protective pain behaviors are viewed as less likable, less dependable, and less likely to return to work. *Pain, 153*(4), 843–849. https://doi.org/10.1016/j.pain.2012.01.007

McCahon, S., Strong, J., Sharry, R., & Cramond, T. (2005). Self-report and pain behavior among patients with chronic pain. *The Clinical Journal of Pain, 21*(3), 223–231.

McDaniel, L. K., Anderson, K. O., Bradley, L. A., Young, L. D., Turner, R. A., Agudelo, C. A., & Keefe, F. J. (1986). Development of an observation method for assessing pain behavior in rheumatoid arthritis patients. *Pain, 24*(2), 165–184.

Melzack, R., & Wall, P. D. (1965). Pain mechanisms: A new theory. *Science, 150*(3699), 971–979.

Moseley, G. L., Nicholas, M. K., & Hodges, P. W. (2004). Pain differs from non-painful attention-demanding or stressful tasks in its effect on postural control patterns of trunk muscles. *Experimental Brain Research, 156*(1), 64–71.

Ohlund, C., Lindstrom, I., Areskoug, B., Eek, C., Peterson, L. E., & Nachemson, A. (1994). Pain behavior in industrial subacute low back pain. Part I. Reliability: Concurrent and predictive validity of pain behavior assessments. *Pain, 58*(2), 201–209.

Parker, J. C., Callahan, C. D., Smarr, K. L., McClure, K. W., Stucky-Ropp, R. C., Anderson, S. K., & Walker, S. E. (1993). Relationship of pain behavior to disease activity and health status in rheumatoid arthritis. *Arthritis Care and Research, 6*(2), 71–77.

Pilowsky, I., & Spence, N. D. (1976). Pain, anger and illness behaviour. *Journal of Psychosomatic Research, 20*(5), 411–416.

Poole, G. D., & Craig, K. D. (1992). Judgments of genuine, suppressed, and faked facial expressions of pain. *Journal of Personality and Social Psychology, 63*(5), 797–805.

Pransky, G., Katz, J. N., Benjamin, K., & Himmelstein, J. (2002). Improving the physician role in evaluating work ability and managing disability: A survey of primary care practitioners. *Disability and Rehabilitation, 24*(16), 867–874. https://doi.org/10.1080/09638280210142176

Prkachin, K. M. (1992). Dissociating spontaneous and deliberate expressions of pain: Signal detection analyses. *Pain, 51*(1), 57–65.

Prkachin, K. M., & Craig, K. (1995). Expressing pain: The communication and interpretation of pain signals. *Journal of Nonverbal Behavior, 19*, 191–205.

Prkachin, K. M., Currie, N. A., & Craig, K. D. (1983). Judging nonverbal expressions of pain. *Canadian Journal of Behavioral Science-Revue Canadienne Des Sciences Du Comportement, 15*(4), 409–421. https://doi.org/10.1037/h0080757

Prkachin, K. M., Hughes, E., Schultz, I., Joy, P., & Hunt, D. (2002). Real-time assessment of pain behavior during clinical assessment of low back pain patients. *Pain, 95*(1–2), 23–30.

Prkachin, K. M., Schultz, I., Berkowitz, J., Hughes, E., & Hunt, D. (2002). Assessing pain behaviour of low-back pain patients in real time: Concurrent validity and examiner sensitivity. *Behaviour Research and Therapy, 40*(5), 595–607.

Prkachin, K. M., Schultz, I. Z., & Hughes, E. (2007). Pain behavior and the development of pain-related disability: The importance of guarding. *The Clinical Journal of Pain, 23*(3), 270–277. https://doi.org/10.1097/AJP.0b013e3180308d28

Rachlin, H. (2010). Pain and behavior. *Behavioral and Brain Sciences, 8*(1), 43–53. https://doi.org/10.1017/S0140525X00019488

Richards, J. S., Nepomuceno, C., Riles, M., & Suer, Z. (1982). Assessing pain behavior: The UAB pain behavior scale. *Pain, 14*(4), 393–398.

Romano, J. M., Jensen, M. P., Turner, J. A., Good, A. B., & Hops, H. (2000). Chronic pain patient-partner interactions: Further support for a behavioral model of chronic pain. *Behavior Therapy, 31*, 415–440.

Romano, J. M., Syrjala, K. L., Levy, R. L., Turner, J. A., Evans, P., & Keefe, F. J. (1988). Overt pain behaviors: Relationship to patient functioning and treatment outcome. *Behavior Therapy, 19*(2), 191–201. https://doi.org/10.1016/s0005-7894(88)80042-x

Romano, J. M., Turner, J. A., Friedman, L. S., Bulcroft, R. A., Jensen, M. P., Hops, H., & Wright, S. F. (1992). Sequential analysis of chronic pain behaviors and spouse responses. *Journal of Consulting and Clinical Psychology, 60*(5), 777–782.

Romano, J. M., Turner, J. A., Jensen, M. P., Friedman, L. S., Bulcroft, R. A., Hops, H., & Wright, S. F. (1995). Chronic pain patient-spouse behavioral interactions predict patient disability. *Pain, 63*(3), 353–360.

Schiavenato, M., & Craig, K. D. (2010). Pain assessment as a social transaction: Beyond the "gold standard". *The Clinical Journal of Pain, 26*(8), 667–676. https://doi.org/10.1097/AJP.0b013e3181e72507

Schultz, I. Z., Crook, J. M., Berkowitz, J., Meloche, G. R., Milner, R., Zuberbier, O. A., & Meloche, W. (2002). Biopsychosocial multivariate predictive model of occupational low back disability. *Spine (Phila Pa 1976), 27*(23), 2720–2725. https://doi.org/10.1097/01.brs.0000035323.16390.b5

Schultz, I. Z., Joy, P. W., Crook, J., & Fraser, K. (2008). Models of diagnosis and rehabilitation in musculoskeletal pain-related occupational disability. In I. Z. Schultz & R. J. Gatchel (Eds.), *Handbook of complex occupational disability claims: Early risk identification, intervention, and prevention*. New York, NY: Springer.

Sullivan, M. J. (2008). Toward a biopsychomotor conceptualization of pain: Implications for research and intervention. *The Clinical Journal of Pain, 24*(4), 281–290. https://doi.org/10.1097/AJP.0b013e318164bb15

Sullivan, M. J., Adams, H., & Sullivan, M. E. (2004). Communicative dimensions of pain catastrophizing: Social cueing effects on pain behaviour and coping. *Pain, 107*(3), 220–226.

Sullivan, M. J., Davidson, N., Garfinkel, B., Siriapaipant, N., & Scott, W. (2009). Perceived injustice is associated with heightened pain behavior and disability in individuals with whiplash injuries. *Psychological Injury and Law, 2*, 238–247.

Sullivan, M. J., & Main, C. (2007). Service, advocacy and adjudication: Balancing the ethical challenges of multiple stakeholder agendas in the rehabilitation of chronic pain. *Disability and Rehabilitation, 29*(20–21), 1596–1603. https://doi.org/10.1080/09638280701618802

Sullivan, M. J., Martel, M. O., Tripp, D., Savard, A., & Crombez, G. (2006a). The relation between catastrophizing and the communication of pain experience. *Pain, 122*(3), 282–288. https://doi.org/10.1016/j.pain.2006.02.001

Sullivan, M. J., Martel, M. O., Tripp, D. A., Savard, A., & Crombez, G. (2006b). Catastrophic thinking and heightened perception of pain in others. *Pain, 123*(1–2), 37–44. https://doi.org/10.1016/j.pain.2006.02.007

Sullivan, M. J., & Neish, N. (2000). Catastrophic thinking and the experience of pain during dental procedures. *The Journal of the Indiana Dental Association, 79*(4), 16–19.

Sullivan, M. J., Thibault, P., Savard, A., Catchlove, R., Kozey, J., & Stanish, W. D. (2006). The influence of communication goals and physical demands on different dimensions of pain behavior. *Pain, 125*(3), 270–277. https://doi.org/10.1016/j.pain.2006.06.019

Sullivan, M. J., Thorn, B., Haythornthwaite, J. A., Keefe, F., Martin, M., Bradley, L. A., & Lefebvre, J. C. (2001). Theoretical perspectives on the relation between catastrophizing and pain. *The Clinical Journal of Pain, 17*(1), 52–64.

Sullivan, M. J., Tripp, D., & Santor, D. (2000). Gender differences in pain and pain behavior: The role of catastrophizing. *Cognitive Therapy and Research, 24*, 121–134.

Tait, R. C., & Chibnall, J. T. (1997). Physician judgments of chronic pain patients. *Social Science & Medicine, 45*(8), 1199–1205.

Tang, N. K., Salkovskis, P. M., Poplavskaya, E., Wright, K. J., Hanna, M., & Hester, J. (2007). Increased use of safety-seeking behaviors in chronic back pain patients with high health anxiety. *Behaviour Research and Therapy, 45*(12), 2821–2835. https://doi.org/10.1016/j.brat.2007.05.004

Thibault, P., Loisel, P., Durand, M. J., Catchlove, R., & Sullivan, M. J. (2008). Psychological predictors of pain expression and activity intolerance in chronic pain patients. *Pain, 139*(1), 47–54. https://doi.org/10.1016/j.pain.2008.02.029

Verplanken, B., & Faes, S. (1999). Good intentions, bad habits, and effects of forming implementation intentions on healthy eating. *European Journal of Social Psychology, 29*, 591–604.

Vlaeyen, J. W., & Linton, S. J. (2000). Fear-avoidance and its consequences in chronic musculoskeletal pain: A state of the art. *Pain, 85*(3), 317–332.

Waddell, G. (1998). *The back pain revolution*. London, England: Churchill Livingstone.

Waddell, G., Newton, M., Henderson, I., Somerville, D., & Main, C. J. (1993). A fear-avoidance beliefs questionnaire (FABQ) and the role of fear-avoidance beliefs in chronic low back pain and disability. *Pain, 52*(2), 157–168.

Wall, P. (1999). *Pain: The science of suffering*. London, England: Weidenfeld & Nicolson.

Watson, P. J., Booker, C. K., Main, C. J., & Chen, A. C. (1997). Surface electromyography in the identification of chronic low back pain patients: The development of the flexion relaxation ratio. *Clinical Biomechanics (Bristol, Avon), 12*(3), 165–171.

Williams, A. (2002). Facial expression of pain: An evolutionary account. *Behavioral and Brain Sciences, 25*, 439–488.

Chapter 6
When, How, and Why Do We Express Pain?

Miriam Kunz, Kai Karos, and Tine Vervoort

Abstract The experience of pain is typically accompanied by various verbal and nonverbal behavioral expressions that help to inform our social environment about our pain. These expressions range from verbal reports (e.g., "I feel pain in my shoulder that is quite strong") to nonverbal expressions, like moaning and facial grimacing. Depending on the situational context, however, as well as on previous learning experiences, personality traits and our affective state, the way we express pain can vary substantially. In the present chapter we give an in-depth overview of the complex psychosocial factors that affect when, how and why we express pain.

Keywords Social context · Facial expression of pain · Pain vocalization · Social display rules · Threat

The experience of pain is typically accompanied by a certain set of verbal and nonverbal behavioral expressions. These expressions range from verbal reports (e.g., "I feel pain in my shoulder that is quite strong") to nonverbal expressions, like moaning and facial grimacing. While some pain behaviors (e.g., body posture) may serve a protective function (i.e., by limiting pain or further harm), other forms of verbal and nonverbal pain expressions (e.g., facial expression) mainly serve the purpose of informing our social environment about our inner state, namely the experience of pain. Why we want to inform our social environment about our pain

M. Kunz (✉)
Department of General Practice and Elderly Care Medicine, University of Groningen,
University Medical Center Groningen, Groningen, The Netherlands
e-mail: m.kunz@umcg.nl

K. Karos
Research Group on Health Psychology, KU Leuven, Leuven, Belgium

T. Vervoort
Department of Experimental-Clinical and Health Psychology, Ghent University,
Ghent, Belgium

© Springer International Publishing AG, part of Springer Nature 2018
T. Vervoort et al. (eds.), *Social and Interpersonal Dynamics in Pain*,
https://doi.org/10.1007/978-3-319-78340-6_6

and the way we inform them can certainly vary. An illustrative example of *how* and *why* we might express pain can be found at football (or soccer) matches. When football players are hit by an opposing player, one can often observe them falling to the ground, dramatically clutching the affected body part, rolling about, powerfully grimacing and groaning. Despite these dramatic displays of gruesome pain, the players often recover miraculously within a few seconds and continue playing as if nothing had happened. Reasons for the dramatic pain displays might include—besides experiencing strong pain—that football players hope to draw attention to a potential wrong-doing of the opposing player and as a result draw a game-changing free-kick or penalty.

This chapter discusses the different forms of verbal and nonverbal pain expressions and how these different forms are interrelated, underlying motives for why we express pain, and factors which influence the way we express pain to our environment. The main focus is on nonverbal forms of pain expressions which have been shown to be most powerful in signifying pain to others (Hadjistavropoulos et al., 2011).

How Do We Express Pain?

Pain is considered "an unpleasant sensory and emotional experience associated with actual or potential tissue damage, or described in terms of such damage" (IASP, 1979). Thus, pain is by definition a subjective experience and only becomes accessible by being expressed. But how do we express pain? Pain is expressed via different nonverbal and verbal channels that include facial expressions, body movements, as well as (paralinguistic) vocalizations that can be nonverbal (e.g., moaning) or verbal ("I am in pain"). Indeed, only the expression of pain in its verbal and nonverbal forms makes pain accessible to the social environment or, in other words, to the "audience" of that expression. In clinical settings, the verbal report is the most often used form of pain assessment. In contrast, nonverbal forms of pain expressions often do not play an important role in clinical pain assessment; although nonverbal expressions surely have a great impact on psychosocial interactions and on clinical decision-making.

Verbal Expressions

Clinical pain assessment typically relies on subjective estimates of pain, using numerical or verbal scales (Jensen & Karoly, 2001). For example, when using a numerical scale, individuals might be asked to estimate their pain by providing a rating on a scale from 0 to 10, where 0 equals "no pain" and 10 is the "worst pain you can imagine." When using such a scale to express one's pain, one has to quantify as well as average one's pain experience over time (e.g., the last hours or previous week) and over situations (e.g., walking, sitting down, picking something up or doing the household). These numerical rating scales are easy to administer and are often used for clinical pain assessment, especially for the assessment of acute pain intensity (e.g., post-surgery). In case of more complex chronic pain conditions, the McGill Pain Questionnaire (Melzack, 1975; Melzack & Katz, 2001) is frequently used. Here, patients can describe not only the intensity but also the quality of their pain experience, by choosing from a list of adjectives those that best describe their pain (e.g., throbbing, pinching, burning). Given that the expression of pain via verbal report is not only easily accessible, but also allows the person in pain to differentially describe their experience, its potential causes and options for dealing with the pain, it is not surprising that self-report is viewed as the gold standard for pain assessment. However, despite all its advantages, self-report of pain also has several disadvantages. For one, it is dependent on cognitive, especially language capability and thus not available to individuals with language deficits, like patients with dementia (Kunz, Scharmann, Hemmeter, Schepelmann, & Lautenbacher, 2007), patients with aphasia, infants and toddlers (see Chap. 17) as well as individuals with intellectual disabilities (Defrin et al., 2015). Moreover, the verbal report is less reflexive/automatic compared to nonverbal pain expressions (e.g., facial expression) and therefore, might be more prone to self-report biases (Schiavenato & Craig, 2010) (see also Chap. 5). Accordingly, nonverbal forms of pain expression are not only of relevance when self-report is not available but also in situations when the credibility of the self-report might be questionable or when more reflex-like responses are of interest (Craig, Versloot, Goubert, Vervoort, & Crombez, 2010).

Nonverbal Expressions

Nonverbal expressions of pain are usually divided into three groups, namely body postures/movements, paralinguistic vocalizations and facial expressions (Craig et al., 2010). This division into three distinct groups of nonverbal expressions is also apparent in observational pain assessment scales used to assess pain in nonverbal individuals (e.g., patients with dementia), like PAINAD (Warden, Hurley, & Volicer, 2003), PACSLAC (Chan, Hadjistavropoulos, Williams, & Lints-Martindale, 2014), or PAIC (Corbett et al., 2014). Among the three groups, the facial expression of pain has been studied most extensively. This mirrors research activities in the field of emotion expressions, with extensive research having been conducted in the field of facial expressions of emotions, whereas body postures and vocalizations during emotions have just recently become of research interest (Kunz, 2015).

Expressing Pain via Body Movements

Although it is unquestionable that the experience of pain is typically accompanied by body movements (Walsh, Eccleston, & Keogh, 2014), little research has thus far been conducted to classify or describe body movements accompanying pain.

Reasons for the lack of research might stem from the complexity and great interindividual variability of bodily movements accompanying pain as well as from the lack of instruments to objectively assess them. Within the group of nonverbal behavioral responses to pain, body movements are believed to primarily serve a pain management or pain protection function (Prkachin, 1986; Williams, 2002). For example, rubbing and holding the affected body part or cautious, rigid approaches to movement mainly serve the purpose of protecting the self from further noxious input and to promote pain relief as well as healing. In contrast, the other two forms of nonverbal pain expression (facial expression and vocalization) are believed to primarily serve a communicative function (Prkachin, 1986). Given that bodily movements accompanying pain may not primarily serve a communicative function, the variability and complexity of body movements seems less surprising. In other words; because body movements associated with pain may not mainly serve a communicative purpose, they may not need to be as distinct or as definable as facial expressions of pain or pain vocalizations. In line with this, Walsh et al. (2014) found that pain is not expressed via one single prototypical movement but rather via a combination of different movements that when paired with contextual cues can become a distinctive indicator for pain. This lack of a single pain-prototypical body movement is not surprising considering that the origin of pain, the quality of pain and the body areas/body parts being affected can vary immensely and therefore, body movements aiming at reducing or controlling the pain should also vary greatly. Nevertheless, although body movements are assumed to primarily serve protective functions, they can also be communicative, since they can be picked up as pain-indicative behaviors by others thus, serving the potential to also communicate (voluntarily or involuntarily) to others that one is in pain (Walsh et al., 2014).

Given the diversity of pain-indicative body movements, several authors have used an approach, where they do not try to define an overall pain-typical set of body movements, but instead tried to characterize body movements that are indicative for one specific type of pain (e.g., lung cancer pain (Wilkie, Keefe, Dodd, & Copp, 1992), back pain (Keefe & Block, 1982), and rheumatoid arthritis (McDaniel et al., 1986)). However, despite the enormous diversity among pain-indicative body movements, there seem to be some body movements that have repeatedly been observed across different types of pain and that might be pain-indicative for various types of pain. These body movements are guarding (abnormally slow, stiff, interrupted or rigid movement), bracing (a stiff, static position), and rubbing the painful area (Walsh et al., 2014).

Expressing Pain via Vocalization

So far, very little is known about paralinguistic vocalization changes occurring during pain. Although it is acknowledged that pain experiences are accompanied by nonverbal vocalizations and although vocalization items—such as crying, shouting, groaning—are included in nearly all observational scales for pain assessment in patients with dementia (Herr, Bjoro, & Decker, 2006; Zwakhalen, Hamers,

Abu-Saad, & Berger, 2006), studies that have tried to investigate these pain-indicative vocalizations using specialized tools are lacking. Around three decades ago
several attempts were made to analyze and characterize pain vocalization in infants,
with a special focus on pain cries (see overview by Craig, Gilbert-MacLeod, &
Lilley, 2000). It was reported that pain cries could be differentiated from cries due
to anger or fear because pain cries were longer, the intensity was greater and there
was a higher percentage of dysphonation (blurring of harmonies) (Johnston &
O'Shaugnessy, 1987). However, it has been questioned whether pain cries indeed
have discrete features that help to differentiate them from cries due to other types of
negative affective states. It seems that pain cries in infants are not really qualitatively
different from other types of cries but just differ quantitatively, due to a higher level
of arousal due to pain. Thus, it remains unclear whether the observed features of
pain cries in infants are indicative of a distinct type of affective state (namely pain)
or only of different degrees of a negative affective arousal (Craig et al., 2000).

These findings on pain vocalizations in infants are difficult to transfer to adults
or even to children, given the anatomical maturing of the vocal chords, vocal tract,
throat, mouth, lips and tongue. Studies on pain vocalizations in adults are mostly
missing so far. In one recent pilot study, Lautenbacher, Salinas-Ranneberg, Niebuhr,
and Kunz (2017) have investigated objective acoustic-phonetic characteristics like
loudness (i.e., acoustic-energy level) and pitch (i.e., F0, Hz) and whether they
qualify to detect and grade different pain intensities. More precisely, they studied
the production of different vowels while participants immersed their hand in hot
water that elicited non-painful as well as painful sensations. The authors found that
those vowels that were best approximations to moaning and groaning (vowels "u"
and the central vowel "schwa") showed a significant increase in pitch and loudness
during pain. Moreover, changes in these vocal parameters also significantly
predicted concurrent changes in subjective pain ratings. These are promising results;
however, more studies are needed that study a broader set of voice parameters, like
further acoustic parameters of source (i.e., voice-quality exponents like spectral
emphasis/tilt) and filter (i.e., formant) characteristics during pain, in order to provide
a more precise characterization of vocalizations due to pain. Likewise, further
research is needed to examine the specific communicative value of discrete pain
vocalizations and whether these are truly discriminatively indicative of pain or just
indicative of a stronger intensity of a negative affective state; as has been suggested
for pain vocalizations in infants.

Expressing Pain via Facial Responses

As stated above, facial expressions of pain have been studied most extensively.
Especially in the last two decades a considerable number of studies have been
conducted that tried to capture the prototypical facial expression of pain and examine
which biopsychosocial factors affect the extent and specific ways in which we
facially express pain. Reasons why research on pain behavior has predominantly
focused on facial expressions of pain include that facial expressions are readily

accessible, highly plastic and are believed to be the most specific pain behavior in humans (Williams, 2002). Research endeavors on facial expression of pain also mirror research activities in the field of emotion expression which have largely focused on facial displays.

When investigating facial responses to pain, nearly all studies have employed the Facial Action Coding System (FACS; Ekman & Friesen, 1978), which is based on anatomical analysis of visible facial movements. These facial movements are categorized as so-called Action Units (AUs). The FACS lists 44 different AUs; each AU being based on discrete movements of specific muscles or, in a few cases, on groups of muscles of the face. FACS analyses of facial expressions are not carried out in real-time but instead the videotaped facial expressions are coded in slow-motion and stop-frame feedback. FACS-coders, who undergo approximately 100–200 h of training (Ekman & Friesen, 1978), identify which AUs are displayed, their onset and offset and their intensity during specified time intervals. Not only is FACS training rather long but FACS coding itself is also very time-consuming, thus making FACS analyses difficult to use in clinical settings. For research purposes, however, the FACS has enabled us to better describe and understand specific facial responses occurring during the anticipation or experience of pain.

Using the FACS, it has been shown that facial activity during pain is not unspecific grimacing but conveys pain-specific information (Hadjistavropoulos et al., 2011; Williams, 2002). Evidence for this can be mainly taken from two sources. First, despite some variability, there seems to be a subset of facial movements that repeatedly occur across different types of pain (ranging from different types of experimental pain induction procedures to clinical pain (Prkachin, 1992; Prkachin & Solomon, 2008)) as well as across individuals (male/female (Kunz, Gruber, & Lautenbacher, 2006); young/old (Kunz, Mylius, Schepelmann, & Lautenbacher, 2008)). This subset of facial movements indicative of pain includes the following facial movements: tightening of the muscles surrounding the eyes (AU6_7), furrowed brows (AU4), raising the upper lip/nose wrinkling (AU9_10), opening of the mouth (AU25_26_27) and eye closure (AU43) (Kunz & Lautenbacher, 2014; Prkachin, 1992; Prkachin & Solomon, 2008). Images of these facial movements are displayed in Fig. 6.1. The combination of these facial movements is often referred to as the "prototypical facial expression of pain." Second, when actors are taught to display this subset of "pain-prototypical" facial movements, observers can recognize pain among other emotions above chance level (Simon, Craig, Gosselin, Belin, & Rainville, 2008).

However, it is important to keep in mind that despite the evidence that these key facial movements reliably occur during pain, this by no means implies that a fixed uniform facial expression of pain can be observed across diverse situations within and between individuals (Craig, Prkachin, & Grunau, 2011). Instead, the frequencies of occurrence of these key movements during pain usually range from 10 to 60% (Kunz, Chen, Lautenbacher, Vachon-Presseau, & Rainville, 2011; Kunz & Lautenbacher, 2014; Kunz, Rainville, & Lautenbacher, 2011). Therefore, the likelihood that all four key facial movements occur simultaneously or in other words the likelihood that an individual experiencing pain displays the complete "prototypical

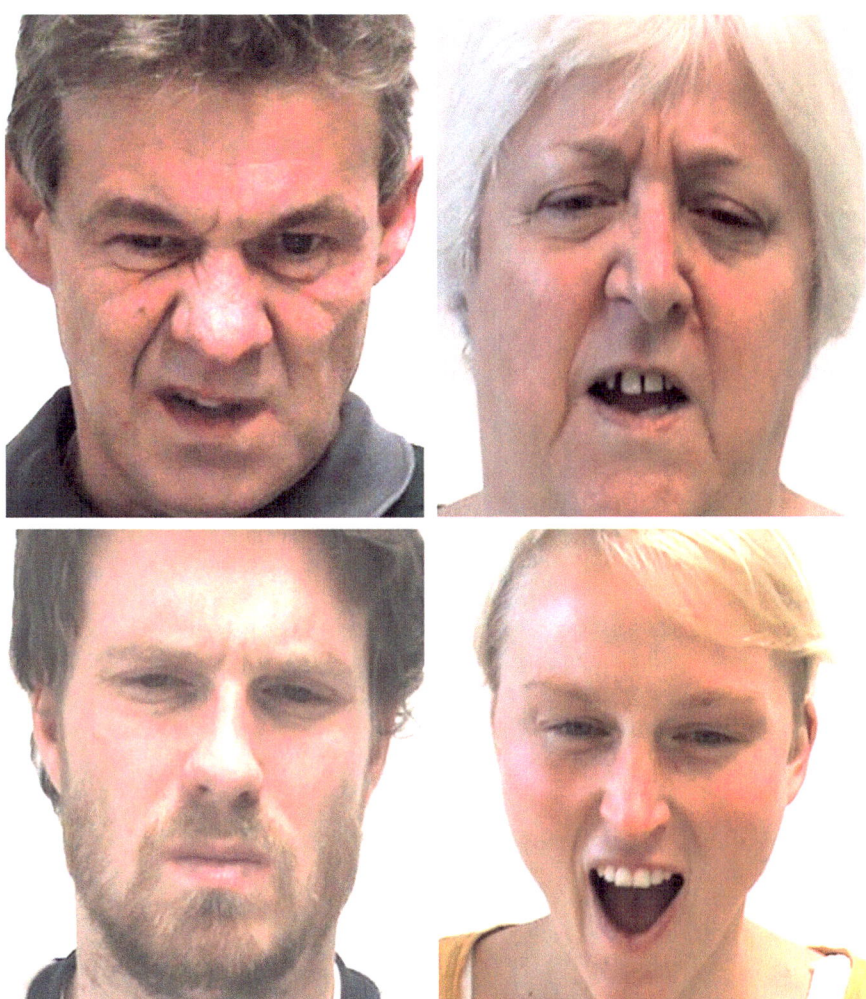

Fig. 6.1 Examples of facial expressions of pain

expression of pain" is very low. Rather, individuals often display only parts of this subset, sometimes even blending it with a limited range of other facial movements (e.g., smiling (Hale & Hadjistavropoulos, 1997; Kunz, Peter, Huster, & Lautenbacher, 2013; Kunz, Prkachin, & Lautenbacher, 2009)). We recently demonstrated in a training study that observers were better in detecting facial expressions of pain after they learned about different facial activity patterns of pain compared to a group that was only trained to recognize the "prototypical expression of pain" (Kunz & Lautenbacher, 2015). These different facial activity patterns are composed of different combinations of facial movements (Kunz & Lautenbacher, 2014). These are tightening of the muscles surrounding the eyes that is either paired (1) with furrowed brows or (2) with wrinkled nose, (3) or with an opened mouth. These different facial activity patterns all have one facial movement in common, namely the tightening of the muscles surrounding the eyes (AU6_7). This facial movement is indeed the most frequent and thus possibly the most important facial movement occurring in the context of pain (Craig et al., 2011). Moreover, the tightening of the muscles surrounding the eyes is also the single facial movement that helps observers to differentiate the very similar facial expressions of pain and disgust; which is critically important for clinical assessment since facial expressions of pain and of disgust are very frequently mistaken for each other (Kunz, Prkachin, & Lautenbacher, 2013).

Last but not least, it is also important to mention that a considerable percentage of individuals (approximately 15–25%) do not show any visible facial responses during the experience of pain although they do report moderate to even strong pain intensities (Kunz & Lautenbacher, 2014). Overall, the threshold of facial expressions of pain is much higher than the subjective pain threshold (Craig et al., 2011). Prkachin and Craig (1995) referred to the facial expression of pain as a late signaling system since we tend to only express pain when it has reached a moderate or strong intensity, and even then individuals might not facially express it. Reasons for stoic expressions (e.g., social display rules) are discussed below. Interestingly, individuals are often not aware of their stoic facial responses during pain (as well as other facial expressions of emotions (see for example Barr & Kleck, 1995)), and overestimate the degree to which they express pain via the face. This is important to keep in mind when judging pain based on facial expressions, since this indicates that individuals might be experiencing pain although they do not show any pain-related facial activity and that a "stoic-face" is not necessarily incompatible with the experience of pain.

Correlation Between the Different Pain Expression Forms

One might ask why we express pain via so many different channels and whether these different channels transmit exactly the same type of information content to our social environment. When clinicians started to be interested in using nonverbal forms of expression to assess pain in nonverbal individuals (e.g., patients with dementia), many believed that the facial expression of pain might serve as a 1:1 substitute for the compromised self-report (Lautenbacher & Kunz, 2017). However, empirical as well as theoretical reasons speak against the assumption that each form of pain expression simply mirrors another form. The term "facial expression of pain" is actually already misleading because it suggests a unidirectional processing—with the subjective experience evolving first and the facial expression following after. However, the pain response system mostly runs in parallel, with mutual influences between the subjective experience and its different forms of verbal and nonverbal expressions. Moreover, each form of pain expression is only able to capture certain aspects of the multidimensional pain experience. Neither can a pain rating on a scale from 0–10 capture the complex multidimensionality of pain (Schiavenato & Craig, 2010), nor can a few facial muscle movements or few vocal parameters. Thus, it is not surprising that correlations between self-report ratings and facial expressions of pain are small in most studies (Kunz, Mylius, Schepelmann, & Lautenbacher, 2004). It seems that each form of pain expression constitutes an independent source of information for observers, which might help them to identify certain aspects of the multidimensional pain experience (Craig et al., 2011; Kunz, Chen, et al., 2011; Kunz, Rainville, & Lautenbacher, 2011). Which aspect of pain is conveyed via which communication channel has yet to be unraveled. Accordingly, disregarding nonverbal pain expressions as valid pain indicators simply because of a weak correlation with self-reported pain ratings is based on an erroneous conclusion.

Why Do We Express Pain

The main reason why we express pain is to solicit help, support, and empathy responses from our social environment in a situation of distress and potential danger. Moreover, it is also believed that the expression of pain (especially via facial responses and nonverbal vocalizations) serves the purpose of alerting others (Hadjistavropoulos et al., 2011; Williams, 2002) to potential danger. Given that both the gaining of help and support from others as well as warning others of potential danger seem crucial for survival (of the person in pain or his/her social environment) it is believed that evolution played an important role in bringing about the expression of pain (Williams, 2002; see also Chap. 1). Indeed, at least with regard to the facial expression of pain, it has been shown that is not a learned but a mostly inborn behavior that is already displayed by infants (Grunau & Craig, 1987; Grunau, Johnston, & Craig, 1990) as well as by congenitally blind individuals (Kunz, Faltermeier, & Lautenbacher, 2012).

Evidence supporting the assumption that the expression of pain serves the purpose of eliciting empathy and social support from one's social environment can be found in various studies. For instance, multiple studies have examined the impact of observing another's facial pain expressions on the observer (see also Chaps. 11 and 12). Using imaging studies, it has been repeatedly shown that the observation of pain behaviors, and particularly observation of facial expressions of pain, activates largely similar brain responses in the observer as the direct experience of pain itself (see Chap. 8). This suggests that observing pain automatically references the self, potentially signaling threat to one's own physical integrity (Yamada & Decety, 2009) and motivates avoidance behavior. However, this motivation for avoidance behavior is counterbalanced by social roles and social rules (e.g., as a health care professional it is my role to care for the patient) as well as by social bonds (e.g., between parents and the child) that make caregiving behavior more likely than not.

Three different but related dimensions have commonly been distinguished when depicting the impact of pain expression upon observing others: first, the *detection and discrimination* of available (pain) information; second, the *meaning* attached to what has been observed; third, the *behavioral responses* of the observer (Prkachin & Craig, 1995; Prkachin, Solomon, & Ross, 2007). Specific characteristics of the observer (e.g., parent) may influence both attention to pain cues and interpretation of these pain cues, thereby having an impact upon caregiving behavior (Hadjistavropoulos, Craig, Grunau, & Whitfield, 1997). In line with the cognitive-affective model of pain, in which the interruptive function of pain is central (Eccleston & Crombez, 1999), evidence has shown that individuals who perceive pain as highly threatening (i.e., engage in high levels of catastrophizing) are more attentive to the pain signals of others, estimate the pain of others to be more severe and/or interpret others' experiences more negatively (Goubert, Vervoort, Cano, & Crombez, 2009), and engage in various helping behaviors aimed at reducing, avoiding or escaping the other's pain. This dynamic is particularly evident in parent-child dyads, where parental attention towards child pain and associated distress when anticipating/ observing their child's pain motivates behaviors to restrict the child's pain exposure (Caes, Vervoort, Eccleston, & Goubert, 2012; Caes, Vervoort, Eccleston, Vandenhende, & Goubert, 2011). Research with healthy school children (Caes et al., 2012) and children with chronic pain (Caes et al., 2011) finds that parental distress contributes to increased restriction of experimentally induced child pain and painful physical activity. Although empathetic observer behaviors that aim at restricting or controlling the others' pain exposure might be adaptive in the short term, evidence suggests these responses have, particularly in the context of long term or inescapable pain, maladaptive consequences for the person in pain; catastrophizing thoughts in caregivers, such as parents (but also spouses) are associated with higher levels of functional disability, pain intensity, and emotional distress in the person suffering pain (Cano, 2004; Goubert, Eccleston, Vervoort, Jordan, & Crombez, 2006).

When Do We Express Pain

The ability to solicit support from others in the social environment may have stress-, pain- or fear-reducing properties and hence serve protective social functions (Prkachin & Craig, 1995). Facial expressions of pain may be particularly salient in this regard (Hadjistavropoulos et al., 1997; Williams, 2002). However, while the expression of pain seems to have mostly positive consequences; there are individuals or certain situations when pain is not expressed but when the experience of pain is accompanied by stoic expressions. How can that be? Why do we sometimes tend to not express our pain and/or why does pain expression vary across different situations and within and between individuals? In the following, we will discuss different psychosocial factors that have been found to impact "when" we express pain. Especially the impact of learning via observation and operant conditioning will be described. Moreover, the role of social rules (social display rules) that govern when (in which social context) and how we express pain will be discussed. And lastly, we will touch upon the impact of interpersonal/social threat.

Learning of Social Display Rules

Based on empirical findings, it is acknowledged that facial expressions of pain are a product of both innate (hardwired) as well as of social learning effects (Hadjistavropoulos et al., 2011). This means that facial responses become modifiable across early and late childhood through social learning experiences (Hadjistavropoulos et al., 2011). In line with this notion, studies have indicated that children, from an early age on, are able to modulate their expression of pain and distress (Buss & Kiel, 2004) and that they do so for a variety of reasons. Children's pain expression may vary, in part by the way a child is socialized to think about pain and behave when in pain (Craig, Stanford, Fairbairn, & Chambers, 2006; Fearon, McGrath, & Achat, 1996; Zeman & Garber, 1996)—learning that may be influenced by a broader set of cultural display rules (Gnepp & Hess, 1986). Facial expression of pain is particularly susceptible to social learning effects. Whereas young children tend to show vigorous facial expressions of pain, older children and adults seem to have learned to effectively downregulate their facial expressions of pain (Larochette, Chambers, & Craig, 2006). In line with this finding, a functional imaging study demonstrated that a low degree of facial expressiveness to pain was associated with higher activation in frontostriatal structures (Kunz, Chen, et al., 2011; Kunz, Rainville, & Lautenbacher, 2011). Given that these frontostriatal structures are known to be involved in motor inhibition, this finding suggests that low expressive individuals actively suppress their facial expression of pain (Kunz, Chen, et al., 2011; Kunz, Rainville, & Lautenbacher, 2011). A similar suggestion stems from a recent study that showed a close correlation between facial expressions of pain and the ability to inhibit automatic motor movements (Anti-saccade task), with low inhibitory ability being associated with stronger expressions of pain (Karmann, Lautenbacher, & Kunz, 2015). When trying to interpret these findings, it seems reasonable that individuals learn to intentionally suppress the facial display of negative affect (including pain) following culturally/socially learned "display rules." These display rules represent social norms about when, where, and how one should express affective states (Ekman, Sorenson, & Friesen, 1969). These social display rules are learned already at a young age. Children are aware of the interpersonal ramifications of expressing their pain and base their decisions to express, hide or even dissemble their pain on the type of response they expect to receive following a pain disclosure. For example, children as young as 9 years old report being less likely to express pain in front of a peer than in presence of their parent because they perceive peers to be less accepting of pain displays and responding more negatively than parents (Zeman & Garber, 1996). Children may also hide their pain because of other-protective reasons (Crombez & Eccleston, 2002) like not wanting to worry or upset their parents (Larochette et al., 2006). Accordingly, facially responding to pain would be the "default" which individuals learn to suppress due to social/cultural demands (e.g., "big boys don't cry," "don't be a sissy").

Further evidence for the assumption that social learning impacts the degree to which we express pain was found in a study on operant conditioning of facial expressions of pain (Kunz, Rainville, & Lautenbacher, 2011). In a within subject design, participants were in one block reinforced over a series of trials whenever they displayed facial expressions of pain and in another block were reinforced for not expressing their pain via the face (stoic expression). The operant conditioning led to strong changes in the expression of pain. Positive reinforcement of facial expressions of pain resulted in a significant increase in facial expression, whereas the positive reinforcement of a stoic expression resulted in a strong decrease in facial expressions during noxious stimulation. Thus, it is plausible that we learn when to express pain based on the reactions of our peers, parents, family and friends (responding by reinforcing or punishing our expression of pain) when and how we should express our pain. See also Chap. 13 for more details on the effect of operant reinforcement on pain.

Social Presence

Regardless of the social situation (i.e., who is present when experiencing pain), it has been shown that pain is expressed via the same set of facial movements. Thus, the elements of the facial language used to express pain remain unaltered by social situations and thereby stay constantly recognizable (Karmann, Lautenbacher, Bauer, & Kunz, 2014). However, the *degree* of facial expressiveness is strongly affected by the social situation, social presence in particular.

Social presence affects pain displays from an early age on. For instance, when studying facial expressions of pain in children it was found that children facially display pain to a higher degree in the presence of their parents, whereas they suppress their communication of pain in the presence of a stranger (Vervoort et al., 2008; Zeman & Garber, 1996). Similar findings in pediatric samples have been observed when comparing parental presence to situations where no one is observing (Vervoort et al., 2011). Studies in adults reveal comparable findings. In particular, studies have demonstrated that the expression of pain is much more stoic when individuals are tested in the presence of an unfamiliar observer compared to being alone or being in the presence of a loved one (Karmann et al., 2014; Kleck et al., 1976; Vlaeyen et al., 2009). The more stoic expression of pain in the presence of a stranger is likely due to the fact that expressing one's pain freely could be interpreted as a sign of weakness and vulnerability (Williams, 2002) and thus, as stated in more detail above—we have learned to inhibit our expression. In contrast, expressing one's pain freely in the presence of a loved one seems beneficial since sympathetic observers might faster be able to identify painful experiences and therefore the possibility of receiving help is elevated. Thus, the learned inhibition of facial expressions of pain seems to be disinhibited/released in the presence of a familiar or loved one.

Interestingly, the effect of the social situation on the expression of pain also seems to be dependent on different *intraindividual* factors. For one, the sex of the person seems to play a role. In the presence of a stranger, women were found to decrease their facial expression of pain much more than men did (Karmann et al.,

2014). This finding is well in line with previous findings on sex differences in social display rules. In front of strangers, females—compared to males—seem to express positive affective states, like happiness, facially, and tend to conceal negative ones like anger (Davis, 1995; LaFrance, Hecht, & Paluck, 2003).

Moreover, the tendency to catastrophize about pain has also been found to play a role, not only in understanding the level of pain expression (see Chap. 5), but also in understanding the impact of social presence. Specifically, the studies described above on child facial pain expression as a function of social presence (Vervoort et al., 2008, 2011) revealed a significant *moderation* effect of the child's pain catastrophizing. In particular, Vervoort et al. (2008) demonstrated that children showed increased facial pain expression in presence of their parent rather than a stranger, but *only* when the child reported infrequent or low levels of catastrophic thoughts about pain. For high catastrophizing children, an *indiscriminate* pattern of facial pain display was found. High catastrophizers' facial pain expression was equally pronounced regardless of the relational status of the observer; they expressed as much pain in presence of their parent as in presence of a stranger. These findings suggest that high catastrophizing children may have difficulty suppressing pain expression and identify others, even those from whom help or care is uncertain, more easily as potential deliverers of care. Similar findings were observed when comparing parental presence with being alone (see Vervoort et al., 2011); high catastrophizing children showed equally high levels of facial display of pain, regardless of social context, whereas low catastrophizing children showed higher levels of facial display in presence of their parent than when alone.

Pain Expression in Unsafe or Threatening Environments

As mentioned previously, one of the main motivations to express pain is to solicit help and support from others and possibly alert them to approaching danger. However, both evolutionary theory and social learning theory would predict that there are certain environments where it is not advantageous to express pain (see also Chap. 1 and Williams, 2002). We would expect that pain expression is reduced when we are surrounded by individuals who are unlikely to offer help or even might take advantage of us when in a state of vulnerability (e.g., someone who intentionally tries to cause harm or take resources from us) as this would be disadvantageous for survival. Above-noted findings that children express less pain in presence of a stranger compared to parental presence are in line with this notion (Vervoort et al., 2008). Furthermore, the above-described findings on operant conditioning of pain expressions (Kunz, Chen, et al., 2011; Kunz, Rainville, & Lautenbacher, 2011) would likewise predict that pain expression is inhibited following punishment (e.g., when expressing vulnerability is met with further harm, see also Chap. 13). In other words, we might expect higher levels of pain expression in a safe social context (e.g., in the presence of family, friends or caregivers) but reduced pain expression when the social context is perceived to be threatening (e.g., in the presence of adversaries) or in ambiguous situations (e.g., in the presence of strangers).

There is only limited empirical research to date testing this prediction. Some evidence comes from studies in rodents. In one influential study by Langford et al. (2006), pain behavior in mice was investigated when in the presence of either a stranger mouse, a cagemate, a sibling, or in isolation. Findings of this study indicated that mice expressed significantly less pain when in the presence of a stranger mouse compared to all other conditions, most likely because the presence of a stranger is a source of social stress. This result was later replicated in a second study, and seemed to be specific for same-sex male dyads (Langford et al., 2011). What about humans? A study by Williams, Gallagher, Fidalgo, and Bentley (2016) used agent-based modelling to study whether exploitation of injured agents would lead to reductions in pain expression. They found that pain expression indeed was reduced almost to zero when expressing vulnerability was met with exploitation across numerous iterations, providing support for the evolutionary prediction that expressing vulnerability can be associated with costs and if these costs are high enough, expression will be reduced. In addition, there is a single experimental study in humans which investigated the effect of social threat on facial pain expression and pain reports (Peeters & Vlaeyen, 2011). In this study, social threat was manipulated by leading participants to believe that others were willing to inflict varying levels of pain upon them. While an earlier study had found that intentional pain is associated with increased pain reports (Gray & Wegner, 2008), this study was the first to demonstrate that social threat can lead to a dissociation between pain reports and facial pain expression. Specifically, findings demonstrated that while subjective pain reports were indeed higher in the threatening social context, facial display of pain was reduced.

As mentioned in Chap. 1, it is still a matter of debate whether pain expression is actively suppressed in an unsafe environment or whether suppression of pain expression is the norm and is only released when in a safe environment. The finding that pain expression is commonly suppressed in the presence of strangers, who are not actively threatening, seems to indicate the latter. Moreover, we recently conducted a study (Karmann et al., 2016) where we used repetitive transcranial magnetic stimulation (rTMS) to decrease the excitability of the medial prefrontal cortex and to investigate its effect on facial expressiveness during pain. Given the prominent role of the prefrontal cortex in suppressing facial expressions of pain (Kunz, Chen, et al., 2011; Kunz, Rainville, & Lautenbacher, 2011), we expected that reducing the activity of the prefrontal cortex (via rTMS) would result in a disinhibition of facial expressions of pain, and thus in increased facial responses. This is exactly what we found (Karmann et al., 2016). Decreasing prefrontal activity resulted in increased facial expressions of pain, which supports the notion that—due to socialization—suppression of pain expressions seems to be the default; and that this suppression is released when in safe environments.

The idea that pain expression is reduced in threatening or unsafe environments has important implications for clinical practice. For instance, experiences of pain in threatening social environments might create a double burden for the sufferer. One such example might be bullying, which is highly prevalent and frequently involves not only psychological but also physical assault (Salmivalli, 2010; Vanderbilt & Augustyn, 2010). Based on the arguments outlined above, experiences of bullying are highly threatening social experiences often involving intentional pain by one or more assailants and might lead not only to worsened pain outcomes including a higher chance for the development of chronic pain (Fekkes, Pijpers, Fredriks, Vogels, & Verloove-Vanhorick, 2006; Voerman et al., 2015), but at the same time reduced expression of pain to protect oneself from more bullying. This might have detrimental consequences for the sufferer, as others (including the bullies) would likely underestimate the pain that is caused, thus, further exacerbating the problem.

Along similar lines, if pain is only adequately expressed in safe environments, it should be in our best interest to create safe interpersonal environments in clinical practice to lay the groundwork for adequate treatment of acute and chronic pain. Unfortunately, as is also discussed in Chap. 12, we have ample reason to believe that clinical settings are frequently not perceived as safe. Especially chronic pain patients are often met with doubt, judgment, stigmatization, invalidation and accusations of deception (Cohen, Quintner, Buchanan, Nielsen, & Guy, 2011; De Ruddere & Craig, 2016; Williams, 2016). At the same time, we know that pain is commonly underestimated by lay observers and experienced clinicians (Kappesser, Williams, & Prkachin, 2006; Kappesser & Williams, 2008). Based on the arguments put forward in the present chapter, this underestimation might at least be partly due to suppressed pain expression in an environment that is not perceived as safe. It should therefore be in our best interest to create a supportive and safe environment for individuals suffering from acute and chronic pain, where expression of vulnerability is encouraged rather than questioned (also see Chap. 13 for a discussion of the Intimacy Process Model), as only such an environment will provide a chance for adequate pain assessment and subsequent treatment.

Future Research

In the present chapter we have given an in-depth overview of the complex psychosocial factors that affect when, how and why we express pain. This complexity is further increased by the different channels via which we express pain (verbal, facial expression, vocalizations, body movements/postures) and which are often differently impacted by psychosocial factors. So far, most studies have only focused on one or two pain expression channels, and thus more multichannel approaches are needed that help us to grasp more comprehensively how pain expression is differentially affected by psychosocial factors. Moreover, pain expression is a dynamic communication process. This dynamic nature of it has mostly been neglected in the study designs so far; with the majority of studies focussing either on how social settings affect the expression of pain (focussing on the person in pain) or on how facial expressions of pain affect the observer. However in order to better understand when, how and why we express pain, we need to study the dynamics of pain expression by studying both the person expressing pain as well as the social interactant, their relationship, their behavioral responses across time, their learning history and their psychological characteristics.

References

Barr, C. L., & Kleck, R. E. (1995). Self-other perception of the intensity of facial expressions of emotion: Do we know what we show? *Journal of Personality and Social Psychology, 68*, 608.

Buss, K. A., & Kiel, E. J. (2004). Comparison of sadness, anger, and fear facial expressions when toddlers look at their mothers. *Child Development, 75*, 1761–1773.

Caes, L., Vervoort, T., Eccleston, C., & Goubert, L. (2012). Parents who catastrophize about their child's pain prioritize attempts to control pain. *Pain, 153*(8), 1695–1701.

Caes, L., Vervoort, T., Eccleston, C., Vandenhende, M., & Goubert, L. (2011). Parental catastrophizing about child's pain and its relationship with activity restriction: The mediating role of parental distress. *Pain, 152*(1), 212–222.

Cano, A. (2004). Pain catastrophizing and social support in married individuals with chronic pain: The moderating role of pain duration. *Pain, 110*(3), 656–664.

Chan, S., Hadjistavropoulos, T., Williams, J., & Lints-Martindale, A. (2014). Evidence-based development and initial validation of the pain assessment checklist for seniors with limited ability to communicate-II (PACSLAC-II). *The Clinical Journal of Pain, 30*(9), 816–824.

Cohen, M., Quintner, J., Buchanan, D., Nielsen, M., & Guy, L. (2011). Stigmatization of patients with chronic pain: The extinction of empathy. *Pain Medicine, 12*(11), 1637–1643.

Corbett, A., Achterberg, W., Husebo, B., Lobbezoo, F., de Vet, H., Kunz, M., … de Waal, M. (2014). An international road map to improve pain assessment in people with impaired cognition: The development of the Pain Assessment in Impaired Cognition (PAIC) meta-tool. *BMC Neurology, 14*(1), 229.

Craig, K. D., Gilbert-MacLeod, C. A., & Lilley, C. M. (2000). Bioevolutionary perspectives on the functional value of cry. In R. Barr, B. Hopkins, & J. A. Green (Eds.), *Crying as a sign, a symptom, and a signal: clinical, emotional and developmental aspects of infant and toddler crying* (Vol. 152, p. 23). New York, NY: Cambridge University Press.

Craig, K. D., Prkachin, K. M., & Grunau, R. V. E. (2011). The facial expression of pain. In D. C. Turk & R. Melzack (Eds.), *Handbook of pain assessment* (3rd ed., pp. 117–133). New York, NY: Guilford Press.

Craig, K. D., Stanford, E. A., Fairbairn, N. S., & Chambers, C. T. (2006). Emergent pain language communication competence in infants and children. *Enfance, 58*(1), 52–71.

Craig, K. D., Versloot, J., Goubert, L., Vervoort, T., & Crombez, G. (2010). Perceiving pain in others: Automatic and controlled mechanisms. *The Journal of Pain, 11*(2), 101–108.

Crombez, G., & Eccleston, C. (2002). To express or suppress may be function of others' distress. *Behavioral and Brain Sciences, 25*(4), 457–458.

Davis, T. L. (1995). Gender differences in masking negative emotions: Ability or motivation? *Developmental Psychology, 31*(4), 660.

De Ruddere, L., & Craig, K. D. (2016). Understanding stigma and chronic pain: A-state-of-the-art review. *Pain, 157*(8), 1607–1610.

Defrin, R., Amanzio, M., de Tommaso, M., Dimova, V., Filipovic, S., Finn, D. P., … Kunz, M. (2015). Experimental pain processing in individuals with cognitive impairment: Current state of the science. *Pain, 156*(8), 1396–1408.

Eccleston, C., & Crombez, G. (1999). Pain demands attention: A cognitive–affective model of the interruptive function of pain. *Psychological Bulletin, 125*(3), 356.

Ekman, P., Sorenson, E. R., & Friesen, W. V. (1969). Pan-cultural elements in facial displays of emotion. *Science, 164*(3875), 86–88.

Ekman, P. E., & Friesen, W. V. (1978). *Facial action coding system*. Palo Alto, CA: Consulting Psychologists Press.

Fearon, I., McGrath, P. J., & Achat, H. (1996). 'Booboos': The study of everyday pain among young children. *Pain, 68*(1), 55–62.

Fekkes, M., Pijpers, F. I., Fredriks, A. M., Vogels, T., & Verloove-Vanhorick, S. P. (2006). Do bullied children get ill, or do ill children get bullied? A prospective cohort study on the relationship between bullying and health-related symptoms. *Pediatrics, 117*(5), 1568–1574.

Gnepp, J., & Hess, D. L. (1986). Children's understanding of verbal and facial display rules. *Developmental Psychology, 22*(1), 103.

Goubert, L., Eccleston, C., Vervoort, T., Jordan, A., & Crombez, G. (2006). Parental catastrophizing about their child's pain. The parent version of the Pain Catastrophizing Scale (PCS-P): A preliminary validation. *Pain, 123*(3), 254–263.

Goubert, L., Vervoort, T., Cano, A., & Crombez, G. (2009). Catastrophizing about their children's pain is related to higher parent–child congruency in pain ratings: An experimental investigation. *European Journal of Pain, 13*(2), 196–201.

Gray, K., & Wegner, D. M. (2008). The sting of intentional pain. *Psychological Science, 19*(12), 1260–1262.

Grunau, R. V., & Craig, K. D. (1987). Pain expression in neonates: Facial action and cry. *Pain, 28*(3), 395–410.

Grunau, R. V., Johnston, C. C., & Craig, K. D. (1990). Neonatal facial and cry responses to invasive and non-invasive procedures. *Pain, 42*(3), 295–305.

Hadjistavropoulos, H. D., Craig, K. D., Grunau, R. E., & Whitfield, M. F. (1997). Judging pain in infants: Behavioural, contextual, and developmental determinants. *Pain, 73*(3), 319–324.

Hadjistavropoulos, T., Craig, K. D., Duck, S., Cano, A., Goubert, L., Jackson, P. L., … Fitzgerald, T. D. (2011). A biopsychosocial formulation of pain communication. *Psychological Bulletin, 137*(6), 910.

Hale, C. J., & Hadjistavropoulos, T. (1997). Emotional components of pain. *Pain Research and Management, 2*(4), 217–225.

Herr, K., Bjoro, K., & Decker, S. (2006). Tools for assessment of pain in nonverbal older adults with dementia: A state-of-the-science review. *Journal of Pain and Symptom Management, 31*(2), 170–192.

International Association for the Study of Pain (IASP). (1979). Pain terms: A list with definitions and notes on usage. *Pain, 6*, 249–252.

Jensen, M. P., & Karoly, P. (2001). Self-report scales and procedures for assessing pain in adults. In D. Turk & R. Melzack (Eds.), *Handbook of pain assessment* (pp. 15–34). New York, NY: Guilford Press.

Johnston, C. C., & O'Shaugnessy, D. (1987). Acoustical attributes of infant pain cries: Discriminating features. *Pain, 30*, S233.

Kappesser, J., & Williams, A. C. D. C. (2008). Pain judgements of patients' relatives: Examining the use of social contract theory as theoretical framework. *Journal of Behavioral Medicine, 31*(4), 309–317.

Kappesser, J., Williams, A. C. D. C., & Prkachin, K. M. (2006). Testing two accounts of pain underestimation. *Pain, 124*(1), 109–116.

Karmann, A. J., Lautenbacher, S., Bauer, F., & Kunz, M. (2014). The influence of communicative relations on facial responses to pain: Does it matter who is watching? *Pain Research and Management, 19*(1), 15–22.

Karmann, A. J., Lautenbacher, S., & Kunz, M. (2015). The role of inhibitory mechanisms in the regulation of facial expressiveness during pain. *Biological Psychology, 104*, 82–89.

Karmann, A. J., Maihöfner, C., Lautenbacher, S., Sperling, W., Kornhuber, J., & Kunz, M. (2016). The role of prefrontal inhibition in regulating facial expressions of pain: A repetitive transcranial magnetic stimulation study. *The Journal of Pain, 17*(3), 383–391.

Keefe, F. J., & Block, A. R. (1982). Development of an observation method for assessing pain behavior in chronic low back pain patients. *Behavior Therapy, 13*(4), 363–375.

Kleck, R. E., Vaughan, R. C., Cartwright-Smith, J., Vaughan, K. B., Colby, C. Z., & Lanzetta, J. T. (1976). Effects of being observed on expressive, subjective, and physiological responses to painful stimuli. *Journal of Personality and Social Psychology, 34*(6), 1211.

Kunz, M. (2015). Behavioural/facial markers of pain, emotion, cognition. In G. Pickering & S. Gibson (Eds.), *Pain, emotion and cognition* (pp. 123–133). Cham, Switzerland: Springer International Publishing.

Kunz, M., Chen, J. I., Lautenbacher, S., Vachon-Presseau, E., & Rainville, P. (2011). Cerebral regulation of facial expressions of pain. *Journal of Neuroscience, 31*(24), 8730–8738.

Kunz, M., Faltermeier, N., & Lautenbacher, S. (2012). Impact of visual learning on facial expressions of physical distress: A study on voluntary and evoked expressions of pain in congenitally blind and sighted individuals. *Biological Psychology, 89*(2), 467–476.

Kunz, M., Gruber, A., & Lautenbacher, S. (2006). Sex differences in facial encoding of pain. *The Journal of Pain, 7*(12), 915–928.

Kunz, M., & Lautenbacher, S. (2014). The faces of pain: A cluster analysis of individual differences in facial activity patterns of pain. *European Journal of Pain, 18*(6), 813–823.

Kunz, M., & Lautenbacher, S. (2015). Improving recognition of pain by calling attention to its various faces. *European Journal of Pain, 19*(9), 1350–1361.

Kunz, M., Mylius, V., Schepelmann, K., & Lautenbacher, S. (2004). On the relationship between self-report and facial expression of pain. *The Journal of Pain, 5*(7), 368–376.

Kunz, M., Mylius, V., Schepelmann, K., & Lautenbacher, S. (2008). Impact of age on the facial expression of pain. *Journal of Psychosomatic Research, 64*(3), 311–318.

Kunz, M., Peter, J., Huster, S., & Lautenbacher, S. (2013). Pain and disgust: The facial signaling of two aversive bodily experiences. *PLoS One, 8*(12), e83277.

Kunz, M., Prkachin, K., & Lautenbacher, S. (2009). The smile of pain. *Pain, 145*(3), 273–275.

Kunz, M., Prkachin, K., & Lautenbacher, S. (2013). Smiling in pain: Explorations of its social motives. *Pain Research and Treatment, 2013*, e128093.

Kunz, M., Rainville, P., & Lautenbacher, S. (2011). Operant conditioning of facial displays of pain. *Psychosomatic Medicine, 73*(5), 422–431.

Kunz, M., Scharmann, S., Hemmeter, U., Schepelmann, K., & Lautenbacher, S. (2007). The facial expression of pain in patients with dementia. *Pain, 133*(1), 221–228.

LaFrance, M., Hecht, M. A., & Paluck, E. L. (2003). The contingent smile: A meta-analysis of sex differences in smiling. *Psychological Bulletin, 129*(2), 305.

Langford, D. J., Crager, S. E., Shehzad, Z., Smith, S. B., Sotocinal, S. G., Levenstadt, J. S., … Mogil, J. S. (2006). Social modulation of pain as evidence for empathy in mice. *Science, 312*(5782), 1967–1970.

Langford, D. J., Tuttle, A. H., Briscoe, C., Harvey-Lewis, C., Baran, I., Gleeson, P., … Mogil, J. S. (2011). Varying perceived social threat modulates pain behavior in male mice. *The Journal of Pain, 12*(1), 125–132.

Larochette, A. C., Chambers, C. T., & Craig, K. D. (2006). Genuine, suppressed and faked facial expressions of pain in children. *Pain, 126*(1), 64–71.

Lautenbacher, S., & Kunz, M. (2017). Facial pain expression in dementia: A review of the experimental and clinical evidence. *Current Alzheimer Research, 14*(5), 501–505.

Lautenbacher, S., Salinas-Ranneberg, M., Niebuhr, O., & Kunz, M. (2017). Phonetic characteristics of vocalizations during pain. *Pain Reports, 2*(3), e597.

McDaniel, L. K., Anderson, K. O., Bradley, L. A., Young, L. D., Turner, R. A., Agudelo, C. A., & Keefe, F. J. (1986). Development of an observation method for assessing pain behavior in rheumatoid arthritis patients. *Pain, 24*(2), 165–184.

Melzack, R. (1975). The McGill Pain Questionnaire: Major properties and scoring methods. *Pain, 1*(3), 277–299.

Melzack, R., & Katz, J. (2001). *The McGill Pain Questionnaire: Appraisal and current status*. New York, NY: Guilford Press.

Peeters, P. A., & Vlaeyen, J. W. (2011). Feeling more pain, yet showing less: The influence of social threat on pain. *The Journal of Pain, 12*(12), 1255–1261.

Prkachin, K. M. (1986). Pain behaviour is not unitary. *Behavioral and Brain Sciences, 9*(4), 754–755.

Prkachin, K. M. (1992). The consistency of facial expressions of pain: A comparison across modalities. *Pain, 51*(3), 297–306.

Prkachin, K. M., & Craig, K. D. (1995). Expressing pain: The communication and interpretation of facial pain signals. *Journal of Nonverbal Behavior, 19*(4), 191–205.

Prkachin, K. M., & Solomon, P. E. (2008). The structure, reliability and validity of pain expression: Evidence from patients with shoulder pain. *Pain, 139*(2), 267–274.

Prkachin, K. M., Solomon, P. E., & Ross, J. (2007). Underestimation of pain by health-care providers: Towards a model of the process of inferring pain in others. *CJNR (Canadian Journal of Nursing Research), 39*(2), 88–106.

Salmivalli, C. (2010). Bullying and the peer group: A review. *Aggression and Violent Behavior, 15*(2), 112–120.

Schiavenato, M., & Craig, K. D. (2010). Pain assessment as a social transaction: Beyond the "gold standard". *The Clinical Journal of Pain, 26*(8), 667–676.

Simon, D., Craig, K. D., Gosselin, F., Belin, P., & Rainville, P. (2008). Recognition and discrimination of prototypical dynamic expressions of pain and emotions. *Pain, 135*(1), 55–64.

Vanderbilt, D., & Augustyn, M. (2010). The effects of bullying. *Paediatrics and Child Health, 20*(7), 315–320.

Vervoort, T., Caes, L., Trost, Z., Sullivan, M., Vangronsveld, K., & Goubert, L. (2011). Social modulation of facial pain display in high-catastrophizing children: An observational study in schoolchildren and their parents. *Pain, 152*(7), 1591–1599.

Vervoort, T., Goubert, L., Eccleston, C., Verhoeven, K., De Clercq, A., Buysse, A., & Crombez, G. (2008). The effects of parental presence upon the facial expression of pain: The moderating role of child pain catastrophizing. *Pain, 138*(2), 277–285.

Vlaeyen, J. W., Hanssen, M., Goubert, L., Vervoort, T., Peters, M., van Breukelen, G., … Morley, S. (2009). Threat of pain influences social context effects on verbal pain report and facial expression. *Behaviour Research and Therapy, 47*(9), 774–782.

Voerman, J. S., Vogel, I., Waart, F., Westendorp, T., Timman, R., Busschbach, J. J. V., … Klerk, C. (2015). Bullying, abuse and family conflict as risk factors for chronic pain among Dutch adolescents. *European Journal of Pain, 19*(10), 1544–1551.

Walsh, J., Eccleston, C., & Keogh, E. (2014). Pain communication through body posture: The development and validation of a stimulus set. *Pain, 155*(11), 2282–2290.

Warden, V., Hurley, A. C., & Volicer, L. (2003). Development and psychometric evaluation of the Pain Assessment in Advanced Dementia (PAINAD) scale. *Journal of the American Medical Directors Association, 4*(1), 9–15.

Wilkie, D. J., Keefe, F. J., Dodd, M. J., & Copp, L. A. (1992). Behavior of patients with lung cancer: Description and associations with oncologic and pain variables. *Pain, 51*(2), 231–240.

Williams, A. C. d. C. (2002). Facial expression of pain, empathy, evolution, and social learning. *Behavioral and Brain Sciences, 25*(4), 475–480.

Williams, A. C. d. C. (2016). Defeating the stigma of chronic pain. *Pain, 157*(8), 1581–1582.

Williams, A. C. d. C., Gallagher, E., Fidalgo, A. R., & Bentley, P. J. (2016). Pain expressiveness and altruistic behavior: An exploration using agent-based modeling. *Pain, 157*(3), 759.

Yamada, M., & Decety, J. (2009). Unconscious affective processing and empathy: An investigation of subliminal priming on the detection of painful facial expressions. *Pain, 143*(1), 71–75.

Zeman, J., & Garber, J. (1996). Display rules for anger, sadness, and pain: It depends on who is watching. *Child Development, 67*(3), 957–973.

Zwakhalen, S. M., Hamers, J. P., Abu-Saad, H. H., & Berger, M. P. (2006). Pain in elderly people with severe dementia: A systematic review of behavioural pain assessment tools. *BMC Geriatrics, 6*, 3.

Chapter 7
Automatic, Objective, and Efficient Measurement of Pain Using Automated Face Analysis

Zakia Hammal and Jeffrey F. Cohn

Abstract Pain typically is measured by patient self-report, but self-reported pain is difficult to interpret and may be impaired or in some circumstances not possible to obtain. Automatic, objective assessment of pain from video or camera input is emerging as a powerful alternative. We review the current state of the art in automatic, objective assessment of pain from video or camera input and the databases that have made progress in this area possible. Because most efforts have involved facial expression of pain, we emphasize that in our review. We discuss current challenges and prospects to advance automatic assessment of the occurrence and intensity of pain for research and clinical use.

Keywords Automatic · Objective measurement of pain · Facial expression · Pain intensity

Introduction

Pain is a source of human suffering and lost productivity, a symptom and consequence of numerous disorders, and a contributing factor in medical and surgical treatment. Yet standard clinical assessments of pain are limited primarily to subjective reports from patients, family members, or clinicians. Visual analog scales (VAS) are a frequent example. Because they are reproducible, efficient, and can be used in a variety of settings, they are widely used. While convenient and useful, VAS and other subjective ratings have notable limitations. These include

Z. Hammal
The Robotics Institute, Carnegie Mellon University, Pittsburgh, PA, USA
e-mail: zhammal@andrew.cmu.edu

J. F. Cohn (✉)
University of Pittsburgh, Pittsburgh, PA, USA
e-mail: jeffcohn@pitt.edu

© Springer International Publishing AG, part of Springer Nature 2018   121
T. Vervoort et al. (eds.), *Social and Interpersonal Dynamics in Pain*,
https://doi.org/10.1007/978-3-319-78340-6_7

idiosyncratic use, inconsistent metric properties across scale dimensions (extreme pain in one context may be only intermediate in another), reactivity to suggestion, susceptibility to impression management and deception, and differences between clinicians' and sufferers' conceptualizations of pain (Chambers, Reid, Craig, McGrath, & Finley, 1998; Craig, Korol, & Pillai, 2002; Prkachin, Solomon, Hwang, & Mercer, 2001). For infants, young children, patients with certain neurological or psychiatric impairments, and many patients in postoperative care or transient states of consciousness, ratings are not even possible. Given individual differences among patients, their families, and healthcare providers, pain often is poorly assessed, underestimated, and inadequately treated (Craig, 2009). To improve assessment of pain and guide treatment, reliable, valid, and efficient assessment of the onset, intensity, and pattern of occurrence of pain is necessary.

To achieve this goal, automatic face analysis (AFA) is emerging as a powerful option. AFA enables graded pain measurement from video and camera input at video rate (25–30 f/s or faster). AFA is poised to greatly contribute to the reliability, validity, and efficiency of pain assessment at relatively little cost. Widespread adoption of AFA could lead to uniform yet individualized management of pain and a more efficient utilization of healthcare for pain sufferers. For research and clinical practice, AFA offers the prospect of an objective and qualitative tool with which to investigate pain and evaluate the efficacy and response to treatment of pharmaceutical and surgical treatments, physical therapy, and other interventions.

AFA for pain research and clinical use has been achieved by several interrelated advances. The first was Darwin's (Darwin, 1872/1998) insight that facial expression communicates information about pain and motivational and emotional states more broadly. Second, seminal work by Ekman and colleagues provided a method to reliably annotate the facial actions observed by Darwin. That method was the Facial Action Coding System, known as FACS (Ekman & Friesen, 1978; Ekman, Friesen, & Hager, 2002). Third, Prkachin, Craig, and their colleagues used FACS to discover and validate rigorous pain-related facial measures of pain (Craig, Prkachin, & Grunau, 2001; Craig, Prkachin, & Grunau, 2010; Prkachin, 1992; Prkachin & Solomon, 2008). The Prkachin and Solomon Pain Intensity scale (PSPI: Prkachin & Solomon, 2008), for instance, measures the occurrence and intensity of pain as revealed in the face. Fourth was AFA, which made possible automatic measurement of facial actions related to pain, PSPI scores of pain intensity, and novel measures of pain, such as the velocity of changes in pain intensity. A fifth advance proved critical to the advancement of AFA. That was the creation and distribution of well-annotated video recordings of pain experience. Without appropriate data with which to train automated measures of pain occurrence and intensity, well-validated AFA for pain measurement could not exist. This chapter reviews the discovery of facial indicators of pain, current status of AFA and its application to pain, and the databases that have made possible automatic detection of the occurrence, intensity, and dynamics of pain. We consider current challenges and prospects for clinical and research use of AFA for pain measurement.

Fig. 7.1 Left: Muscles of the face (Clemente, 1997). Middle: Action units and corresponding muscles used in calculating PSPI. **AU4**: corrugator supercilli (brow lowerer). **AU6**: orbicularis oculi pars orbitalis (cheek raiser). **AU9**: levator labii superioris alaquae nasi (nose wrinkler). **AU10**: levator labiii superioris (upper lip raiser). **AU25**: depressor labii inferioris or orbicularis oris (lips parted). **AU43**: levator palpebrae superioris; orbicularis occuli, pars palpebralis (eyes closed)

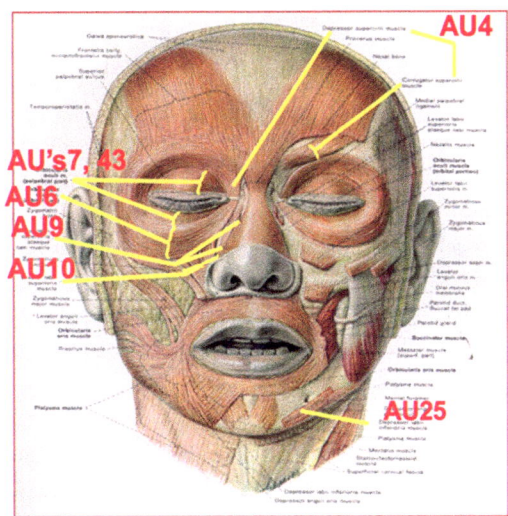

Facial Actions That Communicate Pain

Significant efforts have been made in human behavioral studies to identify reliable and valid facial indicators of pain (Craig et al., 2001; Prkachin & Solomon, 2008). The most comprehensive approaches require labeling of anatomically based facial actions by highly trained human coders using the Facial Action Coding System (FACS) (Cohn, Ambadar, & Ekman, 2007; Ekman et al., 2002). The current version of FACS specifies 30+ anatomically based action units (AUs) and a large number of action descriptors for which the anatomic basis is not yet known. Each AU describes the action of one or in some cases a few facial muscles. For instance, AU6 refers to contraction of the outer portion of the orbicularis oculi muscle, which raises the cheeks and AU10 refers to contraction of the levator labii superioris, which wrinkles the nose. Both AUs frequently co-occur in pain. AUs are sufficiently detailed that individually or in combinations they can describe nearly all-possible facial expressions.

Seminal work by Craig, Prkachin, and their colleagues (Craig, Hyde, & Patrick, 1991; Craig et al., 2001; Prkachin, 1992; Prkachin & Solomon, 2008) identified AUs related to pain. Although there is some variability in the AUs that have been found to be associated with pain across studies, several appear routinely in the literature. These are: brow-lowering (AU4), cheek-raising (AU6), eyelid tightening (AU7), nose wrinkling (AU9), upper-lip raising (AU10), oblique lip raising (AU12), horizontal lip stretching (AU20), lip parting (AU25), jaw dropping (AU26), mouth stretching (AU27) and eye-closure (AU43) (Craig et al., 2001; Prkachin, 1992) (see Fig. 7.1). Except for AU43, which is binary, the intensity of each of these AUs can be measured on a six-point ordinal scale (0 = absent, 1 = trace, 2 = slight, 3 = pronounced, 4 = severe, and 5 = maximum) as provided by FACS.

Prkachin found that a subset of these actions—brow lowering (AU4), orbital tightening (AU6 and AU7), levator labii contraction (AU9 and AU10), and eye closure (AU43)—corresponded to the intensity of pain experience (Prkachin, 1992). In a follow-up study, Prkachin and Solomon proposed the Prkachin and Solomon pain intensity (PSPI) metric as the sum of the intensities of these AUs (see Fig. 7.1) (Prkachin & Solomon, 2008). The PSPI metric is defined as:

$$
\begin{aligned}
\text{Pain} = \ & \text{Intensity of} \left(\text{AU4} \right) + \text{intensity of} \left(\text{AU6 or AU7,whichever is larger} \right) \\
& + \text{intensity of} \left(\text{AU9 or AU10,whichever is larger} \right) + \text{intensity} \left(\text{AU43} \right).
\end{aligned}
$$

The PSPI metric discriminates among 16 pain intensity levels and is the only metric that can delimit pain intensity on a frame-by-frame basis. Until recently, skilled application of the PSPI required over a hundred hours of training and certification in FACS and approximately an hour or more per minute of video to manually annotate video. A more recent version (Rash, Prkachin, Solomon, & Campbell, n.d.) has reduced training time to within 10–15 h, which still is considerable. The intensive time required to manually annotate video using the PSPI makes it ill-suited for real-time applications and clinical use.

Automated Measurement of Facial Expression of Pain

Automated face analysis (AFA) addresses the need for objective, valid, and efficient measurement of pain from video or camera input (e.g., from a webcam). Processing can be performed on an ordinary laptop at video frame rate.

AFA consists of several steps. Face shape, facial features (e.g., eyes and mouth), and appearance (e.g., texture or furrowing of the skin) are detected in each frame of the video input. Face shape and appearance then are aligned to a normalized, or canonical view, so that variation in head orientation to the camera (i.e., pose) does not confound measurement. Discriminative features then are extracted from the aligned face shape or appearance and inputted to a classifier or regressor to learn associations between features and pain score occurrence or intensity. The following sections give an overview of each of these steps.

Tracking and Alignment of Face Shape and Appearance

Face and facial feature tracking and alignment consist of fitting a predefined face shape and appearance model to an image. This can be done using a variety of approaches (e.g., active appearance models (AAM) (Cootes, Edwards, & Taylor,

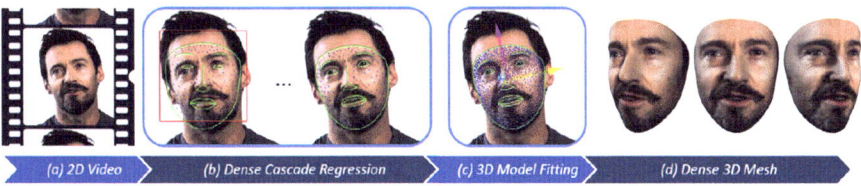

Fig. 7.2 Iterative model fitting and alignment of face image from video (Jeni, Cohn, & Kanade, 2016). A dense cascade regression is used to detect the face, fit a predetermined model, and iteratively adjust model parameters to improve the model's fit. The face then is aligned to a canonical view, typically a frontal view as shown in the second image from the right. Other views are possible (e.g., first and third images from the right). The iterative model fitting and alignment are fully automatic

2001), constrained local models (CLM) (Saragih, Lucey, & Cohn, 2011), 3D CLM (Baltrusaitis, Robinson, & Morency, 2012), supervised descent method (SDM) (Zhang & De la Torre, 2015), and related methods (Jeni et al., 2016)). The first of these approaches, AAMs, are semiautomatic using person-specific methods that must first be customized for each participant for face and facial features tracking. For each participant, approximately 3% of video frames must be manually labeled to learn an AAM, prior to the fully automatic tracking phase. Because qualified personnel are required for training AAMs before they can be applied to a new face, they are not ideal for general use.

More recent approaches to face tracking are well suited for general use. Approaches referred to as CLM (constrained local model), 3D CLM, and SDM (supervised descent method) are fully automatic and person independent. They may be used with previously unknown faces. These methods are thus better suited to research and clinical use for which time-intensive person-specific methods may not be feasible.

For all these approaches, the predefined models are deformed iteratively to fit the actual face and facial expression. Each optimization step predicts improved model parameters to obtain the closest possible match to the face. An example of iterative improvements in a face model and subsequent alignment to a canonical view can be seen in Fig. 7.2 (from Jeni et al., 2016). The example shown is fully automatic. The registered, or aligned, shape and appearance correspond to synthesized shape and appearance images in which non-rigid variations due to head pose (i.e., translation, rotation, and scale) were automatically removed (see Fig. 7.2c). The resulting normalized shape refers to the x- and y- coordinates of the N vertex points (66 in the case of the AAMs model) leading to a vector of Nx2 dimensional features (Lucey et al., 2012).

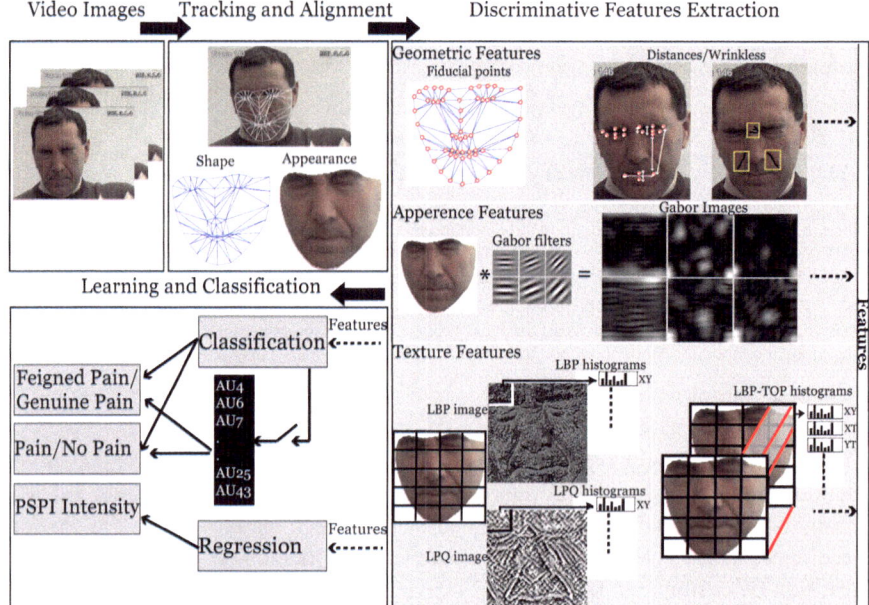

Fig. 7.3 Overview of automated face analysis (AFA) to detect occurrence and intensity of pain and discrimination between genuine and feigned pain

Discriminative Features Extraction

Discriminative features encode changes in normalized facial shape and appearance with representations that afford invariance to illumination, registration error, and variability across subjects. Several types of discriminative features have been used for pain assessment from facial expression. We describe the three main approaches in the following sections.

Geometric Features

Geometric features refer to predefined sets of geometrical distances between facial landmarks (i.e., eyes, eyebrows, mouth, and nose). These geometrical distances measure changes in displacement between fiduciary points (i.e., nodes of the "face mesh") around permanent facial features as shown in Fig. 7.3. As an example, the displacement between points around the upper and lower eyelids decreases to zero during blinks and eye closures. Geometric distances, however, lack robustness to errors in face alignment (Chew et al., 2012), and fail to represent changes in appearance that are highly discriminative for pain expression. For instance, nasal root wrinkles (i.e., AU4) that occur in pain may produce little change in the shape of facial features but produce changes in the texture of the skin around the nose.

Without attention to appearance and texture features, some pain related facial deformations might be difficult or impossible to detect.

Appearance and Texture Features

Appearance and texture features characterize changes in texture of the face. Among the most used appearance and texture based features for pain assessment are local descriptors. Examples include Gabor and Log-Normal filters, Local Binary Patterns (LBP), and Local Phase Quantization (LPQ) (see Fig. 7.3). Because appearance and texture features are robust to variation in illumination, scale, and registration error, they are highly discriminative for facial expression recognition in comparison with geometric features (Chew et al., 2012).

Gabor and Log-Normal filters (Hammal & Cohn, 2012; Hammal & Massot, 2011; Littlewort, Bartlett, & Lee, 2009) are referred to as biologically inspired because they resemble the function of cells in mammalian visual cortex. They represent frequency and orientation variation in texture images. The magnitude of facial appearance deformations (e.g., strong or soft appearance of nasal root wrinkles) can be measured directly in the energy-based representation by the magnitude of energy appearing in the face relative to a relaxed state (see Fig. 7.2).

LBPs characterize a local texture pattern with a binary code obtained by thresholding a neighborhood of pixels with the gray value of its center pixel (Ojala et al., 1996; Ojala, Pietikainen, & Maenpaa, 2002). A face texture can thus be described with a histogram of LBP codes (see Fig. 7.3). LBPs are computationally inexpensive (i.e., fast to compute), which make them well suited for clinical adaptations. LPQ is based on quantizing the Fourier transform phase in local neighborhoods. Similar to an LBP, an LPQ describes a local neighborhood with an integer (see Fig. 7.3). Local histograms simply count LPQ patterns to describe the face texture (Ojansivu & Heikkila, 2008).

While appearance and texture features most often are extracted from individual video frames without respect to their order, they may also be extracted and ordered for contiguous frames. The former case is referred to as spatial sampling; the latter is referred to as spatiotemporal sampling because the timing of changes in facial appearance is represented. Spatiotemporal representations of spatial LBP and LPQ are referred to as LBP-TOP and LPQ-TOP, respectively. LBP-TOP and LPQ-TOP combine changes in motion and appearance together to describe the spatiotemporal pattern/changes of facial texture (i.e., dynamic facial texture) (Pietikäinen, 2010; Zhao & Pietikäinen, 2007). Dynamic facial textures are characterized by a set of volumes in space and time. The neighborhood of each pixel is thus defined in terms of three-dimensional space-by-time volumes, referred to as textons. Textons may be extracted into histograms to characterize the spatiotemporal changes in facial expression of pain (see Fig. 7.3). Preliminary work suggests that spatiotemporal representations yield higher accuracy than spatial representations for pain assessment (Bartlett, Littlewort, Frank, & Lee, 2014; Yang et al., 2016).

Learning and Classification

The final step in automatic measurement of pain is classification. A classifier is an algorithm (or a mathematical function) that maps input data to an output category. In the case of pain assessment, the input data are the discriminative features and the output categories are pain scores. To learn associations between features and pain scores, the extracted discriminative features are input to sets of classifiers. Among the most used classifiers for pain assessment (and action unit detection more generally) are support vector machines (SVMs) (Ashraf et al., 2009; Bartlett et al., 2014; Hammal & Cohn, 2012; Littlewort et al., 2009; Lucey et al., 2012). SVMs are binary classifiers that attempt to find the hyperplane (a decision boundary in a high-dimensional space) that maximizes the margin between positive and negative observations for a specified class (e.g., pain vs. no-pain) (Vapnik, 1995, 1998). Other classification strategies include regression techniques (Florea, Florea, & Vertan, 2014; Kaltwang, Rudovic, & Pantic, 2012), heteroscedastic conditional ordinal random fields (Rudovic, Pavlovic, & Pantic, 2013), multiple instance learning with boosting (Sikka, Dhall, & Bartlett, 2014), random forests (Werner et al., 2016), and, more recently, deep learning using Recurrent Convolutional Neural Networks (RCNN) (Zhou, Hong, Su, & Zhao, 2016).

Deep-learning approaches, such as CNN, markedly differ from other approaches. While other approaches for classification, such as SVM, learn association between a priori discriminative features (e.g., Gabor features) and pain scores, deep learning learns features empirically by integrating feature learning and classification over multiple iterations (LeCun, Bengio, & Hinton, 2015). For action unit detection, deep learning has achieved higher accuracy than other approaches and may be more generalizable to new data (Ghosh et al., 2015; Jaiswal et al., 2016). Because deep learning has yet to be applied more broadly to pain detection, its benefits for evaluating pain occurrence and intensity are still to be evaluated.

After the training phase, a classifier's performance is evaluated by testing the accuracy of its predictions for new test examples (new observations). To avoid over fitting or spurious correlation, an iterative k-fold cross-validation is used. K-fold cross-validation is a classifier's validation technique. It involves multiple rounds of training, tuning, and testing on independent subsets of data. That is, data are partitioned into k (e.g., 5 or 10) folds, or subsamples. On each round of cross-validation, the classifier is trained using all but one of the folds. The predictions of the optimized classifier then are tested through extrapolation to the final fold. This process is repeated k times until the classifiers have been tested on all folds. Performance is assessed by calculating the average results from the k different test sets.

Performance may be quantified using a variety of metrics. Accuracy refers to the percentage of correct agreements. While appealing, accuracy can be difficult to interpret when data are skewed. For events that rarely occur, a high level of agreement may mask very low agreement for instances in which one or the other method fails to detect an event when the other does. Other metrics include F1 and ROC. F1 is the geometric mean of precision and recall and is affected by skew. ROC quantifies the relation between true and false positives. Girard and Cohn recommend

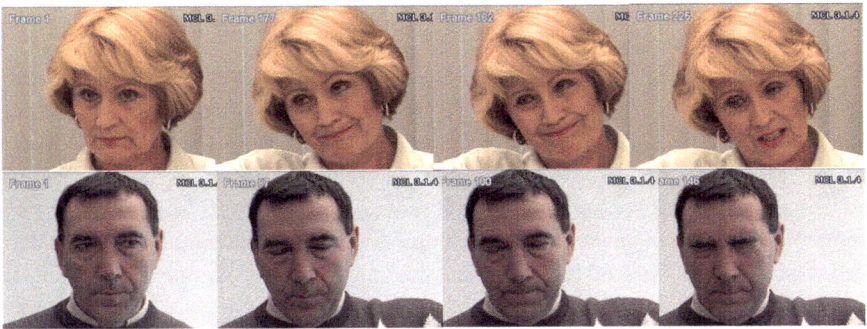

Fig. 7.4 Examples of image sequences from the UNBC-McMaster Pain Archive database (Lucey, Cohn, Matthews, et al., 2011; Lucey, Cohn, Prkachin, et al., 2011; Lucey et al., 2012)

kappa for binary data (e.g., occurrence/non-occurrence of pain), weighted kappa for ordinal data (e.g., PSPI scores), and ICC for continuous data (Girard & Cohn, 2016). Kappa and weighted kappa quantify agreement while adjusting for chance, but are influenced by imbalanced data (Brennan & Prediger, 1981; Shrout & Fleiss, 1979). ICC can quantify consistency as well as agreement; both are relevant for continuous measures. When studies use different metrics or skew varies, comparisons across studies are problematic.

Facial Expression of Pain: Databases for Automatic Pain Assessment

To learn the association between discriminative features and pain occurrence or intensity, ample, well-annotated video from diverse participants responding to varied pain elicitors or conditions are necessary for training and testing the classifiers. In the following, we distinguish between databases that are publicly available (or soon to be available) and those that are not. Publically available databases may be used by different researchers, which makes possible direct comparisons between different methods. The databases vary with respect to participants' characteristics, type of pain, type of labels (e.g., behavioral observation or self-report of pain intensity), and available demographics (e.g., age, ethnicity) and measures.

Publicly Available Pain Databases

UNBC-McMaster Shoulder Pain Archive (Pain Archive)

The Pain Archive (Lucey, Cohn, Matthews, et al., 2011; Lucey, Cohn, Prkachin, Solomon, & Matthews, 2011; Lucey et al., 2012) was the first effort to address the need for well-annotated facial expression recordings of participants with acute pain.

Participants, self-identified as having a problem with shoulder pain, were recruited from physiotherapy clinics and by advertisements. Participants suffered from arthritis, bursitis, tendonitis, subluxation, rotator cuff injuries, impingement syndromes, bone spur, capsulitis, and dislocation. The participants were video-recorded during abduction, flexion, and internal and external rotation of their affected and unaffected shoulders.

The Pain Archive is composed of 200 sequences from 25 different participants (66 female) in the active condition (see Fig. 7.4). For each video sequence, the distribution includes 66 AAM tracked landmarks at frame-by-frame level (fiducial points around the eyes, eyebrows, and mouth, see section "Automated Measurement of Facial Expression of Pain") and several types of per-frame annotation. Expert-labeled FACS codes were scored on a 0–5 ranking of intensity. Intercoder percent agreement as calculated by the Ekman–Friesen formula (Ekman & Friesen, 1978) was 95%. Self-reported pain intensity and observer's ratings of pain intensity (OPI) were annotated at the sequence level. Offline observer ratings were performed on a 6-point Likert-type scale that ranged from 0 (no pain) to 5 (strong pain). To assess interobserver reliability of the OPI pain ratings, a second rater independently rated 210 randomly selected videos. The Pearson correlation between the observers' OPI was 0.80, which represents high interobserver reliability. The Pain Archive is the most widely used dataset for automatic pain detection and intensity measurement from facial expression (see section "State of the Art in Automatic Detection of Occurrence and Intensity of Pain").

BioVid Heat Pain

The BioVid Heat Pain Database (BioVid) (Walter et al., 2013) is a multimodal pain database of acute heat-induced pain in healthy participants. Four intensities of heat-induced pain were administered. Pain intensity was calibrated according to each participant's pain threshold (i.e., feeling of heat turns into pain) and pain tolerance (i.e., pain becomes intolerable). For each participant, each of the four pain intensities was stimulated 20 times in randomized order and used as ground truth for the corresponding videos. For each stimulus, the maximum temperature was held for 4 s, alternating with pauses of 8–12 s. The distributed portion of BioVid is composed of 87 participants that range in age from 18 to 65 years. For each participant, BioVid includes baseline (20 samples with no pain) and 4×20 pain intensities. For each sample, participants were video-recorded using synchronized cameras at 30 fps and Microsoft Kinect camera (see Fig. 7.5), which measures depth information. Each video is 5.5 s in duration. Unlike Pain Archive, BioVid lacks behavioral annotation of facial expression. For each video, ground truth consists of subjective thresholds for heat pain intensity on a 1–4 Likert scale. Because the correspondence of self-reported thresholds and facial expression is unknown, manual annotation of the dataset would greatly increase its value for training facial-based measures of occurrence and intensity of pain.

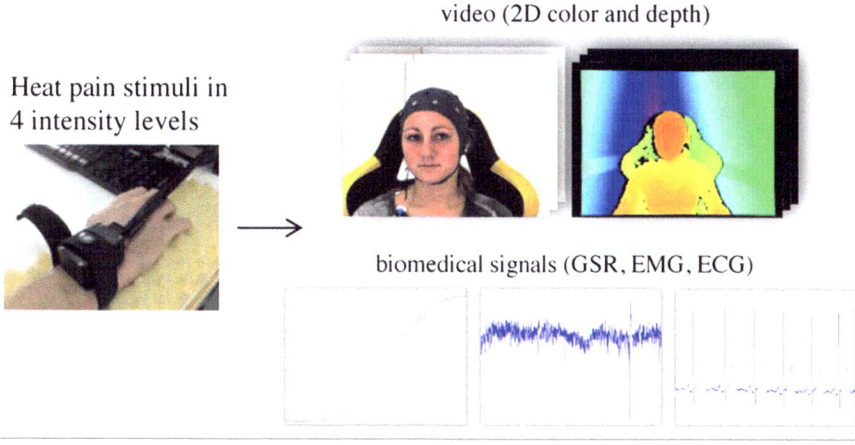

Fig. 7.5 Overview of the data collection of the BioVid Heat Pain Database from Walter et al. (2013)

In addition to video, electrodermal conductance (SCL), electrocardiogram (ECG), electromyogram (EMG), and electroencephalogram (EEG) were recorded and distributed for multimodal pain intensity measurement.

EmoPain

The EmoPain database was collected as part of the Emotion and Pain (EmoPain) project (Aung et al., 2015). EmoPain project is a multidisciplinary collaboration of computer vision and machine learning scientists, clinical psychologists, physiotherapists, and experts in pain management and rehabilitation. A primary goal of the project is the development of an intelligent system that achieves ubiquitous monitoring and assessment of patients' lower back pain (LBP) and related mood and range and quality of movement in a clinical environment (Aung et al., 2015). A secondary goal is to disseminate a multimodal, spontaneous, clinically relevant, well-defined pain database to promote research and development of machine intelligent systems dedicated to the assessment of LBP (Aung et al., 2015).

Participants are 22 adults identified as having LBP for more than 6 months. They were selected from the Pain Management Centre at the National Hospital for Neurology and Neurosurgery in London and through pain charities in London. Participants were recorded while undertaking a series of instructed and non-instructed movements. The movements were considered to reflect traditional scenarios of physiotherapist directed therapy and home-based self-directed therapy for LBP (e.g., sitting, reaching forwards, bending down, and walking). To elicit a range of pain-related behavioral reactions, instructed movements were obtained for two levels of difficulty.

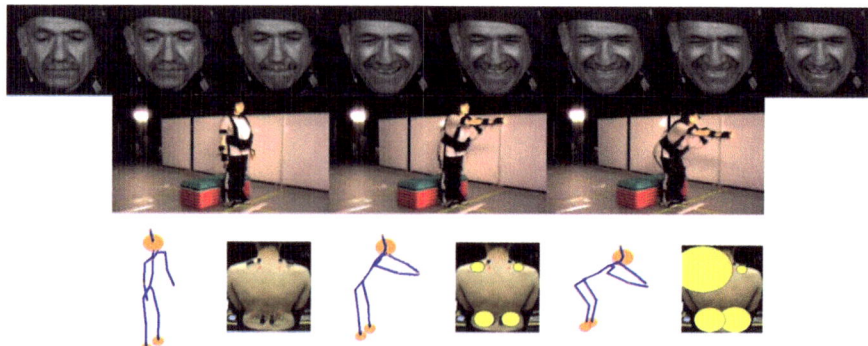

Fig. 7.6 Overview of the data collection of the EmoPain database from Aung et al. (2015). The top row shows video frames from one of the four cameras showing examples of facial expressions of pain. The middle row shows three frames from patient undergoing a reaching forward exercise. The bottom row shows the concurrent motion captured avatar (left) and back muscle activity (right) visualized as circles with radii corresponding to the rectified sEMG amplitude (Aung et al., 2015)

Participants' data consists of four fully synchronized data streams: (1) high resolution multiple-view face videos, (2) head-mounted and fixed microphone recordings, (3) full body 3D motion capture, and (4) electromyographic signals from the upper and lower back muscles (see Fig. 7.6). After each exercise, participants reported their level of pain and anxiety using Likert-type 0–10 scales. Three independent coders also performed Offline observer ratings. Facial expression of pain from video was measured using a joystick device on a continuous scale. These values then were thresholded into a dichotomous variable (i.e., pain vs. no pain) for which interobserver reliability was low. To select a more reliable subset of the data, frames for which only one or two coders detected pain were then omitted from consideration. Interobserver agreement for these frames was higher but still relatively low (Kripendorf's alpha and Fleiss kappa = 0.393). They next used a variant of canonical correlation for which ICC for continuous values was acceptable. The EmoPain database is not publicly available yet and will be released soon for the research community. Given the difficulties with interobserver reliability, caution would be advised in selecting ground truth (i.e., human defined pain score used for training automatic classifiers) from the full EmoPain dataset.

Non-publicly Available Pain Databases

In Littlewort et al. (2009), 26 participants (20 female, all university students) were video-recorded under three experimental ordered conditions: baseline, posed pain, and genuine pain (Littlewort et al., 2009). In a follow-up study (Bartlett et al., 2014), 45 new participants (27 female, all university students) were video-recorded under two ordered conditions: posed pain and genuine pain (Bartlett et al., 2014). In both datasets the pain condition consisted of cold pressor pain induced by immersing participants' arm in cold water. For the baseline and faked pain conditions, the water was 20 °C. For genuine pain the water was 3 °C in (Littlewort et al., 2009) and 5 °C in (Bartlett et al., 2014). For each condition, subjects were instructed to immerse their forearm into the water up to the elbow for 60 s. Participants' facial expressions were recorded using a digital video camera during each condition. In faked pain condition, participants were asked to manipulate their facial expressions so that an "expert would be convinced they were in actual pain." (Bartlett et al., 2014; Littlewort et al., 2009).

In Hammal and Kunz (2012) and Hammal, Kunz, Arguin, and Gosselin (2008), pain video recordings were acquired by a research group working on the relation between facial expressions and the neural networks of pain (Kunz, Chatelle, Lautenbacher, & Rainville, 2008). The videos were recorded during a study on the relation between pain catastrophizing and facial responsiveness of pain in healthy, pain-free individuals (Kunz et al., 2008). Forty subjects (twenty female) were video-recorded. Pain was induced experimentally by means of a Peltier-based, computerized thermal stimulator with a 3×3 cm^2 contact probe attached to the participants' left lower leg. Baseline temperature was always set to 38 °C. One non-painful (1 °C below the individual pain threshold) and two painful thermal stimuli (2–3 °C above the individual pain threshold) were applied in a random order. The temperature increased from baseline with a heating rate of 4 °C/s to the preset temperatures, remained at a plateau for 5 s and returned to baseline with a rate of 4 °C/s. ISIs varied between 30 and 35 s (Kunz et al., 2008). Participants were video-recorded during the experiments with a video camera placed in front of the participants at a distance of approximately 4 m.

In Sikka et al. (2015), participants consisted of 50 children from 5 to 17 years old of age (average age = 12 years) undergoing laparoscopic appendectomy. Fifty-four participants were boys, thirty-five Hispanic, nine non-Hispanic white, five Asian, and one Native American. Data collection occurred over three study visits: first, within 24 h after appendectomy; second, 1 calendar day after the first visit time lapse of 20 h between visits 1 and 2; and 3, at a follow-up visit 21 days postoperatively. At each study visit, children were video-recorded and self- and parent-rated pain scores were obtained. At visits 1 and 2, nurse ratings of pain also were obtained. Video recordings were during two pain experiences: endogenous pain (during 5 min as a measure of ongoing pain) and exogenous pain (transient pain when manual pressure was exerted at the surgical site for 2, 10-s periods). Pain ratings (self-reported and per-proxy) were obtained using the 0-to-10 Numerical Rating Scale (NRS).

Summary

The publically available Pain Archive, BioVid, and EmoPain databases address the need for annotated facial expression recordings during induced pain. However, these databases are limited to a laboratory environment and focus on a single type of pain elicitor (e.g., unspecified shoulder injury or temperature probe). Pain can have many possible causes (e.g., cardiac conditions and chronic illnesses such as sickle cell disease) that may produce different behavioral responses both within and across modalities. Given the variety of pain experiences, variety of procedures, both experimental and observational, participants, and sensors are needed. Additionally, pain experience and perception could differ by gender, age, and ethnic background (Fillingim, King, Ribeiro-Dasilva, Rahim-Williams, & Riley, 2009; Green et al., 2003; Wandner, Scipio, Hirsh, Torres, & Robinson, 2012). To the best of our knowledge, with the exception of the non-publicly available database collected by Sikka et al. (2015), demographic information is incomplete or lacking. In the future, it would be important to collect participants' demographics (e.g., age, ethnicity) to investigate the variance/invariance of pain experience and measurement across different demographics for a more comprehensive assessment of pain occurrence and intensity.

State of the Art in Automatic Detection of Occurrence and Intensity of Pain

The last decade has witnessed an increasing effort to develop vision-based methods to detect the occurrence and intensity of pain. Most efforts were trained and evaluated on the Pain Archive database (Ashraf et al., 2009; Florea et al., 2014; Hammal & Cohn, 2012; Kaltwang et al., 2012; Lucey, Cohn, Matthews, et al., 2011; Lucey, Cohn, Prkachin, et al., 2011; Lucey et al., 2012; Rudovic et al., 2013; Sikka et al., 2014). A smaller number used the BioVid Heat Pain database (Kachele et al., 2015; Werner et al., 2016; Yang et al., 2016) and non-publicly available databases using induced or feigned pain (Bartlett et al., 2014; Hammal & Kunz, 2012; Hammal et al., 2008; Littlewort et al., 2009) and clinically and well-characterized pain (Sikka et al., 2015). No studies have explicitly trained and tested classifiers on different databases in order to evaluate generalizability of automatic pain assessment across databases. Unless generalizability between separate databases is examined, it remains unknown whether methods developed in one database would be valid in others.

Within one or more of the databases, researchers have automatically detected pain (Ashraf et al., 2009; Lucey et al., 2012; Sikka et al., 2014), differentiated feigned from genuine pain (Bartlett et al., 2014; Littlewort et al., 2009), detected pain intensity (Florea et al., 2014; Hammal & Cohn, 2012; Kaltwang et al., 2012; Rudovic et al., 2013; Sikka et al., 2015), and distinguished pain from expressions of emotion (Hammal & Kunz, 2012). In the following sections, we introduce recent advances in computer vision and machine learning for automatic analysis and recognition of pain occurrence and intensity from facial expression. Due to space limitation, not all work could be included.

Detection of Pain Occurrence

Using the Pain Archive, Ashraf et al. (2009) proposed the first automated approach to detecting pain from digitized video. Using person specific Active Appearance Models (AAMs) they extracted facial shape and appearance, normalized them to remove variation due to head pose (see Fig. 7.2), and inputted them to an SVM classifier to learn presence from absence of pain in each video frame. The obtained frame-by-frame results then were summed to give a cumulative score for each video sequence. They then used a threshold to detect occurrence of pain in video sequences (the threshold was set such that false accept rate equaled false reject rate). To ascertain the utility of the various AAM based representations, they also evaluated the use of shape and/or appearance alone and in combination. Best results were obtained by using both shape and appearance features rather than using only one (Ashraf et al., 2009).

PSPI scores are based on FACS action units (see section "Facial Actions That Communicate Pain"). Expert raters annotate AU intensity at the frame-by-frame level and then the PSPI metric is used to compute pain presence (PSPI > 0) and intensity (PSPI scores). Lucey, Cohn, Matthews, et al. (2011) and Lucey, Cohn, Prkachin, et al. (2011) asked whether automated pain detection needed to follow the same course. That is, to first learn AUs and then use the automatically detected AUs to detect presence from absence of pain. To answer this question, Lucey, Cohn, Matthews, et al. (2011) and Lucey, Cohn, Prkachin, et al. (2011) used a two-step approach, where first ten linear SVMs were trained to detect ten AUs and then fused using a Logistical Linear Regression (Brummer & du Preez, 2005) to detect pain. Similar to Ashraf et al. (2009), the authors compared the performances of appearance and shape features alone and in combination for AUs and pain detection, respectively. Perhaps not surprisingly, they found that fusing AAM based shape and appearance representations together with a Logistical Linear Regression, improved both AU and pain detection.

To address the problem of dealing with multiple segments of pain or no pain within video sequences, Sikka and colleagues (Sikka et al., 2014) proposed a multisegment multi-instance learning (MS-MIL) framework for pain detection. Each video was represented as a bag containing multiple segments of varying durations. The segments were generated via multiple clustering of a sequence or running a multiscale temporal scanning window. The extracted BoW representation was used to train the classifier to determine whether pain is present or absent in a given video sequence.

Most approaches to pain detection seek to determine only whether pain is present or absent in a given video frame or across a video sequence. Hammal and colleagues were one of the first to detect pain among the six basic facial expressions (multiclass classification (pain vs. six basic facial expressions) rather than two-alternative forced choice classification (pain vs. no pain)) (Hammal & Kunz, 2012; Hammal et al., 2008). The authors proposed a hybrid machine learning approach based on the Transferable Belief Model (TBM: a generalization of the Bayesian model). The proposed model is based on the dynamic fusion of geometric distances, appearance features around the wrinkle areas (the deepening of transient facial features), and the context information for the dynamic recognition of pain in a video sequence (Hammal & Kunz, 2012; Hammal et al., 2008). Experimental results, on two-alternative forced-choice and on eight-alternative forced choice bases, showed good classification rates for both tasks.

Discrimination Between Feigned and Genuine Pain

An important problem in medical practice often is to distinguish between genuine and feigned pain. Using the non-publicly available feigned and genuine pain database described above, Bartlett, Littlewort, and colleagues (Bartlett et al., 2014; Littlewort et al., 2009) investigated the problem of automatically recognizing feigned from genuine pain from facial expressions. The authors employed a two-stage approach. In the first stage, 20 linear SVMs were trained separately to detect the presence of 20 AUs at the fame-by-frame level (Bartlett et al., 2014). This data was then passed to a second stage, in which classifiers were trained to detect genuine pain from faked pain using window-based statistics (Littlewort et al., 2009). To do so, each video was organized into overlapping segments of 500 frames. For each segment, a set of five statistics was measured to characterize each of the 20 detected AU and used to train an SVM classifier to dissociate presence from absence of pain. Another SVM was trained to recognize genuine from feigned facial expression of pain.

In a following study Bartlett et al. (2014) proposed a Bag of Temporal Features (BoTF) descriptor instead of the window-based statistics to condense the 20 action units detected during the first stage. Two sets of descriptors were employed: one set described the dynamics of facial movement events and another set described the intervals between events (interval between AUs). The extracted BoTF descriptors were then used to train an SVM to discriminate genuine from feigned pain videos.

In a both studies (Bartlett et al., 2014; Littlewort et al., 2009), the authors asked whether classifiers could discriminate genuine from feigned pain better than human observers could. Using the same data, they found that classifiers were far more accurate than naïve observers (Bartlett et al., 2014; Littlewort et al., 2009) and briefly trained observers (Bartlett et al., 2014). They interpreted the classifier's better accuracy to their ability to use the dynamics of behavior that were missed by human observers (Bartlett et al., 2014). This interpretation is not altogether satisfying, however, in that both humans and computer viewed the same videos.

Measurement of Pain Intensity

Most approaches to pain detection seek to determine only whether pain is present or absent in a given video frame or across multiple video frames. We often are interested, however, in the intensity of pain. Hammal and Cohn (2012), extended previous efforts for the measurement of four pain scores from the PSPI metric (i.e., none (PSPI = 0), trace (PSPI = 1), weak (PSPI = 2), and strong (PSPI >= 3)). For each video frame, AAMs were first used to track and register rigid and non-rigid face motion (Lucey et al., 2012). Based on this information, the canonical appearance of the face (CAPP) was extracted for each frame (see Fig. 7.3). CAPP features were then rescaled to 96 × 96 pixels and passed through a set of Log-Normal filters of 7 frequencies and 15 orientations (Hammal & Cohn, 2012; Hammal & Massot, 2011). The extracted spatial face representation was then aligned as a vector of 9216 features used by four SVMs trained separately for the automatic measurement of four pain intensity levels.

Kaltwang et al. (2012) extended previous efforts by comparing shape and appearance based features for the measurement of 16 pain intensity scores from the PSPI at the frame-by-frame level. The authors compared several approaches: The 66 AAM based facial landmarks available with the Pain Archive database (Lucey, Cohn, Matthews, et al., 2011; Lucey, Cohn, Prkachin, et al., 2011; Lucey et al., 2012); Discrete Cosine Transform coefficients (DCT) (Ahmed, Natarajan, & Rao, 1974); and Local Binary Patterns (LBP) (Ojala et al., 2002). For each set of features, a separate Relevance Vector Regression (RVR) (Tipping, 2001) was trained. The outputs of the RVRs trained using different feature sets were then combined in two ways: first, by computing the mean estimate of the regressors, and second, by using the outputs of separate regressors as an input to another RVR, which gives a single estimate for pain intensity. The combination of appearance features (DCT and LBP) led to the best performance for pain intensity measurement (compared to the separately trained RVRs or shape appearance features).

Werner et al. (2016) proposed an automatic system for the recognition of five self-reported BioVid Heat Pain intensity scores. For each video frame, 49 facial landmarks and the 6 degrees of rigid head pose were automatically tracked. Similarly to Hammal et al. (2008) and Hammal and Kunz (2012), the 49 facial landmarks were converted to a small set of geometrical distances (e.g., distances between brows and eyes). Using the tracked facial landmarks they calculated the mean gradient magnitude within a set of rectangular regions around the nasolabial folds and the nasal root wrinkles areas (see Fig. 7.3). By extracting the visual features (distances, head pose, and mean gradient) at each frame of the video, a time series representation was obtained for the entire video. The velocity (first derivative) and acceleration (second derivative) of each smoothed time series were then computed. A set of 16 condensed statistical features was then extracted from each time series (e.g., mean, median, range) and concatenated to one feature vector to train a Random Forest classifier (Ho, 1995, 1998) for pain intensity measurement.

Early approaches to pain intensity detection investigated either spatial features or spatiotemporal features on different databases. To assess the efficiency of the temporal information (compared to the spatial information) for pain intensity measurement, Yang et al. (2016) compared both approaches on the Pain Archive and BioVid Heat Pain databases. The authors compared three spatial local descriptors (e.g., LBP) against their spatiotemporal form that takes into account the video dynamics (e.g., LBP-TOP) for pain intensity levels. Sixty-eight fiducial points were first automatically detected and used to crop and align the participants' faces for each frame. Using the aligned faces, the spatial and spatiotemporal appearance-based features (using Three Orthogonal Planes, i.e., TOP), such as local binary patterns (LBP and LBP-TOP, respectively), local phase quantization (LPQ and LPQ-TOP, respectively) and binarized statistical image features (BSIF and BSIF-TOP, respectively), were extracted for each image and video, respectively (see example in Fig. 7.3). The resulting discriminative features were then combined and used as the input of a set of SVMs trained separately to detect the presence and absence of pain and pain intensity, respectively. For both pain detection (two-alternative forced-choice classification) and pain intensity estimation (multiclass choice classification), the authors used the one-vs-one strategy, where one SVM is trained for each pair of classes (Yang et al., 2016). A mean voting method was then applied to obtain the final decision. For all three different local appearance-based discriminative features (LBP, LPQ, and BSIF) the corresponding spatiotemporal forms (LBP-TOP, LPQ-TOP, and BSIF-TOP) achieved better performance for both pain classification and pain intensity measurement. These results highlight the importance of temporal information for automatic measurement of pain occurrence and intensity.

Almost all work in pain detection has been in adults. Pain in children and especially in infants, is an important problem (Rajasagaram, Taylor, Braitberg, Pearsell, & Capp, 2009; Singer, Gulla, & Thode, 2002; Zhou, Roberts, & Horgan, 2008). Infants are unable to report pain and pain is difficult to assess by self-report in children. Pain more often is assessed by proxy—by parents or clinicians and is underestimated. One of the few efforts to automatically detect pain in children is that of Sikka and Bartlett and their colleagues (Sikka et al., 2015). For each video sequence, 14 AUs were detected using the model proposed by Littlewort et al. (2009). For each detected AU, a set of statistics (e.g., mean, 75th percentile, and 25th percentile) was used as discriminative features to assess pain intensity in two separate regression-based approaches (a first for the detection of presence from absence of pain, and a second for the estimation of pain intensity). Regression-based estimates of pain intensity were compared with child, parent, and nurse ratings. Automatic detection of presence from absence of pain demonstrated good-to-excellent accuracy in both ongoing and transient pain conditions (Sikka et al., 2015). Similarly, automatic detection of pain intensity demonstrated strong correlations with patient self-reported pain intensity and parent-equivalent estimation of children's pain intensity after appendectomy. This initial effort suggests the feasibility of automatic measurement of pain in children.

All of the approaches to date have used a priori features, such as shape and Gabor filters. An exception is a recent effort to use a deep-learning based approach in which feature representations and classifiers are learned simultaneously. Zhou et al. (2016) proposed a regression framework based on Recurrent Convolutional Neural Networks (RCNN) for automatic frame-by-frame PSPI pain intensity estimation. The normalized AAM-based appearance was used within a sliding window to predict pain intensity of each frame by considering sufficiently large historical frames while limiting the scale of the parameters within the model (Zhou et al., 2016).

Challenges and Future Directions

With few exceptions (e.g., Sikka et al., 2015), most previous efforts in automatic assessment of pain are limited to data collected in a laboratory environment and focus on a single modality (e.g., face), and a single type of pain elicitor (e.g., unspecified shoulder injury (Ashraf et al., 2009; Hammal & Cohn, 2012; Kaltwang et al., 2012; Lucey, Cohn, Matthews, et al., 2011; Lucey, Cohn, Prkachin, et al., 2011; Lucey et al., 2012; Rudovic et al., 2013; Sikka et al., 2014) or temperature probe (Bartlett et al., 2014; Hammal & Kunz, 2012; Hammal et al., 2008; Littlewort et al., 2009; Walter et al., 2013; Werner et al., 2016)). However, pain can have many possible causes (e.g., spinal stenosis, rotator cuff tear, cardiac conditions, or chronic illnesses such as low back pain) that may produce multiple behavioral responses both within and across modalities (e.g., facial expression, head, and body postures/ movements). Pain can be acute, as a result of an injury (e.g., touching a burning ember), or chronic (e.g., pain that persists after an injury heals). Behavioral pain responses may well differ between acute and chronic pain. For instance, acute pain is likely associated with faster onset. Presence of other people and context further influence the experience and expression of pain. Pain is thus a complex subjective experience that may have varied indicators, which influence its communication to others. A machine-based method should take such factors into consideration.

With few exceptions (Werner et al., 2016; Yang et al., 2016), most efforts for pain detection to date have been semiautomatic. That is, they have used AAMs, which must first be trained separately for each participant. More recent approaches to facial feature tracking and representation (e.g., CLM and SDM) are fully automatic and have strong concurrent validity with person-dependent AAMs. These are robust as well to skin color, non-frontal view, and head movement up to about ±60° from frontal (Jeni et al., 2016; Zhang & De la Torre, 2015). These innovations will contribute toward making pain detection and intensity measurement feasible for clinical use.

Temporal Dynamics

The focus has been on detection of pain occurrence and intensity in individual video frames or in short segments of video. This emphasis on static images or subset of images is consistent with approaches to AU detection more generally, in which temporal information is infrequently used (Corneanu, Oliu, Cohn, & Escalera, 2015). However, pain communication is dynamic. Pain onset may be gradual or abrupt. Differences in timing may be critical in detecting fake versus actual pain. Dynamics of pain warrants explicit attention not only because they may improve pain detection but because they further our understanding of the pain experience.

Fully Automatic Multimodal Pain Assessment

Pain is communicated through different modalities (Arif et al., 2010; Garrett, Happ, Costello, & Fried-Oken, 2007; Gélinas, Arbour, Michaud, Vaillant, & Desjardins, 2011; Monroe & Mion, 2012; Payen et al., 2001). For this reason, efforts are needed to extend technologies in computer vision and machine learning beyond facial expression to include body and head movement, speech, and paralinguistic communication related to pain experience.

Head and body movements have proven critical to the communication of emotion (Hammal & Cohn, 2014; Hammal, Cohn, & George, 2014; Hammal, Cohn, Heike, & Speltz, 2015; Hammal, Cohn, & Messinger, 2015), and monitoring of post-surgery pain of cognitively impaired elders (Arif et al., 2010). In physical medicine and rehabilitation, specific body movements and postural patterns can reveal emotional conflict, stress responses, and the capacity to relax (Haugstad et al., 2006; Joshi, Dhall, Goecke, & Cohn, 2013; Karg et al., 2014; Kleinsmith & Bianchi-Berthouze, 2013; Kvale, Ljunggren, & Johnsen, 2003; Vlaeyen & Linton, 2000; Zagyapan, Iyem, Kurkcuoglu, Pelin, & Tekindal, 2012). Body language is an important behavioral index of pain in patients with moderate to severe cognitive impairments, and those who have difficulty communicating verbally (de Knegt et al., 2013; Warden, Hurley, & Volicer, 2003).

Vocal features related to affect recognition (El Ayadi, Kamel, & Karray, 2011; Scherer, 2003; Schuller, Batliner, Steidl, & Seppi, 2011) and depression severity (Cummins, Epps, & Ambikairajah, 2013; Williamson et al., 2013; Yang et al., 2013) have been identified. With respect to pain, nonverbal (e.g., screaming, sounds of distress) and verbal (e.g., "ouch," "owie") pain vocalizations (Arif et al., 2010; de Knegt et al., 2013) have proven clinically useful for pain detection in young children and others with limited linguistic abilities (Dubois, Bringuier, Capdevilla, & Pry, 2008). There is strong likelihood that automatic analysis of acoustic characteristics of vocal expression can contribute to pain detection and understanding.

Automatic multimodal measurement affords potentially rich sets of behavioral features to include in automatic measurement of the occurrence and intensity of pain. Newer databases that include multimodal measures, such as EmoPain and BioVid make this development possible. Efforts in this direction will enable the objective measurement and monitoring of pain intensity in clinical, family, and work environments.

Interpersonal Influence and Context

Pain is a complex psychological and physiological experience that requires consideration of social and communicative displays between patients, healthcare givers, and families. Interpersonal conceptualization of pain requires a consideration of both the ways in which pain is expressed in a given context and the reactions of others (Coll, Gregoire, Latimer, Eugene, & Jackson, 2011; Craig, 2009; Craig, Prkachin, et al., 2010; Craig, Versloot, Goubert, Vervoort, & Crombez, 2010). Perception of pain in others elicits behavioral and emotional responses (Coll et al., 2011; Craig, Prkachin, et al., 2010; Craig, Versloot, et al., 2010). These responses influence the experience and communication of the person in pain (Hadjistavropoulos et al., 2011). Pain communication is thus influenced by a number of contextual, social, and psychological factors that include the personality of the individual (Peters & Vancleef, 2008), previous experiences with pain (Hofle, Hauck, Engel, & Senkowski, 2012), and preexisting relationships between healthcare providers and the person in pain. It will be important to include such factors in further research.

To date, little attention has been applied to how automatic pain detection may vary between men and women, people of different racial and ethnic backgrounds, or context, to name just a few factors. Further, little is known about the extent to which automated measures may be generalized from one type of data to another. For research and clinical use, we will want to know that methods developed in one or another dataset may be applied to others with confidence. Research has begun in this direction with potential to significantly impact both research and clinical use.

Acknowledgments This work was supported by the National Institute of Nursing Research of the National Institutes of Health under Award Number R21NR016510. The content is solely the responsibility of the authors and does not necessarily represent the official views of the National Institutes of Health.

References

Ahmed, N., Natarajan, T., & Rao, K. R. (1974). Discrete cosine transform. *IEEE Transactions on Computers, 23*, 90–93.

Arif, M., Grap, M. J., Munro, C. L., Lyon, D. E., Sessler, D. C. N., & Cohn, J. F. (2010). Facial expression and pain in the critically-ill, non-communicative patient: State of science review. *Intensive and Critical Care Medicine, 26*, 343–352.

Ashraf, A. B., Lucey, S., Cohn, J. F., Chen, T., Prkachin, K. M., & Solomon, P. E. (2009). The painful face: Pain expression recognition using active appearance models. *Image and Vision Computing, 27*, 1788–1796.

Aung, M. S. H., Kaltwang, S., Romera-Paredes, B., Martinez, B., Singh, A., Cella, M., ... Bianchi-Berthouze, N. (2015). The automatic detection of chronic pain-related expression: Requirements, challenges and a multimodal dataset. *IEEE Transactions on Affective Computing, 7*, 435–451.

Baltrusaitis, T., Robinson, P., & Morency, L. P. (2012). 3D constrained local model for rigid and non-rigid facial tracking. In *IEEE CVPR*.

Bartlett, M., Littlewort, G., Frank, M., & Lee, K. (2014). Automated detection of deceptive facial expressions of *Pain. Current Biology, 24*(7), 738–743.

Brennan, R. L., & Prediger, D. J. (1981). Coefficient kappa: Some uses, misuses, and alternatives. *Educational and Psychological Measurement, 41*, 687–699.

Brummer, N., & du Preez, J. (2005). Application-independent evaluation of speaker detection. *Computer Speech and Language, 20*, 230–275.

Chambers, C. T., Reid, G. J., Craig, K. D., McGrath, P. J., & Finley, G. A. (1998). Agreement between child and parent reports of pain. *The Clinical Journal of Pain, 14*, 336–342.

Chew, S. W., Lucey, P., Lucey, S., Saragih, J. M., Cohn, J. F., Matthews, I., & Sridharan, S. (2012). In the pursuit of effective affective computing: The relationship between features and registration. *IEEE Transactions on Systems, Man, and Cybernetics, Part B, 42*(4), 1–12.

Clemente, C. D. (1997). *Anatomy: A regional atlas of the human body* (4th ed.). Baltimore, MD: Williams & Wilkins.

Cohn, J. F., Ambadar, Z., & Ekman, P. (2007). Observer-based measurement of facial expression with the facial action coding system. In J. A. Coan & J. J. B. Allen (Eds.), *Handbook of emotion elicitation and assessment, Oxford University Press series in affective science* (pp. 203–221). New York, NY: Oxford University Press.

Coll, M. P., Gregoire, M., Latimer, M., Eugene, F., & Jackson, P. L. (2011). Perception of pain in others: Implications for caregivers. *Pain Management, 1*(3), 257–265.

Cootes, T., Edwards, G., & Taylor, C. (2001). Active appearance models. *IEEE Transactions on Pattern Analysis and Machine Intelligence, 23*(6), 681–685.

Corneanu, C., Oliu, M., Cohn, J. F., & Escalera, S. (2015). Survey on RGB, thermal, and multimodal approaches for facial expression analysis: History, trends, and affect-related applications. *IEEE Transactions on Pattern Analysis and Machine Intelligence, 38*, 1548–1568.

Craig, K. D. (2009). A social communications model of pain. *Canadian Psychology/Psychologie canadienne, 50*, 22–32. doi:10.1037/a0014772

Craig, K. D., Hyde, S. A., & Patrick, C. J. (1991). Genuine, suppressed and faked facial behavior during exacerbation of chronic low back pain. *Pain, 46*(2), 161–171.

Craig, K. D., Korol, C. T., & Pillai, R. R. (2002). Challenges of judging pain in vulnerable infants. *Clinics in Perinatology, 29*, 445–457.

Craig, K. D., Prkachin, K. M., & Grunau, R. V. E. (2001). The facial expression of pain. In D. C. Turk & R. Melzack (Eds.), *Handbook of pain assessment* (2nd ed.). New York, NY: Guilford Press.

Craig, K. D., Prkachin, K. M., & Grunau, R. V. E. (2010). The facial expression of pain. In D. C. Turk & R. Melzack (Eds.), *Handbook of pain assessment* (3rd ed.). New York, NY: Guilford Press.

Craig, K. D., Versloot, J., Goubert, L., Vervoort, T., & Crombez, G. (2010). Perceiving pain in others: Automatic and controlled mechanisms. *The Journal of Pain, 11*(8), 101–108.

Cummins, N., Epps, J., & Ambikairajah, E. (2013). Spectro temporal analysis of speech affected by depression and psychomotor retardation. In *IEEE ICASSP* (pp. 7542–7546).

Darwin, C. (1872/1998). *The expression of the emotions in man and animals* (3rd ed.). New York, NY: Oxford University Press.

de Knegt, N. C., Pieper, M. J., Lobbezoo, F., Schuengel, C., Evenhuis, H. M., Passchier, J., & Scherder, E. J. (2013). Behavioral pain indicators in people with intellectual disabilities: A systematic review. *Journal of Pain, 14*(9), 885–896.

Dubois, A., Bringuier, S., Capdevilla, X., & Pry, R. (2008). Vocal and verbal expression of postoperative pain in preschoolers. *Pain Management Nursing, 9*(4), 160–165.

Ekman, P., & Friesen, W. V. (1978). *Facial action coding system*. Palo Alto, CA: Consulting Psychologists Press.

Ekman, P., Friesen, W. V., & Hager, J. C. (2002). *Facial action coding system*. Salt Lake City, UT: Research Nexus, Network Research Information.

El Ayadi, M., Kamel, M. S., & Karray, F. (2011). Survey on speech emotion recognition: Features, classification schemes, and databases. *Pattern Recognition, 44*(3), 572–587.

Fillingim, R. B., King, C. D., Ribeiro-Dasilva, M. C., Rahim-Williams, B., & Riley, J. L. (2009). Sex, gender, and pain: A review of recent clinical and experimental findings. *The Journal of Pain, 10*(5), 447–485.

Florea, C., Florea, L., & Vertan, C. (2014). Learning pain from emotion: Transferred HoT data representation for pain intensity estimation. In *ECCV Workshop on ACVR*, Zurich, Switzerland.

Garrett, K. L., Happ, M. B., Costello, J. R., & Fried-Oken, M. B. (2007). AAC in the intensive care unit. In D. R. Beukelman, K. L. Garrett, & K. M. Yorkston (Eds.), *Augmentative commu-*

nication strategies for adults with acute or chronic medical conditions. Baltimore, MD: Paul H. Brookes.

Gélinas, C., Arbour, C., Michaud, C., Vaillant, F., & Desjardins, S. (2011). Implementation of the critical-care pain observation tool on pain assessment/management nursing practices in an intensive care unit with nonverbal critically ill adults: A before and after study. *International Journal of Nursing Studies, 48*(12), 1495–1504.

Ghosh, S., Laksana, E., Scherer, S. & Morency, L.-P. (2015) *A multi-label convolutional neural network approach to cross-domain action unit detection*, presented at the Affective Computing and Intelligent Interaction, Xi'an, China, 2015.

Girard, J. M., & Cohn, J. F. (2016). A primer on observational measurement. *Assessment, 23*(4), 404–413.

Green, C. R., Anderson, K. O., Baker, T. A., Campbell, L. C., Decker, S., Fillingim, R. B., ... Vallerand, A. H. (2003). The unequal burden of pain: Confronting racial and ethnic disparities in pain. *Pain Medicine, 4*(3), 277–294.

Hadjistavropoulos, T., Craig, K. D., Duck, S., Cano, A., Goubert, L., Jackson, P. L., ... Fitzgerald, T. D. (2011). A biopsychosocial formulation of pain communication. *Psychological Bulletin, 137*(6), 910–939.

Hammal Z., & Cohn J. F. (2012, October 23–25). Automatic detection of pain intensity. In *Proc. 14th ICMI*, 47–52, Santa Monica, CA.

Hammal, Z., & Cohn, J. F. (2014, November 12–16). Intra- and interpersonal functions of head motion in emotion communication. In *RFMI in Conjunction with the 16th ACM International Conference on Multimodal Interaction ICMI 2014*, Istanbul, Turkey.

Hammal, Z., Cohn, J. F., & George, D. T. (2014). Interpersonal coordination of head motion in distressed couples. *IEEE Transactions on Affective Computing, 5*(2), 155–167.

Hammal, Z., Cohn, J. F., Heike, C., & Speltz, M. L. (2015, September 21–24). What can head and facial movements convey about positive and negative affect? In *The 6th Biannual Humaine Association Conference on Affective Computing and Intelligent Interaction (ACII 2015)*, Xi'an, China (Best Paper Award).

Hammal, Z., Cohn, J. F., & Messinger, D. (2015). Head movement dynamics during normal and perturbed mother-infant interaction. *IEEE Transactions on Affective Computing, 6*(4), 361–370.

Hammal, Z., & Kunz, M. (2012). Pain monitoring: A dynamic and context-sensitive system. *Pattern Recognition, 45*(4), 1265–1280.

Hammal, Z., Kunz, M., Arguin, M., & Gosselin, F. (2008, September 22–24). Spontaneous pain expression recognition in video sequences. In *Proc. BCS Int'l Conf. on Visions of Computer Science (BCS-Visions 2008)*, Imperial College, London, England.

Hammal, Z., & Massot, C. (2011). Gabor-like image filtering for transient feature detection and global energy estimation applied to multi-expression classification. In P. Richard & J. Braz (Eds.), *Communications in computer and information science (CCIS 229)* (pp. 135–153). Heidelberg, Germany: Springer.

Haugstad, G. K., Haugstad, T. S., Kirste, U. M., Leganger, S., Wojniusz, S., Klemmetsen, I., & Malt, U. F. (2006). Posture, movement patterns, and body awareness in women with chronic pelvic pain. *Journal of Psychosomatic Research, 61*(5), 637–644.

Ho, T. K. (1995, August 14–16). Random decision forests (PDF). In *Proceedings of the 3rd International Conference on Document Analysis and Recognition* (pp. 278–282), Montreal, QC.

Ho, T. K. (1998). The random subspace method for constructing decision forests. *IEEE Transactions on Pattern Analysis and Machine Intelligence, 20*(8), 832–844.

Hofle, M., Hauck, M., Engel, A. K., & Senkowski, D. (2012). Viewing a needle pricking a hand that you perceive as yours enhances unpleasantness of pain. *Pain, 153*(3), 1074–1081.

Jaiswal, S., & Valstar, M. F. (2016) *Deep learning the dynamic appearance and shape of facial action units*, presented at the Winter Conference on Applications of Computer Vision (WACV), Lake Placid, USA, 2016.

Jeni, L. A., Cohn, J. F., & Kanade, T. (2016). Dense 3D face alignment from 2d video for real-time use. *Image Vision and Computing, 58*, 13–24.

Joshi, J., Dhall, A., Goecke, R., & Cohn, J. (2013, September 2–5). Relative body part movement for automatic depression analysis. In *Proc. 5th ACII*, Geneva, Switzerland.

Kachele, M., Thiam, P., Amirian, M., Werner, P., Walter, S., Schwenker, F., & Palm, G. (2015). Multimodal data fusion for person-independent, continuous estimation of pain intensity. In L. Iliadis & C. Jayne (Eds.), *Engineering applications of neural networks, Communications in computer and information science* (Vol. 517, pp. 275–285). Berlin, Germany: Springer.

Kaltwang, S., Rudovic, O., & Pantic, M. (2012). Continuous pain intensity estimation from facial expressions. In G. Bebis et al. (Eds.), *Proceedings of the 8th International Symposium on Advances in Visual Computing, ISVC 2012, LNCS* (Vol. 7432, pp. 368–377). Heidelberg, Germany: Springer.

Karg, M., Samadani, A. A., Gorbert, R., Kuhnlenz, K., Hoey, J., & Kulic, D. (2014). Body movements for affective expression: A survey of automatic recognition and generation. *IEEE Transactions on Affective Computing, 4*(4), 341–359.

Kleinsmith, A., & Bianchi-Berthouze, N. (2013). Affective body expression perception and recognition: A survey. *IEEE Transactions on Affective Computing, 4*(1), 15–33.

Kunz, M., Chatelle, C., Lautenbacher, S., & Rainville, P. (2008). The relation between catastrophizing and facial responsiveness to pain. *Pain, 140*, 127–134.

Kvale, A., Ljunggren, A. E., & Johnsen, T. B. (2003). Examination of movement in patients with long-lasting musculoskeletal pain: Reliability and validity. *Physiotherapy Research International, 8*, 36–52.

LeCun, Y., Bengio, Y., & Hinton, G. (2015). Deep learning. *Nature, 521*(7553), 436–444.

Littlewort, G., Bartlett, M., & Lee, K. (2009). Automatic coding of facial expressions displayed during posed and genuine pain. *Image and Vision Computing, 27*(12), 1741–1844.

Lucey, P., Cohn, J. F., Matthews, I., Lucey, S., Sridharan, S., Howlett, J., & Prkachin, K. M. (2011). Automatically detecting pain in video through facial action unit recognition. *Systems, Man, and Cybernetics, Part B, 41*(3), 664–674.

Lucey, P., Cohn, J. F., Prkachin, K. M., Solomon, P., Chew, S., & Matthews, I. (2012). Painful monitoring: Automatic pain monitoring using the UNBC-McMaster shoulder pain expression archive database. *Image and Vision Computing, 30*(3), 197–205.

Lucey, P., Cohn, J. F., Prkachin, K. M., Solomon, P., & Matthews, I. (2011). Painful data: The UNBC-McMaster shoulder pain expression archive database. In *IEEE International Conference on Automatic Face and Gesture Recognition (FG2011)*, Santa Barbara, CA.

Monroe, T. B., & Mion, L. C. (2012). Patients with advanced dementia: How do we know if they are in pain? *Geriatric Nursing, 33*(3), 226–228.

Ojala, T., Pietikäinen, M., & Harwood, D. (1996). A comparative study of texture measures with classification based on feature distributions. *Pattern Recognition, 29*(1), 51–59.

Ojala, T., Pietikainen, M., & Maenpaa, T. (2002). Multiresolution gray-scale and rotation invariant texture classification with local binary patterns. *IEEE Transactions on Pattern Analysis and Machine Intelligence, 24*, 971–987.

Ojansivu, V., & Heikkila, J.. (2008). Blur insensitive texture classification using local phase quantization. In *Proceedings on international conference on image and signal processing* (pp. 236–243).

Payen, J. F., Bru, O., Bosson, J. L., Lagrasta, A., Novel, E., Deschaux, I., … Jacquot, C. (2001). Assessing pain in critically ill sedated patients by using a behavioral pain scale. *Critical Care Medicine, 29*(12), 2258–2263.

Peters, M. L., & Vancleef, L. M. G. (2008). The role of personality traits in pain perception and disability. *Reviews in Analgesia, 10*, 11–21.

Pietikäinen, M. (2010). Local binary patterns. *Scholarpedia, 5*(3), 9775.

Prkachin, K. M. (1992). The consistency of facial expressions of pain: A comparison across modalities. *Pain, 51*, 297–306.

Prkachin, K. M., Solomon, P., Hwang, T., & Mercer, S. R. (2001). Does experience influences judgments of pain behaviour? Evidence from relatives of pain patients and therapists. *Pain Research & Management, 6*, 105–112.

Prkachin, K. M., & Solomon, P. E. (2008). The structure, reliability and validity of pain expression: Evidence from patients with shoulder pain. *Pain, 139*, 267–274.

Rajasagaram, U., Taylor, D. M., Braitberg, G., Pearsell, J. P., & Capp, B. A. (2009). Paediatric pain assessment: Differences between triage nurse, child and parent. *Journal of Paediatrics and Child Health, 45*(4), 199–203.

Rash, J. A., Prkachin, K. M., Solomon, P. E., & Campbell, T. A. (n.d.). *Assessing the efficacy of a manual-based intervention for improving the detection of facial pain expression: The index of facial pain expression* (Unpublished manuscript).

Rudovic, O., Pavlovic, V., & Pantic, M. (2013). Automatic pain intensity estimation with heteroscedastic conditional ordinal random fields. In *Proceedings of the 9th Int'l Symposium on Advances in Visual Computing, ISVC, Part II, Greece, LNCS* (Vol. 8034, pp. 234–243). Heidelberg, Germany: Springer.

Saragih, J., Lucey, S., & Cohn, J. F. (2011). Deformable model fitting by regularized landmark mean shift. *International Journal of Computer Vision, 91*(2), 200–215.

Scherer, K. R. (2003). Vocal communication of emotion: A review of research paradigms. *Speech Communication, 40*, 227–256.

Schuller, B., Batliner, A., Steidl, S., & Seppi, D. (2011). Recognizing realistic emotions and affect in speech: State of the art and lessons learnt from the first challenge. *Speech Communication, 53*(9/10), 1062–1087. Special Issue: Sensing Emotion and Affect – Facing Realism in Speech Processing.

Shrout, P. E., & Fleiss, J. L. (1979). Intraclass correlations: Uses in assessing rater reliability. *Psychological Bulletin, 86*, 420–428.

Sikka, K., Ahmed, A., Diaz, D., Goodwin, M., Craig, K., Bartlett, M., & Huang, J. (2015). Automated assessment of children's post-operative pain using computer vision. *Pediatrics, 136*, 124–131.

Sikka, K., Dhall, A., & Bartlett, M. (2014). Weakly supervised pain localization and classification with multiple segment learning. *Image and Vision Computing, 32*(10), 659–670.

Singer, A. J., Gulla, J., & Thode, H. C., Jr. (2002). Parents and practitioners are poor judges of young children's pain severity. *Academic Emergency Medicine, 9*(6), 609–612.

Tipping, M. E. (2001). Sparse Bayesian learning and the relevance vector machine. *The Journal of Machine Learning Research, 1*, 211–244.

Vapnik, V. (1995). *The nature of statistical learning theory*. New York, NY: Springer-Verlag.

Vapnik, V. (1998). *Statistical learning theory*. New York, NY: John Wiley & Sons.

Vlaeyen, J. W. S., & Linton, S. J. (2000). Fear-avoidance and its consequences in muscle skeleton pain: A state of the art. *Pain, 85*(3), 317–332.

Walter, S., Gruss, S., Ehleiter, H., Tan, J., Traue, H., Werner, P., ... Moreira da Silva, G. (2013) The BioVid Heat Pain Database: Data for the advancement and systematic validation of an automated pain recognition system. In *2013 Proceedings of IEEE International Conference on Cybernetics.*

Wandner, L. D., Scipio, C. D., Hirsh, A. T., Torres, C. A., & Robinson, M. E. (2012). The perception of pain in others: How gender, race, and age influence pain expectations. *The Journal of Pain, 13*(3), 220–227.

Warden, V., Hurley, A. C., & Volicer, L. (2003). Development and psychometric evaluation of the pain assessment in advanced dementia scale. *Journal of the American Medical Directors Association, 4*(1), 9–15.

Werner, P., Al-Hamadi, A., Limbrecht-Ecklundt, K., Walter, S., Gruss, S., & Traue, H. (2016). Automatic pain assessment with facial activity descriptors. *IEEE Transactions on Affective Computing, 8*, 286–299.

Williamson, J. R., Quatieri, T. F., Helfer, B. S., Horwitz, R., Daryush, B. Y., & Mehta, D. (2013). Vocal biomarkers of depression based on motor incoordination. In *Proc. ACM AVEC* (pp. 41–48).

Yang, Y., Fairbairn, C., & Cohn, J. F. (2013). Detecting depression severity from vocal prosody. *IEEE Transactions on Affective Computing, 4*(2), 142–150.

Yang, R., Tong, S., López, M. B., Boutellaa, E., Peng, J., Feng, X., & Hadid, A. (2016, December). On pain assessment from facial videos using spatio-temporal local descriptors. In *IPTA* (pp. 1–6).

Zagyapan, R., Iyem, C., Kurkcuoglu, A., Pelin, C., & Tekindal, M. A. (2012). *The relationship between balance, muscles, and anthropomorphic features in young adults.* Cairo, Egypt: Hindawi Publishing Corporation, Anatomy Research International.

Zhao, G., & Pietikäinen, M. (2007). Dynamic texture recognition using local binary patterns with an application to facial expressions. *IEEE Transactions on Pattern Analysis and Machine Intelligence, 29*(6), 915–928.

Zhang, X., & De la Torre, F. (2015). Global supervised descent method. In *Proceedings of the IEEE International Conference on Computer Vision.*

Zhou, H., Roberts, P., & Horgan, L. (2008). Association between self-report pain ratings of child and parent, child and nurse and parent and nurse dyads: Meta-analysis. *Journal of Advanced Nursing, 63*(4), 334–342.

Zhou, J., Hong, X., Su, F., & Zhao, G. (2016). Recurrent convolutional neural network regression for continuous pain intensity estimation in video. In *IEEE CVPR Workshop of Affect "in-the-Wild"* (pp. 84–92).

Part III
The Neuroscience of Interpersonal Pain Dynamics

Chapter 8
The Neural Signature of Empathy for Physical Pain … Not Quite There Yet!

Marie-Pier B. Tremblay, Aurore Meugnot, and Philip L. Jackson

Abstract The perception and evaluation of other's pain has been largely used in social neuroscience as a paradigm to study human empathy. Thanks to the growing attention given to this concept over the last 15 years, the cerebral bases of empathy in the context of physical pain are increasingly well documented. The aim of this chapter is to provide a critical overview of the most recent evidence while fostering discussion about the extent to which the cerebral changes associated with empathy can lead to a specific signature of this key process of social interactions. The authors firstly clarify the complex definition of empathy and its principal components, and make a clear distinction between pain perception in others, empathy and the behavioral outputs that can follow. Secondly, the cerebral networks underlying the distinct, yet interacting, components of empathy for physical pain are defined. Lastly, recent work on the factors that are likely to modulate empathy and these cerebral networks is discussed. The study of brain function has advanced our understanding of empathy in the context of physical pain considerably, but the complexity of this often fleeting process, especially in healthcare, is such that multiple levels of analysis will be needed to fully uncover its mysteries.

Keywords Empathy · Factors modulating empathy · Physical pain · Neuroimaging · Shared-representation network · Mentalizing network · Emotional regulation network

M.-P. B. Tremblay · P. L. Jackson (✉)
École de Psychologie, Université Laval, Québec, QC, Canada

Centre interdisciplinaire de recherche en réadaptation et intégration sociale, Québec, QC, Canada

Centre de recherche de l'Institut universitaire en santé mental de Québec, Québec, QC, Canada
e-mail: Philip.Jackson@psy.ulaval.ca

A. Meugnot
Centre interdisciplinaire de recherche en réadaptation et intégration sociale, Québec, QC, Canada

Centre de recherche de l'Institut universitaire en santé mental de Québec, Québec, QC. Canada

149

Abbreviations

ACC   Anterior cingulate cortex
AI   Anterior insula
aMCC   Anterior midcingulate cortex
CIP   Congenital insensitivity to pain
dACC   Dorsal anterior cingulate cortex
DLPFC   Dorsolateral prefrontal cortex
EEG   Electroencephalography
fMRI   Functional magnetic resonance imaging
IFG   Inferior frontal gyrus
IPL   Inferior parietal lobule
LPP   Late positive potential
MEP   Motor evoked potentials
mPFC   Medial prefrontal cortex
OFC   Orbitofrontal cortex
PCC   Posterior cingulate cortex
preSMA   Pre-supplementary motor area
pSTS   Posterior superior temporal sulcus
S1   Primary somatosensory cortex
S2   Secondary somatosensory cortex
TMS   Transcranial magnetic stimulation
TPJ   Temporoparietal junction
vmPFC   Ventromedial prefrontal cortex

Introduction

Imagine yourself sitting on your front porch, enjoying a cold drink and watching people passing by on the street. You see two people riding their bicycles and, as you look more closely at them, you see that one hits a pothole and falls to the ground. Different versions of this scenario will be illustrated in order to demonstrate different key concepts that will be used throughout this chapter. First, imagine that the two people on the bicycles are kids, and you quickly realize they are your son and one of his friends. As you are watching them coming back home, your child's friend falls. You run over to him to help and comfort him; he is crying because he says that his knee hurts and you notice some blood trickling down his leg. Even if his injury is minor, you understand his pain and you feel bad about it. To a certain degree, you share a part of his pain. In fact, your reaction would be interpreted as *empathic*. Second, in this same example, switch the roles and imagine that it was your son who fell off his bike and got hurt. In this situation, because (we assume) you love and care for him so much, you might feel distressed and your reaction would no doubt be much stronger than in the first example; perhaps even a bit disproportionate considering the seriousness of the event. According to the conceptualization used in this chapter (see later for a detailed definition of empathy), your reaction towards your son could not be qualified as empathic but rather one mostly characterized by sympathy, as you would most likely feel the same emotion as your son and share his distress. Third, visualize that the two people on their bicycle are two adults and you recognize one of them as the bully who used to tease you about your ginger hair in high school, needless to say that you did not particularly like him. While you are watching him, he suddenly falls on the pavement. Although you perceive that he is in pain, you do not feel the same urge to run to him in order to check that he is fine, even if you did not necessarily wish him such bad luck. Thus, perceiving pain in others might trigger an empathic response and prosocial behaviors in some instances, but this reaction is far from universal, because other reactions (e.g., distress or detachment) could also stem from a situation as the one portrayed here. The first and second examples depict respectively the difference between an *empathic reaction* followed by a *prosocial behavior* and a nonoptimal empathic reaction, engendering distress caused by an inadequate regulation of your own emotional response to the other's pain. The contrast between the first and third example illustrates a more rudimentary, albeit complex, distinction between *empathy* and *pain perception*, as well as the importance of the relation between the observer and the person experiencing pain. In fact, perception of pain in others and the empathy, which may or may not emerge from it, are two processes that are sometimes confounded, and, as this distinction is of great importance, the peculiarity of these concepts will first be established. The distinction between *empathy* and *prosocial behaviors* will also be drawn.

Perception of Others' Pain vs. Empathy for Physical Pain in Others   Pain is an unpleasant subjective experience that emerges from the interaction of sensory, emotional, affective, cognitive and social components, and is associated with actual or potential tissue damage (Coll, Grégoire, Latimer, Eugene, & Jackson, 2011; Loeser & Treede, 2008). Thus, the perception of others' pain includes a rapid and efficient decoding phase in which the observer learns of a person's pain through different cues (e.g., facial expressions, vocal expressions) in order to appraise it (e.g., pain severity and intensity) (Craig, 2009; Goubert et al., 2005). While detecting and evaluating someone else's pain, the observer assigns a certain level of psychological affects and distress to the other. Perceiving the pain of someone often, but not always, involves empathy. This strong association led to the reductionist conception that seeing pain in others amounts to "pain empathy," but the distinction between these concepts is of great importance, especially as pain observation tasks have been largely used in experimental paradigms to study empathy. The later requires one to perceive the emotion of the other, and then to understand and share that emotion to a certain degree (Decety & Jackson, 2004). As such, it is plausible that perceiving pain in others does not automatically trigger empathy, but perhaps constitutes a step towards it, and maybe towards prosocial behaviors (Coll et al., 2011; Yamada & Decety, 2009).

The aim of this chapter is foremost to depict the current literature on empathy for others' pain from a neuroscience perspective. First, a definition of empathy will be drawn, as consensus is still lacking (Batson, 2009). Second, the cerebral responses associated with distinct components of empathy in the context of physical pain will be portrayed and, finally, recent advances concerning the factors known to modulate the cerebral response of empathy will be explicated. More than a decade of cognitive neuroscience research has contributed to the beginning of a quest to find a neural signature of empathy for others' pain (e.g., Krishnan et al., 2016). However, as exciting this may be, the expectations towards finding such a cerebral signature in a near future should be moderated. The last decade has seen important neuroimaging methodologic and analytic improvements, leading to a rapid growth in the knowledge base, but we are not quite there yet.

Empathy: A Unique, Yet Complex Concept

Despite some discrepancy in the scientific literature regarding what exactly the concept of empathy means, most authors refer to the capacity to perceive, understand, represent, and share, to a certain degree, someone else's mental states and feelings (Decety & Jackson, 2004). Empathy is a unique, complex and multifactorial human faculty that emerges through social interactions (Gerdes, Segal, & Lietz, 2010; Marcoux & Jackson, 2012). Importantly, a prerequisite to empathy is *self-consciousness*, as a person must distinguish between himself and the other, to avoid confusion between his or her own feelings and the other's. Then, to be empathic, an individual must have: (1) the emotional capacity to share the affective experience of others (i.e., affective component); (2) the cognitive ability to understand his or her perspective (i.e., cognitive component) (Melloni, Lopez, & Ibanez, 2014); and (3) varying regulatory processes that contribute to the ability to find some balance between the other two components. While a majority of authors agree that these components are needed for empathy, some accentuate the role, hierarchy and importance of one over the others (e.g., de Waal & Preston, 2017).

Affective Resonance The affective component of empathy allows an individual to represent what the other feels based on what he would feel in a similar situation (Decety & Jackson, 2004). This *affective resonance* is the core of the *shared representations theory*, which postulates that the perception of other's behavior automatically activates the neural and cognitive substrates underpinning the direct experience of that behavior (Decety & Jackson, 2004; Decety & Sommerville, 2003; Prinz, 1997). This resonance to someone's pain relies on an automatic activation of the observer's own experience of pain, i.e., the motor, sensory, and emotional representations when experiencing a similar state and situation (Decety & Jackson, 2004; Jeannerod, 2001; Preston & De Waal, 2002). Therefore, the activation of shared representations would be associated with an automatic, unconscious response to the observer's sensorimotor and affective states (i.e., sensations and emotions) (Preston & de Waal, 2002). The concept of shared representation in the case of empathy for physical pain has been largely supported by the finding of similar cerebral patterns activated during both direct and vicarious experience of pain (Botvinick et al., 2005;

Jackson, Rainville, & Decety, 2006; Keysers & Gazzola, 2010; Singer et al., 2004). For instance, in the situation mentioned above, seeing a child seated on the ground and crying because his knee hurts would evoke the representations of the hard impact with the ground if you fell off your own bike and the unpleasant pain you would feel on your knee. Even today, many studies are still interpreted on the basis of this theory, even though the extent to which one's own representation and someone else's share similar neural substrate is increasingly being questioned (Krishnan et al., 2016; Van Overwalle & Baetens, 2009; Zaki, Wager, Singer, Keysers, & Gazzola, 2016).

Perspective-Taking   The cognitive component of empathy, sometimes referred to as *perspective-taking* or *mentalizing* or even *theory of mind*, is the controlled and deliberate ability to impute emotions, intentions, beliefs, and desires to someone else in order to predict his or her behavior (Decety & Jackson, 2004; Frith & Frith, 2006). According to that theory, empathy requires mental flexibility to be able to adopt and understand others' subjective perspective in order to infer their feelings. As such, mentalizing relies on controlled processes, as the ability to take another's perspective requires some mental effort (Decety & Jackson, 2004; Goubert et al., 2005).

Emotion Regulation   Even though affective resonance and mentalizing constitute the principal components of empathy, mechanisms of *emotion regulation* are also needed, so that a person is not overwhelmed by others' emotions and does not experience distress (Decety & Jackson, 2004; Decety, Jackson, & Brunet, 2007). A recent study showed that acute stress was linked with an increased cerebral response in the regions underlying affective resonance with others' pain. The authors also reported a stronger activation in regions associated with emotion regulation in the stress group compared with controls. They interpreted these results as indicating a greater (yet unsuccessful) involvement of regulatory mechanisms to modulate this automatic sharing with others' pain (Tomova et al., 2016). Thus, the *emotion regulation* component seeks an equilibrium between the affective and cognitive components of empathy. There are different models conceptualizing emotion regulation mechanisms and most agree that these strategies can be classified as goal-oriented, need-oriented and person-oriented (e.g., Gross & Thompson, 2007; Koole, 2009; Morawetz, Bode, Derntl, & Heekeren, 2017).

Behavioral Expression of Empathy   To some authors, empathy refers simply to an automatic affective mechanism (i.e., emotion resonance), whereas for others it requires more controlled cognitive processes (i.e., perspective-taking; see de Waal & Preston, 2017 for a recent discussion). In this chapter, empathy implies the combination of all the processes previously mentioned; they are all interconnected and necessary to evoke empathy (Decety & Jackson, 2004). Moreover, some authors, including us, also put emphasis on the behavioral output of the different components of empathy (e.g., helping behaviors; Goubert et al., 2005). As such, empathy implies that someone resonates, takes the perspectives of the other, but also means to act for the good of another person. In the context of pain, this means that empathy will drive the need to alleviate the pain of the other. Thus, even if measuring the behavioral expression of empathy is not always easy or feasible, it remains one of the most important markers of this complex process. Note, however, that some helping behaviors might stem from other motivations than empathy. For instance, in the above mentioned example, you ran to your son's friend to help him when he injured himself. You could be running to help him ease his pain because he is obviously uncomfortable with it, which would be a behavioral output of empathy, but you could also do it because it is socially expected for a parent to act like that; the latter would not constitute a behavioral output of empathy (Jackson, Eugène, & Tremblay, 2015). Therefore, the optimal measure of empathy would be based not only on the overt behavior of a seemingly caring person, but also on the underlying cognitive and affective processes.

Brain Activation in Empathy

Over the last decade, many studies in the field of social neuroscience have addressed this topic, thus greatly advancing knowledge about the cerebral basis of empathy for others' physical pain and, at the same time, improving the global comprehension of this multidimensional concept. The study of the brain responses underlying empathy is mainly realized through negative emotions or states, such as pain, whereas little is known about empathy for positive emotions. Because pain is very effective at evoking empathy many experimental paradigms use it to assess empathy. In fMRI studies, empathy for pain is usually assessed while the participant lies in the scanner watching body parts (i.e., hands or feet) in painful situations or facial expressions of pain. What is asked to the participants may vary. For instance some studies require the participants to evaluate the pain they perceived in the stimuli on a visual analog scale, whereas others ask for the help needed by the person in pain. Furthermore, in some studies, the participant has nothing to do except watch the painful stimuli. This allows the identification of different networks underlying the components of empathy; namely, the shared-representation network (i.e., affective component), the mentalizing network (i.e., cognitive component) and the different networks involved in emotion regulation.

Shared-Representation Network The neural basis of empathy gained interest after the discovery that the physical experience of pain shares a cerebral basis with the observation of someone else's pain. More precisely, the core networks underlying the experience of physical pain, named the "*pain matrix*," have been widely studied by multiple techniques (e.g., functional magnetic resonance imaging, electroencephalography, transcranial magnetic stimulation). The principal regions of this pain matrix are: primary and secondary somatosensory cortices (S1; S2), thalamus, anterior insula (AI), anterior cingulate cortex (ACC), and medial prefrontal cortex (mPFC; Garcia-Larrea & Peyron, 2013; Lamm, Decety, & Singer, 2011).

Different components of pain are processed by different groups of structures in this pain matrix (Treede, Kenshalo, Gracely, & Jones, 1999). For instance, S1 and S2 are involved in the sensory-discriminative dimension of pain, as they allow someone to perceive the pain's location and intensity. The AI and the ACC are related to the affective component of pain, whereas the mPFC is linked with the cognitive integration of pain (Apkarian, Hashmi, & Baliki, 2011; Baliki et al., 2006). In recent years, a myriad of authors have argued that the relationship between behaviors and the brain is complex and that a specific function cannot be assigned to a unique brain region, thus questioning the idea that some areas of the brain uniquely process physical pain (e.g., Kucyi & Davis, 2016; Rogachov, Cheng, Erpelding, Hemington, & Crawley, 2016; Wager et al., 2013). Despite this emerging controversy surrounding the *pain matrix*, it is still relevant to mention this neural network because, as argued earlier, parts of many regions of the pain matrix are also activated in the affective component of empathy. These regions and the network in which they are included are referred to as the *shared-representation network* or *affective resonance* or *salience network*. To simplify, the unique expression "shared-representation network" will be used to refer to this network (Fan, Duncan, de Greck, & Northoff, 2011). This network comprises the inferior parietal lobule, the posterior superior temporal sulcus (pSTS), the AI, the thalamus, the medial orbitofrontal cortex (mOFC), the inferior frontal gyrus, the premotor cortex, the somatosensory cortex, the dorsolateral prefrontal cortex (DLPFC) and the mACC/dACC (Hynes, Baird, & Grafton, 2006; Jackson, Rainville, & Decety, 2006; Lamm et al., 2011; Nummenmaa, Hirvonen, Parkkola, & Hietanen, 2008; Shamay-Tsoory, 2009; Singer et al., 2004; Zaki & Oschner, 2012). Among these cerebral regions, some are associated with the sensory-discrimination experience of pain (i.e., the somatosensory cortex, the medial and dorsal ACC, the supplementary motor area, the periaqueductal gray matter, the amygdala and the inferior frontal gyrus); others with the affective-motivational dimension of pain (i.e., ACC and AI) (Akitsuki & Decety, 2009; Avenanti, Bueti, Galati, & Aglioti, 2005; Corradi-Dell'Acqua, Hofstetter, & Vuilleumier, 2011; Corradi-Dell'Acqua, Tusche, Vuilleumier, & Singer, 2016; Jackson, Brunet, Meltzoff, & Decety, 2006; Lamm et al., 2011; Lamm, Batson, & Decety, 2007; Singer et al., 2004). The DLPFC is of particular importance as it is related to the recognition of facial expressions of emotions (Conson et al., 2015; Wang, Wang, Hu, & Li, 2014). The AI and ACC are systematically activated in empathy for pain, and therefore they are considered key regions for the affective component of empathy. The AI is involved in personal emotional processing, but also in the processing of other's people feelings along with the OFC (Kurth, Zilles, Fox, Laird, & Eickhoff, 2010; Price, 2010). The OFC is also involved in facial emotion recognition (Heberlein, Padon, Gillihan, Farah, & Fellows, 2008; Willis, Palermo, McGrillen, & Miller, 2014). As for the ACC, this region is involved in emotional processing and resolution of conflicts, specifically the dACC is associated with the processing of aversive and emotionally conflicting stimuli (Baumgartner, Fischbacher, Feieraben, Lutz, & Fehr, 2009; Liu et al., 2007). Figure 8.1, Panel (a) depicts these two regions of the shared-representation network.

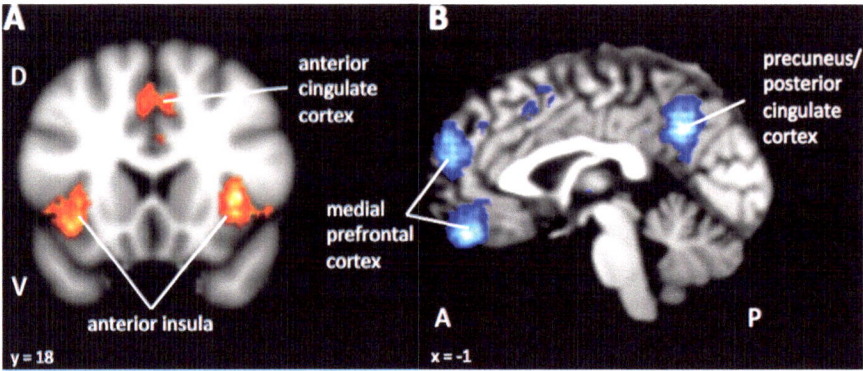

Fig. 8.1 The main networks underlying empathy for pain. Panel (**a**) depicts the most important brain regions included in the *shared-representation network* or *salience network*: the anterior cingulate cortex and the anterior insula. The image was retrieved using the keyword "Salience network" from term-based meta-analyses in Neurosynth (neurosynth.org; 60 studies, forward inference, threshold = 5) and was modified using Mango (http://rii.uthscsa.edu/mango/). Panel (**b**) represents some of the brain regions included in the *mentalizing network*: the medial prefrontal cortex, the precuneus, and the posterior cingulate cortex. Note that the temporal poles and the temporoparietal junction are also key regions in this network even if they do not appear on this panel. The image was retrieved using the keyword "Mentalizing" from term-based meta-analyses in Neurosynth (neurosynth.org; 124 studies, forward inference, threshold = 5) and was modified using Mango (http://rii.uthscsa.edu/mango/). *A* anterior, *D* dorsal, *P* posterior, *V* ventral

While some authors strongly support the notion of the shared-representation network (e.g., Corradi-Dell'Acqua et al., 2011; Corradi-Dell'Acqua et al., 2016), other researchers in social neuroscience are beginning to question the simplicity of this perspective. For instance, using a multivariate pattern analysis, some researchers suggest that even if similar brain regions are activated in both observed and experienced pain, the pattern of these activations indicates separate modifiability, suggesting different brain representations of these two concepts (Krishnan et al., 2016). However, studies on the shared-representation network based on multivariate pattern analysis need to be extended to a variety of experimental stimuli, before enabling an overview of what is actually shared or not between the brain representations of self- and other's pain perception (Zaki et al., 2016; see also Chap. 9, "On the Overlap Between Physical and Social Pain" for a similar discussion about a shared-representation network between physical pain and social pain). Overall, it is important to point out that the sole activity of the shared-representation network does not automatically imply an empathic response, because emotional resonance without the more controlled process of mentalizing cannot be considered as empathy per se (Jackson et al., 2015).

Mentalizing Network There is a set of cerebral regions mostly involved in the cognitive component of empathy, often called the *mentalizing network*. This network mostly involves the temporal poles, the temporoparietal junction (TPJ), the precuneus and the posterior cingulate cortex, the septal area and the medial part of the prefrontal cortex (mPFC) (Amodio & Frith, 2006; D'Argembeau et al., 2007; Morelli & Lieberman, 2013; Van Overwalle & Baetens, 2009; Zaki & Oschner, 2012). The TPJ is an important region of the mentalizing network as it plays a crucial role in the differentiation between self and other and is involved in reasoning about others' perspectives and emotional states (Decety & Lamm, 2007; Donaldson, Rinehart, & Enticott, 2015; Frith & Frith, 2006; Geng & Mangun, 2011; Geng & Vossel, 2013; Samson, Apperley, Chiavarino, & Humphreys, 2004; Saxe & Kanwisher, 2003). The temporal poles are useful in generating semantic and emotional contexts from the social experiences of an individual (Frith, 2007; Völlm et al., 2006). The mPFC is involved in empathic judgments and in mentalizing tasks requiring an individual to infer others' mental states, as well as inferences about their beliefs and intentions (Amodio & Frith, 2006; D'Argembeau et al., 2007; Frith, 2007; Frith & Frith, 2006; Saxe, 2006; Van Overwalle & Baetens, 2009). Figure 8.1, Panel (b) shows some of these brain regions crucial to the mentalizing network.

Interestingly, this network shares neural substrates with the *default-mode network*, which is mostly activated in resting-state studies when a person is not engaging in a specific activity, thinks about him/herself and has nothing to do (i.e., no task) (Buckner, Andrews Hanna, & Schacter, 2008; Li, Mai, & Liu, 2014; Mars et al., 2012). The overlap between the default-mode network and the mentalizing network, particularly in the mPFC and the TPJ, is not surprising as thinking about oneself and social cognition tasks both require an individual to think and understand one's feelings, beliefs and intentions (Mars et al., 2012). Some authors have even suggested the idea that the fundamentally social basis of human nature would be reflected in brain function, even while resting, and this so-called social brain would be a prerequisite to accomplishing more complex tasks (Schilbach, Eickhoff, Rotarska-Jagiela, Fink, & Vogeley, 2008).

Emotion Regulation Networks It is generally acknowledged that the two previously discussed networks are at the core of empathy for pain, and therefore fewer studies have focused on the cerebral response underlying emotion regulation in the context of empathy for pain. A meta-analysis (Morawetz et al., 2017) described a neural model of emotion regulation based on three different networks: attentional deployment, knowledge and appraisal, and body and response system. The attentional deployment network is engaged in tasks where an individual distracts himself from a given situation, or on the contrary concentrates on its emotional content (Gross & Thompson, 2007). This network involves mostly brain regions that are in the core network of attention, comprising the right AI and the preSMA (Morawetz et al., 2017). The knowledge and appraisal network is involved in situations where an individual tries to alter the emotional significance of a situation (e.g., reappraisal, perspective taking; Gross & Thompson, 2007). It involves mostly prefrontal regions (i.e., DLPFC, DMPFC, VLPFC), and also the TPJ (Morawetz et al., 2017). Finally, the body and response system is invoked when one tries to alter the experience of an emotional situation, through different mechanisms (e.g., thought suppression) (Gross & Thompson, 2007). The brain network underlying this system is supported by many regions, including but not limited to, the left VLPFC and right TPJ, as it is involved in complex cognitive functions (Morawetz et al., 2017). However, the distinction between emotion regulation for different types of emotions is not clear (Ochsner & Gross, 2005), making it hard to identify the networks specifically involved in emotion regulation during empathy for pain. Nonetheless, attentional distraction, which could be used as an emotion regulation strategy would diminish the aversion of pain. This reduction would be expected to be reflected in brain activity, notably with a diminished activation in some regions of the pain matrix (e.g., insula, ACC, thalamus, mPFC) (Ochsner & Gross, 2005).

To summarize, empathy is a multifaceted concept that relies on three major networks underlying its principal components; namely, the shared-representation network for the affective component (i.e., affective sharing), the mentalizing network for the cognitive component (i.e., perspective-taking) and, lastly, the networks underlying emotion regulation, essential for an optimal empathic response. An important question arises from the body of literature surrounding the brain response that underlies empathy: even though there is strong evidence supporting the shared-representation and the mentalizing networks, can we predict a person's empathy on the basis of the brain response to another's pain? Moreover, can we infer a person's empathy for others' physical pain on the sole foundation of the structure and activity of his or her brain? The complexity of this question emerges not only from the intricacy of the brain, but also from the fact that, even though we know about the networks underlying empathy for the physical pain of others, this activity can be modulated by a variety of factors related to the person in pain, the observer and the context.

Factors Modulating the Cerebral Activations Associated with Empathy for Pain

Studies highlighting how individual and social factors may influence the empathic brain response to others' pain are commonly classified in three categories: *factors related to the person in pain*, those linked to the *observer*, and those associated to the *contextual factors* in which pain is observed (see previous reviews on this topic; e.g., Coll et al., 2011). The most recent brain imaging findings are presented below, focusing on factors related to the observer and the context, which have been studied more extensively.

Besides driving forward the theoretical models of empathy for physical pain, these studies are of critical importance in clinical settings, because empathy is at the core of quality care, despite being highly challenging for caregivers (Del Canale et al., 2012; Rakel et al., 2009). In fact, the distressing situations that people have to cope with daily may lead health professionals to compassion fatigue, emotional distress, and even burnout (Gleichgerrcht & Decety, 2013; Latimer et al., 2017). Such negative outcomes to being empathic may paradoxically put caregivers in a state that reduces the likelihood of displaying empathy in the long run (Bonvicini et al., 2009; Feighny, Monaco, & Arnold, 1995).

The Suffering Person The brain response to others' pain is influenced by the *individual characteristics* of the person in pain, such as the gender (Simon, Craig, Miltner, & Rainville, 2006) or the intensity of a painful facial expression (Budell, Jackson, & Rainville, 2010). Using fMRI, Budell et al. (2010) investigated brain responses of healthy participants while they rated the level of pain expressed in video clips displaying actors producing facial expressions of three different levels (mild, moderate, and strong) of pain. In a control condition, participants were scanned while observing the same video clips, but they were asked to focus on the facial movements rather than the meaning of the emotion expressed. The neural response associated with pain evaluation was sensitive to different intensities of pain expression, as demonstrated by increased brain responses related to the amount of pain perceived in others in the pain matrix (e.g., ACC and AI), as well as in certain areas of the mPFC (associated with mentalizing). Moreover, some areas engaged in action observation (e.g., vIPL) were strongly activated in the pain evaluation condition, demonstrating that their functional role is not limited to the processing of facial movements, but may also include a more "in-depth" processing, namely the extraction of the expression meaning.

The Observer The neural response of empathy for physical pain is also modulated by the observer's *personal characteristics* such as gender (i.e., women generally show stronger brain activations than men in the different brain networks of empathy for physical pain; Preis, Schmidt-Samoa, Dechent, & Kroener-Herwig, 2013; Yang, Decety, Lee, Chen, & Cheng, 2009), culture (Cheon et al., 2011, 2013), one's own pain while perceiving others' pain (e.g., Meng et al., 2013) or empathy deficits (for a review see Lockwood, 2016). Using fMRI, Cheon et al. (2011) scanned Korean and American participants while observing photos depicting either Koreans or Caucasian-Americans in an emotionally painful or neutral situation. Compared to Caucasian-American participants, Korean participants reported experiencing greater empathy and showed stronger activity in the left TPJ (a key region in mentalizing) for in-group compared to out-group members. Moreover, a growing amount of evidence suggests that individuals with empathy deficits such as autism spectrum disorders, psychopathy (Lockwood, 2016) and schizophrenia (Gonzalez-Liencres, Brown, Tas, Breidenstein, & Brüne, 2016; Vistolli, Lavoie, Sutliff, Jackson, & Achim, 2017), showed atypical brain patterns when viewing others in pain. For instance, there is evidence that adolescents and adults with extreme levels of psychopathic traits show a reduced neural responses to others' pain in regions related to affective resonance (i.e., AI, IFG, ACC and amygdala), when compared with healthy controls (Decety, Chen, Harenski, & Kiehl, 2013; Decety, Skelly, & Kiehl, 2013; Marsh et al., 2013; Meffert, Gazzola, den Boer, Bartels, & Keysers, 2013). The literature is much more heterogeneous regarding the neural changes in empathy for pain response in people with autism spectrum disorders, with evidence for normal (Hadjikhani et al., 2014), increased (Gu et al., 2015) and decreased activation (Fan, Chen, Chen, Decety, & Cheng, 2014) in brain regions involving affective resonance compared with healthy controls. Overall, the investigation of the cerebral response of empathy for physical pain in people presenting deficits to one or more components provides new insight into these disorders. A better understanding of the underlying networks and their dysfunction is crucial to highlight how empathy and helping behaviours that stem from it are processed in the brain, and more practically, to provide insight into the development of strategies and interventions to reduce the impact of empathy deficits.

Self-Pain Experience   The role of self-pain experience in empathy for physical pain has also aroused a large amount of attention among neuroscientists. For instance, investigations of congenital amputees (Aziz-Zadeh, Sheng, Liew, & Damasio, 2012) or individuals with congenital insensitivity to pain (CIP; Danziger, Faillenot, & Peyron, 2009) have provided excellent opportunities to examine whether the lack of self-pain experiences modulates the neural representation of others' pain. These studies have aimed notably at assessing whether the representation of vicarious pain in the brain might be grounded in one's own pain experience and underlying cerebral organization. Danziger et al. (2009) used fMRI to explore the brain correlates of empathy for physical pain in CIP patients, compared with healthy controls, when observing video-clips depicting others in pain. Consistent with previous results (Danziger, Prkachin, & Willer, 2006), CIP patients' ratings of pain intensity were lower when viewing body parts in painful situations, while pain ratings did not differ for painful facial expression. At first glance, the CIP patients showed a similar pattern of brain activations compared with controls, regardless of whether the painful event depicted painful situation of body parts or facial expression of pain. Regardless of the group, there were no correlations between brain activation to painful facial expressions and pain-intensity ratings. Nevertheless, the cerebral activations could reflect different processes in the two groups. For instance, although AI and ACC engagement may reflect the emotional processing of vicarious pain in both groups, it is likely to be related to an automatic affective resonance, as this mechanism is believed to be shaped by one's previous pain experiences (Decety & Jackson, 2004). While self-pain representations are lacking in CIP patients, the AI and ACC activations may be associated with cognitive processes, thus allowing the CIP patients to access a vicarious representation of pain unpleasantness. Moreover, in the CIP patients (but not in controls) brain responses to facial expression of pain in the vmPFC and to pictures of body parts in painful situations in the vPCC were strongly and positively correlated with empathy traits, underlying a potential link between these areas and empathic abilities.

The contribution of self-pain experience processes in empathy for physical pain has also been examined in a study on placebo analgesia in healthy subjects (Rütgen et al., 2015). The participants were scanned while they received, or witnessed another person receiving painful or non-painful electrical stimulation, before and after undergoing a placebo analgesia protocol. The participants experiencing placebo analgesia reported decreased self-pain as well as decreased empathy for pain compared with controls. This decrease was associated with reduced activation of emotional processing of pain areas (AI and midcingulate cortex) reflecting affective resonance. Overall, this study adds evidence that, in healthy persons, the understanding of another's pain level engages the mental representation of self-pain experiences.

Exposure to Others' Pain   Some studies have also highlighted how previous experience with others' pain may modulate the actual cerebral response to others' pain. In a seminal study using fMRI, Cheng et al. (2007) were the first to investigate the cerebral responses of empathy for pain in relation to a person's experiences. They demonstrated different patterns of brain activation in areas associated with empathy for others' pain in acupuncturists compared to controls, when they were observing pictures of a needle puncturing the skin (painful events) or a cotton tip touching the skin (non-painful events; Cheng et al., 2007). Acupuncturists showed less activation than controls in the AI and the aMCC/dACC, suggesting a reduced affective resonance in their cerebral response when viewing someone having a needle puncturing the skin. The authors also reported a decrease in the mPFC that they interpreted in association with the underestimation of vicarious pain, as a potential self-protective bias that would dampen the affective resonance to others' pain to prevent the acupuncturists from emotional contagion of their patients' distress.

In the same vein, other authors have specifically examined the effect of pain over-exposure on the brain response to vicarious pain. The amount of exposure to pain cues is considered as one of the main source of the patients' pain underestimation by physicians or nurses (Prkachin, Solomon, & Ross, 2007). Therefore, this factor appears critical if one wants to address the issue of healthcare professionals' well-being and medical empathy. Healthcare workers routinely deal with suffering in every form, which could definitely be stressful and exhausting, and sometimes an obstacle to responding empathically to suffering patients. In fact, pain overexposure could lead to remaining detached (or desensitized) to others' pain, causing a general underestimation of patients' pain (Halpern, 2012; Neumann et al., 2011). This behavior would be a way to regulate the emotional distress triggered by the observation (or sharing) of someone's pain (Prkachin et al., 2007). Understanding the cerebral impact of pain exposure on the perception of others' pain may help decipher the relationship between pain overexposure and pain underestimation, as well as their link with the different components of empathy (i.e., affective resonance, perspective-taking, emotion regulation). In an experimental study using EEG, Coll, Grégoire, Prkachin, and Jackson (2016) examined the neural changes underlying repeated exposure to someone in pain. They measured behavioral (pain detection task) and event-related-potential responses of healthy adults who were either repeatedly exposed to facial expressions of pain or to neutral facial expressions. As in previous behavioural studies (e.g., Prkachin, Mass, & Mercer, 2004; Prkachin & Rocha, 2010), the participants were less inclined to consider moderate expressions of pain as painful after being exposed to intense expressions of pain. Most notably, this effect was associated with a decrease in the Late Positive Potential (LPP) response to pain expressions following exposure to intense pain compared with participants exposed to neutral expressions. This result was interpreted as an alteration of the cerebral responses to the pain of others, which would indicate that the repeated exposure to vicarious pain leads to a decrease in the perceived salience of pain expressions (i.e., low-level attentional processes implied in others' pain perception). Furthermore, correlation analysis showed a relation between self-reported empathic concern and the LPP response in the control group, but not in the exposure group. In accordance with Cheng et al. (2007), this result suggested that repeated exposure to pain in others might affect the regulation of vicarious pain responses. Although it remains experimental, this study pinpoints the critical impact that a repeated exposure to suffering may have on the perception of others' pain, as well as on its brain mechanisms, at least in the short term. Therefore, it appears highly relevant to further understand its effects on people who are regularly exposed to others' pain, over several years.

Moreover, in a recent fMRI study, Jackson et al. (2017) compared the brain activity pattern of pediatric intensive care nurses (i.e., people who are exposed to babies' pain on a daily basis) and a control group of health workers (e.g., social workers, pharmacists) when watching clips of babies undergoing painful or non-painful procedures or clips of adults with chronic shoulder pain (from the UNBC-McMaster Shoulder Pain database; see Lucy, Cohn, Prkachin, Solomon, & Matthrews, 2011). Consistent with a previous study revealing overestimation of babies' pain in non-pediatric healthcare professionals (Latimer, Jackson, Johnston, & Vine, 2011), pediatric nurses scored the pain of infants and adults significantly higher than other health workers. The fact that they perceived higher pain than non-expert controls even in adults, for whom they have no specific expertise, may suggest that the specialized training they received in the pediatric field generalizes to adult patient or even that they are more sensitive to other's pain overall. Analysis of fMRI data yielded a significantly lower activation of brain regions associated with affective resonance (e.g., left IFG/AI, right thalamus) and emotion regulation (e.g., mPFC) in pediatric nurses when observing infants in pain compared with controls, while the neural response related to the observation of adults in pain did not vary between the two groups. Correlation analysis also revealed that the relatively reduced activation in the left IFG/AI in nurses was proportional to the number of years of experience in the neonate care unit. Note, however, that the differences in brain response were not correlated with ratings of others' pain. The authors suggested that the lower activation of IFG/AI and thalamus indicates a *neural habituation* or *blunting* following repeated pain exposure. This result is consistent with a recent neuroimaging study showing that repeated exposure to hand stimuli in painful situations was associated with a reduced neural response in brain regions including the AI (Preis, Kröner-Herwig, Schmidt-Samoa, Dechent, & Barke, 2015). Contrary to the study of Cheng et al. (2007) with acupuncturists, the pediatric nurses showed a lower activation in the mPFC compared with the controls when viewing infants' pain. This result is congruent with their higher infant pain ratings and would suggest lesser emotion regulation (i.e., lack of a self-protective bias) in nurses when they are exposed to babies' pain. These results are quite different from those obtained by Cheng et al. (2007), suggesting that the cerebral impact of vicarious pain is specific to the kind of pain and to the type of patient that healthcare professionals encounter in their practice.

The Context, and the Interaction Between the Sufferer and the Observer   The *affective link* between the observer and the person in pain is one of the first factors that were shown to be a strong modulator of the neural response to vicarious pain (Singer et al., 2006). In this original study, Singer et al. (2006) measured brain responses when individuals empathized with the pain of someone they liked or disliked (based on a prior session where they interacted in a competitive game). Male participants showed significantly less empathic activity (affective resonance) for people they disliked compared with ones they liked, while there were no marked difference in women. *Ethnicity* is also a well-known factor that influences the empathic brain response for physical pain (Avenanti, Sirigu, & Aglioti, 2010; Contreras-Huerta, Baker, Reynolds, Batalha, & Cunnington, 2013; Mathur, Harada, Lipke, & Chiao, 2010; Riečanský, Paul, Kölble, Stieger, & Lamm, 2015; Xu, Zuo, Wang, & Han, 2009). In the study by Contreras-Huerta et al. (2013), for example, the brains of Caucasian participants were scanned using fMRI while they were watching video clips of Asian or Caucasian people receiving either a painful (syringe needle) or non-painful (cotton-bud) touch on the left or right cheek. After each clip, they rated how painful each stimulus looked on a 4-point scale. Results revealed no significant differences in the pain ratings regarding the ethnic group. Interestingly, the neural empathic responses revealed a greater activation in the left insular cortex when observing painful touch to the faces of same-ethnicity people compared with other-ethnicity people.

Responsibility   Using fMRI, Cui, Abdelgabar, Keysers, and Gazzola (2015) examined whether brain responses to dynamic facial expressions of pain are influenced by the observer's responsibility for the pain in someone he or she is observing. The participant and a confederate performed a difficult task simultaneously, while the participant was in the scanner. The task consisted of displaying a central target letter flanked by distractors and the two players had to press the button corresponding to the central letter. If one of them or both erred in the task, the confederate received a noxious shock. In some trials the participant or the confederate was fully responsible for the other's electric stimuli, while in some trials they both shared the responsibility for their own pain. The participants were seeing the confederate being shocked via a video-feed depicting her facial expressions. The author also scanned the participants' brains while they were delivered noxious and innocuous electric stimuli to the right hand in order to localize regions involved in the self-pain experience (i.e., pain matrix). The regions of the functionally localized pain-matrix of the participants (including the middle temporal gyrus around the superior temporal sulcus, the inferior frontal gyrus, ACC, AI, amygdala, striatum, and right superior frontal gyrus) showed stronger activations for conditions in which the witnessed pain was entirely due to the participant's mistake compared with those where the confederate or both individuals had erred. This "boosted" activation in areas of the *shared-representation* network suggests a stronger affective reaction to pain in others when the observer witnesses a pain he/she had caused.

Sense of Control In another study, De Coster, Andres, and Brass (2014) tested whether the sense of exerting control over the hand of someone else may change the corticospinal excitability evoked by viewing this hand receiving painful stimulation. In a preliminary *action* phase, the sense of control was manipulated (De Coster, Verschuere, Goubert, Tsakiris, & Brass, 2013). In an imitative paradigm, a hand displayed on a screen imitated participants, giving them the sense of having control over this hand. In a non-imitative condition, the hand performed non-matching movements. After being imitated or not by this hand, the participants observed the hand receiving painful stimulation. During this *pain observation* phase, motor evoked potentials (MEPs) induced by transcranial magnetic stimulation (TMS) were measured in the right dominant hand of participants. The result revealed that when participants did not exert control over the hand that received painful stimulation (i.e., incongruent movements in the preliminary *action* phase), decreased corticospinal excitability was found during pain observation. In contrast, when participants exerted control over the hand that received painful stimulation (i.e., congruent movements in the preliminary *action* phase), increased corticospinal excitability was observed. Moreover this facilitation effect was higher for people who were more strongly affected by others' distress as measured by self-reported distress on the Interpersonal Reactivity Index (IRI; Davis, 1980). Corticospinal excitability changes, consequent to the observation of pain in others, were interpreted as reflecting sensory resonance with another's pain; namely, the sensory aspects of others' painful experience would be mapped onto the motor system of the observer, who would react as if he or she was actually experiencing pain (for experimental evidence of sensorimotor resonance with another's pain see Avenanti et al., 2005). The authors interpreted the motor inhibition as a *freezing* (or *anesthetic*) response reflecting the participants' helplessness to prevent the other from receiving painful stimulation (i.e., the participant has no control over the hand he/she is seeing). In contrast, increasing control-induced motor facilitation may be interpreted as the preparation of an avoidance response (i.e., the participant has the illusion of commanding the other's hand in order to avoid the painful stimulation).

These two studies (Cui et al., 2015; De Coster et al., 2014) are of particular interest from a clinical perspective, as healthcare professionals sometimes have to perform painful medical procedures (e.g., wound care in patients with severe burn injuries; Hoffman et al., 2008; Perry, Heidrich, & Ramos, 1981) and are not always able to ease patients' pain (i.e., a situation where they exert no control on pain). It would be interesting to investigate more specifically people who are regularly exposed to pain, and how the sense of being responsible, or exerting or not exerting control over others' pain may change the functional brain networks underlying empathy for physical pain as well as the empathic reaction to others' pain. In line with this issue, a recent fMRI study (Jensen et al., 2014) demonstrated that physicians' brain activation during a patient-physician interaction while the patient was experiencing pain was modulated by the physician's expectancy of the patient's pain relief.

Conclusion

Although humans may be spontaneously inclined to respond empathically to others' pain, the social neuroscience findings discussed above highlight the evidence that the reaction to someone's pain (at least at the cerebral level) is not a one-to-one relationship and may be modulated by multiple intraindividual and interindividual factors. These factors stem from an individual's characteristics, the suffering person's characteristics, the interaction between the two individuals, as well as contextual events. Despite the many advances in this neuroscientific research domain, we cannot state that all the factors influencing someone's empathy are currently known. Understanding each of these factors and their specific impact on one person's behaviours and cerebral activations may be a difficult task indeed.

More importantly, as already pointed out by Zaki and Oschner (2012), in the field of empathy, the explicit links between the brain and human behaviors are still lacking or unclear in the literature. Even when neuroimaging studies include behavioral estimation of others' pain perception (often ratings of pain intensity on a visual analog scale), the cerebral data are not necessarily associated with behavioral markers, or can even be in opposite directions. Several reasons might explain this apparent lack of convergence. First, some of the behavioral measures have their limitations, as empathy is frequently inferred from pain rating. But what do pain ratings mean in the context of the study of empathy? Higher level of pain ratings has been implicitly interpreted as higher level of empathy, but is that always the case? *Empathic accuracy*, the congruence between the observer's pain rating with the subjective pain rating of the person in pain (see for instance Issner, Cano, Leonard, & Williams, 2012) might be a more relevant behavioral marker of empathy. It directly assesses the ability of the observer to rightly understand the mental state of the other individual, but unfortunately it is not the most used tool in assessing empathy. Second, as it was previously mentioned, there are many factors influencing empathy and the way it is captured at the behavioral and cerebral levels. It is important to consider that these differences actually account for the lack of consistency in the empathy domain. For instance, different tasks or even similar tasks using different stimuli can trigger utterly different behavioral and brain responses. Therefore, it is well known, but sometimes forgotten, how tricky it may be to infer specific cognitive processes based solely on activation in particular brain areas (i.e., *inverse inference problem*; see Poldrack, 2006). So, considering all these points, whether we can determine the level of empathy of an individual, as well as predict his/her response to someone's pain, solely on the brain responses to others' pain, seems a far-reaching goal. As suggested by Preusche and Lamm (2016), the combination of neuroimaging with behavioral and physiological measures of empathy and the reaction to others' suffering (e.g., self-ratings of experienced emotions or observational methods assessing an empathic behavior) is likely the best way to meet the challenge of determining the optimal degree of empathy of an individual in order to favor a prosocial stance while preserving oneself from emotional distress. The specific endeavor to understand the relationship between the cerebral basis of human empathy and social behavior will lead to additional insights, which might help different disciplines to translate this knowledge into practice. This can be achieved by teaching what is empathy—its components, its goals and importance, as well as its costs and pitfalls. It is primordial to teach how to maintain reliable empathic behaviors in professions where this competence is required but may be costly (e.g., health professionals). Ultimately, the knowledge we seek in research would be highly applicable in clinical settings. For instance, the cerebral basis of empathy might prove useful in highlighting and treating the physiopathology of patients suffering from empathy deficits (autism, psychopathy, and schizophrenia).

References

Akitsuki, Y., & Decety, J. (2009). Social context and perceived agency affects empathy for pain: An event-related fMRI investigation. *NeuroImage, 47*(2), 722–734. https://doi.org/10.1016/j.neuroimage.2009.04.091

Amodio, D. M., & Frith, C. D. (2006). Meeting of minds: The medial frontal cortex and social cognition. *Nature Reviews Neuroscience, 7*(4), 268–277.

Apkarian, A. V., Hashmi, J. A., & Baliki, M. N. (2011). Pain and the brain: Specificity and plasticity of the brain in clinical chronic pain. *Pain, 152*(3 Suppl), S49.

Avenanti, A., Bueti, D., Galati, G., & Aglioti, S. M. (2005). Transcranial magnetic stimulation highlights the sensorimotor side of empathy for pain. *Nature Neuroscience, 8*, 955–960. https://doi.org/10.1038/nn1481

Avenanti, A., Sirigu, A., & Aglioti, S. M. (2010). Racial bias reduces empathic sensorimotor resonance with other-race pain. *Current Biology, 20*(11), 1018–1022. https://doi.org/10.1016/j.cub.2010.03.071

Aziz-Zadeh, L., Sheng, T., Liew, S. L., & Damasio, H. (2012). Understanding otherness: The neural bases of action comprehension and pain empathy in a congenital amputee. *Cerebral Cortex, 22*(4), 811–819. https://doi.org/10.1093/cercor/bhr139

Baliki, M. N., Chialvo, D. R., Geha, P. Y., Levy, R. M., Harden, R. N., Parrish, T. B., & Apkarian, A. V. (2006). Chronic pain and the emotional brain: Specific brain activity associated with spontaneous fluctuations of intensity of chronic back pain. *The Journal of Neuroscience, 26*(47), 12165–12173. https://doi.org/10.1523/JNEUROSCI.3576-06.2006

Batson, C. D. (2009). These things called empathy: Eight related but distinct phenomena. In J. Decety & W. Ickes (Eds.), *Social neuroscience. The social neuroscience of empathy* (pp. 3–15). Cambridge, MA: MIT Press.

Baumgartner, T., Fischbacher, U., Feieraben, A., Lutz, K., & Fehr, E. (2009). The neural circuitry of a broken promise. *Neuron, 64*(5), 756–770.

Bonvicini, K. A., Perlin, M. J., Bylund, C. L., Carroll, G., Rouse, R. A., & Goldstein, M. G. (2009). Impact of communication training on physician expression of empathy in patient encounters. *Patient Education and Counseling, 75*, 3–10. https://doi.org/10.1016/j.pec.2008.09.007

Botvinick, M., Jha, A. P., Bylsma, L. M., Fabian, S. A., Solomon, P. E., & Prkachin, K. M. (2005). Viewing facial expressions of pain engages cortical areas involved in the direct experience of pain. *NeuroImage, 25*, 312–319.

Buckner, R. L., Andrews Hanna, J. R., & Schacter, D. L. (2008). The brain's default network. *Annals of the New York Academy of Sciences, 1124*(1), 1–38.

Budell, L., Jackson, P. L., & Rainville, P. (2010). Brain responses to facial expressions of pain: Emotional or motor mirroring? *NeuroImage, 53*(1), 355–363. https://doi.org/10.1016/j.neuroimage.2010.05.037

Cheng, Y., Lin, C. P., Liu, H. L., Hsu, Y. Y., Lim, K. E., Hung, D., & Decety, J. (2007). Expertise modulates the perception of pain in others. *Current Biology, 17*(19), 1708–1713. https://doi.org/10.1016/j.cub.2007.09.020

Cheon, B. K., Im, D. M., Harada, T., Kim, J. S., Mathur, V. A., Scimeca, J. M., … Chiao, J. Y. (2011). Cultural influences on neural basis of intergroup empathy. *NeuroImage, 57*(2), 642–650. https://doi.org/10.1016/j.neuroimage.2011.04.031

Cheon, B. K., Im, D. M., Harada, T., Kim, J. S., Mathur, V. A., Scimeca, J. M., … Chiao, J. Y. (2013). Cultural modulation of the neural correlates of emotional pain perception: The role of other-focusedness. *Neuropsychologia, 51*(7), 1177–1186. https://doi.org/10.1016/j.neuropsychologia.2013.03.018

Coll, M. P., Grégoire, M., Latimer, M., Eugene, F., & Jackson, P. L. (2011). Perception of pain in others: Implication for caregivers. *Pain Management, 1*, 257–265. https://doi.org/10.2217/pmt.11.21

Coll, M. P., Grégoire, M., Prkachin, K., & Jackson, P. L. (2016). Repeated exposure to vicarious pain alters electrocortical processing of pain expressions. *Experimental Brain Research, 234*(9), 2677–2686. https://doi.org/10.1007/s00221-016-4671-z

Conson, M., Errico, D., Mazzarella, E., Giordano, M., Grossi, D., & Trojano, L. (2015). Transcranial electrical stimulation over dorsolateral prefrontal cortex modulates processing of social cognitive and affective information. *PLoS One, 10*(5), e0126448. https://doi.org/10.1371/journal.pone.0126448

Contreras-Huerta, L. S., Baker, K. S., Reynolds, K. J., Batalha, L., & Cunnington, R. (2013). Racial bias in neural empathic responses to pain. *PLoS One, 8*(12). https://doi.org/10.1371/journal.pone.0084001

Corradi-Dell'Acqua, C., Hofstetter, C., & Vuilleumier, P. (2011). Felt and seen pain evoke the same local patterns of cortical activity in insular and cingulate cortex. *The Journal of Neuroscience, 31*, 17996–18006. https://doi.org/10.1523/JNEUROSCI.2686-11.2011

Corradi-Dell'Acqua, C., Tusche, A., Vuilleumier, P., & Singer, T. (2016). Cross-modal representations of first-hand and vicarious pain, disgust and fairness in insular and cingulate cortex. *Nature Communications, 7*. https://doi.org/10.1038/ncomms10904

Craig, K. D. (2009). The social communication model of pain. *Canadian Psychology/Psychologie Canadienne, 50*(1), 22.

Cui, F., Abdelgabar, A. R., Keysers, C., & Gazzola, V. (2015). Responsibility modulates pain-matrix activation elicited by the expressions of others in pain. *NeuroImage, 114*, 371–378. https://doi.org/10.1016/j.neuroimage.2015.03.034

D'Argembeau, A., Ruby, P., Collette, F., Degueldre, C., Balteau, E., Luxen, A., … Salmon, E. (2007). Distinct regions of the medial prefrontal cortex are associated with self-referential processing and perspective taking. *Journal of Cognitive Neuroscience, 19*(6), 935–944. https://doi.org/10.1162/jocn.2007.19.6.935

Danziger, N., Faillenot, I., & Peyron, R. (2009). Can we share a pain we never felt ? Neural correlates of empathy in patients with congenital insensitivity to pain. *Neuron, 29*(2), 203–212. https://doi.org/10.1016/j.neuron.2008.11.023

Danziger, N., Prkachin, K. M., & Willer, J. C. (2006). Is pain the price of empathy? The perception of others' pain in patients with congenital insensitivity to pain. *Brain, 129*(Pt 9), 2494–2507. https://doi.org/10.1093/brain/awl155

Davis, M. H. (1980). A multidimensional approach to individual differences in empathy. *JSAS Catalog of Selected Documents in Psychology, 10*, 85.

De Coster, L., Andres, M., & Brass, M. (2014). Effects of being imitated on motor responses evoked by pain observation: Exerting control determines action tendencies when perceiving pain in others. *The Journal of Neuroscience, 34*(20), 6952–6957. https://doi.org/10.1523/JNEUROSCI.5044-13.2014

De Coster, L., Verschuere, B., Goubert, L., Tsakiris, M., & Brass, M. (2013). I suffer more from your pain when you act like me: Being imitated enhances affective responses to seeing someone else in pain. *Cognitive, Affective, & Behavioural Neuroscience, 13*, 519–532. https://doi.org/10.3758/s13415-013-0168-4

De Waal, F. B. M., & Preston, S. D. (2017). Mammalian empathy: Behavioural manifestations and neural basis. *Nature Reviews Neuroscience*. https://doi.org/10.1038/nrn.2017.72

Decety, J., Chen, C., Harenski, C., & Kiehl, K. A. (2013). An fMRI study of affective perspective taking in individuals with psychopathy: Imagining another in pain does not evoke empathy. *Frontiers in Human Neuroscience, 7*, 489. https://doi.org/10.3389/fnhum.2013.00489

Decety, J., & Jackson, P. L. (2004). The functional architecture of human empathy. *Behavioral and Cognitive Neuroscience Reviews, 3*, 71–100.

Decety, J., Jackson, P. L., & Brunet, E. (2007). The cognitive neuropsychology of empathy. In Dans Farrow, T. & Woodruff, P. (Dir.), Empathy in mental illness (pp. 239–260). New York, NY: Cambridge University Press.

Decety, J., & Lamm, C. (2007). The role of the right temporoparietal junction in social interaction: How low-level computational processes contribute to meta-cognition. *The Neuroscientist, 13*(6), 580–593. https://doi.org/10.1177/1073858407304654

Decety, J., Skelly, L. R., & Kiehl, K. A. (2013). Brain response to empathy-eliciting scenarios involving pain in incarcerated individuals with psychopathy. *JAMA Psychiatry, 70*(6), 638–645. https://doi.org/10.1001/jamapsychiatry.2013.27

Decety, J., & Sommerville, J. A. (2003). Shared representations between self and other: A social cognitive neuroscience view. *Trends in Cognitive Sciences, 7*(12), 527–533. https://doi.org/10.1016/j.tics.2003.10.004

Del Canale, S., Louis, D. Z., Maio, V., Wang, X., Rossi, G., Hojat, M., & Gonnella, J. S. (2012). The relationship between physician empathy and disease complications: An empirical study of primary care physicians and their diabetic patients in Parma, Italy. *Academic Medicine, 87*, 1243–1249. https://doi.org/10.1097/acm.0b013e3182628fbf

Donaldson, P. H., Rinehart, N. J., & Enticott, P. G. (2015). Noninvasive stimulation of the temporoparietal junction: A systematic review. *Neuroscience and Biobehavioral Reviews, 55*, 547–572. https://doi.org/10.1016/j.neubiorev.2015.05.017

Fan, Y., Duncan, N. W., de Greck, M., & Northoff, G. (2011). Is there a core neural network in empathy? An fMRI based quantitative meta-analysis. *Neuroscience & Biobehavioral Reviews, 35*(3), 903–911. https://doi.org/10.1016/j.neubiorev.2010.10.009

Fan, Y. T., Chen, C., Chen, S. C., Decety, J., & Cheng, Y. (2014). Empathic arousal and social understanding in individuals with autism: Evidence from fMRI and ERP measurements. *Social Cognitive and Affective Neuroscience, 9*(8), 1203–1213. https://doi.org/10.1093/scan/nst101

Feighny, K. M., Monaco, M., & Arnold, L. (1995). Empathy training to improve physician-patient communication skills. *Academic Medicine, 70*, 435–436. https://doi.org/10.1097/00001888-199505000-00031

Frith, C. D. (2007). *Making up the mind; how the brain creates our mental world.* Oxford, England: Blackwell.

Frith, C. D., & Frith, U. (2006). How we predict what other people are going to do. *Brain Research, 1079*(1), 36–46. https://doi.org/10.1016/j.brainres.2005.12.126

Garcia-Larrea, L., & Peyron, R. (2013). Pain matrices and neuropathic pain matrices: A review. *Pain, 154*, S29–S43. https://doi.org/10.1016/j.pain.2013.09.001

Geng, J. J., & Mangun, G. R. (2011). Right temporoparietal junction activation by a salient contextual cue facilitates target discrimination. *NeuroImage, 54*(1), 594–601. https://doi.org/10.1016/j.neuroimage.2010.08.025

Geng, J. J., & Vossel, S. (2013). Re-evaluating the role of TPJ in attentional control: Contextual updating? *Neuroscience & Biobehavioral Reviews, 37*(10), 2608–2620. https://doi.org/10.1016/j.neubiorev.2013.08.010

Gerdes, K. E., Segal, E. A., & Lietz, C. A. (2010). Conceptualising and measuring empathy. *British Journal of Social Work, 40*(7), 2326–2343. https://doi.org/10.1093/bjsw/bcq048

Gleichgerrcht, E., & Decety, J. (2013). Empathy in clinical practice: How individual dispositions, gender, and experience moderate empathic concern, burnout, and emotional distress in physicians. *PLoS One, 8*(4), e61526. https://doi.org/10.1371/journal.pone.0061526

Gonzalez-Liencres, C., Brown, E. C., Tas, C., Breidenstein, A., & Brüne, M. (2016). Alterations in event-related potential responses to empathy for pain in schizophrenia. *Psychiatry Research, 241*, 14–21. https://doi.org/10.1016/j.psychres.2016.04.091

Goubert, L., Craig, K. D., Vervoort, T., Morley, S., Sullivan, M. J. L., Williams, A. C., ... Crombez, G. (2005). Facing others in pain: The effects of empathy. *Pain, 118*(3), 285–288. https://doi.org/10.1016/j.pain.2005.10.025

Gross, J. J., & Thompson, R. A. (2007). Emotion regulation: Conceptual foundations. In J. J. Gross (Ed.), *Handbook of emotion regulation* (pp. 3–24). New York, NY: Guilford Press.

Gu, X., Eilam-Stock, T., Zhou, T., Anagnostou, E., Kolevzon, A., Soorya, L., ... Fan, J. (2015). Autonomic and brain responses associated with empathy deficits in autism spectrum disorder. *Human Brain Mapping, 36*, 3323–3338. https://doi.org/10.1002/hbm.22840

Hadjikhani, N., Zürcher, N. R., Rogier, O., Hippolyte, L., Lemonnier, E., Ruest, T., ... Helles, A. (2014). Emotional contagion for pain is intact in autism spectrum disorders. *Translational Psychiatry, 4*(1), e343. https://doi.org/10.1038/tp.2013.113

Halpern, J. (2012). Clinical empathy in medical care. In J. Decety (Ed.), *Empathy: From bench to bedside* (pp. 229–244). Cambridge, MA: MIT Press.

Heberlein, A. S., Padon, A. A., Gillihan, S. J., Farah, M. J., & Fellows, L. K. (2008). Ventromedial frontal lobe plays a critical role in facial emotion recognition. *Journal of Cognitive Neuroscience, 20*, 721–733.

Hoffman, H. G., Patterson, D. R., Seibel, E., Soltani, M., Jewett-Leahy, L., & Sharar, S. R. (2008). Virtual reality pain control during burn wound debridement in the hydrotank. *The Clinical Journal of Pain, 24*(4), 299–304.

Hynes, C. A., Baird, A. A., & Grafton, S. T. (2006). Differential role of the orbitofrontal lobe in emotional versus cognitive perspective-taking. *Neuropsychologia, 44*, 374–383. https://doi.org/10.1016/j.neuropsychologia.2005.06.011

Issner, J. B., Cano, A., Leonard, M. T., & Williams, A. M. (2012). How do I empathize with you? Let me count the ways: Relations between facets of pain-related empathy. *The Journal of Pain, 13*(2), 167–175. https://doi.org/10.1016/j.jpain.2011.10.009

Jackson, P. L., Brunet, E., Meltzoff, A. N., & Decety, J. (2006). Empathy examined through the neural mechanisms involved in imagining how I feel versus how you feel pain. *Neuropsychologia, 44*, 752–761.

Jackson, P. L., Eugène, F., & Tremblay, M.-P. B. (2015). Improving empathy in the care of pain patients. *American Journal of Bioethics – Neuroscience, 6*(3), 25–33. https://doi.org/10.1080/21507740.2015.1047053

Jackson, P. L., Latimer, M., Eugène, F., Macloead, E., Hatfield, T., Vachon-Presseau, E., ... Prkachin, K. M. (2017). Empathy in paediatric intensive care nurses part 2: Neural correlates. *Journal of Advanced Nursing.* https://doi.org/10.1111/jan.13334

Jackson, P. L., Rainville, P., & Decety, J. (2006). To what extent do we share the pain of others? Insight from the neural bases of pain empathy. *Pain, 125*(1–2), 5–9. https://doi.org/10.1016/j.pain.2006.09.013

Jeannerod, M. (2001). Neural simulation of action: A unifying mechanism for motor cognition. *NeuroImage, 14*, S103–S109.

Jensen, K. B., Petrovic, P., Kerr, C. E., Kirsch, I., Raicek, J., Cheetham, A., ... Kaptchuk, T. J. (2014). Sharing pain and relief: Neural correlates of physicians during treatment of patients. *Molecular Psychiatry, 19*(3), 392–398. https://doi.org/10.1038/mp.2012.195

Keysers, C., & Gazzola, V. (2010). Social neuroscience: Mirror neurons recorded in humans. *Current Biology, 20*(8), R353–R354.

Koole, S. L. (2009). The psychology of emotion regulation: An integrative review. *Cognition and Emotion, 23*(1), 4–41.

Krishnan, A., Woo, C. W., Chang, L. J., Ruzic, L., Gu, X., López-Solà, M., ... Wager, T. D. (2016). Somatic and vicarious pain are represented by dissociable multivariate brain patterns. *eLife, 5*, e15166.

Kucyi, A., & Davis, K. D. (2016). The neural code for pain: From single-cell electrophysiology to the dynamic pain connectome. *The Neuroscientist*, 1–18. https://doi.org/10.1177/1073858416667716

Kurth, F., Zilles, K., Fox, P. T., Laird, A. R., & Eickhoff, S. B. (2010). A link between the systems: Functional differentiation and integration within the human insula revealed by meta-analysis. *Brain Structure and Function, 214*, 519–534. https://doi.org/10.1007/s00429-010-0255-z

Lamm, C., Batson, C. D., & Decety, J. (2007). The neural substrate of human empathy: Effects of perspective-taking and cognitive appraisal. *Journal of Cognitive Neuroscience, 19*, 42–58.

Lamm, C., Decety, J., & Singer, T. (2011). Meta-analytic evidence for common and distinct neural networks associated with directly experienced pain and empathy for pain. *NeuroImage, 54*(3), 2492–2502. https://doi.org/10.1016/j.neuroimage.2010.10.014

Latimer, M., Jackson, P., Johnston, C., & Vine, J. (2011). Examining nurse empathy for infant procedural pain: Testing a new video measure. *Pain Research and Management, 16*(4), 228–233.

Latimer, M., Jackson, P. L., Eugène, F., Macloead, E., Hatfield, T., Vachon-Presseau, E., … Prkachin, K. M. (2017). Empathy in pediatric nurses part 1: Behavioral and psychological correlates. *Journal of Advanced Nursing, 00*, 1–10. https://doi.org/10.1111/jan.13333

Li, W., Mai, X., & Liu, C. (2014). The default mode network and social understanding of others: What do brain connectivity studies tell us. *Frontiers in Human Neuroscience, 8*, 74.

Liu, X., Powell, D. K., Wang, H., Gold, B. T., Corbly, C. R., & Joseph, J. E. (2007). Functional dissociation in frontal and striatal areas for processing of positive and negative reward information. *The Journal of Neuroscience, 27*, 4587–4597.

Lockwood, P. L. (2016). The anatomy of empathy: Vicarious experience and disorders of social cognition. *Behavioural Brain Research, 311*, 255–266. https://doi.org/10.1016/j.bbr.2016.05.048

Loeser, J. D., & Treede, R. D. (2008). The Kyoto protocol of IASP basic pain terminology. *Pain, 137*(3), 473–477.

Lucy, P., Cohn, J. F., Prkachin, K. M., Solomon, P., & Matthrews, I. (2011). Painful data: The UNBC-McMaster shoulder pain expression archive database. In *IEEE International Conference on Automatic Face and Gesture Recognition* (FG2011).

Marcoux, L. A., & Jackson, P. L. (2012). Perspective des neurosciences sociales sur l'influence des différences individuelles et de la psychopathologie sur l'empathie pour la douleur. *Médecin Sciences Amérique, 2*(1), 51–67.

Mars, R. B., Neubert, F. X., Noonan, M. P., Sallet, J., Toni, I., & Rushworth, M. F. (2012). On the relationship between the "default mode network" and the "social brain". *Frontiers in Human Neuroscience, 6*, 189.

Marsh, A. A., Finger, E. C., Fowler, K. A., Adalio, C. J., Jurkowitz, I. T., Schechter, J. C., … Blair, R. J. R. (2013). Empathic responsiveness in amygdala and anterior cingulate cortex in youths with psychopathic traits. *Journal of Child Psychology and Psychiatry, 54*(8), 900–910. https://doi.org/10.1111/jcpp.12063.Empathic

Mathur, V. A., Harada, T., Lipke, T., & Chiao, J. Y. (2010). Neural basis of extraordinary empathy and altruistic motivation. *NeuroImage, 51*(4), 1468–1475.

Meffert, H., Gazzola, V., den Boer, J. A., Bartels, A. A., & Keysers, C. (2013). Reduced spontaneous but relatively normal deliberate vicarious representations in psychopathy. *Brain, 136*(8), 2550–2562. https://doi.org/10.1093/brain/awt190

Melloni, M., Lopez, V., & Ibanez, A. (2014). Empathy and contextual social cognition. *Cognitive, Affective, & Behavioral Neuroscience, 14*(1), 407–425. https://doi.org/10.3758/s13415-013-0205-3

Meng, J., Jackson, T., Chen, H., Hu, L., Yang, Z., Su, Y., & Huang, X. (2013). Pain perception in the self and observation of others: An ERP investigation. *NeuroImage.* https://doi.org/10.1016/j.neuroimage.2013.01.024

Morawetz, C., Bode, S., Derntl, B., & Heekeren, H. R. (2017). The effect of strategies, goals and stimulus material on the neural mechanisms of emotion regulation: A meta-analysis of fMRI studies. *Neuroscience & Biobehavioral Reviews, 72*, 111–128.

Morelli, S. A., & Lieberman, M. D. (2013). The role of automaticity and attention in neural processes underlying empathy for happiness, sadness, and anxiety. *Frontiers in Human Neuroscience, 7*, 160. https://doi.org/10.3389/fnhum.2013.00160

Neumann, M., Edelhäuser, F., Tauschel, D., Fischer, M. R., Wirtz, M., Woopen, C., … Scheffer, C. (2011). Empathy decline and its reasons: A systematic review of studies with medical students and residents. *Academic Medicine, 86*(8), 996–1009.

Nummenmaa, L., Hirvonen, J., Parkkola, R., & Hietanen, J. K. (2008). Is emotional contagion special? An fMRI study on neural systems for affective and cognitive empathy. *NeuroImage, 43*, 571–580.

Ochsner, K. N., & Gross, J. J. (2005). The cognitive control of emotion. *Trends in Cognitive Sciences, 9*(5), 242–249.

Perry, S., Heidrich, G., & Ramos, E. (1981). Assessment of pain by burn patients. *Journal of Burn Care & Research, 2*(6), 322–326.

Poldrack, R. A. (2006). Can cognitive processes be inferred from neuroimaging data? *Trends in Cognitive Sciences, 10*(2), 59–63. https://doi.org/10.1016/j.tics.2005.12.004

Preis, M. A., Kröner-Herwig, B., Schmidt-Samoa, C., Dechent, P., & Barke, A. (2015). Neural correlates of empathy with pain show habituation effects. An fMRI study. *PLoS One, 10*(8), e0137056. https://doi.org/10.1371/journal.pone.0137056

Preis, M. A., Schmidt-Samoa, C., Dechent, P., & Kroener-Herwig, B. (2013). The effects of prior pain experience on neural correlates of empathy for pain: An fMRI study. *Pain.* https://doi.org/10.1016/j.pain.2012.11.014

Preston, S. D., & de Waal, F. B. M. (2002). Empathy: Its ultimate and proximate bases. *Behavioral and Brain Sciences, 25*(1), 1–72.

Preusche, I., & Lamm, C. (2016). Reflections on empathy in medical education: What can we learn from social neurosciences? *Advances in Health Sciences Education, 21*(1), 235–249. https://doi.org/10.1007/s10459-015-9581-5

Price D. D. (2010). Psychological and neural mechanisms of the affective dimension of pain. *Science, 288*(5472), 1769–1772. https://doi.org/10.1126/science.288.5472.1769

Prinz, W. (1997). Perception and action planning. *European Journal of Cognitive Psychology, 9*(2), 129–154. https://doi.org/10.1080/713752551

Prkachin, K. M., Mass, H., & Mercer, S. R. (2004). Effects of exposure on perception of pain expression. *Pain, 111*(1), 8–12. https://doi.org/10.1016/j.pain.2004.03.027

Prkachin, K. M., & Rocha, E. M. (2010). High levels of vicarious exposure bias pain judgments. *The Journal of Pain, 11*(9), 904–909. https://doi.org/10.1016/j.jpain.2009.12.015

Prkachin, K. M., Solomon, P. E., & Ross, J. (2007). La sous-estimation de la douleur par les prestateurs de soins : vers la conception d'un modèle d'inférence pour évaluer la douleur chez autrui. *Canadian Journal of Nursing Research, 39*, 88–106.

Rakel, D. P., Hoeft, T. J., Barrett, B. P., Chewning, B. A., Craig, B. M., & Niu, M. (2009). Practitioner empathy and the duration of the common cold. *Family Medicine, 41*(7), 494. https://doi.org/10.1016/j.bbi.2008.04.014

Riečanský, I., Paul, N., Kölble, S., Stieger, S., & Lamm, C. (2015). Beta oscillations reveal ethnicity ingroup bias in sensorimotor resonance to pain of others. *Social Cognitive and Affective Neuroscience.* https://doi.org/10.1093/scan/nsu139

Rogachov, A., Cheng, J. C., Erpelding, N., Hemington, K. S., & Crawley, A. P. (2016). Regional brain signal variability: A novel indicator of pain sensitivity and coping. *Pain, 157*(11), 2483–2492.

Rütgen, M., Seidel, E. M., Silani, G., Riečanský, I., Hummer, A., Windischberger, C., ... Lamm, C. (2015). Placebo analgesia and its opioidergic regulation suggest that empathy for pain is grounded in self pain. *Proceedings of the National Academy of Sciences, 112*(41), E5638–E5646. https://doi.org/10.1073/pnas.1511269112

Samson, D., Apperley, I. A., Chiavarino, C., & Humphreys, G. W. (2004). Left temporoparietal junction is necessary for representing someone else's beliefs. *Nature Neuroscience, 7*, 499–500.

Saxe, R. (2006). Uniquely human social cognition. *Current Opinion in Neurobiology, 16*, 235–239. https://doi.org/10.1016/j.conb.2006.03.001

Saxe, R., & Kanwisher, N. (2003). People thinking about people: The role of the temporoparietal junction in theory of mind. *NeuroImage, 19*, 1835–1842. https://doi.org/10.1016/S1053-8119(03)00230-1

Schilbach, L., Eickhoff, S. B., Rotarska-Jagiela, A., Fink, G. R., & Vogeley, K. (2008). Minds at rest? Social cognition as the default mode of cognizing and its putative relationship to the "default system" of the brain. *Consciousness and Cognition, 17*(2), 457–467.

Shamay-Tsoory, S. G. (2009). Empathic processing. In J. Dans Decety & W. Ickes (Eds.), *The social neuroscience of empathy* (pp. 215–232). London, England: MIT Press.

Simon, D., Craig, K. D., Miltner, W. H. R., & Rainville, P. (2006). Brain responses to dynamic facial expressions of pain. *Pain, 126*(1), 309–318.

Singer, T., Seymour, B., O'Doherty, J., Kaube, H., Dolan, R. J., & Frith, C. D. (2004). Empathy for pain involves the affective but not sensory component of pain. *Science, 303*(5661), 1157–1162. https://doi.org/10.1126/science.1093535

Singer, T., Seymour, B., O'Doherty, J. P., Stephan, K. E., Dolan, R. J., & Frith, C. D. (2006). Empathic neural responses are modulated by the perceived fairness of others. *Nature, 439*(7075), 466–469. https://doi.org/10.1038/nature04271

Tomova, L., Majdandžić, J., Hummer, A., Windischberger, C., Heinrichs, M., & Lamm, C. (2016). Increased neural responses to empathy for pain might explain how acute stress increases pro-sociality. *Social Cognitive and Affective Neuroscience, nsw146.* https://doi.org/10.1093/scan/nsw146

Treede, R. D., Kenshalo, D. R., Gracely, R. H., & Jones, A. K. (1999). The cortical representation of pain. *Pain, 79*(2), 105–111.

Van Overwalle, F., & Baetens, K. (2009). Understanding others' actions and goals by mirror and mentalizing systems: A meta-analysis. *NeuroImage, 48*(3), 564–584. https://doi.org/10.1016/j.neuroimage.2009.06.009

Vistolli, D., Lavoie, M. A., Sutliff, S., Jackson, P. L., & Achim, A. (2017). fMRI examination of empathy for pain in people with schizophrenia reveals abnormal activation related to cognitive perspective-taking but typical activation linked to affective-sharing. *Journal of Psychiatry and Neuroscience, 42,* 262–272.

Völlm, B. A., Taylor, A. N., Richardson, P., Corcoran, R., Stirling, J., McKie, S., … Elliott, R. (2006). Neuronal correlates of theory of mind and empathy: A functional magnetic resonance imaging study in a nonverbal task. *NeuroImage, 29*(1), 90–98.

Wager, T. D., Atlas, L. Y., Lindquist, M. A., Roy, M., Woo, C.-W., & Kross, E. (2013). An fMRI-based neurologic signature of physical pain. *The New England Journal of Medicine, 368*(15), 1388–1397. https://doi.org/10.1056/NEJMoa1204471

Wang, J., Wang, Y., Hu, Z., & Li, X. (2014). Transcranial direct current stimulation of the dorso-lateral prefrontal cortex increased pain empathy. *Neuroscience, 281C,* 202–207. https://doi.org/10.1016/j.neuroscience.2014.09.044

Willis, M. L., Palermo, R., McGrillen, K., & Miller, L. (2014). The nature of facial expression recognition deficits following orbitofrontal cortex damage. *Neuropsychology, 28*(4), 613–623.

Xu, X., Zuo, X., Wang, X., & Han, S. (2009). Do you feel my pain? Racial group membership modulates empathic neural responses. *The Journal of Neuroscience.* https://doi.org/10.1523/JNEUROSCI.2418-09.2009

Yamada, M., & Decety, J. (2009). Unconscious affective processing and empathy: An investigation of subliminal priming on the detection of painful facial expressions. *Pain, 143*(1), 71–75.

Yang, C. Y., Decety, J., Lee, S., Chen, C., & Cheng, Y. (2009). Gender differences in the mu rhythm during empathy for pain: An electroencephalographic study. *Brain Research, 1251,* 176–184. https://doi.org/10.1016/j.brainres.2008.11.062

Zaki, J., & Oschner, K. N. (2012). The neuroscience of empathy: Progress, pitfalls and promise. *Nature Neuroscience, 15*(5), 675–680.

Zaki, J., Wager, T. D., Singer, T., Keysers, C., & Gazzola, V. (2016). The anatomy of suffering: Understanding the relationship between nociceptive and empathic pain. *Trends in Cognitive Sciences, 20*(4), 249–259.

Chapter 9
On the Overlap Between Physical and Social Pain

Kai Karos

Abstract When asked to name their most negative life events, people often cite an event of loss such as the dissolution of a valued relationship or the death of a loved one. Curiously, such events are often experienced and described as painful. Curiously, the overlap between physical pain and distressing social experiences does not end there. This chapter explores a growing body of social neuroscience and experimental laboratory research that demonstrates a fascinating, dynamic interplay between distressing social experiences such as exclusion and ostracism, and the experience of physical pain.

Keywords Ostracism · Exclusion · Social neuroscience · Social pain · Overlap theory

Introduction

When asked to name their most negative life events, what would people say? The chances are that an experience of loss will be at least one of these events: the end of a romantic relationship, the dissolution of a friendship, the death of a loved one. Indeed, research has shown that three out of four people describe the loss of a close relationship as the single most negative event of their lives (Jaremka, Gabriel, & Carvallo, 2011). In many different languages, such experiences are described as painful and expressions are used that describe physical pain: A *broken* heart, a *painful* breakup, *hurt* feelings, or emotional *scars*. Do these linguistic similarities merely represent a metaphorical curiosity, or does this overlap extend further?

A growing body of research has tried to investigate the overlap between experiences of interpersonal loss and exclusion and physical pain (see Eisenberger, 2012a, 2012b, 2015 for a review). In the literature, such experiences have been referred to

K. Karos (✉)
Research Group on Health Psychology, KU Leuven, Leuven, Belgium
e-mail: Kai.Karos@kuleuven.be

© Springer International Publishing AG, part of Springer Nature 2018   173
T. Vervoort et al. (eds.), *Social and Interpersonal Dynamics in Pain*,
https://doi.org/10.1007/978-3-319-78340-6_9

as experiences of *social pain*. Social pain has been defined as "the unpleasant experience that is associated with actual or potential damage to one's sense of social connection or social value" (Eisenberger, 2012a, p. 421). Although this term has raised considerable controversy, I will use it throughout this chapter in the interest of consistency with the existing literature. The goals of this chapter are to summarize the main predictions of the *overlap theory* of physical and social pain, review empirical evidence in support of these predictions, and highlight common criticisms of this account. Moreover, I will outline future directions for the integration of this line of research in the field of pain research.

The Overlap Theory of Physical and Social Pain

Next to a basic need for safety and physical integrity, humans have a basic need for lasting and supportive social bonds (Baumeister & Leary, 1995; Eisenberger, 2012b). In fact, such bonds can be crucial for well-being and even survival, especially early in life. Consequently, threats to social connections might be just as detrimental to survival as threats to physical integrity. Considering their importance for survival, the detection of threats to both physical and social integrity is of evolutionary importance. Therefore, it has been suggested that the detection of social threat might overlap with the mechanisms responsible for the detection of physical threat (Panksepp, 1998). Due to this overlap, experiences of social pain might indeed feel "painful," which would be adaptive for survival.

The affective component of pain can aid organisms in avoiding threats to physical safety because it serves as a form of punishment and as negative reinforcement for seeking safety. Similarly, painful feelings in response to the threat of exclusion will guide an organism's approach/avoidance responses to different social situations. For instance, one might avoid social interactions that are the source of rejection and exclusion, and seek interactions that provide support and understanding. An additional advantage of an overlap between physical and social pain is the ability to quickly and adequately respond to imminent threat. Physical pain has a strong link with the threat-defense system, which is not only responsible for fast detection of threat but also a quick and appropriate response to it (Gray & McNaughton, 2000). If the experience of social exclusion is indeed linked to pain, exclusion would gain the ability to also capitalize on the threat-defense system for threat detection and response (Macdonald & Leary, 2005).

The overlap theory of physical and social pain (also referred to as the *social pain theory*) makes a number of predictions (Eisenberger, 2012a; Macdonald & Leary, 2005): *First*, the processing of physical and social pain relies on similar mechanisms, specifically with regard to the neural circuitry underlying both kinds of pain. *Second*, as a result of these overlapping underlying mechanisms, there should also be an overlap in sensitivity to social and physical pain. That is, individuals who are more sensitive to one kind of pain should also be more sensitive to the other. *Third,* and perhaps most importantly, an overlap in underlying mechanisms could mean that factors affecting one kind of pain might also affect the other. That is, decreasing or increasing physical pain might similarly affect levels of social pain, and vice versa. In the next section, empirical evidence for each prediction will be reviewed.

Empirical Evidence

Shared Mechanisms

Evidence for shared underlying mechanisms in physical and social pain come from several different fields and include pharmacological, neuropsychological, and neuroimaging evidence.

Pharmacological Evidence

The first empirical evidence for an overlap between social and physical pain comes from animal research and the use of opioids. Panksepp (1998) proposed that the opioid system, which is mainly associated with euphoria and pain relief, may also affect social bonding processes. Indeed, there is some experimental work that supports this idea. The administration of morphine, an opioid agonist which is used for pain relief, also reduces distress following maternal separation in animals. In contrast, naloxone—an opioid *antagonist*—can increase distress following maternal separation (Herman & Panksepp, 1978; Kalin, Shelton, & Barksdale, 1988; Panksepp, Herman, Vilberg, Bishop, & DeEskinazi, 1980).

There are also a few more recent studies conducted in humans, which have investigated the effects of common painkillers such as paracetamol on the experience of distressing social situations. Most notably, Dewall et al. (2010) found that the administration of acetaminophen not only reduced pain reports but also reports of social pain in daily life and reduced neural activity in response to experiences of social rejection. Further, Mischkowski, Crocker, and Way (2016) evaluated the effects of taking paracetamol on the experience of physical pain and empathy for pain in others. The researchers found that paracetamol not only reduces pain in oneself but also reduces empathy in response to others' pain. These studies suggest that agents that are intended to target symptoms of physical pain can also affect interpersonal processes.

Neuropsychological Evidence

The experience of physical pain entails a *sensory* component, which is related to perceptions of the location, quality, and intensity of the sensation, as well as an *affective* component, which is related to feelings of unpleasantness and distress associated with the experience and motivates behavior intended to terminate the

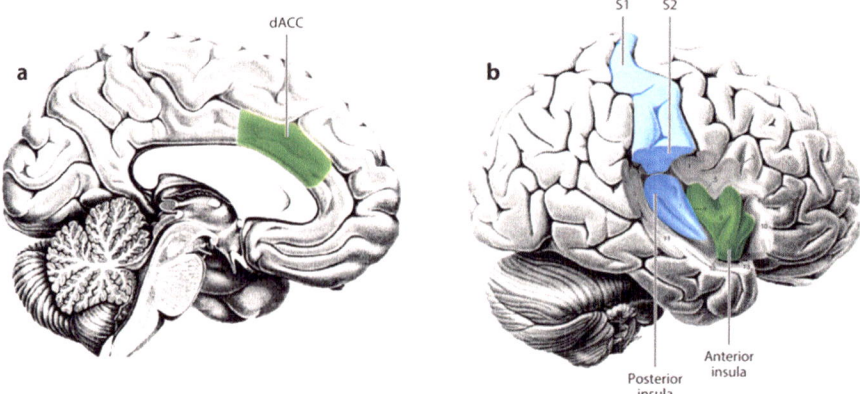

Fig. 9.1 Cortical neural regions associated with the affective and sensory components of pain. The neural regions associated with the affective component of pain (green) include the dorsal anterior cingulate cortex (dACC) (**a**) and the anterior insula (**b**). The neural regions associated with the sensory component of pain (blue) include the posterior insula, primary somatosensory cortex (S1), and secondary somatosensory cortex (S2) (**b**). Reprinted from Eisenberger NI. Social Pain and the Brain: Controversies, Questions, and Where to Go from Here. Annu. Rev. Psychol. 2015;66:601–629. Copyright © 2015 by Annual Reviews

pain (Price, Harkins, & Baker, 1987). Though often highly correlated, these two components of the pain experience can be dissociated and have separate underlying neural correlates: the affective component has been associated with the dorsal anterior cingulate cortex (dACC) and the anterior insula (AI), whereas the sensory component has been linked to the primary and secondary somatosensory cortices (S1, S2) and the posterior insula (PI) (see Fig. 9.1).

As stated before, according to the overlap theory, physical and social pain both motivate behavior intended to avoid and escape from situations that cause pain. Consequently, social pain may share underlying mechanisms concerning the affective component of pain, rather than the sensory components (Eisenberger, 2012b; Eisenberger, Lieberman, & Williams, 2003). That is, social pain should rely on regions such as the dACC and the AI, explaining why physical and social pain cause similar feelings of distress and motivate behavior but are easily distinguished on a sensory level.

Evidence for this overlap comes primarily from lesion studies in humans and animals. For instance, the ACC has also been implicated in separation distress behavior. That is, lesions to the ACC reduce the expression of distress by an infant mammal following mother–infant separation (Hadland, Rushworth, Gaffan, & Passingham, 2003), whereas stimulation of this region leads to increases in expression of distress (Robinson, 1967). In addition, lesions to the ACC in monkeys are associated with a reduction in social interaction and the amount of time spent with other monkeys (Murphy, MacLean, & Hamilton, 1981). In humans, there is anecdotal evidence of a patient who suffered from congenital insensitivity to pain (which is mainly associated with the sensory component of pain) who did report feelings of (social) pain following the death of his sister (Danziger & Willer, 2005).

Neurobiological Evidence

Most neurobiological support for the overlap theory comes from studies focused on neural activation following experiences of social and physical pain using brain imaging techniques such as functional magnetic resonance imaging (fMRI). Before summarizing the empirical evidence, it is important to describe two of the most common paradigms to induce experiences of social pain (more specifically, *social exclusion*) in the lab: The Cyberball paradigm and the Life Alone paradigm. Cyberball is an online ball-tossing game wherein the participant believes he or she is playing with two other participants (Williams & Jarvis, 2006). However, the "others" are actually controlled by the program itself. The experimenter is able to manipulate whether the participant is included or excluded in the ball-tossing game (i.e., whether or not the ball is tossed to the participant). In the Life Alone paradigm, participants fill in a personality questionnaire and then receive feedback that they are likely to have numerous rewarding relationships later in life (*inclusion condition*) or that they will likely end up alone later in life (*exclusion condition*) (Twenge, Baumeister, Tice, & Stucke, 2001). There are also other paradigms to induce feelings of exclusion in the lab, such as having participants be rejected by other "participants" (Baumeister, DeWall, Ciarocco, & Twenge, 2005) or having participants recall an experience of rejection and exclusion (Williams, 2002). However, the Cyberball and Life Alone paradigm are by far the most frequently used.

Several studies have examined the neural activation following experiences of social exclusion and experiences of physical pain. A landmark study by Eisenberger et al. (2003) investigated neural activation while participants played the Cyberball game. They found a pattern of activation that was very similar to the one elicited by physical pain: activity in the dorsal ACC, which has been linked to experiences of physical distress, was also related to self-reported emotional distress following social exclusion (e.g., "I felt rejected"). Moreover, social exclusion also activated the AI which has also been associated with the experience of physical pain. This study has since been replicated a number of times with comparable results (see Eisenberger, 2012b for a review). More subtle cues of rejection can also activate these brain areas: looking at a rejection-themed painting compared to an acceptance-themed painting leads to increased activation in both the dACC and the AI (Kross, Egner, Ochsner, Hirsch, & Downey, 2007). Even videos of disapproving facial expressions can lead to increased activity in the dACC in people who are highly sensitive to social rejection (Burklund, Eisenberger, & Lieberman, 2007).

Cyberball represents a social interaction with strangers, but social exclusion by people we know is arguably even more salient. A few studies have investigated neural activation to rejection from a close other. For example, looking at a photo of an ex-relationship partner following an unwanted breakup versus a friend is associated with increased activity in the dACC and the AI (Fisher, Brown, Aron, Strong, & Mashek, 2010). Another study added a physically painful task to this paradigm and found overlapping neural activation during both tasks (Kross, Berman, Mischel, Smith, & Wager, 2011). Lastly, social pain does not only refer to experiences of exclusion but also to experiences of loss: viewing pictures of a lost loved one (versus a stranger) increased activity in the dACC and the AI (Gündel, O'Connor, Littrell, Fort, & Lane, 2003).

Interestingly, similar patterns of activation are found following anticipation or experience of social evaluation, as well. When participants prepare a speech that is later evaluated by others, activity in the dACC increases (Somerville, Heatherton, & Kelley, 2006). Similarly, when participants are evaluated on an interview, distress following negative evaluation is associated with activity in the dACC (Eisenberger, Inagaki, Muscatell, Byrne Haltom, & Leary, 2011). Lastly, when participants are asked to compare themselves unfavorably with a superior peer, activity in the dACC increases (Takahashi et al., 2009). While the question of how specific these activation patterns are still remains, these studies point to an overlap in neural activation following social and physical pain.

In addition, the activation in the dACC and/or the AI are modulated by several variables that are known to modulate experiences of social pain: low self-esteem (Onoda et al., 2010), anxious attachment (DeWall et al., 2012), and interpersonal sensitivity (Macdonald, 2006) increase activation of these brain areas during social exclusion, whereas social support (Masten, Telzer, Fuligni, Lieberman, & Eisenberger, 2012) and avoidant attachment (DeWall et al., 2012) reduce activation. These findings again demonstrate that the dACC and the AI play an important role in the processing of distress associated with experiences of social exclusion. However, it should be noted that in many of these studies brain activity was not correlated with self-reported distress ratings. Therefore, the exact relationship between self-reported distress and the activity in the dACC and the AI is still speculative.

In sum, a range of aversive interpersonal situations such as exclusion and loss are associated with activation in several pain-related neural regions. Although this research points to an overlap in neural circuitry underlying physical and social pain, it is currently unclear how specific this pattern of activation is, and what its boundary conditions are (e.g., which kinds of interpersonal situations result in similar activation patterns?).

Shared Sensitivity

One of the implications of an overlap between physical and social pain is that individuals who are more sensitive to one kind of pain should also be more sensitive to the other kind of pain. This implication is especially relevant for clinical practice, as it would mean that sensitization to physical pain (which seems to play an important role in the transition from acute to chronic pain) might be associated with a sensitization to painful social situations as well, and vice versa.

In fact, there is some evidence for this assumption from clinical research. For instance, it has been shown that patients suffering from chronic pain were also more fearful and avoidant of social interactions and situations (Asmundson, Norton, & Jacobson, 1996). In addition, higher daily pain reports are associated with higher levels of anxious attachment and greater rejection sensitivity (Macdonald, 2006). Rejection sensitivity refers to the tendency to anxiously expect, readily perceive, and intensely react to experiences of social rejection. The opposite pattern has also been shown: Individuals with anxious attachment styles or greater rejection sensitivity tend to report more somatic symptoms, including physical pain (Ciechanowski, Walker, Katon, & Russo, 2002; Ehnvall, Mitchell, Hadzi-Pavlovic, Malhi, & Parker, 2009).

One distressing social experience that is characterized by long-term exclusion and ostracism is bullying. Bullying has received surprisingly little attention in the social pain literature. However, over the recent years, there has been an increased interest in the relationship between experiences of childhood bullying and the development of somatic complaints including chronic pain. A meta-analysis by Gini and Pozzoli (2009) found that victims, bullies, and bully-victims (individuals who are both victims and perpetrators of bullying) had a higher risk of developing psychosomatic complaints compared to peers who had not been affected by bullying. The question remains, however, whether bullied children become ill or ill children are more likely to be bullied. A prospective cohort study found that victims of bullying had a higher risk of developing both psychosomatic as well as psychosocial problems later in life. In contrast, only some psychosocial, but not physical, health symptoms preceded bullying victimization (Fekkes, Pijpers, Fredriks, Vogels, & Verloove-Vanhorick, 2006). More specifically, recent studies have investigated whether a history of bullying and abuse is a risk factor for the development of chronic pain. Voerman et al. (2015) found that adolescents who suffered from chronic pain were more likely to be physically and sexually abused by others, reported more family conflict, and were more likely to be bullied. Taken together, this line of research indicates that early childhood experiences of bullying might be a risk factor for the development of chronic pain. Similarly, bullying could be an important target for intervention in childhood and adolescence to prevent the development of psychosomatic complaints in general and chronic pain in particular.

In addition to these clinical studies, experimental research in healthy participants has also revealed a shared sensitivity between physical and social pain. For instance, participants who have a higher sensitivity for experimental pain (i.e., lower self-reported pain unpleasantness thresholds to heat pain) also report more social distress following a Cyberball manipulation (Eisenberger, Jarcho, Lieberman, & Naliboff, 2006). This shared sensitivity has also been shown on a genetic level: Individuals that have a rare form of the *OPRM1* polymorphism, which has been linked to increased sensitivity to physical pain (Chou et al., 2006), also demonstrate higher sensitivity for activity of the dACC and AI in response to experimentally induced social exclusion (Way, Taylor, & Eisenberger, 2009).

In summary, there is clinical and experimental evidence for shared sensitivity to physical and social pain. Considering the clinical importance of this hypothesis, more controlled research is warranted to shed light on the underlying mechanisms that explain this shared sensitivity. In addition, questions can be raised about the specificity and boundary conditions of this overlap.

Interrelationship

Lastly, a consequence of the physical–social pain overlap is that factors that either increase or decrease one kind of pain should have similar effects on the other. This idea leads to interesting predictions such as that traditional painkillers might also affect distress following experiences of social rejection.

There is some clinical support for this assumption that is also fairly well documented in the pain literature: Patients suffering from somatoform pain disorders such as fibromyalgia are also more likely to have experienced early-life social traumas such as emotional abuse or family conflict in general (Brown, Schrag, & Trimble, 2005). Similarly, as mentioned before, victims of childhood bullying are more likely to develop chronic pain later in their lifetime (Fekkes et al., 2006; Gini & Pozzoli, 2009). Moreover, a recent study found that perceived levels of social isolation are a predictor of disability from chronic low back pain (Oliveira et al., 2014). These findings suggest that distressing social experiences might be a risk factor for the development of somatoform disorders later in life.

In addition, there is an interesting line of experimental research investigating whether social pain can directly affect one's perception of physical pain and vice versa. It has been shown that providing participants with failure feedback following an intelligence test increases pain reports during a subsequent cold pressor task (van den Hout, Vlaeyen, Peters, Engelhard, & van den Hout, 2000). Further, several studies that have induced social exclusion in the lab have found an effect on pain sensitivity. For example, playing the Cyberball paradigm led to hypersensitivity to physical pain later (Bernstein & Claypool, 2012), and individuals who are more distressed following social exclusion also report higher physical pain ratings in response to a painful stimulus administered after social exclusion (Eisenberger et al., 2006).

Some experimental studies have found an opposite pattern, however. Imagining yourself alone later in life was associated with reduced sensitivity to physical pain, as indicated by higher pain thresholds and tolerance, as well as emotional insensitivity as indicated by reductions in affective forecasting (the ability to predicts one's own future emotional state) and reduced empathizing with another person's suffering (Bernstein & Claypool, 2012; DeWall & Baumeister, 2006). Even though this finding is unexpected based on the social overlap theory, it does mirror findings from the physical pain literature which have shown both hyperalgesia and analgesia following nociceptive stimulation (Rhudy & Meagher, 2000). One explanation for this dissociation might be the severity of the social distress inflicted, mirroring findings in the physical pain literature. That is, when painful stimulation becomes too great or occurs for too long, painful sensations can become numbed (Bernstein & Claypool, 2012). Similarly, highly intense social exclusion manipulations (such as the Life Alone paradigm) lead to reductions of physical pain, whereas milder forms of social exclusion (such as Cyberball) lead to increases of physical pain.

What about the reverse relationship? Can experiences of physical pain also affect feelings of social distress? It seems that increases in physical pain are associated with increases of social distress. After being exposed to a cold pressor task, participants' feelings of belongingness (e.g., "I felt rejected"), of self-esteem (e.g., "I felt liked"), of control (e.g., "I felt I had control"), and of meaningful existence (e.g., "I felt invisible") were assessed using the Need-Threat Scale (Williams, Cheung, & Choi, 2000). It turned out that participants reported feelings of exclusion and rejection after the pain task, even though no actual experience of exclusion had taken place (Riva, Wirth, & Williams, 2011). In addition, greater inflammatory activity, which is associated with increased physical pain reports, also increases feelings of social disconnection (Eisenberger, Inagaki, Mashal, & Irwin, 2010) and greater activity of the dACC and AI in response to lab-induced social exclusion (Eisenberger, Inagaki, Rameson, Mashal, & Irwin, 2009).

On the other hand, factors that reduce one kind of pain should also reduce the other as well. There is considerable research into the effects of social support on pain, both clinically and experimentally. Higher levels of social support are associated with faster recovery from surgery (Kulik & Mahler, 1989) and reductions in cancer-related pain (Zaza & Baine, 2002). Experimental research shows that pain reports are usually lowered in the presence of a supportive other (Brown, 2003), or when merely looking at the photo of a loved one (Master et al., 2009). These findings are also mirrored in the brain, in that viewing a photo of a loved one or holding their hand reduces activation in the dACC and the AI (Eisenberger et al., 2011; Younger, Aron, Parke, Chatterjee, & Mackey, 2010). However, as mentioned previously, such effects of social support are not specific for physical pain but have been implicated as a protective factor against stress in general (Cohen & McKay, 1984).

Again, this relationship is hypothesized to be bidirectional, so factors reducing physical pain should have a similar effect on the perception of social pain. A double-blind, placebo-controlled study found that administering paracetamol also reduced daily self-reported hurt feelings, and reduced activation of the dACC and the AI in response to experimental inductions of social exclusion (DeWall et al., 2010). However, it should be noted that the very same painkillers have also been shown to reduce the "pain" associated with decision-making (DeWall, Chester, & White, 2015), so the specificity again is questionable.

To summarise, there is some support for the idea that factors that influence one kind of pain also affect the other. Independent from the specificity of these findings and the underlying mechanisms, it is crucial to underline the clinical implications of this line of research: When physical pain is paired with distressing social experiences (as it frequently is), the painful experience may be worsened. Further, addressing distressing social experiences in treatment might have positive side-effects on treating physical pain, as well.

Controversy

The overlap theory of physical and social pain has received increasing empirical interest over the past decade and has also sparked a considerable amount of questions and controversy. In the following part of this chapter I will shortly review the main criticisms of the overlap theory of physical and social pain. In addition, I will address a few critical notes concerning terminology and how the question of whether social pain really is *pain* has possibly distracted us from the core issue.

Neuroscience

A lot of empirical evidence for overlap theory comes from social neuroscience and so it is no surprise that most criticism has focused on the exact role of the dACC and the AI (for a complete review see Eisenberger, 2015). The criticism mainly regards the specificity of the response of the dACC and the AI to distressing social experiences and/or sensations of physical pain.

Originally, when the first study on social exclusion was published in 2003 (Eisenberger et al., 2003), the dACC was primarily considered a region that was implicated in cognitive processes such as conflict monitoring and discrepancy detection, rather than affective processing (Botvinick, Cohen, & Carter, 2004). Consequently, it was suggested that activation in this region in response to social exclusion might not reflect affective distress but rather expectancy violation (namely, to be unexpectedly excluded). However, this view is outdated. A meta-analysis by Shackman et al. (2011) found that the dACC is not only activated by tasks that involve conflict monitoring but also by negative affect (fear, anxiety, anger, etc.) and, most prominently, physical pain. Moreover, some studies have directly tested the expectancy violation account by comparing the neural activation following both exclusion and overinclusion paradigms using the Cyberball paradigm (Kawamoto et al., 2012). According to their reasoning, exclusion and overinclusion violate expectations and should therefore activate the dACC. However, they found that only exclusion, but not overinclusion, activated the dACC and the AI, demonstrating that dACC responses seem to relate more to experienced social distress rather than expectancy violation. Some authors have also suggested that the dACC might function as a neural alarm system, encompassing both discrepancy detection and an affective alarm response (Eisenberger & Lieberman, 2004).

Following the increased evidence that the dACC plays a crucial role in affective processing, especially negative affect, a new criticism arose: Does social exclusion only activate the dACC because *all* negative emotional experiences activate this region? In other words, is there anything specific about distressing social experiences and their overlap with physical pain? Several meta-analyses have investigated neural correlates of each kind of basic emotion. Their results suggest that the dACC is most reliably responsive to fear- and anxiety-inducing tasks (Etkin, Egner, & Kalisch, 2011; Shackman et al., 2011). Although both physical and social pain are a frequent source of anxiety and fear, the question of whether the dACC is specifically activated by threats of physical and social pain or more generally by negative emotions (especially fear and anxiety) is still unanswered.

Lastly, Iannetti, Salomons, Moayedi, Mouraux, and Davis (2013) proposed that common activation of the dACC to physical and social pain reflects the processing of salience (i.e., the contrast between a stimulus and its surroundings). This argument is partly based on the reverse inference problem. That is, just because regions that are associated with physical pain are also activated during distressing social experiences, does not necessarily mean that this processing reflects pain. This assumption depends on the specificity of the brain regions in question. The pattern of activation observed by Eisenberger et al. (2003) during social exclusion has previously been described as involving the so-called "*pain matrix*" because it was consistently activated during nociceptive stimulation in animals and humans, and also correlated with the intensity of stimulation. However, this term is misleading as it is unknown whether these areas are *only* activated during pain or also correspond to other types of stimulation. Moreover, the idea that social exclusion is experienced as painful is exactly based on this reverse inference, namely that one can infer mental states such as pain from brain activity.

As an alternative, Iannetti et al. (2013) propose that the activity is indicative of salience processing. Mouraux, Diukova, Lee, Wise, and Iannetti (2011) studied brain activation following nociceptive (salient) stimulation and nonnociceptive (salient) stimulation. The authors found that various regions of the "pain matrix" (including the dACC) were activated in response to each of the stimuli, and that activation correlated to self-reported salience. Further, more recent research also sheds doubt on the concept that there are specific anatomical regions in the brain that are correlated to pain. For instance, it has recently been proposed that the dynamic nature of pain can be better understood in terms of communication within and among various brain networks (Kucyi & Davis, 2016; Rogachov, Cheng, Erpelding, Hemington, & Crawley, 2016). In addition, other researchers have tried to use machine-learning algorithms to identify a "neurological signature of physical pain" (Wager et al., 2013). The underlying idea is that overlap between social and physical pain in different brain regions might be misleading, because the underlying neural representations might be still nonoverlapping. A study specifically tested this idea and compared the neural representation of both physical pain and social rejection (Woo et al., 2014). Participants experienced painful heat and were presented with photos of ex-partners and friends on separate trials. Using this data, an fMRI pattern classifier was trained to discriminate between pain trials and rejection trials. Their findings challenge the overlap theory of physical and social pain, as the pattern classifier was able to successfully discriminate between pain and rejection with an accuracy between 80–92%. It was concluded that rejection and pain have separate underlying neural representations despite common fMRI activity at the gross anatomical level.

Taken together, most of the criticisms of the overlap theory have focused on the assumption that social pain and physical pain share the same neurological signature. This debate is still ongoing and parallels the current attempt to identify a specific neural signature of physical pain. While it is certainly relevant to examine the predictions made by the overlap theory, the prominent focus on the underlying neuroscience of pain may have distracted researchers from the relevant findings that have emerged from this line of research. In the next section, I will briefly discuss why the terminology of *social pain* in this case might be misleading and how this line of research could be better integrated into the broader pain literature.

Terminology

Research into social pain has received a lot of attention within the field of (social) neuroscience but surprisingly little in the general field of (clinical) pain research. It seems that a lot of resistance and initial controversy concerning the overlap theory may have been caused by the terminology used. The term *social pain* seemed to suggest an overlap in both underlying mechanisms and experiential quality and even though the authors themselves clearly state that "physical pain and social pain are not the same experience" (Eisenberger, 2015, p. 621), the term seemed to challenge our understanding of what pain actually is (and what it is not). Specifically, even though the view of pain as a dualistic, purely biomedical process is outdated (Gatchel, Peng, Peters, Fuchs, & Turk, 2007), this view is still surprisingly prevalent in the public, clinical, and scientific understanding of pain. In fact, the term social pain was coined to refer to the *experiential* overlap between feelings of social rejection and feelings of physical pain and was met with a lot of resistance. Part of the reason might be that we (still) consider physical pain to be more akin to other physical sensations, whereas social pain is understood as a purely affective, emotional response. Part of the resistance to recognizing the importance of this research for the understanding and treatment of pain might stem from our inclination to separate physical pain from other "affective" mental states of suffering, overemphasizing the importance of the sensory component of pain.

This line of research raises the question of which human experiences can and should be labeled as "painful," and for a long time this label has only been accepted in the context of tissue damage. Yet we now know that there can be tissue damage without pain (e.g., in the case of soldiers being wounded in battle) and more importantly, pain without tissue damage, as is often the case in chronic pain (e.g., migraines, fibromyalgia). The current definition of pain recognizes that it is an unpleasant sensory *and* emotional experience, which is associated with actual *or* potential tissue damage, or merely described in such terms (International Association for the Study of Pain, 1994). Similarly, we know that pain is not merely explained in terms of biomedical factors such as tissue damage but also psychological factors (cognitive, affective, sensory) and environmental/social factors (physical, family, friends, medical professionals) leading to a biopsychosocial approach to pain (Gatchel et al., 2007; Hadjistavropoulos et al., 2011). Recently, a proposed update for the definition of pain even specifically recognizes the social dimension next to the sensory, cognitive, and affective dimensions (Williams & Craig, 2016), making the social aspect an integral part of what pain actually is.

So are experiences of social rejection really *painful*? As others have noted, "from an experiential perspective, the critical component of a painful experience may be rooted in the experience of suffering" (Eisenberger, 2015, p. 623) and in this sense there is clearly overlap between physical and social pain. It seems clear that the discussion regarding the relevance of this literature for the field of pain has been sidetracked by the question of whether there is an overlap between physical and social pain and what the exact nature of this overlap might be. This might be partly caused by the terminology used. As an alternative, *social distress* might be a better term as it would avoid the overlap in terminology but at the same time capture the experiential overlap as a distressing experience of suffering.

Integration

Despite the controversy that has arisen around the potential overlap between physical and social pain, the extant literature in this field has profound implications for our understanding of pain that have not yet been fully integrated. First and foremost, at the heart of this line of research and fittingly at the heart of this book, it shows that social context *matters* in our understanding of pain. In fact, the social pain literature provides one of the first empirical investigations into the effect of distressing social experiences on pain. Although there is some empirical research on harnessing social context to improve coping with pain or increase treatment efficacy (e.g., research on the relevance of social support, e.g., Brown, 2003), we know surprisingly little about the effect of maladaptive or distressing social influences on pain.

This is in fact surprising, considering that distressing social experiences seem to be a worryingly common part of suffering from acute and especially chronic pain. Recent research shows that individuals suffering from chronic pain frequently face stigmatization and invalidation by others (Cohen, Quintner, Buchanan, Nielsen, & Guy, 2011; De Ruddere & Craig, 2016; Waugh, Byrne, & Nicholas, 2014), especially so when there is no medical explanation for the pain (De Ruddere, Goubert, Vervoort, Prkachin, & Crombez, 2012). Unfortunately, individuals experiencing acute or chronic pain face stigmatization not only from the general population but also from health-care professionals such as medical students, nursing students, general practitioners, and physiotherapists. Stigmatization has serious consequences such as underestimating pain in patients, especially when medical evidence is absent (Taylor, Skelton, & Butcher, 1985; Teske, Daut, & Cleeland, 1983). Interestingly, a recent study has shown that not only physical pain—but also social pain—is commonly underestimated by others (Nordgren, Banas, & MacDonald, 2011). Moreover, research has shown that patients who suffer from pain without a medical explanation are also socially excluded by others (De Ruddere, Bosmans, Crombez, & Goubert, 2016). This study perfectly fits within the context of the social pain literature and yet these two lines of research have not been integrated. Based on the literature reviewed in this chapter, it is reasonable to expect that these distressing social experiences directly affect pain levels in patients, but experimental research is still scarce.

There is some experimental work that indicates that threatening social environments can negatively affect pain-relevant processes. For instance, a study by Karos,

Meulders, and Vlaeyen (2014) has shown that threatening social stimuli can facilitate learning of pain-related fear, a crucial component in the development and maintenance of chronic pain complaints. An additional study demonstrated that a threatening social environment can increase acute pain reports while at the same time inhibiting painful facial expressions, possibly leading to underestimation of pain in others (Peeters & Vlaeyen, 2011).

Another line of research that has gained increasing interest is the role of perceived injustice in pain (Sullivan et al., 2008). Especially in cases where chronic pain and disability is the consequence of another's error or negligence (e.g., a car crash), beliefs of injustice are common in the patient. In line with the research into social pain, beliefs of injustice have been linked to adverse outcomes such as increased depression, slower recovery from injury, prolonged work disability (Sullivan, Scott, & Trost, 2012; Trost et al., 2015) and elevated pain intensity levels (Trost et al., 2014). Relatedly, when the sufferer perceives pain as intentionally caused by someone else it is perceived as more painful than when it is unintentional (Gray & Wegner, 2008).

Lastly, as mentioned previously, there is increasing evidence that experiences of bullying are common in individuals suffering from chronic pain (Fekkes et al., 2006) and that these experiences are related to more somatic complaints later in life (Gini & Pozzoli, 2009). This line of research is again closely related to the social pain literature, as bullying overlaps with intense experiences of social exclusion. Yet recognition of the importance of distressing social experiences in the development of chronic pain complaints is still surprisingly uncommon.

Taken together, distressing social experiences seem to negatively impact pain and pain-related processes such as recovery from injury and treatment. The social pain literature is another body of literature demonstrating the adverse effects of distressing social experiences (mainly social exclusion) on pain, and yet there is no complete integration of these separate lines of research in the pain literature. While the social pain literature mainly focuses on fundamental research regarding social exclusion and acute pain, there is a growing recognition of various distressing social experiences in patients suffering from chronic pain such as stigmatization, invalidation, injustice and bullying that we are just now paying attention to. It is time to develop an overarching theoretical framework that incorporates different kinds of social experiences and the mechanisms by which they affect pain, and to recognize their importance in the etiology and maintenance of pain complaints. The overlap theory is valuable as it proposes a theoretical framework that aims to explain why distressing social experiences might affect pain and vice versa leading to clear, testable hypotheses that have been reviewed here. However, considering that this theory is relatively mute with regard to chronic pain and common social challenges faced by people suffering from it, it is necessary to expand this theory and integrate other lines of research that have run separately until now.

One possible avenue might come from motivational theories in pain and the recognition that acute and especially chronic pain threaten several basic human needs, especially in the interpersonal domain. First, and directly related to the present chapter, pain can threaten the human need to belong (Baumeister & Leary,

1995). Experiences of ostracism, stigmatization and exclusion which have been associated with pain experiences, have a host of detrimental consequences for physical and mental health in general, and pain in particular (De Ruddere et al., 2016; De Ruddere & Craig, 2016; Williams, 2007). Second, pain can challenge the human need for autonomy and control (Caspar, Desantis, Dienes, Cleeremans, & Haggard, 2016; Vlaeyen, 2015), because it frequently makes the sufferer dependent on others, such as health-care professionals or family members. Loss of control and autonomy, as well as feelings of helplessness, have also been associated with a wide range of detrimental health consequences (Abramson, Seligman, & Teasdale, 1978; Crombez, Eccleston, De Vlieger, Van Damme, & De Clercq, 2008). Lastly, experiences of acute and chronic pain often conflict with the human need for justice and fairness (Miller, 2001), especially when pain is the direct result of someone else's error or negligence (Sullivan et al., 2012). Perceptions of injustice are common and are associated with a whole range of problematic pain outcomes, including increased pain sensitivity, prolonged recovery and anger (McParland, Knussen, & Murray, 2016; Scott et al., 2016; Trost et al., 2015). By highlighting the different interpersonal needs and motivations that are often times threatened by pain experiences, we might be better able to predict how a person suffering from pain might cope with pain and communicate it to others. It will also help us differentiate between different kinds of social experiences (e.g., invalidation, stigmatization, assault) based on the specific need that they threaten in the sufferer. This account would nicely incorporate social context research into a wider motivational perspective, which acknowledges that the motivation to minimize pain and suffering are just one of several, dynamic motivations that are relevant for humans as social beings (Van Damme, Crombez, & Eccleston, 2008; Wiech & Tracey, 2013).

Future Directions

Social experiences in general, and distressing social experiences in particular, can have a profound effect on the way pain is perceived and is dealt with. The overlap theory of physical and social pain has brought welcome attention to the interconnectivity of these two fundamental human experiences that is too often ignored. At the same time, there is still a long way to go. In order to integrate the existing lines of research and produce new hypotheses, there are still several questions that must be answered.

First, it is necessary to investigate the boundary conditions of the relationship between pain and distressing social experiences. The overlap theory of physical and social pain has mainly focused on experiences of social exclusion, since these experiences are the most relevant for our survival in evolutionary terms (Macdonald & Leary, 2005). Yet one can assume that other forms of distressing social experiences, such as bullying or the experience of stigmatization and invalidation, also share characteristics with social exclusion and might overlap in terms of underlying mechanisms. For example, to the best of my knowledge, there is no research that has investigated neural activity during the experience of invalidation or stigmatization. It would be worthwhile to see whether these experiences, which are especially relevant for chronic pain patients (De Ruddere & Craig, 2016), also share an overlap in underlying mechanisms with the processing of pain.

Second, and relatedly, empirical evidence for the overlap theory of social and physical pain has almost exclusively focused on acute pain sensations, mainly in a lab context. Considering the alarming prevalence of chronic pain worldwide (Breivik, Collett, Ventafridda, Cohen, & Gallacher, 2006; Briere & Elliott, 2003), and the importance of social experiences in the development, maintenance and treatment of such complaints (McCracken, 2005; Voerman et al., 2015), it is essential to investigate a potential overlap in underlying mechanisms between distressing social experiences and chronic pain. While recent neuroscience research has tended to abandon the attempt to localize acute pain in distinct regions of the brain and has instead focused on multilevel approaches (Wager et al., 2013) and the pattern of connectivity between different neural areas (Kucyi & Davis, 2016; Rogachov et al., 2016), we still understand very little about neural representations of chronic pain conditions. Research has shown that several chronic pain conditions are associated with spatial, temporal, and anatomical changes (e.g., changes in grey matter volume) and also with activation in neural areas that are commonly not recruited in acute pain (Apkarian, Hashmi, & Baliki, 2011). The question then, is in how far predictions of the overlap theory of social and physical pain are also relevant for chronic pain conditions. Moreover, it is paramount to extend this research into clinical settings as well, to increase ecological validity and better understand distressing social experiences that chronic pain patients face on a daily basis, such as invalidation by others (including care givers) and stigmatization.

Third, there is a great need for new conceptual models that can explain the dynamic interplay between social experiences and the processing of pain. The overlap theory of social and physical pain attempts to explain this interplay based on an overlap in underlying mechanisms but clearly, this is only one of many possible explanations. For instance, a recent meta-analysis (Krahé, Springer, Weinman, & Fotopoulou, 2013) proposed a *free energy framework* to understand the effects of social context on pain. According to this framework, others function as social, predictive signals of threat and safety and thereby affect the salience of a painful stimulus. This theory is elegant in so far as it makes specific predictions for different kinds of social contexts, both distressing and reassuring, and under which circumstances they do or do not affect the perception of pain. Still, the interplay between social context and pain is poorly understood, and we are severely lacking new conceptual frameworks to predict when and how social context can affect pain. New models will need to be multidisciplinary, including social psychology, (social) neuroscience, health psychology and both fundamental and applied pain research.

Fourth, and perhaps most importantly, this line of research should lead to increased recognition, both in research and clinical practice, that pain is a result of biological, psychological *and* social processes, and can only be understood when properly acknowledging all facets of this complex experience (Gatchel et al., 2007). Recent advancements have been made and current research has shed more light on the contribution of social experiences to painful experiences, demonstrating that our social, psychological, and physical worlds are deeply entangled (Macdonald & Leary, 2005). As mentioned before, we are at the verge of including social components alongside sensory, cognitive, and emotional components in our very definition of pain (Williams & Craig, 2016) and hopefully this book as a whole will further contribute to the rising interest and understanding of social processes in pain research and treatment.

References

Abramson, L. Y., Seligman, M. E., & Teasdale, J. D. (1978). Learned helplessness in humans: Critique and reformulation. *Journal of Abnormal Psychology, 87*, 49–74. https://doi.org/10.1037/0021-843X.87.1.49

Apkarian, A. V., Hashmi, J. A., & Baliki, M. N. (2011). Pain and the brain: Specificity and plasticity of the brain in clinical chronic pain. *Pain, 152*(Suppl. 3), S49–S64. https://doi.org/10.1016/j.pain.2010.11.010

Asmundson, G. J. G., Norton, G. R., & Jacobson, S. J. (1996). Social, blood/injury, and agoraphobic fears in patients with physically unexplained chronic pain: Are they clinically significant? *Anxiety, 2*(1), 28–33. https://doi.org/10.1002/(SICI)1522-7154(1996)2:1<28::AID-ANXI4>3.0.CO;2-9

Baumeister, R. F., DeWall, C. N., Ciarocco, N. J., & Twenge, J. M. (2005). Social exclusion impairs self-regulation. *Journal of Personality and Social Psychology, 88*(4), 589–604. https://doi.org/10.1037/0022-3514.88.4.589

Baumeister, R. F., & Leary, M. R. (1995). The need to belong: Desire for interpersonal attachments as a fundamental human motivation. *Psychological Bulletin, 117*(3), 497–529. https://doi.org/10.1037/0033-2909.117.3.497

Bernstein, M. J., & Claypool, H. M. (2012). Social exclusion and pain sensitivity: Why exclusion sometimes hurts and sometimes numbs. *Personality & Social Psychology Bulletin, 38*(2), 185–196. https://doi.org/10.1177/0146167211422449

Botvinick, M. M., Cohen, J. D., & Carter, C. S. (2004). Conflict monitoring and anterior cingulate cortex: An update. *Trends in Cognitive Sciences, 8*(12), 539–546. https://doi.org/10.1016/j.tics.2004.10.003

Breivik, H., Collett, B., Ventafridda, V., Cohen, R., & Gallacher, D. (2006). Survey of chronic pain in Europe: Prevalence, impact on daily life, and treatment. *European Journal of Pain, 10*(4), 287–287. https://doi.org/10.1016/j.ejpain.2005.06.009

Briere, J., & Elliott, D. M. (2003). Prevalence and psychological sequelae of self-reported childhood physical and sexual abuse in a general population sample of men and women. *Child Abuse & Neglect, 27*(10), 1205–1222.

Brown, J. L. (2003). Social support and experimental pain. *Psychosomatic Medicine, 65*(2), 276–283. https://doi.org/10.1097/01.PSY.0000030388.62434.46

Brown, R. J., Schrag, A., & Trimble, M. R. (2005). Dissociation, childhood interpersonal trauma, and family functioning in patients with somatization disorder. *American Journal of Psychiatry, 162*(5), 899–905. https://doi.org/10.1176/appi.ajp.162.5.899

Burklund, L. J., Eisenberger, N. I., & Lieberman, M. D. (2007). The face of rejection: Rejection sensitivity moderates dorsal anterior cingulate activity to disapproving facial expressions. *Social Neuroscience, 2*(3–4), 238–253. https://doi.org/10.1080/17470910701391711

Caspar, E. A., Desantis, A., Dienes, Z., Cleeremans, A., & Haggard, P. (2016). The sense of agency as tracking control. *PLoS One, 11*, 1–16.

Chou, W.-Y., Wang, C.-H., Liu, P.-H., Liu, C.-C., Tseng, C.-C., & Jawan, B. (2006). Human opioid receptor A118G polymorphism affects intravenous patient-controlled analgesia morphine
consumption after total abdominal hysterectomy. *Anesthesiology, 105*(2), 334–337. https://doi.
org/10.1097/00000542-200608000-00016

Ciechanowski, P. S., Walker, E. A., Katon, W. J., & Russo, J. E. (2002). Attachment theory: A
model for health care utilization and somatization. *Psychosomatic Medicine, 64*(4), 660–667.
https://doi.org/10.1097/00006842-200207000-00016

Cohen, M., Quintner, J., Buchanan, D., Nielsen, M., & Guy, L. (2011). Stigmatization of patients
with chronic pain: The extinction of empathy. *Pain Medicine, 12*(11), 1637–1643. https://doi.
org/10.1111/j.1526-4637.2011.01264.x

Cohen, S., & McKay, G. (1984). Social support, stress, and the buffering hypothesis: A theoretical
analysis. In A. Baum, S. E. Taylor, & J. E. Singer (Eds.), *Handbook of psychology and health*.
Hillsdale, NJ: Lawrence Erlbaum. https://doi.org/10.1387/ijdb.082595mg

Crombez, G., Eccleston, C., De Vlieger, P., Van Damme, S., & De Clercq, A. (2008). Is it better to
have controlled and lost than never to have controlled at all? An experimental investigation of
control over pain. *Pain, 137*, 631–639. https://doi.org/10.1016/j.pain.2007.10.028

Danziger, N., & Willer, C.-J. (2005). Tension-type headache as the unique pain experience of a
patient with congenital insensitivity to pain. *Pain, 117*(3), 478–483. https://doi.org/10.1016/j.
pain.2005.07.012

De Ruddere, L., Bosmans, M., Crombez, G., & Goubert, L. (2016). Patients are socially excluded
when their pain has no medical explanation. *The Journal of Pain, 17*(9), 1028–1035. https://
doi.org/10.1016/j.jpain.2016.06.005

De Ruddere, L., & Craig, K. D. (2016). Understanding stigma and chronic pain. *Pain, 157*(8), 1.
https://doi.org/10.1097/j.pain.0000000000000512

De Ruddere, L., Goubert, L., Vervoort, T., Prkachin, K. M., & Crombez, G. (2012). We discount
the pain of others when pain has no medical explanation. *Journal of Pain, 13*(12), 1198–1205.
https://doi.org/10.1016/j.jpain.2012.09.002

DeWall, C. N., & Baumeister, R. F. (2006). Alone but feeling no pain: Effects of social
exclusion on physical pain tolerance and pain threshold, affective forecasting, and
interpersonal empathy. *Journal of Personality and Social Psychology, 91*(1), 1–15. https://doi.
org/10.1037/0022-3514.91.1.1

DeWall, C. N., Chester, D. S., & White, D. S. (2015). Can acetaminophen reduce the pain of
decision-making? *Journal of Experimental Social Psychology, 56*, 117–120. https://doi.
org/10.1016/j.jesp.2014.09.006

Dewall, C. N., Macdonald, G., Webster, G. D., Masten, C. L., Baumeister, R. F., Powell, C., …
Eisenberger, N. I. (2010). Acetaminophen reduces social pain: Behavioral and neural evidence.
Psychological Science, 21(7), 931–937. https://doi.org/10.1177/0956797610374741

DeWall, C. N., Masten, C. L., Powell, C., Combs, D., Schurtz, D. R., & Eisenberger, N. I. (2012).
Do neural responses to rejection depend on attachment style? An fMRI study. *Social Cognitive
and Affective Neuroscience, 7*(2), 184–192. https://doi.org/10.1093/scan/nsq107

Ehnvall, A., Mitchell, P. B., Hadzi-Pavlovic, D., Malhi, G. S., & Parker, G. (2009). Pain during
depression and relationship to rejection sensitivity. *Acta Psychiatrica Scandinavica, 119*(5),
375–382. https://doi.org/10.1111/j.1600-0447.2008.01316.x

Eisenberger, N. I. (2012a). The neural bases of social pain: Evidence for shared representations with physical pain. *Psychosomatic Medicine, 74*(2), 126–135. https://doi.org/10.1097/
PSY.0b013e3182464dd1

Eisenberger, N. I. (2012b). The pain of social disconnection: Examining the shared neural underpinnings of physical and social pain. *Nature Reviews. Neuroscience, 13*(6), 421–434. https://
doi.org/10.1038/nrn3231

Eisenberger, N. I. (2015). Social pain and the brain: Controversies, questions, and where to
go from here. *Annual Review of Psychology, 66*(1), 601–629. https://doi.org/10.1146/
annurev-psych-010213-115146

Eisenberger, N. I., Inagaki, T. K., Mashal, N. M., & Irwin, M. R. (2010). Inflammation and social experience: An inflammatory challenge induces feelings of social disconnection in addition to depressed mood. *Brain, Behavior, and Immunity, 24*(4), 558–563. https://doi.org/10.1016/j. bbi.2009.12.009

Eisenberger, N. I., Inagaki, T. K., Muscatell, K. A., Byrne Haltom, K. E., & Leary, M. R. (2011). The neural sociometer: Brain mechanisms underlying state self-esteem. *Journal of Cognitive Neuroscience, 23*(11), 3448–3455. https://doi.org/10.1162/jocn_a_00027

Eisenberger, N. I., Inagaki, T. K., Rameson, L. T., Mashal, N. M., & Irwin, M. R. (2009). An fMRI study of cytokine-induced depressed mood and social pain: The role of sex differences. *NeuroImage, 47*(3), 881–890. https://doi.org/10.1016/j.neuroimage.2009.04.040

Eisenberger, N. I., Jarcho, J. M., Lieberman, M. D., & Naliboff, B. D. (2006). An experimental study of shared sensitivity to physical pain and social rejection. *Pain, 126*(1–3), 132–138. https://doi.org/10.1016/j.pain.2006.06.024

Eisenberger, N. I., & Lieberman, M. D. (2004). Why rejection hurts: A common neural alarm system for physical and social pain. *Trends in Cognitive Sciences, 8*(7), 294–300. https://doi. org/10.1016/j.tics.2004.05.010

Eisenberger, N. I., Lieberman, M. D., & Williams, K. D. (2003). Does rejection hurt? An FMRI study of social exclusion. *Science (New York, N.Y.), 302*(5643), 290–292. https://doi. org/10.1126/science.1089134

Eisenberger, N. I., Master, S. L., Inagaki, T. K., Taylor, S. E., Shirinyan, D., Lieberman, M. D., & Naliboff, B. D. (2011). Attachment figures activate a safety signal-related neural region and reduce pain experience. *Proceedings of the National Academy of Sciences, 108*(28), 11721–11726. https://doi.org/10.1073/pnas.1108239108

Etkin, A., Egner, T., & Kalisch, R. (2011). Emotional processing in anterior cingulate and medial prefrontal cortex. *Trends in Cognitive Sciences, 15*(2), 85–93. https://doi.org/10.1016/j. tics.2010.11.004

Fekkes, M., Pijpers, F. I. M., Fredriks, A. M., Vogels, T., & Verloove-Vanhorick, S. P. (2006). Do bullied children get ill, or do ill children get bullied? A prospective cohort study on the relationship between bullying and health-related symptoms. *Pediatrics, 117*(5), 1568–1574. https://doi.org/10.1542/peds.2005-0187

Fisher, H. E., Brown, L. L., Aron, A., Strong, G., & Mashek, D. (2010). Reward, addiction, and emotion regulation systems associated with rejection in love. *Journal of Neurophysiology, 104*(1), 51–60. https://doi.org/10.1152/jn.00784.2009

Gatchel, R. J., Peng, Y. B., Peters, M. L., Fuchs, P. N., & Turk, D. C. (2007). The biopsychosocial approach to chronic pain: Scientific advances and future directions. *Psychological Bulletin, 133*(4), 581–624. https://doi.org/10.1037/0033-2909.133.4.581

Gini, G., & Pozzoli, T. (2009). Association between bullying and psychosomatic problems: A meta-analysis. *Pediatrics, 123*(3), 1059–1065. https://doi.org/10.1542/peds.2008-1215

Gray, J. A., & McNaughton, N. (2000). *The neuropsychology of anxiety*. Oxford, England: Oxford University Press.

Gray, K., & Wegner, D. M. (2008). The sting of intentional pain. *Psychological Science, 19*(12), 1260–1262. https://doi.org/10.1111/j.1467-9280.2008.02208.x

Gündel, H., O'Connor, M.-F., Littrell, L., Fort, C., & Lane, R. D. (2003). Functional neuroanatomy of grief: An fMRI study. *American Journal of Psychiatry, 160*(11), 1946–1953. https://doi. org/10.1176/appi.ajp.160.11.1946

Hadjistavropoulos, T., Craig, K. D., Duck, S., Cano, A., Goubert, L., Jackson, P. L., … Fitzgerald, T. D. (2011). A biopsychosocial formulation of pain communication. *Psychological Bulletin, 137*(6), 910–939. https://doi.org/10.1037/a0023876

Hadland, K., Rushworth, M. F., Gaffan, D., & Passingham, R. (2003). The effect of cingulate lesions on social behaviour and emotion. *Neuropsychologia, 41*(8), 919–931. https://doi. org/10.1016/S0028-3932(02)00325-1

Herman, B. H., & Panksepp, J. (1978). Effects of morphine and naloxone on separation distress and approach attachment: Evidence for opiate mediation of social affect. *Pharmacology Biochemistry and Behavior, 9*(2), 213–220. https://doi.org/10.1016/0091-3057(78)90167-3

Iannetti, G. D., Salomons, T. V., Moayedi, M., Mouraux, A., & Davis, K. D. (2013). Beyond metaphor: Contrasting mechanisms of social and physical pain. *Trends in Cognitive Sciences, 17*(8), 371–378. https://doi.org/10.1016/j.tics.2013.06.002

Jaremka, L. M., Gabriel, S., & Carvallo, M. (2011). What makes us feel the best also makes us feel the worst: The emotional impact of independent and interdependent experiences. *Self and Identity, 10*(1), 44–63. https://doi.org/10.1080/15298860903513881

Kalin, N. H., Shelton, S. E., & Barksdale, C. M. (1988). Opiate modulation of separation-induced distress in non-human primates. *Brain Research, 440*(2), 285–292. https://doi.org/10.1016/0006-8993(88)90997-3

Karos, K., Meulders, A., & Vlaeyen, J. W. S. (2014). Threatening social context facilitates pain-related fear learning. *The Journal of Pain, 16*(3), 214–225. https://doi.org/10.1016/j.jpain.2014.11.014

Kawamoto, T., Onoda, K., Nakashima, K., Nittono, H., Yamaguchi, S., & Ura, M. (2012). Is dorsal anterior cingulate cortex activation in response to social exclusion due to expectancy violation? An fMRI study. *Frontiers in Evolutionary Neuroscience, 4.* https://doi.org/10.3389/fnevo.2012.00011

Krahé, C., Springer, A., Weinman, J. a., & Fotopoulou, A. (2013). The social modulation of pain: Others as predictive signals of salience—a systematic review. *Frontiers in Human Neuroscience, 7*(July), 386. https://doi.org/10.3389/fnhum.2013.00386

Kross, E., Berman, M. G., Mischel, W., Smith, E. E., & Wager, T. D. (2011). Social rejection shares somatosensory representations with physical pain. *Proceedings of the National Academy of Sciences, 108*(15), 6270–6275. https://doi.org/10.1073/pnas.1102693108

Kross, E., Egner, T., Ochsner, K., Hirsch, J., & Downey, G. (2007). Neural dynamics of rejection sensitivity. *Journal of Cognitive Neuroscience, 19*(6), 945–956. https://doi.org/10.1162/jocn.2007.19.6.945

Kucyi, A., & Davis, K. D. (2016). The neural code for pain: From single-cell electrophysiology to the dynamic pain connectome. *The Neuroscientist.* https://doi.org/10.1177/1073858416667716

Kulik, J. A., & Mahler, H. I. (1989). Social support and recovery from surgery. *Health Psychology, 8*(2), 221–238. https://doi.org/10.1037/0278-6133.8.2.221

Macdonald, G. (2006). Does physical pain augment anxious attachment? *Journal of Social and Personal Relationships, 23*(2), 291–304. https://doi.org/10.1177/0265407506062481

Macdonald, G., & Leary, M. R. (2005). Why does social exclusion hurt? The relationship between social and physical pain. *Psychological Bulletin, 131*(2), 202–223. https://doi.org/10.1037/0033-2909.131.2.202

Masten, C. L., Telzer, E. H., Fuligni, A. J., Lieberman, M. D., & Eisenberger, N. I. (2012). Time spent with friends in adolescence relates to less neural sensitivity to later peer rejection. *Social Cognitive and Affective Neuroscience, 7*(1), 106–114. https://doi.org/10.1093/scan/nsq098

Master, S. L., Eisenberger, N. I., Taylor, S. E., Naliboff, B. D., Shirinyan, D., & Lieberman, M. D. (2009). A picture's worth: Partner photographs reduce experimentally induced pain. *Psychological Science, 20*(11), 1316–1318. https://doi.org/10.1111/j.1467-9280.2009.02444.x

McCracken, L. M. (2005). Social context and acceptance of chronic pain: The role of solicitous and punishing responses. *Pain, 113*(1–2), 155–159. https://doi.org/10.1016/j.pain.2004.10.004

McParland, J. L., Knussen, C., & Murray, J. (2016). The effects of a recalled injustice on the experience of experimentally induced pain and anxiety in relation to just-world beliefs. *European Journal of Pain.* https://doi.org/10.1002/ejp.862

Merskey, H., & Bogduk, N. (1994). *Classification of chronic pain: Descriptions of chronic pain syndromes and definitions of pain terms* (2nd ed.). International Association for the Study of Pain: Seattle.

Miller, D. T. (2001). Disrespect and the experience of injustice. *Annual Review of Psychology, 52,* 527–553.

Mischkowski, D., Crocker, J., & Way, B. M. (2016). From painkiller to empathy killer: Acetaminophen (paracetamol) reduces empathy for pain. *Social Cognitive and Affective Neuroscience, 217,* nsw057. https://doi.org/10.1093/scan/nsw057

Mouraux, A., Diukova, A., Lee, M. C., Wise, R. G., & Iannetti, G. D. (2011). A multisensory investigation of the functional significance of the "pain matrix". *NeuroImage, 54*(3), 2237–2249. https://doi.org/10.1016/j.neuroimage.2010.09.084

Murphy, M., MacLean, P., & Hamilton, S. (1981). Species-typical behavior of hamsters deprived from birth of the neocortex. *Science, 213*(4506), 459–461. https://doi.org/10.1126/science.7244642

Nordgren, L. F., Banas, K., & MacDonald, G. (2011). Empathy gaps for social pain: Why people underestimate the pain of social suffering. *Journal of Personality and Social Psychology, 100*(1), 120–128. https://doi.org/10.1037/a0020938

Oliveira, V. C., Ferreira, M. L., Morso, L., Albert, H. B., Refshauge, K. M., & Ferreira, P. H. (2014). Patients' perceived level of social isolation affects the prognosis of low back pain. *European Journal of Pain (London, England), 19,* 538–545. https://doi.org/10.1002/ejp.578

Onoda, K., Okamoto, Y., Nakashima, K., Nittono, H., Yoshimura, S., Yamawaki, S., … Ura, M. (2010). Effects of trait self-esteem on social pain by ostracism and activation of anterior cingulate cortex. *Clinical Neurophysiology, 121*(7), e34. https://doi.org/10.1016/j.clinph.2010.02.145

Panksepp, J. (1998). *Affective neuroscience: The foundations of human and animal emotions.* New York, NY: Oxford University Press. Retrieved from https://books.google.nl/books?id=qqcRGagyEuAC

Panksepp, J., Herman, B. H., Vilberg, T., Bishop, P., & DeEskinazi, F. G. (1980). Endogenous opioids and social behavior. *Neuroscience & Biobehavioral Reviews, 4*(4), 473–487. https://doi.org/10.1016/0149-7634(80)90036-6

Peeters, P. a. M., & Vlaeyen, J. W. S. (2011). Feeling more pain, yet showing less: The influence of social threat on pain. *The Journal of Pain, 12*(12), 1255–1261. https://doi.org/10.1016/j.jpain.2011.07.007

Price, D. D., Harkins, S. W., & Baker, C. (1987). Sensory-affective relationships among different types of clinical and experimental pain. *Pain, 28*(3), 297–307. https://doi.org/10.1016/0304-3959(87)90065-0

Rhudy, J. L., & Meagher, M. W. (2000). Fear and anxiety: Divergent effects on human pain thresholds. *Pain, 84*(1), 65–75. https://doi.org/10.1016/S0304-3959(99)00183-9

Riva, P., Wirth, J. H., & Williams, K. D. (2011). The consequences of pain: The social and physical pain overlap on psychological responses. *European Journal of Social Psychology, 41*(6), 681–687. https://doi.org/10.1002/ejsp.837

Robinson, B. (1967). Vocalization evoked from forebrain in Macaca mulatta. *Physiology & Behavior, 2*(4), 345–354. https://doi.org/10.1016/0031-9384(67)90050-9

Rogachov, A., Cheng, J. C., Erpelding, N., Hemington, K. S., & Crawley, A. P. (2016). Regional brain signal variability: A novel indicator of pain sensitivity and coping. *Pain, 157*(11), 2483–2492.

Scott, W., McEvoy, A., Garland, R., Bernier, E., Milioto, M., Trost, Z., & Sullivan, M. (2016). Sources of injustice among individuals with persistent pain following musculoskeletal injury. *Psychol. Inj. Law, 9,* 6–15. https://doi.org/10.1007/s12207-015-9249-8

Shackman, A. J., Salomons, T. V., Slagter, H. A., Fox, A. S., Winter, J. J., & Davidson, R. J. (2011). The integration of negative affect, pain and cognitive control in the cingulate cortex. *Nature Reviews Neuroscience, 12*(3), 154–167. https://doi.org/10.1038/nrn2994

Somerville, L. H., Heatherton, T. F., & Kelley, W. M. (2006). Anterior cingulate cortex responds differentially to expectancy violation and social rejection. *Nature Neuroscience, 9*(8), 1007–1008. https://doi.org/10.1038/nn1728

Sullivan, M. J. L., Adams, H., Horan, S., Maher, D., Boland, D., & Gross, R. (2008). The role of perceived injustice in the experience of chronic pain and disability: Scale development and validation. *Journal of Occupational Rehabilitation, 18*(3), 249–261. https://doi.org/10.1007/s10926-008-9140-5

Sullivan, M. J. L., Scott, W., & Trost, Z. (2012). Perceived injustice: A risk factor for problematic pain outcomes. *The Clinical Journal of Pain, 28*(6), 484–488. https://doi.org/10.1097/AJP.0b013e3182527d13

Takahashi, H., Kato, M., Matsuura, M., Mobbs, D., Suhara, T., & Okubo, Y. (2009). When your gain is my pain and your pain is my gain: Neural correlates of envy and schadenfreude. *Science, 323*(5916), 937–939. https://doi.org/10.1126/science.1165604

Taylor, A. G., Skelton, J. A., & Butcher, J. (1985). Nursing duration of pain condition and physical pathology as determinants of nurses' assessments of patients in pain. *Pain, 21*(2), 206–207. https://doi.org/10.1016/0304-3959(85)90317-3

Teske, K., Daut, R. L., & Cleeland, C. S. (1983). Relationships between nurses' observations and patients' self-reports of pain. *Pain, 16*(3), 289–296. https://doi.org/10.1016/0304-3959(83)90117-3

Trost, Z., Agtarap, S., Scott, W., Driver, S., Guck, A., Reynolds, M., … Warren, A. M. (2015). Perceived injustice after traumatic injury: Associations with pain, psychological distress, and quality of life outcomes 12 months after injury. *Rehabilitation Psychology, 60*(3), 213–221. https://doi.org/10.1037/rep0000043

Trost, Z., Scott, W., Lange, J. M., Manganelli, L., Bernier, E., & Sullivan, M. J. (2014). An experimental investigation of the effect of a justice violation on pain experience and expression among individuals with high and low just world beliefs. *European Journal of Pain (United Kingdom), 18*(3), 415–423. https://doi.org/10.1002/j.1532-2149.2013.00375.x

Twenge, J. M., Baumeister, R. F., Tice, D. M., & Stucke, T. S. (2001). If you can't join them, beat them: Effects of social exclusion on aggressive behavior. *Journal of Personality and Social Psychology, 81*, 1058–1069. https://doi.org/10.1037/0022-3514.81.6.1058

Van Damme, S., Crombez, G., & Eccleston, C. (2008). Coping with pain: A motivational perspective. *Pain, 139*, 1–4. https://doi.org/10.1016/j.pain.2008.07.022

van den Hout, J. H., Vlaeyen, J. W. S., Peters, M. L., Engelhard, I. M., & van den Hout, M. A. (2000). Does failure hurt? The effects of failure feedback on pain report, pain tolerance and pain avoidance. *European Journal of Pain (London, England), 4*(4), 335–346. https://doi.org/10.1053/eujp.2000.0195

Vlaeyen, J. W. S. (2015). Learning to predict and control harmful events: Chronic pain and conditioning. *Pain, 156*(Suppl), S86–S93. https://doi.org/10.1097/j.pain.0000000000000107

Voerman, J. S., Vogel, I., De Waart, F., Westendorp, T., Timman, R., Busschbach, J. J. V., … De Klerk, C. (2015). Bullying, abuse and family conflict as risk factors for chronic pain among Dutch adolescents. *European Journal of Pain (United Kingdom), 19*(10), 1544–1551. https://doi.org/10.1002/ejp.689

Wager, T. D., Atlas, L. Y., Lindquist, M. A., Roy, M., Woo, C.-W., & Kross, E. (2013). An fMRI-based neurologic signature of physical pain. *New England Journal of Medicine, 368*(15), 1388–1397. https://doi.org/10.1056/NEJMoa1204471

Waugh, O. C., Byrne, D. G., & Nicholas, M. K. (2014). Internalized stigma in people living with chronic pain. *Journal of Pain, 15*(5), 550.e1–550.e10. https://doi.org/10.1016/j.jpain.2014.02.001

Way, B. M., Taylor, S. E., & Eisenberger, N. I. (2009). Variation in the μ-opioid receptor gene (OPRM1) is associated with dispositional and neural sensitivity to social rejection. *Proceedings of the National Academy of Sciences, 106*(35), 15079–15084. https://doi.org/10.1073/pnas.0812612106

Wiech, K., & Tracey, I. (2013). Pain, decisions, and actions: A motivational perspective. *Frontiers in Neuroscience, 7*, 1–12. https://doi.org/10.3389/fnins.2013.00046

Williams, A. C. d. C., & Craig, K. D. (2016). Updating the definition of pain. *Pain, 157*(11), 2420–2423.

Williams, K. D., Cheung, C. K. T., & Choi, W. (2000). Cyberostracism: Effects of being ignored over the internet. *Journal of Personality and Social Psychology, 79*, 748–762. https://doi.org/10.1037/0022-3514.79.5.748

Williams, K. D. (2002). *Ostracism: The power of silence*. New York, NY: Guilford Press.

Williams, K. D., & Jarvis, B. (2006). Cyberball: A program for use in research on interpersonal ostracism and acceptance. *Behavior Research Methods, 38*(1), 174–180. Retrieved from http://www.ncbi.nlm.nih.gov/pubmed/16817529

Williams, K. D. (2007). Ostracism. *Annual Review of Psychology, 58*, 425–452. https://doi.org/10.1146/annurev.psych.58.110405.085641

Woo, C.-W., Koban, L., Kross, E., Lindquist, M. A., Banich, M. T., Ruzic, L., … Wager, T. D. (2014). Separate neural representations for physical pain and social rejection. *Nature Communications, 5*(May), 5380. https://doi.org/10.1038/ncomms6380

Younger, J., Aron, A., Parke, S., Chatterjee, N., & Mackey, S. (2010). Viewing pictures of a romantic partner reduces experimental pain: Involvement of neural reward systems. *PLoS One, 5*(10), e13309. https://doi.org/10.1371/journal.pone.0013309

Zaza, C., & Baine, N. (2002). Cancer pain and psychosocial factors. *Journal of Pain and Symptom Management, 24*(5), 526–542. https://doi.org/10.1016/S0885-3924(02)00497-9

Chapter 10
Bridging the Gap Between People and Animals: The Roots of Social Behavior and Its Relationship to Pain

Erinn L. Acland, Navdeep K. Lidhar, and Loren J. Martin

Abstract Pain is considered a personal experience, but it is rarely private. Individuals' responses to pain function to communicate distress to others in the environment, eliciting emotional reactions and caregiving actions that in turn impact the sufferer's pain experience. In animals, these behaviors are considered empathy-like and indicative of a complex social framework. Laboratory experiments on animals and humans have shown that social context can have direct effects on the expression of pain. In this review, we discuss the foundations of social behavior in animal models, how they relate to empathy, and highlight shared neural mechanisms between pain and social behaviors.

Keywords Empathy · Pain · Animal model · Emotional contagion · Human · Neuroscience · Oxytocin · Prosocial behavior · Helping behavior · Familiarity

Introduction

The experience of empathy has a profound effect on the way we as humans perceive ourselves, so much so that the term "humanity" is synonymous with compassion. Our ability to understand and share emotions with one another not only affects our ability to gain resources and procreate, but heavily influences the laws and policies that govern our societies. Empathy is considered a crucial component of successful

---

Author contributed equally with all other contributors. Erinn L. Acland and Navdeep K. Lidhar

E. L. Acland · N. K. Lidhar
Department of Psychology, University of Toronto Mississauga, Mississauga, ON, Canada

L. J. Martin (✉)
Department of Psychology, University of Toronto Mississauga, Mississauga, ON, Canada

Department of Cell Systems and Biology, University of Toronto Mississauga, Mississauga, ON, Canada
e-mail: lj.martin@utoronto.ca

cooperative and prosocial behaviors and those that lack it tend to have difficulty forming and maintaining social relationships (De Waal, 2008). Distress, considered a key empathy-evoking emotion due to its association with potential threats and pain, is often used to study empathy processes in nonhuman animals. Empathy behaviors range in complexity from mimicking to active helping behaviors, but are most apparent when two individuals share the same emotional state including fear, stress or pain (Sivaselvachandran, Acland, Abdallah, & Martin, 2016). Elementary processes of empathy, such as emotional contagion, sympathy, and prosociality, provide the building blocks for the development of more complex empathetic processes found in humans. Determining the intention behind empathy-related behaviors in animals is difficult; however, researching these behaviors is fundamental to improving the understanding of our evolutionary adaptiveness and the development of complex social behaviors in humans.

Here, we take a broad comparative view of social behaviors as they relate to parental care, altruism, and empathy. By doing so, we highlight the complexity and richness of animal social behavior so that the intricacies of using animals to study social dynamics and their interaction with pain can be fully appreciated. We consider possible environmental and social pressures that may have led to the natural selection of these behaviors in animals and discuss parallel behaviors in humans. We then delve into the neural mechanisms that engage sociality so that we may establish causal relationships between seeing others in pain and responding appropriately (i.e., helping, consoling etc.), which only helps to further our understanding of the physiology behind empathy and pain processing. Finally, we believe that the true benefit of studying simple emotional behaviors in nonhuman animals is that they will allow us to better understand the complex social processes that are influenced by physical and emotional pain. This will be crucial for making appropriate conclusions about the functioning of empathy and affiliation in humans.

Parental Care in Nonhumans

Humans have a long developmental period, making parental behaviors pivotal for the successful growth and survival of offspring. The ability to understand and act on the needs of young is conserved across a diverse number of species; even creatures with limited cognitive capacities exhibit forms of parental care. Some insects will deposit eggs in protected areas, engage in high-risk behaviors that directly compromise the health and survival of the parent, spin silk around their brood to protect against predators and weather or physically guard offspring by sitting on top of them and fanning their wings in response to potential predators (Edgerly, 1988; Hanelová & Vilímová, 2013). Among invertebrates, care is primarily provided by the females, and seldom do males care for young alone (Tallamy, 1984). However, biparental and communal care can be advantageous for species that have especially low rates of reproductive success. One example of this is the burying beetle, which displays both maternal and paternal care behaviors. To feed their young, burying beetles drag a small vertebrate carcass into a protected lair, lay their eggs on the carcass and then regurgitate predigested carrion to the larvae. Male burying beetles are such competent parents that when the female is removed from a brood, males are just as successful at raising the young as single females or co-parents (Jenkins, Morris, & Blackman, 2000). However, unless the female died or abandoned the brood there is no significant benefit to having the male present, except in threatening or predatory situations. Male beetle intruders easily take over a nest guarded by a single female, but not when a parenting male is present. Thus, male burying beetles alter their behavior based on competition for resources, showing a capacity for behavioral plasticity. This demonstrates that there can be vast variability of care within a single cognitively "simple" species. Regardless, the argument can be put forth that behaviors in insects are not reflective of human behavior, which is why the vast majority of research studying empathy-related processes use nonhuman mammalian models.

Several rodent species employ co-parenting strategies, such as the California mouse, southern bamboo rat, the Mongolian gerbil, and prairie vole (Bamshad, Novak, & de Vries, 1994; Clark & Galef, 2000; Silva, Vieira, & Izar, 2008). To demonstrate the potential benefits of co-parenting in rodents, Cantoni and Brown (1997) assessed whether single or paired California mice would successfully raise more pups. When male and female mice co-parented, four times as many pups were reared over a period of about 2.5 months when compared to an individual female parent. Some primate studies have also shown that having two parents can not only provide more resources for young, but also increase protection from physical threats (Buchan, Alberts, Silk, & Altmann, 2003; Huchard et al., 2012). Similarly, co-parenting benefits are found in humans, where children raised by two parents are more successful in school, and have lower risks of psychiatric disease, suicide, injury, and addiction (Downey, 1994; Weitoft, Hjern, Haglund, & Rosén, 2003).

An entirely separate issue is the rearing of nongenetically related offspring. Species that live in large cooperative groups will sometimes share the responsibility of raising offspring since communal care increases survival for all of the group's offspring due to the improved care and protection they receive. An example of a species that practices communal care is the African wild dog, where 25% of non-breeding members of a pack will provide care to unrelated pups (McNutt, 1996). A more extreme version of communal caring is in colonies of social wasps that have multiple unrelated queens reproducing (Queller et al., 2000). This means that the nonreproducing worker wasps care for unrelated offspring, which has no apparent self-benefit. This seemingly maladaptive behavior may persist due to delayed advantages, where a few subordinates may eventually transition into the role of queen, a status position where they reap the rewards of the hierarchy.

The complete adoption of an unrelated youth is a rare empathetic behavior among animals, since it has no direct evolutionary advantage or benefit for the fostering parent. In humans, adoptive behaviors are commonly motivated by empathy for an unrelated child that is in dire conditions or not being able to have one's own children, but still having the profound urge to become a parent. It would be an impossible feat to argue that nonhuman animals make these same types of value judgments, so why do some animal species display adoptive behavior? Experimentally, it has been shown that animals, such as mice, raise non-kin as their own. From an evolutionary perspective, this is disadvantageous because resources become split between genetically related and unrelated pups, which decreases the probability that related offspring will survive. However, in mice, adoptive behavior may persist—not out of empathy or altruism, but because rodent mothers cannot differentiate foreign pups from their own (Cicirello & Wolff, 1990; Pillay, 2000).

Voluntary adoptive behaviors have been observed in primates, dolphins, seals, gulls and penguins (Graves & Whiten, 1980; Howells et al., 2009; Jouventin, Barbraud, & Rubin, 1995; Riedman & Le Boeuf, 1982). Additionally, several studies have shown that many primate species recognize their own offspring, yet they still display adoptive behaviors suggesting that they understand that the adopted infant is not their own (Buchan et al., 2003; Charpentier, Peignot, Hossaert-McKey, & Wickings, 2007; Parr & de Waal, 1999). It has even been reported that macaques kidnap the infants of others, showing a very strong motivation to provide maternal care, even when the individual is unrelated (Maestripieri, 1993; Schino et al., 1993; Silk, 1980). In one particularly exceptional case of adoption, researchers observed a group of wild capuchin monkeys adopt a marmoset infant (Izar et al., 2006). The adopted marmoset became fully integrated into the capuchin social group over a period of 11 months and all members showed pronounced tolerance towards the cross-species member. In many species, virgin females avoid and even act aggressively towards newborns, thus cases of adoptive behavior tend to be restricted to postpartum females (Holman & Goy, 1980; Richards, 1966). These cases of adoption demonstrate that there are robust motivational mechanisms behind infant care that are conserved across many species and are not unique to humans.

Parental care has clear benefits for increasing offspring success, and having multiple caregivers is especially important when developmental periods are long, there are a small number of offspring per birth, and/or when environmental pressures and resource competition is high. Parsing out the mechanisms behind the development of these nurturing behaviors can be tricky due to the limitations inherent in human research. Thus, most investigations of genetic and motivational mechanisms are done using social rodent models.

Neural Mechanisms of Parental Care

The neuropeptide oxytocin has stood out as a key player in parent-infant bonding and care behaviors in mice, rats, prairie voles, sheep, and primates (Dulac, O'Connell, & Wu, 2014; Holman & Goy, 1995; Kendrick, Keverne, & Baldwin, 1987; Maestripieri, Hoffman, Anderson, Carter, & Higley, 2009; McCarthy, 1990; Olazabal & Young, 2006; Pedersen, Ascher, Monroe, & Prange, 1982). For instance, female prairie voles with higher oxytocin receptor binding in the nucleus accumbens exhibit more infant care behaviors—licking, hovering, retrieval—all of which were decreased with an oxytocin receptor antagonist (Olazabal & Young, 2006; see

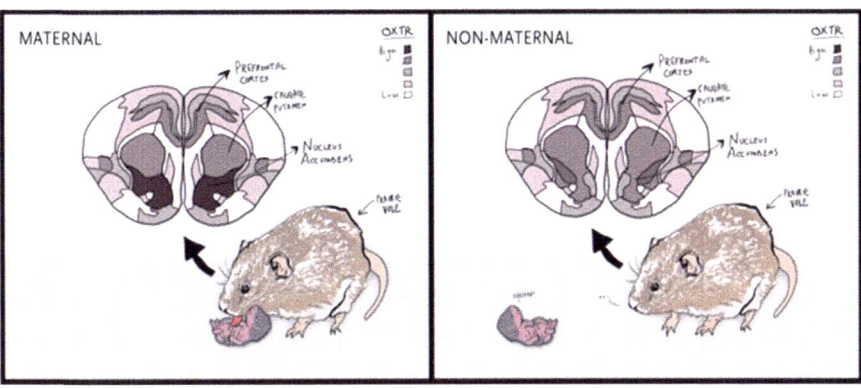

Fig. 10.1 Female prairie voles with higher oxytocin receptor density in the nucleus accumbens (shell subregion) display more maternal behaviors (hovering and licking) when compared with voles that display muted maternal behaviors towards pups. See Olazabal and Young, for the original data. Illustration by E.L.A.

Fig. 10.1). Additionally, female mice who typically show infanticidal behavior were less likely to kill pups when administered oxytocin and oxytocin receptor null mutant mice showed impaired abilities to care for their offspring (McCarthy, 1990; Takayanagi et al., 2005). It is suspected that oxytocin affects cortical processing of auditory distress signals from pups, which enables pup retrieval in maternal rats (Marlin, Mitre, D'amour, Chao, & Froemke, 2015). In humans, oxytocin plasma levels in pregnant and new mothers have been significantly associated with positive affect, affectionate touch, and infant checking (Feldman, Weller, Zagoory-Sharon, & Levine, 2007). Additionally, human research has shown that people with a less effective variant of the oxytocin gene (AA/AG) have lower levels of sensitive responsiveness to toddlers (Bakermans-Kranenburg & van IJzendoorn, 2008).

Whether oxytocin affects paternal behaviors is less clear and reports on the subject are mixed. In California mice, higher oxytocin plasma levels were not related to paternal care behaviors or infanticide (Gubernick, Winslow, Jensen, Jeanotte, & Bowen, 1995). Conversely, another study showed that infant care behaviors in non-monogamous male mice were completely extinguished by knocking out a gene involved in oxytocin secretion ($CD38^{-/-}$). Interestingly, males with intact or rescued CD38 did not display any parental behaviors if their female counterparts lacked the CD38 gene (Akther et al., 2013). This raises the question of whether intact oxytocin-related maternal cues are necessary for the elicitation of paternal behaviors in rodents and perhaps even other mammals. In human males, plasma oxytocin has been associated with increased positive parent-child social interactions, but these data are correlational and do not clarify the role of oxytocin in human paternal behaviors (Feldman, Gordon, & Zagoory-Sharon, 2011). Further complicating matters, a recent study found that measuring free oxytocin in human plasma/serum vastly underestimates total amount of circulating oxytocin, suggesting past studies using these methods should be interpreted with caution (Brandtzaeg et al., 2016).

In addition to this, most human studies assessing the effects of either enhancing or blocking oxytocin are done using intranasal spray. The exact concentration that passes into the brain remains unclear and conclusions are difficult to draw based on these studies. We have only begun to understand how oxytocin relates to empathic abilities at the genetic, molecular and neural circuit level. However, these types of investigations can only be causally assessed in animal models and we discuss some of these key findings below (see Sivaselvachandran et al., 2016, for a more detailed review).

In addition to oxytocin, the neuropeptide arginine vasopressin (AVP) has received considerable attention for its role in paternal care behaviors. Expression of AVP-immunoreactive fibers and receptors in the lateral septum of male prairie voles and California mice has been associated with parental behavior (Bamshad et al., 1994; Bester-Meredith, Young, & Marler, 1999). In male meadow and prairie voles, an injection of AVP increased crouching over and contact behavior with pups, suggesting that AVP mediates some paternal care behaviors (Parker & Lee, 2001; Wang, Ferris, & De Vries, 1994). Furthermore, central blockade of vasopressin receptors during mating prevented normal pair bonding and paternal care (Winslow, Hastings, Carter, Harbaugh, & Insel, 1993). This would indicate that AVP affects general bonding behaviors in male voles including mate and infant care. The human literature concerning AVP and parental behavior remains unclear; however, it has been found that the *AVPR1A* vasopressin receptor gene polymorphism R3 significantly predicted outcomes in partner bonding (e.g., affiliative interactions, perceived marital problems, and marital status) in male, but not female participants (Winslow et al., 1993). The literature has yet to present a concrete narrative, but suggests that vasopressin and oxytocin both have effects on parental prosocial behaviors and that these behaviors are conserved among mammals.

Altruism and Helping Behavior

Altruistic acts are highly praised in human societies. However, the fact that these actions are viewed as especially positive means that they are not expected from all or even most people and drastically vary between individuals. Animal behaviors are generally considered "altruistic" when an action reduces the actor's short-term fitness to increase the fitness of another, regardless of whether the benefit for the recipient was the goal of the act. The motivation behind performing altruistic acts could be due to the release of rewarding neurochemicals, such as how infant suckling releases oxytocin in mothers (Nagasawa, Okabe, Mogi, & Kikusui, 2012). Psychological escape from observing pain may also be a motivating factor, whereby the helper is trying to alleviate their own distress rather than the target's (Silberberg et al., 2014).

Social rodents are able to clearly recognize pain and distress and have been shown to respond to that distress with emotional contagion, helping, or consoling behaviors (Sivaselvachandran et al., 2016). In laboratory studies, rats will press a lever to lower a suspended rat, help a soaked conspecific or free a trapped cagemate (Ben-Ami Bartal, Decety, & Mason, 2011; Rice & Gainer, 1962; Sato, Tan, Tate, & Okada, 2015). Helping behavior displayed by rats occurs significantly more when the conspecific is in distress, and when given the option between a treat and helping a distressed cagemate, most rats help their cagemate prior to retrieving the treat (Sato et al., 2015). Interestingly, rats that have been previously helped by a conspecific are subsequently faster and more likely to help rats that have previously helped them or distressed rats that they have no prior experience with, suggesting that rats' past experiences can affect future altruistic acts. However, if a rat has learnt that a particular conspecific does not help them when they are distressed, they will be less likely in the future to help that particular rat, especially when the task increases in difficulty (Schneeberger, Dietz, & Taborsky, 2012). These experiments suggest that rats not only show reciprocal and generalized altruism but are also affected by the distress of another rat and the costs of performing a particular task. Some of the most striking examples from the animal literature on targeted helping and altruism can be found within elephant and dolphin social groups. Following distress vocalizations by an elephant, fellow elephants will increase physical contact and vocal communication—a type of consoling behavior—that relieves distress among the herd (Plotnik & de Waal, 2014). Elephants also physically assist individuals that have fallen and have even have been observed removing darts or spears that have been shot at members of their herd (Schulte, 2000). Similarly, dolphins perform pushing and lifting behaviors on unwell conspecifics, which effectively raises them to the surface in order to breathe (Kuczaj et al., 2015).

Pain behaviors signal that an individual may need help, which is a useful communication tool for cooperative groups. However, some may exploit injured individuals by stealing food, or usurping social position (Mogil, 2009). A recent study using a computer simulation showed how environmental and social pressures may shape pain expressiveness and altruistic behavior (Williams, Gallagher, Fidalgo, & Bentley, 2016). The suppression of pain behaviors was beneficial when the cost of displaying these behaviors was high, in particular when simulated agents were vulnerable as in predator-prey situations. However, the outright display of pain behavior was favored when the cost of giving help was low, which would be consistent with female mice approaching others in pain (Langford et al., 2010) or elephants gathering around a distressed herd member (Plotnik & de Waal, 2014). Contrary to evolutionary theories of empathy, altruistic behaviors persisted even when pain expressions were nonexistent, costs of helping were increased, or when the benefits of helping were reduced, whereas increasing frequency of injuries effectively abolished altruism and pain expression (Williams et al., 2016). If we are to believe this model of altruistic evolution, the widespread nature of helping behaviors that occur within a species may be dependent mostly on how dangerous an environment is and how high the cost is to help.

Social and Sex Factors in Empathy-Related Processes

Friends Versus Foes

The ability to feel an emotion that another is experiencing (emotional contagion) is a key underlying principle of empathy. In mice, pain contagion was first reported by Langford et al. (2006), who showed that a pain stimulus experienced in the presence of a cagemate—also in pain—elicited more pain behavior than when tested alone or in the presence of a stranger mouse in pain. The researchers reported that mice did not need to be genetically related, only that they needed to be cagemates for at least 21 days in order for the social transfer of pain to occur. Prairie voles also exhibit emotional contagion, whereby fear responses, anxiety-related behaviors, and corticosterone levels mimic those of their distressed cagemate (Burkett et al., 2016). These researchers also found that prairie voles exhibit consoling behaviors based on their social relationships with one another, where a vole will demonstrate increased allogrooming behaviors towards a distressed familiar conspecific, but not a distressed stranger.

Social learning is similarly affected by familiarity, whereby mice and vocal rodents such as *Octodon degus* can learn to associate fear with a particular context through observing a cagemate—but not a stranger—in pain in that context (Jeon et al., 2010; Lidhar, Insel, Dong, & Takehara-Nishiuchi, 2017). *Octodon degus* (highly social Chilean rodents) exposed to painful shocks exhibit different patterns of vocalizations depending on whether a stranger or cagemate is watching. The level of fear behavior exhibited by observer degus correlates with the pattern of vocalization exhibited by the degu in pain. These results indicate that familiarity can affect both the socially learned responses as well as a degus vocal expression of pain or distress (Lidhar et al., 2017). Similarly, rats exposed to a cagemate previously trained to fear a tone, also learn to fear that tone, simply by observing their cagemate's response to the stimuli (Bruchey, Jones, & Monfils, 2010). More complex behaviors such as performing altruistic acts are known to occur in some primate species, but only for in-group members, while most primates display neutral or even aggressive behaviors towards non-group members (De Waal, Aureli, & Judge, 2000; Wilson & Wrangham, 2003). Humans also show more empathy and helping behaviors towards in-group members (similar cultural background, race, wealth, sport teams etc.), even if the in-group is arbitrarily assigned such as being a part of team A or team B in an experimental setting (Stürmer, Snyder, Kropp, & Siem, 2006; Tajfel, Billig, Bundy, & Flament, 1971; Xu, Zuo, Wang, & Han, 2009). A common enemy tends to unite a group, whereby intergroup conflict actually improves affiliative behaviors and cooperation within groups (Bowles, 2009; Radford, 2008). An exception to this trend is the bonobo, who are known for making love, not war, and they display altruistic acts towards non-group members, such as donating food to strangers for no immediate reward (Tan & Hare, 2013).

Why do we feel more empathy for those we perceive to be closer to us? One study found that receiving an electric shock and observing a friend receive a shock activated similar neural patterns—anterior insula, putamen, and supramarginal gyrus—in both the demonstrator and observer. These same patterns were not activated in an observing stranger (Beckes, Coan, & Hasselmo, 2013). Another study found that experimentally increasing empathy—by watching a video of an actor detail an emotional experience—increased physical pain sensitivity in observers even though the two individuals had never met (Loggia, Mogil, & Bushnell, 2008). These findings provide evidence that social bonding is reliant on increasing the overlap of self and other neural representations. The theory is that empathy at its core is experiencing someone else's pain or suffering; however, the more different the "other" is perceived to be, the more difficult it is to understand and imagine what it is like to be that individual. Overall, these studies demonstrate that social relationships and communication of pain states can modulate an individual's experience of pain. The sharing of states based on kinship and social proximity is an elementary form of empathy conserved in a variety of social mammalian species.

Mechanisms of Familiarity Dependent Empathy-Related Behaviors

One of the most valuable things we can learn from animals is how pharmacology and physiology change empathy-related behaviors. We have found that the presence of a stranger impairs pain sensitivity due to an increase in stress hormones. Pharmacologically blocking the stress response allows for the expression of pain empathy behaviors for strangers in both mice and people (Martin et al., 2015). Along the same vein, higher plasma levels of the stress hormone corticosterone impaired helping behavior in rats; however, treatment with an anxiolytic reduced helping behavior (Bartal et al., 2016). This suggests that there may be a "just right" amount of stress required to optimize helping behaviors, which would be similar to performance-based areas of human cognition (Cassady & Johnson, 2002). In humans, inducing psychosocial stress in individuals can increase trust and sharing with others (von Dawans, Fischbacher, Kirschbaum, Fehr, & Heinrichs, 2012) and anticipating an electric shock increased helping behavior, but only when both participants were awaiting similar fates (Hayden, Jackson, & Guydish, 1984). However, there has yet to be a study in animals or humans looking at exactly how much stress is optimal for encouraging empathy-related processes.

Oxytocin has been found to not only be necessary for the display of certain parental care behaviors, but also has a wide range of effects on both stress and empathy-related processes. During stressful experiences, oxytocin has been associated with an increase in prosocial behaviors and a decrease in stress; however, when in the presence of hostile or unsupportive contacts oxytocin may amplify the stress response (Taylor, 2006). Similarly, human studies have shown that oxytocin increases empathy for pain, threat, and economic loss, but only among in-group members (Bartz et al., 2010; Hein, Silani, Preuschoff, Batson, & Singer, 2010).

Recent animal work has shown that oxytocin has complex effects on the processing of social information and neural network integration. The hippocampus, in particular plays a key role in the integration of social information. Electrophysiological recordings of rat hippocampal interneurons reveal that oxytocin specifically enhances spike timing and reduces background noise (Owen et al., 2013), indicating that oxytocin improves the salience of information by increasing the signal-to-noise ratio in neural circuits. In mice, oxytocin receptors in the medial amygdala have been found to be necessary for social recognition, which may play a role in the familiarity bias observed across empathy-related behaviors (Dumais, Alonso, Bredewold, & Veenema, 2016). These studies indicate that oxytocin's function may be more related to increasing attention towards social cues whether positive or negative versus indiscriminately increasing prosociality.

Research has also shown that species of carnivores' and primates' neocortices correlate with their social group size, indicating a larger neocortex is helpful or even necessary for living in more complex social groups (Dunbar & Bever, 1998). For instance, wild savannah baboons live in communal groups, thus male savannah baboons have developed the ability to recognize their own offspring, which allows them to provide selective support to them during conflicts (Buchan et al., 2003). Neocortex size is also predictive of deception rate in primates, suggesting it is required for higher order empathy processes such as perspective taking and theory of mind (Byrne & Corp, 2004). One experiment showed that particular neurons in the anterior cingulate fire when rhesus monkeys either share or give rewards to other monkeys, further solidifying the role of the neocortex in the evolution of complex prosocial behaviors (Chang, Gariepy, & Platt, 2013).

Alpha Versus Beta

In animal social groups, dominance hierarchies are formed when members compete for preferential access to resources and mating opportunities, which provides the top-ranking members enhanced reproductive success and a greater share of food. To become an alpha, often aggressive and violent strategies are employed, which are prototypical antisocial behaviors. Even though this social strategy yields success in certain areas, it is associated with impairments in social learning and emotional sensitivity. For instance, following the observation of biting flies attacking a conspecific, subordinate mice show enhanced learning of fly avoidance behaviors (Kavaliers, Colwell, & Choleris, 2005) allowing them to detect and/or escape from potentially threatening situations more readily than their dominant counterparts. Subordinate mice are also more likely to approach a conspecific in pain compared to dominant mice, suggesting that they are more attuned to social cues (Watanabe, 2014). Subordinate animals tend to have more physical and psychological stressors due to a lack of predictability and control over the social environment; however, their enhanced emotional sensitivity and social learning may be advantageous for navigating and responding to various social and threat cues.

Whether social rank directly impacts pain sensitivity remains unclear. Several studies have looked at the whether the response to an acute pain test would be affected by social rank; when mice were tested in the absence of their subordinate/dominant counterpart, one study found that subordinate mice displayed more acute pain behavior, another study showed the exact opposite effect, and a different study showed no effect of social rank at all (Aghajani et al., 2013; Andre et al., 2005; Gioiosa, Chiarotti, Alleva, & Laviola, 2009). These studies used various pain stimuli and different strains/rodents making it difficult to draw conclusions from their data. What has been shown is that the pain an animal experiences can potentially alter social rank. For instance, one study showed that prolonged pain increases submissive behaviors in dominant rats (Monassi, Bandler, & Keay, 2003). This may serve a protective role by limiting aggressive encounters in situations where the probability of successfully "*winning*" a fight is low. Recent evidence in humans suggests that our empathy for pain in others is shaped by relative positions within a social hierarchy. Observing painful stimulation applied to a perceived lower ranking individual induced robust activation of emotion-related brain regions (anterior insula and anterior medial cingulate cortex), whereas these empathic brain activations were significantly attenuated when painful stimulation was applied to a higher ranking individual (Feng et al., 2016). This would suggest that humans display reduced empathy for those that are perceived to be higher in social rank; this bias may be particularly evident in societies that have developed booming industries based around criticizing and judging those with the highest social status.

Female Versus Male

Considerable evidence from human and animal studies suggests that sex plays a role in physiological and social responses to stressful situations. In particular, males have been shown to exhibit a "fight-or-flight" response to stress, whereas females display a more prosocial "tend and befriend" response. The "tend and befriend" model proposed by Taylor et al. (2000) suggests that under conditions of stress, female, but not male mammals have a tendency to care for their young and engage in social interactions. For example, female mice demonstrate higher social approach behaviors towards conspecifics in pain compared to males; an effect that does not seem to be dependent on oxytocin (Langford et al., 2010). Female rats also demonstrate significantly faster responses in helping trapped cagemates compared to males (Ben-Ami Bartal et al., 2011). Similarly, ewes (female sheep), but not rams have been shown to express more attentive behaviors towards lambs that were recovering from a painful surgical procedure (Hild, Andersen, & Zanella, 2010).

Human females have also been shown to demonstrate higher trait empathy compared to males (Baron-Cohen & Wheelwright, 2004). Undoubtedly, socialization factors account for much of this difference, but there is evidence that other factors, such as hormonal differences, play a role as has been suggested in human and animal studies. Fetal testosterone levels have been found to be inversely correlated with many childhood and adolescent social behaviors, including empathy (Chapman et al., 2006), eye contact (Lutchmaya, Baron-Cohen, & Raggatt, 2002) and quality of social relationships (Knickmeyer, Baron-Cohen, Raggatt, & Taylor, 2005). An investigation by Langford et al. (2011) revealed that male mice in pain display stressed-induced analgesia (SIA) when in the presence of a stranger male mouse. However, in the presence of a castrated stranger, male mice did not exhibit altered pain behavior. This indicates that the social threat of a stranger mouse, which results in SIA, occurs via a testosterone-dependent mechanism. Interestingly, human work demonstrates that testosterone administration in females impairs functional connectivity between critical brain areas for the expression of empathy (Bos et al., 2016; Van Honk et al., 2011). As females naturally express low levels of testosterone and higher trait empathy, this may explain the sexually dimorphic empathy behaviors exhibited across species.

Distinct physiological mechanisms may also help explain how social behavior differs between sexes. Differential binding patterns in key social brain structures may suggest competing processes between females and males. Male rats exhibit higher oxytocin release during a social interaction in the posterior bed nucleus of the stria terminalis (pBNST), a sexually dimorphic brain region important in regulating social behaviors (Dumais, Alonso, Immormino, Bredewold, & Veenema, 2016). Oxytocin release in the central amygdala is similar between male and female rats and has been associated with maternal and intermale aggression (Bosch, Meddle, Beiderbeck, Douglas, & Neumann, 2005; Calcagnoli et al., 2015; Consiglio, Borsoi, Pereira, & Lucion, 2005; Lubin, Elliot, Black, & Johns, 2003). However, when oxytocin receptors are blocked in the central amygdala, male rats' interest in conspecifics is reduced, while females' social interest behavior remains unchanged (Dumais, Alonso, Bredewold, & Veenema, 2016). This indicates that the activation of oxytocin receptors in the central amygdala plays a causal role in male rodents' social interest in other males, however, it appears to have no effect on female social behavior. In female mice, oxytocin mRNA expression increases during estrus, which subsequently downregulates available peripheral oxytocin, resulting in more social interactions and approach behavior (Caligioni & Franci, 2002). Careful dissections of the neural mechanisms responsible for these sex-related differences have revealed increased neural activation in the amygdala and medial prefrontal cortex of males, but not females following a social interaction with a distressed cagemate (Mikosz, Nowak, Werka, & Knapska, 2015). Further, when it comes to inducing monogamous mate bonding in prairie voles, males require exposure to vasopressin, while oxytocin release is crucial for females (Insel & Hulihan, 1995). Neonatal oxytocin exposure in female, but not male, prairie voles leads to later increases in mate-guarding behaviors, which is a crucial component of pair bonding (Bales & Carter, 2003). Complicating matters further, early environmental factors can differentially affect male and female development. For instance, female rats that received high levels of licking and grooming as pups had increased oxytocin receptor binding in the central nucleus of the amygdala and BNST. Alternatively, male pups that received more nurturing behaviors had higher vasopressin receptor binding in the amygdala as adults, suggesting that maternal care has a sex-specific effect on neural development (Francis, Young, Meaney, & Insel, 2002). Altogether, these findings point towards a highly interconnected system between sex hormones, receptor expression and sexually dimorphic neural activation that alter empathy related behaviors. Currently, research on the neural mechanisms of empathy has been conducted almost exclusively in male rodents, thus more research is needed with respect to females before these data can be generalized to humans.

Shared Pathways of Empathy-Related Processes and Pain

The prompt recognition of distress and pain in others is highly adaptive for animals that live in social groups, since it can alert other animals to current or potential threats. In social mammals, empathy and pain processes appear closely linked, whereby when one is affected, the other is also affected. For instance, μ-opioid receptors have been implicated in the expression of maternal behaviors. Several studies have shown that administering μ-opioid agonists to female mice or rats reduces maternal behaviors and reversal of this behavior can be achieved through administration of opioid antagonists (Felicio, Mann, & Bridges, 1991; Ladd et al., 2000; Mann, Kinsley, & Bridges, 1991). One of the possible mediators of this relationship between the pain pathway and caring behaviors is oxytocin. It has been found that morphine significantly delays the birth of rats and decreases their oxytocin plasma levels, which can be reversed through administration of naloxone (an opioid antagonist). This phenomenon has also been found in primates, such as one field study that showed that wild rhesus macaques with a particular variant (G allele) of the μ-opioid receptor gene (OPRM1) had higher oxytocin levels when lactating and also prevented their infants from separating from them more often (Higham et al., 2011). Not only that, humans with this G allele of OPRM1 also report having more emotional pain when rejected by social partners (Way, Taylor, & Eisenberger, 2009). In male mice, when a gene encoding for endogenous opioids is deleted ($enk^{-/-}$), mice show hyperalgesia during an acute pain test, but also increased aggressive and anxious behaviors (Konig, Zimmer, Steiner, & Holmes, 1996). Conversely, knocking out a gene associated with the pain pathway ($NK1^{-/-}$) reduces the amount a male will attack a stranger mouse (De Felipe et al., 1998). These studies would suggest that pain-related genes are intimately involved with the expression of both prosocial and antisocial behaviors.

Not only have pain mechanisms been found to affect empathy-related behaviors and oxytocin, but conversely, oxytocin has also been found to affect pain expression. Social interaction in mice enhances pain thresholds, a phenomenon that is partially mediated by activation of the endogenous opioid system (D'Amato & Pavone, 1996). In one systematic review of animal experiments, it was found that 29 out of 33 studies showed that oxytocin increased pain tolerance, concluding that oxytocin was analgesic for acute animal pain (Rash, Aguirre-Camacho, & Campbell, 2014). They also looked at nine human studies and found similar findings, although more reliability in methodology would be required before appropriate conclusions can be made. Other studies have shown that oxytocin's analgesic effect is medi-ated—in part—by endogenous opioids, such that administering naloxone can block its effect, yet an oxytocin receptor antagonist does not (Uvnasmoberg, Bruzelius, Alster, & Lundeberg, 1993). Additional evidence by Schorscher-Petcu et al. (2010) suggested that oxytocin-induced analgesia was not controlled by oxytocin recep-tors, but required vasopressin-1A receptors in the dorsal root ganglia. Overall, these findings indicate that while oxytocin is involved with a range of social and affiliative behaviors, it is also integral to the modulation of pain by activating other receptor systems. Using animal models we can begin to understand the complex intercon-nected physiological systems that underlie empathetic processes and the modula-tion of pain processing. The literature suggests that the experience and expression of mammalian care behaviors are intimately associated with pain pathways.

The anterior cingulate cortex (ACC) is one brain area, in particular that has been implicated in both pain and empathy processes. For instance, reported feelings of empathy for a loved one in pain correlate with activation in the anterior insula and ACC (Singer et al., 2004). Additionally, a painful pinprick or watching another undergo the same experience correlated with activity in the right dorsal ACC, indi-cating some of the same pain pathways are activated when an individual experi-ences pain or empathizes with another's pain (Lloyd, Di Pellegrino, & Roberts, 2004). To substantiate a more causal link between the ACC and empathy-related processes, Kim, Mátyás, Lee, Acsády, and Shin (2012) assessed whether activating (electrical stimulation) or inactivating (lidocaine injections) empathy-linked brain regions in mice would affect socially mediated learning. They found that the right side of the ACC and both hemispheres of the thalamic nuclei were necessary for mice to learn fear behaviors through observation of another mouse's behaviors. Studies attempting to pinpoint the cellular mechanisms involved in this circuitry have revealed that oxytocin receptors in the ACC are necessary for consoling responses in prairie voles (Burkett et al., 2016). Furthermore, $Ca_v1.2$ Ca^{2+} channels and dopamine D_2 receptors in the ACC have been found to affect the expression of observational fear learning and pain behaviors in rodents (Jeon et al., 2010; Kim et al., 2014). These findings support a role for the ACC in both pain experience and negative empathy-related processes within both humans and rodents alike.

Summary

Understanding the full complexity of human empathy from a basic mechanistic perspective is challenging, and it can be argued that within this domain we are unique as a species (Buchan et al., 2003). However, it is hard to imagine that empa-thy—a characteristic so basic to the identity of the human species—came into exis-tence only when our lineage split off from that of the apes. Empathy processes appear to have evolved in order to motivate protection-related behaviors against physical harm of an offspring or a social group. The ability to effectively detect and transfer information about pain and threats is likely one of the strongest influencers of empathy and social development, which may explain why many social and pain neural pathways overlap. Maternal and paternal care behaviors have been reported in animals from insects to primates, showing the ubiquitous benefits of attending to and defending offspring, especially when resource and/or mating competition are high. The ability to empathize improves cooperation and prosocial behaviors, which increases the evolutionary pressure of empathy trait selection on species that benefit from communal group living. Caution should be exercised as to not over interpret nonhuman social behaviors that do not support human data. The mechanisms behind empathy-related behavior seem to be largely conserved among mammals making them useful models for understanding the neural mechanisms behind empathy-related behaviors.

Human research is limited by its inability to provide definitive evidence of cause-and-effect relationships. The most effective method for supporting correlative and speculative human data is to study nonhuman animals so that the variables are under fine control and can be altered systematically. It is still hotly debated whether animals have the ability to experience empathy, and although this is difficult to assess, we have summarized some convincing literature reporting that a broad range of animals possess at least basic forms of empathy, such as emotional contagion. Beyond this, altruistic behaviors found to be normal in other species, such as sacrificing one's own reproductive success in order to improve the fitness of unrelated individuals, are relatively rare in humans. Not all prosocial behaviors require empathy and determining the internal motivations behind these behaviors is impossible to establish in nonhuman animals. However, just because we may not be able to identify whether a behavior is motivated by selfish or selfless goals does not mean that studying them cannot tell us something about how social and affiliative behaviors evolved and how they function on a mechanistic level.

References

Aghajani, M., Mahdavi, M. R. V., Najafabadi, M. K., Ghazanfari, T., Azimi, A., Soleymani, S. A., & Dust, S. M. (2013). Effects of dominant/subordinate social status on formalin-induced pain and changes in serum proinflammatory cytokine concentrations in mice. *PLoS One, 8*, e80650.

Akther, S., Korshnova, N., Zhong, J., Liang, M. K., Cherepanov, S. M., Lopatina, O., ... Higashida, H. (2013). CD38 in the nucleus accumbens and oxytocin are related to paternal behavior in mice. *Molecular Brain, 6*, 41.

Andre, J., Zeau, B., Pohl, M., Cesselin, F., Benoliel, J. J., & Becker, C. (2005). Involvement of cholecystokininergic systems in anxiety-induced hyperalgesia in male rats: Behavioral and biochemical studies. *Journal of Neuroscience, 25*, 7896–7904.

Bakermans-Kranenburg, M. J., & van IJzendoorn, M. H. (2008). Oxytocin receptor (OXTR) and serotonin transporter (5-HTT) genes associated with observed parenting. *Social Cognitive and Affective Neuroscience, 3*, 128–134.

Bales, K. L., & Carter, C. S. (2003). Sex differences and developmental effects of oxytocin on aggression and social behavior in prairie voles (*Microtus ochrogaster*). *Hormones and Behavior, 44*, 178–184.

Bamshad, M., Novak, M. A., & de Vries, G. J. (1994). Cohabitation alters vasopressin innervation and paternal behavior in prairie voles (*Microtus ochrogaster*). *Physiology and Behavior, 56,* 751–758.

Baron-Cohen, S., & Wheelwright, S. (2004). The empathy quotient: An investigation of adults with Asperger syndrome or high functioning autism, and normal sex differences. *Journal of Autism and Developmental Disorders, 34,* 163–175.

Bartal, I. B., Shan, H. Z., Molasky, N. M. R., Murray, T. M., Williams, J. Z., Decety, J., & Mason, P. (2016). Anxiolytic treatment impairs helping behavior in rats. *Frontiers in Psychology, 7,* 850.

Bartz, J. A., Zaki, J., Bolger, N., Hollander, E., Ludwig, N. N., Kolevzon, A., & Ochsner, K. N. (2010). Oxytocin selectively improves empathic accuracy. *Psychological Science, 21,* 1426–1428.

Beckes, L., Coan, J. A., & Hasselmo, K. (2013). Familiarity promotes the blurring of self and other in the neural representation of threat. *Social Cognitive and Affective Neuroscience, 8,* 670–677.

Ben-Ami Bartal, I., Decety, J., & Mason, P. (2011). Empathy and pro-social behavior in rats. *Science, 334,* 1427–1430.

Bester-Meredith, J. K., Young, L. J., & Marler, C. A. (1999). Species differences in paternal behavior and aggression in peromyscus and their associations with vasopressin immunoreactivity and receptors. *Hormones and Behavior, 36,* 25–38.

Bos, P. A., Hofman, D., Hermans, E. J., Montoya, E. R., Baron-Cohen, S., & van Honk, J. (2016). Testosterone reduces functional connectivity during the 'reading the mind in the eyes' test. *Psychoneuroendocrinology, 68,* 194–201.

Bosch, O. J., Meddle, S. L., Beiderbeck, D. I., Douglas, A. J., & Neumann, I. D. (2005). Brain oxytocin correlates with maternal aggression: Link to anxiety. *Journal of Neuroscience, 25,* 6807–6815.

Bowles, S. (2009). Did warfare among ancestral hunter-gatherers affect the evolution of human social behaviors? *Science, 324,* 1293–1298.

Brandtzaeg, O. K., Johnsen, E., Roberg-Larsen, H., Seip, K. F., MacLean, E. L., Gesquiere, L. R., … Wilson, S. R. (2016). Proteomics tools reveal startlingly high amounts of oxytocin in plasma and serum. *Scientific Reports, 6,* 31693.

Bruchey, A. K., Jones, C. E., & Monfils, M.-H. (2010). Fear conditioning by-proxy: Social transmission of fear during memory retrieval. *Behavioural Brain Research, 214,* 80–84.

Buchan, J. C., Alberts, S. C., Silk, J. B., & Altmann, J. (2003). True paternal care in a multi-male primate society. *Nature, 425,* 179–181.

Burkett, J. P., Andari, E., Johnson, Z. V., Curry, D. C., de Waal, F. B., & Young, L. J. (2016). Oxytocin-dependent consolation behavior in rodents. *Science, 351,* 375–378.

Byrne, R. W., & Corp, N. (2004). Neocortex size predicts deception rate in primates. *Proceedings of the Royal Society B: Biological Sciences, 271,* 1693.

Calcagnoli, F., Stubbendorff, C., Meyer, N., de Boer, S. F., Althaus, M., & Koolhaas, J. M. (2015). Oxytocin microinjected into the central amygdaloid nuclei exerts anti-aggressive effects in male rats. *Neuropharmacology, 90,* 74–81.

Caligioni, C., & Franci, C. (2002). Oxytocin secretion induced by osmotic stimulation in rats during the estrous cycle and after ovariectomy and hormone replacement therapy. *Life Sciences, 71,* 2821–2831.

Cantoni, D., & Brown, R. E. (1997). Paternal investment and reproductive success in the California mouse, *Peromyscus californicus*. *Animal Behaviour, 54,* 377–386.

Cassady, J. C., & Johnson, R. E. (2002). Cognitive test anxiety and academic performance. *Contemporary Educational Psychology, 27*(2), 270–295.

Chang, S. W., Gariepy, J. F., & Platt, M. L. (2013). Neuronal reference frames for social decisions in primate frontal cortex. *Nature Neuroscience, 16,* 243–250.

Chapman, E., Baron-Cohen, S., Auyeung, B., Knickmeyer, R., Taylor, K., & Hackett, G. (2006). Fetal testosterone and empathy: Evidence from the Empathy Quotient (EQ) and the "reading the mind in the eyes" test. *Social Neuroscience, 1,* 135–148.

Charpentier, M. J., Peignot, P., Hossaert-McKey, M., & Wickings, E. J. (2007). Kin discrimination in juvenile mandrills, Mandrillus sphinx. *Animal Behaviour, 73*, 37–45.

Cicirello, D. M., & Wolff, J. O. (1990). The effects of mating on infanticide and pup discrimination in white-footed mice. *Behavioral Ecology and Sociobiology, 26*, 275–279.

Clark, M. M., & Galef, B. G. (2000). Why some male Mongolian gerbils may help at the nest: Testosterone, asexuality and alloparenting. *Animal Behaviour, 59*, 801–806.

Consiglio, A. R., Borsoi, A., Pereira, G. A., & Lucion, A. B. (2005). Effects of oxytocin micro-injected into the central amygdaloid nucleus and bed nucleus of stria terminalis on maternal aggressive behavior in rats. *Physiology & Behavior, 85*, 354–362.

D'Amato, F. R., & Pavone, F. (1996). Reunion of separated sibling mice: Neurobiological and behavioral aspects. *Neurobiology of Learning and Memory, 65*, 9–16.

De Felipe, C., Herrero, J. F., O'brien, J. A., Palmer, J. A., Doyle, C. A., Smith, A. J., … Hunt, S. P. (1998). Altered nociception, analgesia and aggression in mice lacking the receptor for substance P. *Nature, 392*, 394–397.

De Waal, F. B. M. (2008). Putting the altruism back into altruism: The evolution of empathy. *Annual Review of Psychology, 59*, 279–300.

De Waal, F. B. M., Aureli, F., & Judge, P. G. (2000). Coping with crowding. *Scientific American, 282*, 76–81.

Downey, D. B. (1994). The school performance of children from single-mother and single-father families: Economic or interpersonal deprivation? *Journal of Family Issues, 15*, 129–147.

Dulac, C., O'Connell, L. A., & Wu, Z. (2014). Neural control of maternal and paternal behaviors. *Science, 345*, 765–770.

Dumais, K. M., Alonso, A. G., Bredewold, R., & Veenema, A. H. (2016). Role of the oxytocin system in amygdala subregions in the regulation of social interest in male and female rats. *Neuroscience, 330*, 138–149.

Dumais, K. M., Alonso, A. G., Immormino, M. A., Bredewold, R., & Veenema, A. H. (2016). Involvement of the oxytocin system in the bed nucleus of the stria terminalis in the sex-specific regulation of social recognition. *Psychoneuroendocrinology, 64*, 79–88.

Dunbar, R., & Bever, J. (1998). Neocortex size predicts group size in carnivores and some insectivores. *Ethology, 104*, 695–708.

Edgerly, J. S. (1988). Maternal behaviour of a webspinner (order Embiidina): Mother-nymph associations. *Ecological Entomology, 13*, 263–272.

Feldman, R., Gordon, I., & Zagoory-Sharon, O. (2011). Maternal and paternal plasma, salivary, and urinary oxytocin and parent–infant synchrony: Considering stress and affiliation components of human bonding. *Developmental Science, 14*, 752–761.

Feldman, R., Weller, A., Zagoory-Sharon, O., & Levine, A. (2007). Evidence for a neuroendocrinological foundation of human affiliation plasma oxytocin levels across pregnancy and the postpartum period predict mother-infant bonding. *Psychological Science, 18*, 965–970.

Felicio, L. F., Mann, P. E., & Bridges, R. S. (1991). Intracerebroventricular cholecystokinin infusions block beta-endorphin-induced disruption of maternal behavior. *Pharmacology Biochemistry and Behavior, 39*, 201–204.

Feng, C. L., Li, Z. H., Feng, X., Wang, L. L., Tian, T. X., & Luo, Y. J. (2016). Social hierarchy modulates neural responses of empathy for pain. *Social Cognitive and Affective Neuroscience, 11*, 485–495.

Francis, D. D., Young, L. J., Meaney, M. J., & Insel, T. R. (2002). Naturally occurring differences in maternal care are associated with the expression of oxytocin and vasopressin (V1a) receptors: Gender differences. *Journal of Neuroendocrinology, 14*, 349–353.

Gioiosa, L., Chiarotti, F., Alleva, E., & Laviola, G. (2009). A trouble shared is a trouble halved: Social context and status affect pain in mouse dyads. *PLoS One, 4*, e4143.

Graves, J., & Whiten, A. (1980). Adoption of strange chicks by herring gulls, Larus argentatus L. *Ethology, 54*, 267–278.

Gubernick, D. J., Winslow, J. T., Jensen, P., Jeanotte, L., & Bowen, J. (1995). Oxytocin changes in males over the reproductive cycle in the monogamous, biparental California mouse, *Peromyscus californicus*. *Hormones and Behavior, 29*, 59–73.

Hanelová, J., & Vilímová, J. (2013). Behaviour of the central European Acanthosomatidae (Hemiptera: Heteroptera: Pentatomoidea) during oviposition and parental care. *Acta Musei Moraviae, Scientiae Biologicae, 98*, 433–457.

Hayden, S. R., Jackson, T. T., & Guydish, J. (1984). Helping behavior of females: Effects of stress and commonality of fate. *The Journal of Psychology, 117*, 233–237.

Hein, G., Silani, G., Preuschoff, K., Batson, C. D., & Singer, T. (2010). Neural responses to ingroup and outgroup members' suffering predict individual differences in costly helping. *Neuron, 68*, 149–160.

Higham, J. P., Barr, C. S., Hoffman, C. L., Mandalaywala, T. M., Parker, K. J., & Maestripieri, D. (2011). Mu-opioid receptor (OPRM1) variation, oxytocin levels and maternal attachment in free-ranging rhesus macaques *Macaca mulatta*. *Behavioral Neuroscience, 125*, 131–136.

Hild, S., Andersen, I. L., & Zanella, A. J. (2010). The relationship between thermal nociceptive threshold in lambs and ewe–lamb interactions. *Small Ruminant Research, 90*, 142–145.

Holman, S., & Goy, R. (1980). Behavioral and mammary responses of adult female rhesus to strange infants. *Hormones and Behavior, 14*, 348–357.

Holman, S., & Goy, R. W. (1995). Experiential and hormonal correlates of care-giving in rhesus macaques. In *Motherhood in human and nonhuman primates: Biosocial determinants* (pp. 87–93). Basel, Switzerland: Karger Publishers.

Howells, E. M., Reif, J. S., Bechdel, S. E., Murdoch, M. E., Bossart, G. D., McCulloch, S. D., & Mazzoil, M. S. (2009). A novel case of non-offspring adoption in a free-ranging Atlantic bottlenose dolphin (*Tursiops truncatus*) inhabiting the Indian River Lagoon, Florida. *Aquatic Mammals, 35*, 43–47.

Huchard, E., Charpentier, M. J., Marshall, H., King, A. J., Knapp, L. A., & Cowlishaw, G. (2012). Paternal effects on access to resources in a promiscuous primate society. *Behavioral Ecology, 24*, 229–236.

Insel, T. R., & Hulihan, T. J. (1995). A gender-specific mechanism for pair bonding: Oxytocin and partner preference formation in monogamous voles. *Behavioral Neuroscience, 109*, 782.

Izar, P., Verderane, M. P., Visalberghi, E., Ottoni, E. B., Gomes De Oliveira, M., Shirley, J., & Fragaszy, D. (2006). Cross-genus adoption of a marmoset (*Callithrix jacchus*) by wild capuchin monkeys (*Cebus libidinosus*): Case report. *American Journal of Primatology, 68*, 692–700.

Jenkins, E. V., Morris, C., & Blackman, S. (2000). Delayed benefits of paternal care in the burying beetle Nicrophorus vespilloides. *Animal Behaviour, 60*, 443–451.

Jeon, D., Kim, S., Chetana, M., Jo, D., Ruley, H. E., Lin, S.-Y., … Shin, H.-S. (2010). Observational fear learning involves affective pain system and Cav1.2 Ca2+ channels in ACC. *Nature Neuroscience, 13*, 482–488.

Jouventin, P., Barbraud, C., & Rubin, M. (1995). Adoption in the emperor penguin, *Aptenodytes forsteri*. *Animal Behaviour, 50*, 1023–1029.

Kavaliers, M., Colwell, D. D., & Choleris, E. (2005). Kinship, familiarity and social status modulate social learning about "micropredators" (biting flies) in deer mice. *Behavioral Ecology and Sociobiology, 58*, 60–71.

Kendrick, K., Keverne, E., & Baldwin, B. (1987). Intracerebroventricular oxytocin stimulates maternal behaviour in the sheep. *Neuroendocrinology, 46*, 56–61.

Kim, B. S., Lee, J., Bang, M., Am Seo, B., Khalid, A., Jung, M. W., & Jeon, D. (2014). Differential regulation of observational fear and neural oscillations by serotonin and dopamine in the mouse anterior cingulate cortex. *Psychopharmacology, 231*, 4371–4381.

Kim, S., Mátyás, F., Lee, S., Acsády, L., & Shin, H.-S. (2012). Lateralization of observational fear learning at the cortical but not thalamic level in mice. *Proceedings of the National Academy of Sciences U S A, 109*, 15497–15501.

Knickmeyer, R., Baron-Cohen, S., Raggatt, P., & Taylor, K. (2005). Foetal testosterone, social relationships, and restricted interests in children. *Journal of Child Psychology and Psychiatry, 46*, 198–210.

Konig, M., Zimmer, A. M., Steiner, H., & Holmes, P. V. (1996). Pain responses, anxiety and aggression in mice deficient in pre-proenkephalin. *Nature, 383*, 535.

Kuczaj, S. A., Frick, E. E., Jones, B. L., Lea, J. S. E., Beecham, D., & Scholler, F. (2015). Underwater observations of dolphin reactions to a distressed conspecific. *Learning and Behavior, 43*, 289–300.

Ladd, C. O., Huot, R. L., Thrivikraman, K. V., Nemeroff, C. B., Meaney, M. J., & Plotsky, P. M. (2000). Long-term behavioral and neuroendocrine adaptations to adverse early experience. *Progress in Brain Research, 122*, 81–103.

Langford, D. J., Crager, S. E., Shehzad, Z., Smith, S. B., Sotocinal, S. G., Levenstadt, J. S., … Mogil, J. S. (2006). Social modulation of pain as evidence for empathy in mice. *Science, 312*, 1967–1970.

Langford, D. J., Tuttle, A. H., Briscoe, C., Harvey-Lewis, C., Baran, I., Gleeson, P., … Mogil, J. S. (2011). Varying perceived social threat modulates pain behavior in male mice. *The Journal of Pain, 12*, 125–132.

Langford, D. J., Tuttle, A. H., Brown, K., Deschenes, S., Fischer, D. B., Mutso, A., … Sternberg, W. F. (2010). Social approach to pain in laboratory mice. *Social Neuroscience, 5*, 163–170.

Lidhar, N. K., Insel, N., Dong, J. Y., & Takehara-Nishiuchi, K. (2017). Observational fear learning in degus is correlated with temporal vocalization patterns. *Behavioural Brain Research, 332*, 362–371.

Lloyd, D., Di Pellegrino, G., & Roberts, N. (2004). Vicarious responses to pain in anterior cingulate cortex: Is empathy a multisensory issue? *Cognitive, Affective, & Behavioral Neuroscience, 4*, 270–278.

Loggia, M. L., Mogil, J. S., & Bushnell, M. C. (2008). Empathy hurts: Compassion for another increases both sensory and affective components of pain perception. *Pain, 136*, 168–176.

Lubin, D. A., Elliot, J. C., Black, M. C., & Johns, J. M. (2003). An oxytocin antagonist infused into the central nucleus of the amygdala increases maternal aggressive behavior. *Behavioral Neuroscience, 117*, 195.

Lutchmaya, S., Baron-Cohen, S., & Raggatt, P. (2002). Foetal testosterone and eye contact in 12-month-old human infants. *Infant Behavior and Development, 25*, 327–335.

Maestripieri, D. (1993). Infant kidnapping among group-living rhesus macaques: Why don't mothers rescue their infants? *Primates, 34*, 211–216.

Maestripieri, D., Hoffman, C. L., Anderson, G. M., Carter, C. S., & Higley, J. D. (2009). Mother–infant interactions in free-ranging rhesus macaques: Relationships between physiological and behavioral variables. *Physiology and Behavior, 96*, 613–619.

Mann, P., Kinsley, C., & Bridges, R. (1991). Opioid receptor subtype involvement in maternal behavior in lactating rats. *Neuroendocrinology, 53*, 487–492.

Marlin, B. J., Mitre, M., D'amour, J. A., Chao, M. V., & Froemke, R. C. (2015). Oxytocin enables maternal behaviour by balancing cortical inhibition. *Nature, 520*, 499–504.

Martin, L. J., Hathaway, G., Isbester, K., Mirali, S., Acland, E. L., Niederstrasser, N., … Sapolsky, R. M. (2015). Reducing social stress elicits emotional contagion of pain in mouse and human strangers. *Current Biology, 25*, 326–332.

McCarthy, M. M. (1990). Oxytocin inhibits infanticide in female house mice (*Mus domesticus*). *Hormones and Behavior, 24*, 365–375.

McNutt, J. W. (1996). Adoption in African wild dogs, *Lycaon pictus*. *Journal of Zoology, 240*, 163–173.

Mikosz, M., Nowak, A., Werka, T., & Knapska, E. (2015). Sex differences in social modulation of learning in rats. *Scientific Reports, 5*, 18114.

Mogil, J. S. (2009). Animal models of pain: Progress and challenges. *Nature Reviews Neuroscience, 10*, 283–294.

Monassi, C. R., Bandler, R., & Keay, K. A. (2003). A subpopulation of rats show social and sleep-waking changes typical of chronic neuropathic pain following peripheral nerve injury. *European Journal of Neuroscience, 17*, 1907–1920.

Nagasawa, M., Okabe, S., Mogi, K., & Kikusui, T. (2012). Oxytocin and mutual communication in mother-infant bonding. *Frontiers in Human Neuroscience, 6*, 31.

Olazabal, D., & Young, L. (2006). Oxytocin receptors in the nucleus accumbens facilitate "spontaneous" maternal behavior in adult female prairie voles. *Neuroscience, 141*, 559–568.

Owen, S. F., Tuncdemir, S. N., Bader, P. L., Tirko, N. N., Fishell, G., & Tsien, R. W. (2013). Oxytocin enhances hippocampal spike transmission by modulating fast-spiking interneurons. *Nature, 500*, 458–462.

Parker, K. J., & Lee, T. M. (2001). Central vasopressin administration regulates the onset of facultative paternal behavior in *Microtus pennsylvanicus* (meadow voles). *Hormones and Behavior, 39*, 285–294.

Parr, L. A., & de Waal, F. B. M. (1999). Visual kin recognition in chimpanzees. *Nature, 399*, 647–648.

Pedersen, C. A., Ascher, J. A., Monroe, Y. L., & Prange, A. J. (1982). Oxytocin induces maternal behavior in virgin female rats. *Science, 216*, 648–650.

Pillay, N. (2000). Fostering in the African striped mouse: Implications for kin recognition and dominance. *Acta Theriologica, 45*, 193–200.

Plotnik, J. M., & de Waal, F. B. M. (2014). Asian elephants (*Elephas maximus*) reassure others in distress. *PeerJ, 2*, e278.

Queller, D. C., Zacchi, F., Cervo, R., Turillazzi, S., Henshaw, M. T., Santorelli, L. A., & Strassmann, J. E. (2000). Unrelated helpers in a social insect. *Nature, 405*, 784–787.

Radford, A. N. (2008). Duration and outcome of intergroup conflict influences intragroup affiliative behaviour. *Proceedings of the Royal Society of London B: Biological Sciences, 275*, 2787–2791.

Rash, J. A., Aguirre-Camacho, A., & Campbell, T. S. (2014). Oxytocin and pain: A systematic review and synthesis of findings. *The Clinical Journal of Pain, 30*, 453–462.

Rice, G. E., & Gainer, P. (1962). Altruism in albino rat. *Journal of Comparative and Physiological Psychology, 55*, 123–125.

Richards, M. (1966). Maternal behaviour in the golden hamster: Responsiveness to young in virgin, pregnant, and lactating females. *Animal Behaviour, 14*, 310–313.

Riedman, M. L., & Le Boeuf, B. J. (1982). Mother-pup separation and adoption in northern elephant seals. *Behavioral Ecology and Sociobiology, 11*, 203–215.

Sato, N., Tan, L., Tate, K., & Okada, M. (2015). Rats demonstrate helping behavior toward a soaked conspecific. *Animal Cognition, 18*, 1039–1047.

Schino, G., Aureli, F., D'Amato, F. R., D'Antoni, M., Pandolfi, N., & Troisi, A. (1993). Infant kidnapping and co-mothering in Japanese macaques. *American Journal of Primatology, 30*, 257–262.

Schneeberger, K., Dietz, M., & Taborsky, M. (2012). Reciprocal cooperation between unrelated rats depends on cost to donor and benefit to recipient. *BMC Evolutionary Biology, 12*, 41.

Schorscher-Petcu, A., Sotocinal, S., Ciura, S., Dupre, A., Ritchie, J., Sorge, R. E., … Mogil, J. S. (2010). Oxytocin-induced analgesia and scratching are mediated by the vasopressin-1A receptor in the mouse. *Journal of Neuroscience, 30*, 8274–8284.

Schulte, B. A. (2000). Social structure and helping behavior in captive elephants. *Zoo Biology, 19*, 447–459.

Silberberg, A., Allouch, C., Sandfort, S., Kearns, D., Karpel, H., & Slotnick, B. (2014). Desire for social contact, not empathy, may explain "rescue" behavior in rats. *Animal Cognition, 17*, 609–618.

Silk, J. B. (1980). Kidnapping and female competition among captive bonnet macaques. *Primates, 21*, 100–110.

Silva, R. B., Vieira, E. M., & Izar, P. (2008). Social monogamy and biparental care of the neotropical southern bamboo rat (*Kannabateomys amblyonyx*). *Journal of Mammalogy, 89*, 1464–1472.

Singer, T., Seymour, B., O'Doherty, J., Kaube, H., Dolan, R. J., & Frith, C. D. (2004). Empathy for pain involves the affective but not sensory components of pain. *Science, 303*, 1157–1162.

Sivaselvachandran, S., Acland, E. L., Abdallah, S., & Martin, L. J. (2016). Behavioral and mechanistic insight into rodent empathy. *Neuroscience and Biobehavioral Reviews.*

Stürmer, S., Snyder, M., Kropp, A., & Siem, B. (2006). Empathy-motivated helping: The moderating role of group membership. *Personality and Social Psychology Bulletin, 32*, 943–956.

Tajfel, H., Billig, M. G., Bundy, R. P., & Flament, C. (1971). Social categorization and intergroup behaviour. *European Journal of Social Psychology, 1*, 149–178.

Takayanagi, Y., Yoshida, M., Bielsky, I. F., Ross, H. E., Kawamata, M., Onaka, T., … Nishimon, K. (2005). Pervasive social deficits, but normal parturition, in oxytocin receptor-deficient mice. *Proceedings of the National Academy of Sciences U S A, 102*, 16096–16101.

Tallamy, D. W. (1984). Insect parental care. *Bioscience, 34*, 20–24.

Tan, J., & Hare, B. (2013). Bonobos share with strangers. *PLoS One, 8*, e51922.

Taylor, S. E. (2006). Tend and befriend biobehavioral bases of affiliation under stress. *Current Directions in Psychological Science, 15*, 273–277.

Taylor, S. E., Klein, L. C., Lewis, B. P., Gruenewald, T. L., Gurung, R. A., & Updegraff, J. A. (2000). Biobehavioral responses to stress in females: Tend-and-befriend, not fight-or-flight. *Psychological Review, 107*, 411–429.

Uvnasmoberg, K., Bruzelius, G., Alster, P., & Lundeberg, T. (1993). The antinociceptive effect of nonnoxious sensory stimulation is mediated partly through oxytocinergic mechanisms. *Acta Physiologica Scandinavica, 149*, 199–204.

Van Honk, J., Schutter, D. J., Bos, P. A., Kruijt, A.-W., Lentjes, E. G., & Baron-Cohen, S. (2011). Testosterone administration impairs cognitive empathy in women depending on second-to-fourth digit ratio. *Proceedings of the National Academy of Sciences U S A, 108*, 3448–3452.

von Dawans, B., Fischbacher, U., Kirschbaum, C., Fehr, E., & Heinrichs, M. (2012). The social dimension of stress reactivity acute stress increases prosocial behavior in humans. *Psychological Science, 23*, 651–660.

Wang, Z., Ferris, C. F., & De Vries, G. J. (1994). Role of septal vasopressin innervation in paternal behavior in prairie voles (Microtus ochrogaster). *Proceedings of the National Academy of Sciences U S A, 91*, 400–404.

Watanabe, S. (2014). The dominant/subordinate relationship between mice modifies the approach behavior toward a cage mate experiencing pain. *Behavioural Processes, 103*, 1–4.

Way, B. M., Taylor, S. E., & Eisenberger, N. I. (2009). Variation in the μ-opioid receptor gene (OPRM1) is associated with dispositional and neural sensitivity to social rejection. *Proceedings of the National Academy of Sciences U S A, 106*, 15079–15084.

Weitoft, G. R., Hjern, A., Haglund, B., & Rosén, M. (2003). Mortality, severe morbidity, and injury in children living with single parents in Sweden: A population-based study. *The Lancet, 361*, 289–295.

Williams, A. C. d. C., Gallagher, E., Fidalgo, A. R., & Bentley, P. J. (2016). Pain expressiveness and altruistic behavior: An exploration using agent-based modeling. *Pain, 157*, 759.

Wilson, M. L., & Wrangham, R. W. (2003). Intergroup relations in chimpanzees. *Annual Review of Anthropology, 32*, 363–392.

Winslow, J. T., Hastings, N., Carter, C. S., Harbaugh, C. R., & Insel, T. R. (1993). A role for central vasopressin in pair bonding in monogamous prairie voles. *Nature, 365*, 545.

Xu, X., Zuo, X., Wang, X., & Han, S. (2009). Do you feel my pain? Racial group membership modulates empathic neural responses. *Journal of Neuroscience, 29*, 8525–8529.

Part IV
Effects of Facing Others in Pain

Chapter 11
The Spectrum of Third-Person Pain: From Observation to Action

Kenneth M. Prkachin, M. Erin Browne, and Kimberley A. Kaseweter

Abstract Third-person pain refers to the components and processes engaged when an observer is confronted by another person in pain. The literature that has arisen around this topic has approached it from diverse perspectives, including behavioral theory, social perception, affective science, psychophysiology, social neuroscience, evolutionary psychology, and clinical theory. This chapter begins with a review of the behavioral stimuli to third-person pain and then proceeds to a review of major findings and concepts in the field, organized around a component framework. The components include central nervous responses, autonomic and somatomotor responses, implicit and effortful perceptual and emotional processes, and overt behavior. Core findings and concepts linked to these third-person pain components are reviewed, methodological issues are discussed and areas for future research identified. The vast bulk of literature addressing third-person pain has emphasized prosocial features of the phenomenon. That people do not always respond to others' pain with empathy and helping is emphasized and areas for research into malignant third-person pain reactions are identified.

Keywords Pain · Interpersonal communication · Perception · Empathic response · Social behavior

Gary, a 42-year-old, worked at a tire center. While installing winter tires, he turned to lift one on to the mounting studs but dropped it after suffering a sharp jolt of pain in his lower back. Falling to his knees, he cried out in pain. Coworkers who responded to his cry helped him to a chair in the customer waiting area, where he

K. M. Prkachin (✉)
Department of Psychology, University of Northern British Columbia,
Prince George, BC, Canada
e-mail: Ken.Prkachin@unbc.ca

M. Erin Browne
University of Regina, Regina, SK, Canada

K. A. Kaseweter
University of British Columbia, Okanagan Campus, Kelowna, BC, Canada

© Springer International Publishing AG, part of Springer Nature 2018
T. Vervoort et al. (eds.), *Social and Interpersonal Dynamics in Pain*,
https://doi.org/10.1007/978-3-319-78340-6_11

suffered until his wife came to take him home. Retreating to bed to wait for the pain to subside, Gary experienced a restless night and difficulty getting out of bed the following morning. He was able to get an appointment with his family doctor, who ordered x-rays and wrote a prescription for acetaminophen with codeine. Over the following week the pain diminished and he could move a bit more fluidly. When he returned to work the next week, however, he lasted only until he attempted to lift a tire. He returned to his doctor who declared that he must take 2 weeks off from work. Because the event precipitating Gary's difficulties occurred in the workplace, his doctor completed forms entering him into the workers' compensation system. During his trajectory through that system, Gary volunteered for a research study involving a standardized orthopedic examination. One part required him to walk from an examination table across a room—normally at first, then on his heels, then his toes. A video of that test is remarkable for the behavior Gary displays. He moves tentatively and awkwardly, favoring the affected side of his body. Deep inspirations of air and other paraverbal sounds accompany the limited words he uses to describe his discomfort. With every step, his face is a picture of agony.

One of the authors shows this video of Gary during lectures about pain behaviors. The audiences vary, as do people's reactions to Gary. In some, people are visibly uncomfortable as they watch. Deep sympathy is frequently expressed. Other audiences—especially health-care workers—focus on technical aspects, offering explanations of what may be going on or asking questions about his history and the testing context. Others raise objections or express skepticism. One psychologist who viewed the recording summed up his reaction by saying, "that guy's so full of shit."

This range of reactions to Gary's behavior illustrates two salient facts. First, the experience of pain is often accompanied by distinct changes in behavior, based upon which others perceive and draw inferences about the internal experience of the sufferer. Second, the reactions of others are not uniform. Some are drawn toward behaviors that would be considered prosocial, such as expressions of concern and offers of assistance; some become analytic; some may become hostile and rejecting. Nor is this the gamut of possible reactions to others in pain. In the natural environment, some people may not even notice; others may notice but ignore them. This chapter reviews research and theory into the responses of observers to others in pain—what we have termed "third person" responses to pain (Prkachin, Kaseweter, & Browne, 2015). Episodes of pain commonly occur in the presence of others and in broader social contexts of parenting, health care, sports, political conflict, war, and so on. The sufferer's experience is often registered in behaviors that "broadcast" into a social surround in which others perceive, evaluate, and respond to the sufferer according to an Experience → Encoding → Decoding sequence (Prkachin & Craig, 1994), which then determines subsequent actions on the part of others (Prkachin et al., 2015). The sufferer-observer nexus is transactional: properties of the transaction have an impact on the present and future psychological functioning of the sufferer. Our goal in this chapter is to provide a general framework from which to conceptualize the transactions that take place when someone observes someone else suffering from pain, and when the observer takes action.

The Bases of Third-Person Responses to Pain Before we consider the responses to others' pain, we must first devote some attention to the determinants of those responses. It is axiomatic that we cannot observe another's pain directly. For an observer to respond to someone in pain, he or she must first perceive that the other person is in pain. Evidence that pain is present can derive from observation of distinct natural events such as when a child falls in the street, skinning her knee, or observing an accident or broken limb. In this case, the observer knows or suspects that the person observed is in pain because she knows, based on personal experience and collective understanding, that similar events routinely provoke pain. Third-person pain perception can also derive from information available contextually, such as might occur when a health-care worker reviews a clinical history or the results of laboratory testing showing a kidney stone or ovarian cyst. Although there is an emerging literature that investigates people's responses to natural events involving explicit injury, we are concerned here primarily with responses to behavioral evidence of pain and so it is necessary first to describe and characterize those.

The concept of pain behavior refers to the wide range of things that people can be observed to do when in pain. Revicki et al. (2009) identified 39 specific acts or dispositions, such as irritability, guarded movement or posture, behavioral withdrawal and so on, that people report displaying when they are in pain and this survey did not even include such observable changes as shaking, perspiration, flushing or blushing. These behaviors are adapted to serve several functions (see also, Chap. 5). Some, such as withdrawal from an acute source of pain, terminate or limit tissue damage and promote safety. Some, such as rubbing the affected region, have direct antinociceptive effects, serving to diminish the sensory or affective components of pain. Some, such as social withdrawal and diminished activity, promote healing (Wall, 1979). As Darwin (1955/1872) observed, some, such as perspiring or blanching are indirect consequences of physiological homeostatic processes activated to diminish pain or to subserve efforts to seek safety. Some, such as facial expressions, moaning, and crying do not seem to play a direct role in managing the injury, experience or healing. Rather, they appear to be adapted for communicating to others something about the current state and likely future behavior of the individual (Fridlund, 1994; Prkachin, 1986). Humans also have the benefit of language, which allows relatively precise communication about pain qualities, such as location, temporal features, context, and history.

Of the range of behaviors that could form the basis for third-person perception of and reaction to pain, only self-reports and facial expressions have been employed extensively in empirical studies. Self-reports have been manipulated primarily in vignette studies. Such studies have ordinarily been concerned with documenting the ways in which contextual information about a pain sufferer, such as elements of their medical history or psychological make-up, influence third-person perceptions of the sufferer, including judgments of her pain and subsequent responses and are reviewed in Chap. 12. Much research on third-person reactions to pain has focused on facial expressions. Facial expressions have been of interest because they are ubiquitous and it is possible to obtain ecologically valid samples of them in experimental and natural settings with readily available video recording technology. A wealth of research has characterized the facial actions that occur when people are suffering pain (see Chap. 6). Although there is variation across studies in the facial actions that have been found to be empirically associated with pain, there is substantial agreement that a core set of facial actions involving brow lowering, tightening of the orbicularis oculi and levator labii muscles, and eye closure constitute a relatively discrete expression of pain that shows continuity from the neonatal period to older adulthood (Prkachin, 2009) and even continuity across species (Langford et al., 2010). For these reasons, the empirical research to be described in this chapter relies heavily on studies of the reactions of observers to the pain of others as represented in their facial expressions.

In thinking about responses to others in pain, it is helpful to consider different levels of observation and analysis. Confronted with evidence that someone else is hurting, an observer experiences effects that begin with the registration of that evidence and proceed toward some kind of behavioral response. The transaction does not necessarily end at that point because the observer's behavioral response may have recursive effects on the sufferer. Along the way, an observer's reactions can be assessed at multiple levels, including the central nervous system, the autonomic nervous system, the somatic-motor system, perceptual/interpretive reactions that are more-or-less automatic, perceptual/interpretive reactions that employ more in the way of effortful cognitive resources and, finally, overt behavioral reactions (or proxies to them). Reactions to others in pain have been studied at each of these levels. Historically, research on reactions to others in pain began with studies of autonomic and perceptual/interpretive reactions. Technological and other methodological advances enabled access to a fuller range of phenomena across this continuum. For heuristic purposes, we find it helpful to begin by looking at central nervous responses, proceeding along the continuum to overt behavior.

Central Nervous Responses to Others in Pain Advances in technology that enable observation of dynamic changes in neural activity, such as functional magnetic resonance imaging (fMRI), began to be applied to investigations of the response to others in pain around the turn of the twenty-first century. Such studies expose observers to stimuli depicting another person in pain, while measuring changes in metabolic activity across the whole brain. The stimuli depicting pain vary from study to study. In some, participants observe photographs of people who appear to be about to suffer some kind of painful event, such as crushing a finger in a closing door. In others, participants are shown ecological videos of the facial expressions of people who are known, by independent criteria, to be experiencing pain or of people sustaining actual physical injuries. In yet others, participants are shown videos of actors attempting to represent pain by their facial expressions.

In the earliest study, Singer et al. (2004) performed fMRI while exposing spouses to painful stimulation to the hand. Female members of the dyads also viewed their spouses being exposed to painful and nonpainful stimulation. Observing her partner receiving pain was associated with increased activity in anterior cingulate cortex (ACC) and anterior insula, bilaterally, paralleling activation in the same regions when experiencing pain directly. Botvinick et al. (2005) also showed activation in anterior cingulate and insular cortex during first person pain and when participants observed *only the painful facial expressions* of patients undergoing a painful experience. This finding suggests that it is not necessary for observers to see evidence directly showing or indirectly implying painful injury. Simple exposure to a social signal correlated with the experience of pain is enough. In the years since these earliest studies, a substantial literature has established numerous ways in which first- and third-person pain are associated with activation of overlapping brain circuitry in what Tremblay, Meugnot, and Jackson (Chap. 8, this volume) refer to as a *shared representation network*. As reviewed in Chap. 8, subsequent work has shown that this network interacts with others involved in conscious cognitive processing and emotional self-regulation. Even given the substantial advances that have occurred in this field, our ability to account for the actual behavior of observers to pain based on the understanding of central nervous activity remains primitive.

Autonomic and Somatic-Motor Responses to Others in Pain

Autonomic Responses Well before advances in technology enabled more direct access to central-nervous processes, there was a body of research into the physiological correlates of observing pain in others based on autonomic and somatomotor responses evaluated by peripheral psychophysiological measures. In an early study, Craig (1968) exposed participants to direct, imagined, and vicarious experiences of cold pain. Skin conductance (SC) and heart rate (HR) were measured while participants experienced or imagined cold pressor pain or observed a confederate immerse his arm in ice water. Exposure to vicarious pain produced SC increases but not to the same extent as direct or imaginal exposure. Vicarious pain was also associated with a qualitatively distinct HR deceleration unlike the acceleration associated with direct and imaginal exposure. Although participants ostensibly observed the confederate experiencing pain, it is not clear that the confederate actually displayed pain-related behavior so the relation between the autonomic effects obtained and pain-related behavior is unclear. In a later study, participants observed a confederate ostensibly receiving electric shock (Craig & Lowery, 1969). The confederate moved his arm in a manner consistent with having received a shock. Results from this study were similar, indicating that observing someone *responding* to the pain of electric shock was associated with elevated SC and HR deceleration compared with observing no pain or movement.

Vaughan and Lanzetta (1980) examined autonomic and somatomotor responses of observers to facial expressions of pain. In two studies, observers' SC was measured while they watched a male confederate on a series of trials. On half, the confederate posed a facial expression of pain. Exposure to the confederate's pain expression was associated with sharply elevated SC responses. Altogether, the findings indicated that exposure to another's pain expression instigates acute and relatively stable increases in SC, reflecting sympathetic nervous system arousal.

Block (1981) showed the spouses of chronic pain patients video of the facial expressions of their partners and unrelated others taken during painful and neutral conditions. Videos depicting pain were associated with SC responses of greater magnitude than neutral videos. Individual differences in marital satisfaction predicted SC responses such that spouses reporting better marital relationships also displayed higher SC responses to their spouses' pain behaviour.

There has been curiously little published work on autonomic responses to others since these early studies. In a recent exception, Fusaro, Tieri, and Aglioti (2016) measured SC while participants in a virtual reality environment observed an avatar being exposed to (a) a painful stimulus (penetration of the hand by a needle), (b) a stimulus for tactile pleasure (a caress) or (c) a neutral event. Viewing the avatar from a first-person perspective was associated with greater reported "ownership" of the affected hand than the third-person perspective. While the first-person perspective elicited greater SC responses than the third-person perspective when observing pain, the third-person perspective was still associated with responses that were higher than during exposure to neutral stimulation.

In general, the limited data on autonomic responding to others in pain indicates that SC, a measure determined exclusively by sympathetic drive, tends to increase when an observer perceives pain in another, suggesting that the detection of suffering is both personally salient and linked to stress-arousal. The findings suggest that, although personal experience of pain is most stressful, we nevertheless have an instinctive, automatic visceral response to others' pains, even when we know they are not real. Block's work implicates qualities of the relationship between the observer and the sufferer as potential determinants of individual differences in third-person reactions.

Somatomotor Responses In the studies of responses to pain in others by Vaughan and Lanzetta (1980), reported above, somatomotor measures of facial electromyographic (EMG) activity were also taken. EMG measures were taken from the orbicularis oculi (the region around the eyes), frontalis (the forehead), and masseter (jaw) muscles. Recordings from orbicularis oculi showed increased activity when observing pain, but only during early trials, suggesting a relatively rapid habituation of the unconditioned response. Recordings from frontalis and masseter muscles did not show reliable variation with pain conditions. Given that activation of orbicularis oculi is the action that is most reliably associated with pain (see Chap. 6), this suggests a general tendency toward mimicry when people observe others in pain.

It is also consistent with observations of apparent pain contagion—the tendency to automatically mimic, and synchronize facial expressions, vocalizations, postures and movements with another person and, consequently, to converge emotionally (Hatfield, Rapson, & Le, 2009, pp. 19–20). For example, newborn infants exposed to the cries of other infants in nursery settings are likely to cry themselves. When exposed to recordings of their own crying, or to cry-like sounds recorded from primates, they are not (Martin & Clark, 1982). There have been numerous demonstrations of contagion-like phenomena in studies of human responses to exposure to the emotional behavior of others. For example, when people are exposed to photographs depicting prototypic expressions of emotion, EMG recordings of their own facial responses demonstrate activation patterns that resemble those that produce the modeled expressions (Dimberg, 1990).

Altogether, the literature on autonomic and somatomotor responses suggests that observing others in pain activates automatic changes that mark the salience of suffering and may provide deeper insights into the processes evoked by third-person pain. With respect to the latter, the early findings that vicarious pain is associated with HR deceleration were linked to a broader literature on "attentional bradycardia," with implications for understanding empathy. Similarly, findings of pain mimicry suggest that third-person pain evokes behavioral resonance that is consistent with shared representation models of empathy (Preston, 2007; see also Chap. 8). Considering their potential to provide insight into important processes—in particular individual differences in responses to others pain arising from personality, psychopathology, and experiential differences—and their ready availability, it is curious that there has been a relative dearth of studies into the autonomic and somatomotor correlates of third-person pain.

Perceptual Processes

People naturally perceive pain in others when they observe pain-related behaviors such as facial expressions. The judgments of non-specialist observers shown recordings of pain expressions vary linearly, if suboptimally, with measured differences in the intensity of facial actions (Prkachin, Berzins, & Mercer, 1994). In studies of the ability to detect pain in others, it is often necessary to show subtle examples of pain expression or to significantly diminish viewing time because the use of strong or highly prototypic expressions often results in asymptotically high performance (Prkachin, Mass, & Mercer, 2004). Children as young as 5 years of age make reliable quantitative judgments about others' pain by observing differences in their facial expressions (Deyo, Prkachin, & Mercer, 2004). However, the ease with which observers make such judgments obscures complexities that have been discovered in the processes underlying perception of pain in others.

Preattentive Processing Vervoort, Trost, Prkachin, and Mueller (2013), for example, examined eye-tracking patterns among participants shown photographs of facial expressions of pain or neutral photographs. Participants were readily able to quantify differences in pain apparent in the pain faces. When viewing the photographs as pairs, participants in general tended to orient more quickly to pain than to neutral expressions. However, participants high in the trait of catastrophizing—the tendency to feel threatened and helpless in response to pain—were slower to fixate on pain expressions than low-catastrophizing participants, suggesting a tendency to avoid the threat properties of the pain expressions before being fully aware of what they represent—a preattentive process.

Chiesa, Liuzza, Acciarino, and Agliotti (2015) also reported that others' pain is processed subliminally. Participants were shown images of a neutral facial expression, an image depicting pain and another depicting pleasure. Painful images depicted a face displaying a pain expression being slapped, whereas pleasant images showed a face displaying a pleasant expression being caressed. In a subliminal condition, awareness of the target image was suppressed by presenting a flashing image to the contralateral eye. In a supraliminal condition, both eyes were presented with the respective image. Following presentation, participants rated the pleasantness of neutral Chinese pictographs. Participants in the subliminal condition could not identify the nature of the target stimuli to which they were exposed. Nevertheless, in both subliminal and supraliminal conditions, pictographs were evaluated as significantly less pleasant after exposure to pain images and more pleasant after priming with evidence of pleasure. Moreover, the degree of pleasantness was predicted by a measure of pupillary dilation when watching the pain images.

Similarly, Czekala, Mauguiere, Mazza, Jackson, and Frot (2015) exposed participants to still photographs of facial expressions in a combined backward-forward masking paradigm in which the target stimulus was embedded between expressions that had been averaged and therefore conveyed no clear facial expression. At critical presentation durations, this paradigm has been shown to block the ability to consciously identify the targeted visual stimulus. In one condition, participants' task was to identify a static facial feature: the model's sex. In the other, the task was to identify whether the target expression was of pain. At target presentation durations from 100 to 200 ms, pain expressions were detected more readily than sex. Participants could not, however, reliably indicate whether their decisions were correct, suggesting that they could not report consciously on their perceptual experience. Altogether, the findings complement those of Vervoort et al. and Chiesa et al., suggesting that information about others' pain is processed preattentively and, indeed, is given preferential processing access relative to other important features of faces, such as their sex.

Effortful Perceptual Processes These subtle, implicit processes ultimately converge in a conscious perceptual apprehension that another person is in pain. Third-person pain perception can be thought of as involving two components: a sensory element and an element that predisposes to action.

The sensory element is the simple registration of a conscious, quantitative experience--the perception that the sufferer is expressing pain of a certain intensity. This perception is influenced by two general factors: the objective intensity of the signal and the sensory sensitivity of the observer on the other. Bigger signals (such as those produced by very strong pain or as assessed by objective measurement techniques) will be perceived to be more intense than smaller signals. Observers vary in their acuity, which will also affect their ability to detect indications of third-person pain and the intensity of the perceptual experience.

The predisposition element refers to a host of variables that affect what the observer will do, based on the perceptual experience she has had. Such variables include both intrapersonal motivational states and proclivities and environmental contingencies. For example, think of the case of Gary. Everyone saw the same behavior, but some were more willing to see him as suffering than others, perhaps reflecting individual differences in prosocial traits or the need to be "hard-nosed" and objective.

Sensory and predisposition elements correspond generally to the distinctions that are made in signal detection theory (Swets, 1996) between detectability, discriminability and sensitivity, on the one hand, and decision criteria or response predisposition on the other. Methodologically, psychophysical techniques derived from sensory decision theory or magnitude estimation can be used to separate them.

In our studies, we have made use of variations on a Sensitivity to Expressions of Pain (STEP) test (Prkachin et al., 2004; Rash, Prkachin, & Campbell, 2014). In STEP tests, brief video clips of the facial expressions of patients with shoulder pain are shown. The expressions sampled typically fall into three categories: no pain, and two categories of increasing intensity. This allows comparison of perceptual parameters across a range of expressive intensities and relatively simple calculation of the discrimination of others' pain and of observers' tendencies to be liberal or conservative in imputing pain.

Sensitivity and response predispositions appear to be stable characteristics. For example, the average intercorrelation among measures of sensitivity taken from separate forms of a recent version of the STEP test was 0.57; the average intercorrelation of response predisposition was 0.74 (both $p < 0.001$). Response predisposition (the tendency to be either relatively liberal or conservative in imputing pain to others) was, in fact, significantly more stable than sensitivity.

Influences on the Sensory Component What are the variables that affect the sensory component? As would be expected, the magnitude of the sufferer's pain, as encoded in the behavioral signal, affects the discriminability of third-person pain, whether measured by signal-detection (Prkachin, 1992; Prkachin & Craig, 1985; Rash et al., 2014); or magnitude estimation techniques (Browne, Kaseweter, & Prkachin, 2017; Prkachin et al., 1994).

Relatively few variables have been found to further influence observers' sensitivity to evidence of others' pain. One study showed sex differences: female observers were better than males at detecting pain expressions of moderate intensity (Prkachin et al., 2004), consistent with an older, broader literature identifying a female advantage in decoding nonverbal expressions of affect (Hall, 1978). Similarly, as discussed in Chap. 12, De Ruddere et al. (2011) reported that, when observers found patients unlikeable, they discriminated their pain expressions more poorly than patients who were likeable and controls. This finding is particularly interesting because it suggests that the social impact of the sufferer, as appraised by the observer, can have an influence beyond a simple valuing or devaluing of the individual; that it can affect more fundamental ways in which observers process information relevant to the affective state of the sufferer.

A more characterological construct that has been related to processing of third-person pain is psychopathy—a set of affective and interpersonal traits manifested in a lack of empathy, guilt, callousness, and manipulation of others, among other characteristics. Kaseweter (2015) evaluated sensitivity to facial expressions of pain in a sample of observers who varied in psychopathic traits. Overall psychopathy scores, as measured by the Self-Report Psychopathy Scale (Paulhus, Neumann, & Hare, 2012) were negatively correlated with sensitivity to others' pain. Further analysis suggested that these negative relationships were primarily accounted for by the psychopathic trait of callousness. Similar findings have been reported by Caes et al. (2012). This finding is important as it relates to the fact that responses to others in pain are not uniform and may not be for different reasons. The psychopathic trait of callousness involves indifference to the suffering of others. Whereas much of the research on responses to others' pain implicitly views empathy and prosocial behavior as preeminent, as pointed out elsewhere in this volume (see Chap. 1), reactions to others' pain that are not prosocial not only occur but are in desperate need of further study. Why is it that some people may be highly reactive to, empathic with, and inclined to provide assistance while others may be indifferent or even enthusiastic about inflicting pain? Blair (1995) posited the existence of a violence inhibition mechanism to account for the callous indifference of people with psychopathic traits. According to this concept, agonistic behavior toward others is inhibited by cues to distress. Ordinarily, in agonistic or potentially agonistic dyadic interchanges, infliction of suffering is inhibited or terminated by cues of distress, among which are facial and other expressions of pain (Prkachin, 1992). Consistent with the violence inhibition mechanism hypothesis, the finding that psychopathic callousness is associated with diminished sensitivity to the pain of others identifies an important individual difference variable that goes some way toward accounting for divergence in third-person responses.

Influences on the predisposition to impute pain By contrast with the sensory component, a greater range of variables appear to influence the action component. The most frequently discussed is the so-called underestimation bias—the common finding that observers tasked with estimating the amount of pain experienced by another person tend to provide lower ratings than the sufferer him or herself (Prkachin, Solomon, & Ross, 2007). The simple finding that observers tend to underestimate the pain of others should not be surprising. Browne (2014) has even shown that when observers view *their own* facial expressions during a painful experience, they substantially underestimate their original pain ratings. Pain underestimation is at the heart of the problem of intersubjectivity—how could it be possible for me to know precisely what kind and how much pain you are experiencing, given that we are separate people with separate nervous systems?

More interesting are the systematic differences that have been identified in the tendency to impute pain to others. One of the earliest was the finding that different kinds of experience with the pain of others were associated with different degrees of underestimation. Observers with clinical expertise about pain showed an enhanced underestimation bias, relative to observers with no clinical experience with pain sufferers. By contrast, observers who had lived with a chronic pain sufferer also showed an underestimation effect, but it was diminished (Prkachin, Solomon, Hwang, & Mercer, 2001). These findings suggest that the effects of experience on third-person pain are not uniform—some kinds of experience may decrease the tendency to impute; others may increase it. Consistent experimental evidence shows that, other things being equal, simple repeated exposure to others' pain diminishes its imputation (Prkachin et al., 2004). Naïve observers attempted to distinguish between facial expressions of no pain and mild pain after being exposed to expressions of strong pain or a control condition. Exposure to expressions of strong pain diminished the likelihood of imputing pain to others without influencing observers' abilities to detect pain. Moreover, exposure exerted influence rapidly: viewing only one example of strong pain per trial was sufficient to demonstrate the effect. The exposure effect has been replicated (Grégoire, Coll, Tremblay, Prkachin, & Jackson, 2016; Prkachin & Rocha, 2010) and has been associated with a diminution of the central EEG evoked late positive potential response, suggesting that repeated exposure to pain diminishes the salience or motivational significance of pain expressions (Coll, Grégoire, Prkachin, & Jackson, 2016).

Other contextual and personological variables have been found to relate to pain imputation predispositions. Rash et al. (2014) evaluated third-person pain sensitivity and response predispositions as a function of anxious emotional traits, including trait anxiety and catastrophizing, using a variation of the STEP test. Neither variable related to sensitivity, but both were positively related to pain imputation predispositions. Higher trait anxiety and higher catastrophizing predicted predisposition to impute pain to others. The findings were similar to those of Sullivan, Martel, Tripp, Savard, and Crombez (2006), who employed a different method that does not separate sensitivity from response predisposition.

In summary, the existing literature demonstrates that third-person pain perception is a multidimensional process in which automatic/unconscious and deliberative processes combine in complex ways. These include preattentive, sensory, and predispositional components, whose individual determinants are complex and which set the stage for affective and behavioral responses that may or may not be prosocial.

Emotional Responses: Implicit and Explicit

As the case of Gary illustrates, reactions to others in pain are diverse. For a substantial number of people, evidence of his suffering automatically evokes emotions such as sadness and sympathy. Less common, but occasional automatic emotional reactions include disgust and contempt.

The study of pain expression has been central to the revivification of interest in empathy (see Tremblay et al., Chap. 8). Historically, empathy has been seen as both a cognitive and an emotional process, with cognitively oriented theorists focusing on its component of taking the perspective of the other and emotion-oriented theorists focusing on the component of sharing the emotions. A universally accepted definition of empathy is elusive; however, Preston and de Waal's (2002) definition as any process occurring when the perceived state of one person generates a state that is more applicable to the observed person than to the observer is sufficiently precise, but also sufficiently general to cover most examples that come to mind. In the context of third-person pain, Goubert et al. (2005) characterized empathy as "a sense of knowing the experience of another person with cognitive, affective and behavioural components." It is influenced from the "bottom up" by the observable expressive and instrumental behaviors of the sufferer and the context in which they occur and from the "top down" by characteristics of the observer, such as their past experiences, personal characteristics and so on. Preston and de Waal (2002) offered an account of the proximate mechanisms of empathy in a "perception-action" model (PAM). According to the PAM, when an observer detects the behavior of another person, the perception of that behavior simultaneously activates the observer's own "representation" of the same behavior. A representation is "a pattern of activation in the brain and the body corresponding to a particular state" (Preston, 2007, p. 430). In other words, when an observer perceives that another is in a particular state, such as pain, some component of the observer's own neuromotor-affective response when in that state is activated. Output from such representations "automatically proceeds to motor areas of the brain where supporting affective, physiological and behavioral responses are prepared" (Preston & de Waal, 2002, p. 10), and, unless they are actively inhibited, executed. The discovery of mirror neurons and human mirror neuron systems (Di Pellegrino, Fadiga, Fogassi, Gallese, & Rizzolatti, 1992; Iacoboni & Dapretto, 2006) has suggested one mechanism that could mediate such representations.

That personal experience of emotion can be induced implicitly by observing others in pain is suggested by the results of a recent study by De Coster, Verschuere, Goubert, Tsakiris, and Brass (2013). Participants watched videos showing hands ostensibly being injured in various ways. Similarity with the person whose hand was being observed was manipulated by programming the other's hand to imitate or not imitate the movements of the participant. Later, the videos were presented in a startle probe task in which electromyographic (EMG) recordings were made at the orbicularis oculi muscle when a loud sound was presented (the magnitude of the EMG response to the startle probe is a sensitive marker of negative affect). When the other's hand imitated the participant's hand, the participants rated the other's response to be more unpleasant and their own sensory intensity response to be greater than when imitation did not occur. Interestingly, the startle-probe EMG response was also significantly greater in the imitation condition, suggesting an implicit registration of third-person pain in the form of a personal sense of aversion. The results are consistent with the concept of an implicit empathic response based on a shared-representation mechanism.

Research on differential responses to others in pain among populations with special characteristics allows insights that may not be provided by other means. People with congenital insensitivity to pain (CIP) provide a unique opportunity to evaluate the role of the personal experience of pain in third-person pain. CIP results from an autonomic and sensory neuropathy affecting small nociceptive fibers, and results in a marked lifelong deficit in first-person pain. Danziger, Prkachin & Willer (2006) compared the responses of patients with CIP and healthy controls to depictions of painful injuries and facial expressions of pain. CIP patients tended to give lower ratings of the pain of others experiencing obvious injuries. Their performance identifying facial expressions of pain was indistinguishable from that of controls, indicating that, despite lacking normal personal pain perception, they were able to perceive third-person pain normally when exposed to behavioral evidence. Interestingly, among CIP patients, but not controls, the degree to which they imputed pain to others, whether depicted by evidence of injury or facial expressions, was highly correlated with scores on a self-report measure of emotional empathy (note that the tendency to impute pain is a response predisposition effect; patients and controls did not differ in their sensitivity to others' pain). The finding suggests that the development of emotional empathy may provide a kind of "intersubjective prosthetic," allowing people who recognize that their calibrations of others' experiences are off to recalibrate, and also implies that some components of empathy are effortful. The latter interpretation is also supported by a later fMRI study (Danziger, Faillenot, & Peyron, 2009), showing activation in anterior mid-cingulate cortex and anterior insula among CIP patients that was indistinguishable from controls'. Among CIP patients self-reported empathy was correlated with activity in the ventromedial prefrontal cortex when observing injuries and in the posterior cingulate cortex—regions that are thought to support more complex integration and abstraction processes—when observing facial expressions of pain.

Just as unique insight into the process of third-person pain may be achieved by investigation of people who have never experienced pain personally, studies of people who may experience personal pain when observing others in pain can be informative.

In recent years, interest has emerged in the possibility of pain synesthesia, another apparently automatic phenomenon. Synesthesia is generally defined as "… the elicitation of perceptual experiences in the absence of the normal sensory stimulation" ordinarily responsible for those experiences (Ward & Mattingley, 2006, p. 130); for example, hearing colors or experiencing letters as geometric shapes. Pain synesthesia is said to occur when individuals experience pain when they observe or learn about pain affecting others. Though rare, cases that appear to demonstrate pain synesthesia have been reported (see Fitzgibbon, Giummarra, Georgiou-Karistianis, & Bradshaw, 2010, for a review). They tend to occur in later life and to be acquired (Fitzgibbon et al. 2010). In their survey of 74 amputees with phantom-limb pain, 16% reported that they themselves experienced pain when observing or imagining pain in another person. Recent studies have reported prevalence rates in more representative samples ranging from 6.6% (Vandenbrouke et al., 2013) to 28.7% (Osborn & Derbyshire, 2010).

The variability in reports of its prevalence undoubtedly reflects the emerging nature of the concept coupled with the absence of a commonly accepted standard of assessment. Indeed, skepticism about the existence of the phenomenon is justified until such time as evidence accumulates supporting its validity. In one study supporting its validity, Osborn and Derbyshire (2010) identified a subgroup of people who reported an "actual somatic noxious experience" when they observed still pictures or videos of others experiencing injuries. In a later fMRI test these people showed activation of the anterior midcingulate cortex (aMCC), anterior insula, prefrontal cortex, and S1 and S2 regions. A comparison group of nonresponders showed activation only in aMCC, which was itself significantly lower than that observed among responders. The authors noted the similarity to patterns of CNS activation previously demonstrated to occur reliably in response to first-person pain (i.e., the so-called "pain matrix"); emphasizing, however, that the activation in S1 and S2 was consistent with sensory activation and supportive of the existence of a phenomenon of pain synesthesia.

Although the body of research is not yet sufficient to support pain synesthesia as a valid phenomenon, the available evidence does suggest that further validation studies would be worthwhile and hold promise to advance understanding of third-person pain.

Overt Behavioral Responses

Research on third-person pain has tended to focus on the perceptual and affective processes engaged when observers are confronted with another's pain, their personal and contextual determinants, and associated underlying CNS processes that have become accessible with modern technology. The main point of an approach informed by awareness that pain is a fundamentally social phenomenon is that, in the end, people respond to others in pain in various ways. Our concepts of the processes engaged in the witness to pain should allow us to say something meaningful about how others will actually behave and what the impact of different kinds of response may be for the sufferer in the short- and the long-term.

The specific behavioral changes executed in the context of third person pain are not uniform. As Goubert et al. (2005) have pointed out, the observer's reaction may resemble the sufferer's, but it may differ, depending on characteristics of the observer. In particular, the empathic process may trigger self-oriented personal distress, other-oriented sympathy, or some blend. Aroused self-oriented and other-oriented processes have quite different implications for the subsequent behavior of the observer (see Chap. 4). For example, a self-oriented reaction is likely to elicit behavior aimed toward diminishing personal distress, which may not be particularly helpful to the sufferer or appear altruistic.

Research that would allow more comprehensive and definitive conclusions about specific behavioral responses to others' pain and their consequences has been limited. An exception is the extensive literature that has developed in the study of pediatric pain (see Chaps. 3, 14, 17, and 18), where a focus on the child–caretaker dyad provides a natural and accessible crucible for evaluating the influence of caretaker characteristics on overt responses to the child in pain and of the influence of variations in those responses on the child's behavior and outcomes. Similarly, research on the influence of different styles of emotional communication among couples where one spouse has pain (see Chaps. 13, 16, and 19) has permitted some conclusions to be drawn about the effects of different communication styles on the sufferer. The conclusions must be much more tentative because of the lesser ability to perform true experiments or directly measure behavioral outcomes, in comparison with pediatric studies.

Much of the interest in third-person pain has been driven by its relevance to issues that arise in clinical practice with people in pain. Awareness that pain is inadequately treated in several populations, including children, people with communication disorders and the elderly has raised questions whether the problem lies in insensitivity or indifference to evidence of suffering. Major disparities have been documented in the aggressiveness with which pain is treated as a consequence of the sufferer's sex, racial or ethnic background (Chaps. 20 and 21). Patients who suffer from chronic pain conditions routinely describe how their suffering is ignored, diminished, or denied, and they are met with responses ranging from patronizing to open contempt and hostility. For their part, clinicians who deal with pain sufferers can find theory and evidence that justify seemingly incompatible principles to guide their own behavior in the presence of pain sufferers. Moreover, they are not insensitive to the impact that the routine exposure to the suffering of others may have on their own psychological well-being and behavior.

With respect to this broader issue of what the impact of third-person pain processes have on the actual behavior of the observer, however, the conclusions that we can draw have been largely limited by the practical difficulties associated with performing realistic, in-vivo tests, in which the actual behavior of the observer as well as the short- and long-term impact on the sufferer is measured. To some extent, vignette studies and proxy measures can provide guidance and educated suggestions. For example, Lundquist, Higgins, and Prkachin (2002) showed observers recordings of the behavior of shoulder pain patients displaying low, moderate, and high levels of pain expression under various conditions designed to influence the attributions the observers would make about the causes of pain. Observers were asked to recommend one of two possible choices for treatment, characterized as equally effective, but one being more unpleasant than the other. Observers with an unsupportive attributional style—a tendency to view negative outcomes as controllable—were more likely to recommend the unpleasant treatment when the patient was characterized as not coping well. Similarly, De Ruddere et al. (2011) showed observers video recordings of shoulder pain patients in the context of backstories indicating that there was or was not medical evidence and psychosocial evidence for their pain. The results showed that in the absence of medical evidence for their pain, observers were less inclined to say they would offer help.

The particular issue of racial disparities in pain treatment was examined by Drwecki, Moore, Ward, and Prkachin (2011), who showed undergraduates videos of dark-skinned and light-skinned patients displaying pain expressions of the same intensity. Patients with darker skin color were offered less aggressive treatment than those with lighter skin color and the aggressiveness of treatment offered was mediated by measures of the participants' empathy for the patients. In a second study, they found that the racial bias in treatment aggressiveness was effectively eliminated by a brief perspective-taking intervention that reduced the racial disparity in empathy.

These findings imply that the evaluations observers make about the determinants of a sufferer's pain could have an impact on important decisions made about how to manage that pain, to the good or the detriment of the sufferer. Although they accord reasonably with common sense and common accounts of the experience of pain patients, the implication must be tempered by the fact that the outcomes measured were not actual decisions about treatment by a person in a position to make a recommendation. This highlights the artificial nature of the methodology, but points to the kinds of real-life scenarios that need to be modeled and challenge the creativity of researchers to find paradigms to support more realistic modeling.

One example of a paradigm that goes beyond self-report and comes closer to modeling actual clinical scenarios was employed by Coll, Grégoire, Eugène, and Jackson (2017). Health-care providers and controls without experience with pain completed a measure of emotional empathy. They were then shown photographs of the pain expressions of pain patients drawn from the UNBC-McMaster archive (Prkachin & Solomon, 2008). Participants were shown the peak-pain expression and required to decide how much help they would offer, understanding that the more help they gave, the more the patient's pain would be reduced. Offering help came at a price—it would increase their workload and actually lengthen the time of the experimental task. Results showed that the more personal distress the observers reported to the suffering of others the less willing they were to help. Health-care providers, who reported significantly less personal distress than controls, offered more help on this behavioral task with real (though limited) personal costs.

Pain expression and the ability to perceive pain in others coevolved in a social context. Although much current thought about the implications of third-person pain processes focuses on pain as it occurs in a clinical context, it warrants emphasis that there are other important settings in which people are hurt and others are present where an understanding of the processes of third person pain are likely to have implications for the behavior of the observer and the outcome for the pain sufferer. These include settings such as childrearing, sport, criminal justice, and situations that arise in military and security contexts.

Whereas it is customary to think that the natural response to the suffering of others is the motivation of prosocial helping behavior there are times when the response of the observer is anything but helpful or prosocial. Deliberate infliction of pain on others is a common theme in human history. Undoubtedly, it is less a feature of contemporary society than it has been historically (Pinker, 2011); nevertheless, the field of criminal justice exists in part to deal with the fact that some people hurt others deliberately or through indifference. Moreover, the persistence of barbaric acts and revival of torture in the twenty-first century (O'Mara, 2015) and support for it among significant segments of the population indicates that there are some who are inured to suffering and indeed there are others who seem to relish in it.

What distinguishes those for whom exposure to the suffering of others is a matter of indifference and even pleasure from those for whom it elicits responses consistent with "other-oriented" responses of sympathy and approach or "self-oriented" responses of distress and avoidance described by Goubert et al. (2005)? What can the study of third-person pain tell us about how to identify them and what to do? One suggestion comes from the finding that people with antisocial traits of callousness appear to be deficient at detecting evidence of pain in others (Caes et al., 2012; Kaseweter, 2015). If the proclivity toward inflicting harm on others is ordinarily inhibited by signals of distress, as implied by the Violence Inhibition Mechanism hypothesis and numerous observations in ethology, then the behavior of individuals lacking the ability to detect those signs would lack a natural shut-off mechanism. If true, then, based on evidence that sensitivity to pain in others can be assessed as early as middle childhood it is conceivable that assessment tools could be developed and employed for early identification of those tendencies, with potential implication for early identification or counseling.

Conclusion

As the subtitle to this book emphasizes, we don't suffer alone. Along with the ability to communicate features of our internal experiences of pain by way of adapted behavioral signals, evolution has conferred the ability to be personally affected by those signals in a variety of ways that have impact on our own behavior and, by way of reciprocal effects, on the behavior and experience of the sufferer. Research into the processes of third-person pain has identified central nervous, autonomic, somatomotor, perceptual and affective processes to the extent that we presently have a reasonable idea of the general processes involved when an observer is exposed to another person in pain. Our ability to predict the outcome of those processes, in terms of the actual behavior likely to be engaged in when an observer apprehends that someone else is in pain lags behind our understanding of the general processes, in part because of the limited development of ecologically valid tests and realistic proxies of those behaviors, but also, in part, because the requisite studies have not been performed. Returning to Gary and the kinds of reactions that observers have to his display, what are the behaviors likely to follow on the part of those who experience personal distress from seeing him as opposed to those who are dismissive of his display (or those, yet to be observed, who enjoy his display of suffering), and what are the likely effects on his future experience and behavior?

References

Blair, R. J. R. (1995). A cognitive developmental approach to morality: Investigating the psychopath. *Cognition, 57*, 1–29.
Block, A. (1981). An investigation of the response of the spouse to chronic pain behavior. *Psychosomatic Medicine, 43*, 415–422.

Botvinick, M., Jha, A. P., Bylsma, L. M., Fabian, S. A., Solomon, P. E., & Prkachin, K. M. (2005). Viewing facial expressions of pain engages cortical areas involved in the direct experience of pain. *NeuroImage, 25*, 312–319.

Browne, M. E. (2014). *Self-perception of affect expression*. M.Sc. thesis, University of Northern British Columbia.

Browne, M. E., Kaseweter, K. A., & Prkachin, K. M. (2017). *Nonverbal expression and self-perception of pain: The influence of catastrophizing, alexithymia and personal experience* (Unpublished manuscript).

Caes, L., Uzieblo, K., Crombez, G., De Ruddere, L., Vervoort, T., & Goubert, L. (2012). Negative emotional responses elicited by the anticipation of pain in others: Psychophysiological evidence. *Journal of Pain, 13*, 467–476.

Chiesa, P. A., Liuzza, M. T., Acciarino, A., & Agliotti, S. M. (2015). Subliminal perception of others' physical pain and pleasure. *Experimental Brain Research, 233*, 2373–2382. https://doi.org/10.1007/s00221-015-4307-8

Coll, M.-P., Grégoire, M., Eugène, F., & Jackson, P. L. (2017). Neural correlates of prosocial behavior towards persons in pain in healthcare providers. *Biological Psychology, 128*, 1–10.

Coll, M.-P., Grégoire, M., Prkachin, K. M., & Jackson, P. L. (2016). Repeated exposure to vicarious pain alters electrocortical processing of pain expressions. *Experimental Brain Research*. https://doi.org/10.1007/s00221-016-4671-z

Craig, K. D. (1968). Physiological arousal as a function of imagined, vicarious, and direct stress experiences. *Journal of Abnormal Psychology, 73*, 513–520.

Craig, K. D., & Lowery, H. J. (1969). Heart-rate components of conditioned vicarious autonomic responses. *Journal of Personality and Social Psychology, 11*, 381–387.

Czekala, C., Mauguiere, F., Mazza, S., Jackson, P. L., & Frot, M. (2015). My brain reads pain in your face, before knowing your gender. *Journal of Pain, 16*, 1242–1352. https://doi.org/10.1016/j.pain.2015.09.006

Danziger, N., Faillenot, I., & Peyron, R. (2009). Can we share a pain we never felt? Neural correlates of empathy in patients with congenital insensitivity to pain. *Neuron, 61*, 203–212. https://doi.org/10.1016/j.neuron.2008.11.023

Danziger, N., Prkachin, K. M., & Willer, J.-C. (2006). Is pain the price to pay to feel empathy? *Brain, 129*, 2494–2507.

Darwin, C. (1955). *The expression of the emotions in man and animals*. New York, NY: Philosophical Library. (Originally published in 1872).

De Coster, L., Verschuere, B., Goubert, L., Tsakiris, M., & Brass, M. (2013). I suffer more from your pain when you act like me: Being imitated enhances affective responses to seeing someone else in pain. *Cognitive Affective and Behavioral Neuroscience, 13*, 519–532. https://doi.org/10.3758/s13415-013-0168-4

De Ruddere, L., Goubert, L., Prkachin, K. M., Stevens, M. A. L., Van Ryckeghem, D. M. L., & Crombez, G. (2011). When you dislike patients, pain is taken less seriously. *Pain, 152*, 2342–2347.

Deyo, K., Prkachin, K. M., & Mercer, S. R. (2004). Development of sensitivity to facial expressions of pain. *Pain, 107*, 16–21.

Di Pellegrino, G., Fadiga, L., Fogassi, L., Gallese, V., & Rizzolatti, G. (1992). Understanding motor events: A neurophysiological study. *Experimental Brain Research, 91*, 176–180.

Dimberg, U. (1990). Facial electromyography and emotional reactions. *Psychophysiology, 27*, 481–494.

Drwecki, B. B., Moore, C. F., Ward, S. E., & Prkachin, K. M. (2011). Reducing racial disparities in pain treatment: The role of empathy and perspective-taking. *Pain, 152*, 1001–1006.

Fitzgibbon, B. M., Enticott, P. G., Rich, A. N., Giummarra, M. J., Georgiou-Karistianis, N., Tsao, J. W., … Bradshaw, J. L. (2010). High incidence of 'synaesthesia for pain' in amputees. *Neuropsychologia, 48*, 3675–3678.

Fitzgibbon, B. M., Giummarra, M. J., Georgiou-Karistianis, N., Enticott, P. G., & Bradshaw, J. L. (2010). Shared pain: From empathy to synaesthesia. *Neuroscience and Biobehavioral Reviews, 34*, 500–512.

Fridlund, A. J. (1994). *Human facial expression: An evolutionary view.* San Diego, CA: Academic Press.

Fusaro, M., Tieri, G., & Aglioti, S. M. (2016). Seeing pain and pleasure on self and others: Behavioral and psychophysiological reactivity in immersive virtual reality. *Journal of Neurophysiology, 116*, 2656–2662. https://doi.org/10.1152/jn.00489.2016

Goubert, L., Craig, K. D., Vervoort, T., Morley, S., Sullivan, M. J. L., Williams, A. C. d. C., … Crombez, G. (2005). Facing others in pain: The effects of empathy. *Pain, 118*, 285–288.

Grégoire, M., Coll, M.-P., Tremblay, M. P. B., Prkachin, K. M., & Jackson, P. L. (2016). Repeated exposure to others' pain reduces vicarious pain intensity estimation. *European Journal of Pain.* https://doi.org/10.1002/ejp.888

Hall, J. A. (1978). Gender effects in decoding nonverbal cues. *Psychological Bulletin, 85*, 845–857.

Hatfield, E., Rapson, R. L., & Le, Y. L. (2009). Emotional contagion and empathy. In J. Decety & W. Ickes (Eds.), *The social neuroscience of empathy* (pp. 19–30). Boston, MA: MIT Press.

Iacoboni, M., & Dapretto, M. (2006). The mirror neuron system and the consequences of its dysfunction. *Nature Reviews Neuroscience, 7*, 942–951.

Kaseweter, K. A. (2015). *Insensitivity to suffering.* M.Sc. thesis, University of Northern British Columbia.

Langford, D. J., Bailey, A. L., Chanda, M. L., Clarke, S. E., Drummond, T. E., Echols, S., … Mogil, J. S. (2010). Coding of facial expressions of pain in the laboratory mouse. *Nature Methods, 7*, 447–449.

Lundquist, L. M., Higgins, N. C., & Prkachin, K. M. (2002). Accurate pain detection is not enough: Contextual and attributional style biasing factors in patient evaluation and treatment choice. *Journal of Applied Biobehavioral Research, 7*, 114–132.

Martin, G. B., & Clark, R. D. (1982). Distress crying in neonates: Species and peer specificity. *Developmental Psychology, 18*, 3–9.

O'Mara, S. (2015). *Why torture doesn't work. The neuroscience of interrogation.* Cambridge, MA: Harvard University Press.

Osborn, J., & Derbyshire, S. W. G. (2010). Pain sensation evoked by observing injury in others. *Pain, 148*, 268–274.

Paulhus, D. L., Neumann, C. S., & Hare, R. D. (2012). *Manual for the self-report psychopathy (SRP) scale.* Toronto, ON: Multi-Health Systems.

Pinker, S. (2011). *The better angels of our nature. Why violence has declined.* New York, NY: Penguin.

Preston, S. D. (2007). A perception-action model for empathy. In T. Farrow & P. Woodruff (Eds.), *Empathy in mental illness* (pp. 428–447). New York, NY: Cambridge University Press.

Preston, S. D., & de Waal, F. B. M. (2002). Empathy: Its ultimate and proximate bases. *Behavioral and Brain Sciences, 25*, 1–72.

Prkachin, K. M. (1986). Pain behavior is not unitary. *Behavioral and Brain Sciences, 9*, 754–755.

Prkachin, K. M. (1992). Dissociating deliberate and spontaneous expressions of pain. *Pain, 51*, 57–65.

Prkachin, K. M. (2009). Assessing pain by facial expression: Facial expression as nexus. *Pain Research and Management, 14*, 53–58.

Prkachin, K. M., Berzins, S., & Mercer, S. (1994). Encoding and decoding of pain expressions: A judgement study. *Pain, 58*, 253–259.

Prkachin, K. M., & Craig, K. D. (1985). Influencing nonverbal expressions of pain: Signal detection analyses. *Pain, 21*, 399–409.

Prkachin, K. M., & Craig, K. D. (1994). Expressing pain: The communication and interpretation of facial pain signals. *Journal of Nonverbal Behavior, 19*, 191–205.

Prkachin, K. M., Kaseweter, K. A., & Browne, M. E. (2015). Understanding the suffering of others: The sources and consequences of third-person pain. In G. Pickering & S. Gibson (Eds.), *Pain, emotion and cognition: A complex nexus* (pp. 53–72). New York, NY: Springer.

Prkachin, K. M., Mass, H., & Mercer, S. R. (2004). Effects of exposure on perception of pain expression. *Pain, 111*, 8–12.

Prkachin, K. M., & Rocha, E. M. (2010). High levels of vicarious exposure bias pain judgements. *Journal of Pain, 11*, 904–909.

Prkachin, K. M., Solomon, P., Hwang, T., & Mercer, S. R. (2001). Does experience affect judgements of pain behaviour? Evidence from relatives of pain patients and health-care providers. *Pain Research and Management, 6*, 105–112.

Prkachin, K. M., Solomon, P. A., & Ross, A. J. (2007). The underestimation of pain among health-care providers. *Canadian Journal of Nursing Research, 39*, 88–106.

Prkachin, K. M., & Solomon, P. E. (2008). The structure, reliability and validity of pain expression: Evidence from patients with shoulder pain. *Pain, 139*, 267–274.

Rash, J. A., Prkachin, K. M., & Campbell, T. S. (2014). Observer trait anxiety is associated with response predisposition to patient facial pain expression independent of pain catastrophizing. *Pain Research and Management, 20*, 39–45.

Revicki, D. A., Chen, W.-H., Harnam, N., Cook, K. G., Amtmann, D., Callahan, L. G., … Keefe, F. J. (2009). Development and psychometric analysis of the PROMIS pain behavior item bank. *Pain, 146*, 158–169.

Singer, T., Seymour, B., O'Doherty, J., Kaube, H., Dolan, R. J., & Frith, C. D. (2004). Empathy for pain involves the affective but not sensory components of pain. *Science, 303*, 1157–1162.

Sullivan, M. J. L., Martel, M. O., Tripp, D. A., Savard, A., & Crombez, G. (2006). Catastrophic thinking and heightened perception of pain in others. *Pain, 123*, 37–44.

Swets, J. A. (1996). *Signal detection theory and ROC analysis in psychology and diagnosis: Collected papers*. Mahwah, NJ: Lawrence Erlbaum Associates.

Vandenbrouke, S., Crombez, G., Van Ryckeghem, D. M. L., Brass, M., Van Damme, S., & Goubert, L. (2013). Vicarious pain while observing another in pain: An experimental approach. *Frontiers in Human Neuroscience, 7*(Article 265), 1–13. https://doi.org/10.3389/fnhum.2013.00265

Vaughan, K. B., & Lanzetta, J. T. (1980). Vicarious instigation and conditioning of facial expressive and autonomic responses to a model's expressive display of pain. *Journal of Personality and Social Psychology, 38*, 909–923.

Vervoort, T., Trost, Z., Prkachin, K., & Mueller, S. C. (2013). Attentional processing of other's facial display of pain: An eye tracking study. *Pain, 154*, 836–844.

Wall, P. A. (1979). On the relation of injury to pain: The John J. Bonica lecture. *Pain, 6*, 253–264.

Ward, J., & Mattingley, J. B. (2006). Synaesthesia: An overview of contemporary findings and controversies. *Cortex, 42*, 129–136.

Chapter 12
Facing Others in Pain: Why Context Matters

Lies De Ruddere and Raymond Tait

Abstract Judging pain in another is challenging, largely because pain is a subjective phenomenon to which observers have no direct access. Despite this ambiguity, inferences often are made that can drive important clinical decisions, such as estimating another's pain intensity, with significant implications for patient treatment and outcomes. This chapter focuses upon the influence of the context upon observer cognitive, emotional, and behavioral responses toward others in pain. In doing so, we consider context in its broadest form: characteristics of the patient/person in pain, the observer, and the situation, as well as elements of the reported pain experience, itself. Despite the increased understanding of and appreciation for the role of context in observer judgments, knowledge of how context, judgment, and treatment outcomes interact remains sketchy and in need of translational research. Such research is needed if we are to build our current base of knowledge and translate that knowledge into improved approaches to the assessment and treatment of patients in pain.

Keywords Pain · Observer responses · Context influences · Patient characteristics · Observer characteristics · Situational factors · Pain experience

Introduction

> To have great pain is to have certainty, to hear that another person has pain, is to have doubt. (Scarry, 1985, pp. 6–7)

L. De Ruddere (✉)
Department of Experimental-Clinical and Health Psychology, Ghent University,
Ghent, Belgium
e-mail: Lies.DeRuddere@Ugent.be

R. Tait
Department of Psychiatry and Behavioral Neuroscience, Saint Louis University School of Medicine, St. Louis, MO, USA

© Springer International Publishing AG, part of Springer Nature 2018   241
T. Vervoort et al. (eds.), *Social and Interpersonal Dynamics in Pain*,
https://doi.org/10.1007/978-3-319-78340-6_12

Cognitive, Affective, and Behavioral Responses of Observers Toward Others in Pain

It is a good thing that we, social beings, generally do not suffer in silence. When we experience that unpleasant and distressing phenomenon that we call pain, we are lucky if we are surrounded by supportive caregivers, relatives, friends, and/or colleagues. Consider, for example, a situation in which you cut your finger with a knife while preparing food at home. It is very likely that the other people in your house will respond solicitously. Your partner could react with some "pain talk" like "that must have hurt!" Your children could offer some help, e.g., by providing a plaster/band-aid; or your father or mother could offer a seat if you feel lightheaded.

Although we might think that individuals automatically react in a supportive and soothing way to others in pain, this may not always be the case, even if the intentions are good. Consider again the situation in which you cut your finger. This time, your partner tells you, "oh my dear … that is a bad wound … I hope it won't get infected! … You may lose your finger… Do you want some pain killers?" While these comments may be intended as support, they certainly are not soothing. Alternatively, perhaps, others in the house react very differently—imagine that your partner shouts, "how can you be so stupid?" or your children react with laughter, or your father or mother accuses you of exaggerating your pain. These three different scenarios, in which the painful injury is the same, demonstrate that a painful situation can become quite complex, due to the interpersonal dynamics that are involved. While the only factor that differs across the scenarios is the reactions of others, you presumably would feel quite different in each.

The latter examples, while trivial, clearly show that pain is inherently an interpersonal and social experience, characterized by an individual in pain communicating his/her experience to others, who then react to him/her. This interpersonal dynamic is well articulated by Hadjistavropoulos et al. (2011) as a three-step process that involves the individual's subjective experience of pain (step A), an internal experience that then is encoded by the individual into expressive pain behaviors (e.g., self-reports, facial expressions or bodily pain behaviors) (step B), and the decoding of these expressive pain behaviors by an observer (step C). During this decoding phase, observers may make different inferences about the individual's pain experience (e.g., pain intensity) that then occasions different responses toward the person in pain. (See also Chap. 2 for a more elaborate reading on the pain communications model of Hadjistavropoulos and colleagues).

The empathy model for pain, formulated by Goubert and colleagues (Goubert et al., 2005; Goubert, Craig, & Buysse, 2009), provides a related heuristic framework that focuses specifically on observer responses toward another individual's pain (see Fig. 12.1). The model identifies three distinct dimensions of an observer's response that are closely related to each other: (1) the cognitive response, defined as "a sense of knowing the experience of the other in pain" (e.g., an observer's estimates of another's pain), (2) the emotional response, for example sympathy or distress felt for the patient, and (3) the behavioral response, for example helping or

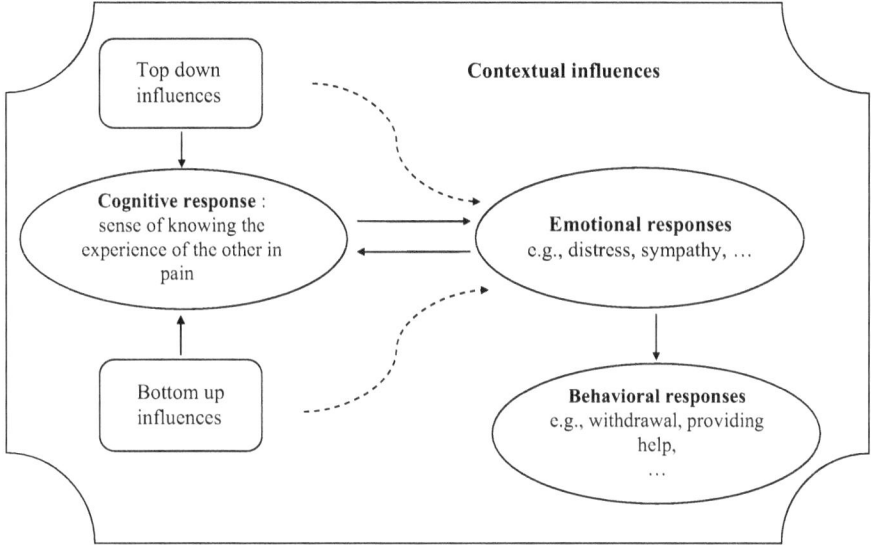

Fig. 12.1 The empathy model in the context of pain (adapted from Goubert et al., 2005)

avoidance behavior. As shown in Fig. 12.1, the empathy model for pain also recognizes that observers' responses are influenced by top-down variables (i.e., variables related to the observer), bottom-up variables (i.e., variables related to the person in pain), and contextual variables (i.e., variables related to the context). In their model for pain judgment, Tait, Chibnall, and Kalauokalani (2009) provided an extensive overview of research findings supporting the influential role of patient, provider, and situational factors upon observer judgments of others' pain. Remarkably, they conclude that much of the information that we think is closely related to the experience of another's pain, such as the absence versus presence of supporting medical evidence, has little association with the severity of the person's actual pain experience. This underscores the importance of considering contextual factors that impact the process of judging another's pain.

Those contextual factors are crucial to consider from both a scientific and a clinical point of view. As reflected in the research described above, judging pain in another is challenging, largely because the pain experience is a subjective phenomenon to which observers have no direct access. Despite this ambiguity, inferences (i.e., cognitive responses), such as estimates of another's pain intensity, often are made that can drive important clinical decisions with significant implications for patient outcomes. To date, there is little research into *why* and *when* observer's responses are beneficial or detrimental to such outcomes. For example, one might assume that higher pain estimates are related to better therapeutic treatments, but those estimates may result in excessive medication prescriptions or in medication overuse by the patient. Similarly, one might expect that more helping behavior from observers is related to better outcomes in patients. However, patients do not always benefit from (well-intended) social support from others (McClure et al., 2013).

While it is beyond the scope of the present chapter to evaluate the beneficial or harmful consequences of observers' responses to pain, the chapter will address the impact of contextual variables on observer biases in judgments, including those made by both clinicians and the lay public.

This chapter focuses upon the influence of the context upon observer cognitive, emotional, and behavioral responses toward others in pain. In doing so, we will consider context in its broadest form. Thus, the following sections will examine how observer judgments are affected by characteristics of the patient/person in pain, the observer, and the situation, as well as elements of the reported pain experience, itself.

Characteristics of Patients

Relative to the pain empathy model of Goubert and colleagues (Goubert et al., 2005, 2009), characteristics of patients reflect the bottom-up variables impacting observer responses toward the patient with pain. In what follows, we will discuss several bottom-up influences which have been shown to systematically influence observer responses. While we mainly focus upon the cognitive response, i.e., pain estimates, we also consider the emotional and behavioral responses of the observer. In particular, we will give a brief overview of the impact of the patient's sociodemographic information, likability, physical attractiveness, coping style, and pain behavior on observer responses.

Sociodemographic Variables

Gender Considerable research has found that both lay observers (e.g., Hadjistavropoulos, McMurtry, & Craig, 1996; Martel, Thibault, & Sullivan, 2011; Robinson & Wise, 2003; Sullivan, Martel, Tripp, Savard, & Crombez, 2006) and health care practitioners (Raftery, Smith-Coggins, & Chen, 1995) attribute more pain to female patients, compared to male patients. The picture is more ambiguous when the impact of patient gender on observers' treatment behaviors is considered. Some studies support the latter interpretation: in an observational study, Hooper, Comstock, Goodwin, and Goodwin (1982) found that physicians communicate more effectively (such as providing clearer information) and also use more empathic skills (such as acknowledging the patient's emotional problems) when interacting with female patients than with male patients. Similarly, in a vignette study with computer-simulated patients, Hirsch and colleagues found that female patients with pain complaints are more likely to be referred to a pain specialist by clinicians and trainees, although this effect was only found with clinicians and trainees who were significantly influenced by the patient's gender (Hirsh, Hollingshead, Matthias, Bair, & Kroenke, 2014). With regard to the prescription of pain medication, two retrospective studies based upon patient care reports have shown that females are less likely than males to receive analgesics (Lord, Cui, & Kelly, 2009; Michael, Sporer, & Youngblood, 2007). Other studies, however, reach different conclusions: the prospective cohort study of Raftery and colleagues, for example, indicated that female patients received more and stronger analgesics than male patients (Raftery et al., 1995), while others find that there is no gender difference in treatments and analgesic use when female and male patients with non-cancer related pain were asked about their treatment and medication use (Turk & Okifuji, 1999).

As already noted by Bernardes and Lima (2011), research into the influence of patient gender upon observer responses, to date, has been descriptive, with mixed results. They propose, instead, that future research be guided by a clear theoretical or heuristic framework in order to develop better insight into the mechanisms through which patient gender impacts observer responses. Considered within a contextual framework, researchers might study the moderating effects of the observer's gender (Hirsh et al., 2014; Safdar et al., 2009), the severity of the pain report (Safdar et al., 2009), and/or the presence or absence of medical evidence (Bernardes & Lima, 2011).

Age In contrast to the considerable research on gender biases in observer responses, research into age-related biases is limited. In general, observers' pain estimates increase with patient age (Hadjistavropoulos, LaChapelle, Hale, & MacLeod, 2000). However, it is not clear that these higher pain estimates occasion better treatment of older people in pain. In fact, older patients with pain are more likely to be undertreated (Cleeland, 1998). Although the effectiveness of pain treatment, of course, depends on the treatment decisions of clinicians, other factors typically related to older adults probably are of importance. For example, older patients might be less likely to seek treatment for their pain because they believe that pain is just part of the aging process (Jones et al., 2016). Similarly, ageism is a persistent problem that can impact clinical care (Butler, 1969), often manifested in a tendency for providers to also view symptoms such as pain as simply a part of aging. Finally, neurocognitive decline in older adults also can complicate pain care, especially given the predisposition of older adults to underestimate levels of pain severity when asked to recall recent past experience (Chibnall & Tait, 2001).

Race/Ethnicity A substantial body of research attests to the influence of a third sociodemographic variable, a patient's race/ethnicity, on observer responses. One of the most investigated topics with regard to patient race is the difference in observer responses to Caucasian and non-Caucasian patients, particularly African Americans. Compared to the pain of Caucasian patients, the pain of African American patients is more likely to be underestimated (Staton et al., 2007) and undertreated by health care practitioners (Green et al., 2003; Todd, Samaroo, & Hoffman, 1993). Although more limited, research on other racial/ethnic populations (e.g., Hispanic whites) reflects a similar trend (Todd et al., 1993). For example, Cleeland et al. (1994) reported that minority patients with cancer pain (primarily black and Hispanic patients) were more likely to receive inadequate analgesia than nonminority patients.

Taken together, research into the impact of patients' race on observer responses suggests that race-related biases potentially disadvantage minorities. However, to our knowledge, none of the abovementioned studies took into account the race of the observer of the patient in pain, which we might expect to moderate the impact of patient race, along with other variables, such as a clinician's level of experience with the treatment of chronic pain (Hirsh et al., 2014).

Patient Likability, Physical Attractiveness, and Coping Style
Evaluating objects or individuals in terms of their valence (positive versus negative), a phenomenon known as automatic evaluation (Bargh, Chaiken, Raymond, & Hymes, 1996), is fundamental to many models of evaluation in social psychology (Tesser & Martin, 1996). Nevertheless, research into the role of a patient's valence on observers' pain estimates is sparse. There is limited preliminary, vignette-based evidence for the role of a patient's likability on observer pain estimates. For example, Chibnall and Tait asked participants to read written vignettes about liked and disliked patients; they demonstrated that observers attributed less pain and disability to disliked than to liked patients, suggesting that the symptoms of negatively valued patients were discounted (Chibnall & Tait, 1995). Similar results, derived from a vignette methodology with videos of actual patients, have been reported by De Ruddere et al. (2011). They found that observers were less sensitive toward the pain of 'disliked' than toward the pain of 'liked' patients. Furthermore, when patients were expressing high intensity pain, observers attributed lower pain to disliked patients than to liked patients.

While the latter research suggests a straightforward relationship between the likability of patients and observers' responses to them, other research suggests that the matter may be more complicated. For example, a vignette study found that, contrary to expectations, physicians attributed more distress and disability to agitated and hostile patients than to less agitated, cooperative patients (Tait & Chibnall, 1997): The authors speculated that the experimental manipulation influenced physician attributions of pain-related distress, rather than the patient's likability. Research on physical attractiveness also yields findings that seem inconsistent with the likability hypothesis. In particular, physically unattractive patients are believed to experience more pain than attractive patients by both lay observers (Hadjistavropoulos et al., 2000; Hadjistavropoulos, Craig, Hadjistavropoulos, & Poole, 1996) and health care practitioners (Hadjistavropoulos, Ross, & Von Baeyer, 1990). Clearly, results such as those described above suggest that the relationship between observer responses to a patient and a patient's likability and/or attractiveness is not linear. In some instances, a positive valence occasions a more generous view of a patient's symptoms, while in other instances the opposite relationship emerges.

While not explicitly linked to likability, the results of research on observer reactions to patients who cope differently with pain are relevant to this discussion. In particular, lay observers have been found to attribute more pain to patients with a presumed adaptive coping style (i.e., reinterpreting, distracting, and/or ignoring pain) than to patients with a presumed maladaptive coping style (i.e., catastrophizing, praying, and hoping) (MacLeod, LaChapelle, & Hadjistavropoulos, 2001).

Also health care practitioners (nurses) seem to feel more negatively about patients that they perceived to cope less well with their pain (i.e., they evaluate these patients as unpopular and demanding) (Salmon & Manyande, 1996). It may be that observers responded positively to chronic pain patients whom they deemed to be working hard to manage their physical condition effectively.

Patient Pain Behavior

The patient's pain behavior is an important cue for both lay observers (Chibnall & Tait, 1995; De Ruddere et al., 2011) and health care providers (De Ruddere et al., 2014; Ferrell, Eberts, McCaffery, & Grant, 1991; Kappesser, Williams, & Prkachin, 2006) to make inferences about the patient's pain experience. When we think of a pain patient, we think of a person who behaves in way that differs from the behavior of a person who is pain-free. Based upon an evolutionary perspective, pain serves as an alarm signal to warn the individual that the body is in risk of being damaged or injured. Accordingly, individuals in pain *behave* in a way that limits the risk of further injury, a *protective* function of pain behavior. However, pain behaviors may serve other functions as well, such as pain management (e.g., rubbing, stretching) and communication (e.g., displaying pain so as to get help from others). The following sections provide a brief overview of the communicative impact of different types of pain behaviors (i.e., facial pain expression, bodily pain behaviors, and (verbal) pain reports).

Facial pain expressions—in contrast to bodily pain behaviors and self-reports of pain—are often conceived as an automatic pain response that is less prone to voluntary control (Williams, 2002). Abundant research indicates that a patient's facial pain expression is a highly influential, bottom-up variable impacting observer responses (Williams, 2002). In general, the level of the patient's facial pain expression positively relates to both lay (Vervoort et al., 2011) and professional observer (Hadjistavropoulos et al., 1990) pain estimates, as well as their sympathy for the patient (De Ruddere, Goubert, Vervoort, Prkachin, & Crombez, 2012) and their inclination to help (De Ruddere et al., 2012). Although less investigated, the patients' full body pain behavior also has been shown to relate to higher pain estimates by both lay observers (De Ruddere et al., 2012; De Ruddere, Goubert, Stevens, Amanda, & Crombez, 2013; Hadjistavropoulos et al., 1990; Sullivan, Martel, et al., 2006; Vervoort et al., 2011) and health care practitioners (De Ruddere et al., 2014), as well as to more sympathy (De Ruddere, Goubert, Stevens, et al., 2013; De Ruddere, Goubert, Vervoort, Kappesser, & Crombez, 2013) and more inclination to help (De Ruddere, Goubert, Stevens, et al., 2013; De Ruddere, Goubert, Vervoort, et al., 2013). While experimental research indicates that patients' facial pain expressions may be more influential than full body pain behaviors (Martel et al., 2011), full body pain behaviors might be a more robust indicator of pain in clinical settings.

Besides the main effect of the patients' expressive pain behaviors on observer responses, considerable evidence has accrued for the moderating effect of nonverbal pain behaviors relative to other variables that can influence observers' responses to a person in pain. Expressive pain behaviors signal pain to others very powerfully (Sullivan, Thibault, et al., 2006) and, therefore, may upregulate or downregulate the effects of other variables on observer pain estimates (see for example De Ruddere et al., 2011; De Ruddere, Goubert, Stevens, et al., 2013; De Ruddere, Goubert, Vervoort, et al., 2013; Tait et al., 2009).

In contrast to facial pain expression and bodily pain behaviors, self-reports of pain are generally considered more conscious expressions and, hence, more susceptible to goal-directed self-representation (e.g., eliciting a helping response from others). At the same time, although criticized (e.g., Schiavenato & Craig, 2010), patients' self-reports also are considered the gold standard of pain assessment when, for example, decisions have to be made regarding doses of pain medication. Those assessments can be based on verbal descriptions, using adjectives such as sharp, cold, crushing, cool, and aching, or they can be based on numerical and/or visual analog scales. Of course, visual analog and the numerical rating scales are most often used (Williams, 2004). In the following section, where we attend to research involving pain characteristics, we will consider the impact of a patient's reported pain severity upon observer responses in greater depth.

Characteristics of Pain

As noted above, judgments of and responses to a person in pain can be colored by a range of factors, defined here as context. Many of the patient factors that can influence observer judgments were described in the previous section. This section focuses on the characteristics of pain, itself, focusing on three elements: (1) its severity, particularly whether it is reported to be of low, moderate, or high intensity; (2) its extent, reflecting both how widely the pain is distributed, as well as the relationship between the reported pain distribution and the expected dermatomes; and (3) its duration, particularly whether the pain is of an acute or chronic nature. The following sections describe how each of these elements can influence how others see a person in pain.

Pain Severity

As noted previously, self-reports of pain are not only subjective but also subject to multiple influences. For example, Weissman and Haddox (1989) found that patients with pain who experience undertreatment inflate their reports of pain severity in order to prompt more aggressive treatment. Of course, as symptom inflation often is interpreted by health care professionals as drug-seeking behavior that is consistent with bona fide addiction, such inflation often occasions a response that is opposite to that which is sought. Another example involves claimants reporting high levels of pain severity who also seek financial compensation for damages for pain following an injury—such circumstances can raise questions about whether the reported symptoms are valid or inflated in order to maximize financial gain.

Of course the latter examples are germane only to persons who report pain of relatively high severity. They serve to raise questions about the effects of reported pain severity, itself, on the judgments of others. Interestingly, the seminal study that examined the effects of increasing levels of reported pain severity on observer/provider pain estimates was conducted in a hospital setting with patients reporting pain from cancer, a condition widely recognized as painful (Grossman, Sheidler, Swedeen, Mucenski, & Piantadosi, 1991). In this study, pain severity ratings provided by patients were categorized (high, medium, low) and compared with those provided by hospital staff (nurses, residents, oncology fellows). Correlations between patient and provider ratings were highest for patients reporting low levels of pain and progressively lower for patients reporting moderate and high levels of pain severity, respectively. In fact, for patients reporting pain of high severity, agreements between patients and nurses was reached in only 7% of the cases, reflecting substantial disagreement between patient and provider ratings and, of course, pain underestimation among providers. Similar tendencies to discount pain levels have been documented in other clinical settings, as well, including the Emergency Department (Marquié et al., 2003) and the postoperative suite (Sjöström, Haljamäe, Dahlgren, & Lindström, 1997; Sommer et al., 2008).

The effects on observer judgments of progressive pain severity levels also have been studied experimentally, through vignette-based methodologies. Not surprisingly, the experimental literature is consistent with the clinical literature described above. In fact, the tendency to discount pain reported at high levels of severity has been demonstrated among undergraduates (Chibnall & Tait, 1995), medical students (Chibnall, Tait, & Ross, 1997), physicians (Tait & Chibnall, 1997), and the lay public (Tait, Chibnall, House, & Biehl, 2016).

Pain Distribution

The distribution of pain has long been a standard part of the assessment of patients with chronic pain (e.g., Melzack, 1975), typically assessed through the administration of "pain drawings"—an outline of a human figure on which the patient is to indicate where pain is felt, as well as its sensory qualities (Carron & Rowlingson, 1981). Subsequently, those drawings were evaluated for selected characteristics, including not only pain extent, but also its distribution (e.g., dermatomal vs. nondermatomal). Indeed, systems were developed to assess pain drawings against pain distribution standards that assigned "penalty points" to features of a drawing that violated those standards, such as drawings where pain was shown outside the boundaries of the human figure (Ransford, Douglas, & Mooney, 1976). Drawings that accrued high levels of penalty points were deemed to reflect "psychological involvement" in the pain condition, raising questions about the validity of the pain report. Not only has subsequent research questioned that interpretation of pain drawings (Von Baeyer, Bergstrom, Brodwin, & Brodwin, 1983), but research also has shown that widespread pain frequently is associated with high levels of disability and distress, independent of the penalty points associated with the pain distribution (Tait, Chibnall, & Margolis, 1990).

While there is evidence that pain drawings can be a valuable tool to evaluate persons with chronic pain conditions in both clinical and epidemiologic settings (Carnes, Ashby, & Underwood, 2006; Gerhardt, Hartmann, Blumenstiel, Tesarz, & Eich, 2014), they also continue to see use in clinic settings as a screening and/or prognostic tool for psychological distress/involvement (Andersen et al., 2010; Carnes et al., 2006). Further, some studies continue to endorse the use of pain drawings as a means of identifying patients with "nonorganic" pain that are likely to respond poorly to treatment (Hayashi et al., 2015) despite limited evidence to support such use (Carnes et al., 2006) Unfortunately, as existing research has focused on the use of such instruments in clinical settings, there are no studies that provide empirical data on direct studies of the effects of varying features of pain drawings on provider judgments, a topic that could benefit from such attention.

Acute Versus Chronic Pain

Characteristics of acute pain are widely recognized as different from those of chronic pain. Typically, definitions of each rely somewhat arbitrarily on their temporal qualities: pain is considered acute when it has been present for less than 3 months, often characterized by clear physiological damage, while chronic pain is considered to persist beyond the normal healing time (International Association for the Study of Pain Task Force on Taxonomy, 1994; Turk & Okifuji, 2001). Of course, relative to chronic pain, there are several variations: chronic pain can be either chronic-recurrent (e.g., migraine headache) or chronic-continuous. Beyond the temporal dimension, however, Table 12.1 demonstrates the other substantial features that distinguish acute from chronic pain.

Given the differences in the characteristics of patients with acute and those with chronic pain, it is not surprising that the literature that has examined observer attitudes toward acute and chronic pain patients has found significant differences between the groups. For example, an early study asked nurses to provide pain estimates and treatment approaches toward patients with acute or chronic pain (Taylor, Skelton, & Butcher, 1984). Nurses significantly discounted their estimates of pain severity for chronic pain patients relative to those with acute pain. While attitudes and treatment approaches demonstrated more complex patterns, those patterns also showed that patients with chronic pain were seen in a consistently negative light. A similar pattern was found in another early study involving nurses (Teske, Daut, & Cleeland, 1983). In that study, nurses were asked to estimate levels of patient pain

Table 12.1 Distinctions between acute and chronic pain (from Tait, 1983, p. 10)

Acute	Chronic
Symptomatic	Disease in itself
Biologically useful	Little biological utility
Induces anxiety	Induces depression
Opioids indicated—under-treatment a concern	Opioid use less clear
Little addiction potential	Polyaddiction potential
Pathologic origin recognized	Pathologic origin unclear—often complex interaction
Cure likely	Little likelihood of cure

severity, and those ratings were compared with actual patient ratings. While there was a consistently significant discrepancy between ratings, such that nurses underestimated pain severity relative to patients, the discrepancy was significantly greater for patients with chronic pain conditions.

More recent literature largely supports the findings of the latter studies, although direct comparisons of attitudes toward the two patient groups have been lacking (likely because of the obvious nature of such differences). Instead, more current research documents the negative attitudes that are prevalent toward chronic pain patients. Such evidence is found not only on the patient side (Upshur, Bacigalupe, & Luckmann, 2010; Werner & Malterud, 2003), but also on the physician side (Epstein et al., 2006). For example, the Album and Westin (2008) study ranked physician specialties relative to the "prestige" of the illness that they treated: diseases such as chronic pain that were more subjective in nature ranked at the bottom of the list, while those with objective medical evidence and that were life-threatening (e.g., myocardial infarction) ranked at the top. Hence, the findings are consistent— patients with chronic pain are vulnerable to negative stereotypes that may undermine symptom assessment and pain management.

There is substantial qualitative evidence, consistent with the above research, showing that individuals with chronic pain commonly perceive themselves to be stigmatized by others (De Ruddere & Craig, 2016; Holloway, Sofaer-Bennett, & Walker, 2007). For example, patients with chronic pain do not feel believed by their relatives (Monsivais, 2013), friends (Toye & Barker, 2010), colleagues and even romantic partners (Holloway et al., 2007). They believe practitioners think their pain is exaggerated (Nguyen, Turner, Rydell, Maclehose, & Harlow, 2013) or imagined (Werner & Malterud, 2003) and they feel blamed (Slade, Molloy, & Keating, 2009), misled (Toye & Barker, 2012), and even dismissed by health care providers (Dewar, White, Posade, & Dillon, 2003).

Hence, on both the provider and the patient side, there is abundant evidence of negative stereotypes and stigmatization of chronic pain. The mechanism underlying these findings might involve the presence of absence of clear physiological damage that might explain the patient's pain experience. In the following section about situational influences on observers' responses toward others in pain, we focus in more depth on the influence of the absence versus the presence of medical evidence upon observer responses toward others' pain.

Situational Features

While many features of a person's pain condition can impact how he/she is seen by another, an observer's judgments of a person in pain are influenced by more than characteristics of the patient or of the pain, itself. Indeed, a substantial literature has arisen around situational factors that can influence how a person in pain is perceived. This section examines the research findings associated with three situational factors: (1) the presence/absence of medical evidence supporting a pain report, (2) the presence/absence of psychosocial stress factors and/or comorbidities, and (3) whether the person in pain is involved in compensation and/or litigation involving a pain condition.

Medical Evidence

From the perspective of the observer, there is considerable research indicating that observers take the pain of patients with medically unexplained pain less seriously than the pain of patients with medically explained pain (De Ruddere & Craig, 2016). Much of the literature is based on vignette-based methodologies in which a hypothetical person/patient in pain is characterized with varying levels of supporting medical evidence, typically in the context of other factors that also are systematically varied. While this approach provides several methodological advantages (e.g., control over the experimental manipulations of interest, randomization of subjects), it also has limitations, including the questionable relevance of experimental findings to the "real world" (e.g., clinical) settings. While the latter considerations must be weighed in evaluating the accumulating literature, the consistency and volume of the evidence presented below demonstrates the weight of supporting medical evidence in influencing observers' judgments.

Early evidence regarding the importance of a medical explanation for the pain as a validating factor was found in studies of college students (Chibnall & Tait, 1995; Tait & Chibnall, 1994). In both studies, each using clinical vignettes, patients with chronic low back pain that were presented with supporting medical diagnostic findings were seen by students as having higher levels of pain, pain-related disability, and emotional distress than patients without supporting evidence. The 1995 study, which differed from the first through its manipulation of pain severity (high vs. low) as an independent variable and the inclusion of personality measures as dependent variables, showed that the medical evidence effect was most pronounced among patients reporting pain at high severity levels. Further, it showed that patients without supporting medical evidence were viewed as more likely to be dishonest, complaining, weak, and lazy. Of course, these data were derived from college students, a group likely to be relatively naïve in regard to such health conditions as chronic pain.

More recently, De Ruddere and colleagues asked individuals from the general population to watch videos of patients with chronic low back pain (De Ruddere, Goubert, Stevens, et al., 2013; De Ruddere, Goubert, Vervoort, et al., 2013) or shoulder pain (De Ruddere et al., 2012) who performed several pain inducing movements. Again, the information about the presence or absence of medical evidence was manipulated by means of a vignette methodology. Similar to the findings referenced above, the researchers found that lay observers attributed less pain to the patients, as well as less sympathy and less inclination to help, when patients presented with pain in the absence of supporting medical evidence. Finally, De Ruddere, Bosmans, Crombez, and Goubert (2016) found that lay observers were less inclined to interact with patients when their pain could not be medically explained; they also found that patients with medically unexplained pain were seen as less socially desirable than patients with medically explained pain.

Observer biases related to the presence or absence of supporting medical evidence apply not only to college students and members of the general population. Indeed, considerable research has indicated that health care practitioner inferences of and responses to patient pain are influenced by medical evidence. For example, a study of practicing internists showed that physician ratings of pain severity were influenced by the presence or absence of supporting medical evidence (Tait & Chibnall, 1997): patients with such evidence were judged to have more pain and disability than those without. A similar pattern emerged for a study involving medical students (Chibnall et al., 1997): patients with supporting medical evidence were credited with higher levels of pain and pain-related disability than were patients without such evidence. Interestingly, in the latter study the medical evidence effect did not offset a general trend for medical students to discount high levels of reported pain: even with medical evidence, medical students discounted the pain of patients who reported very severe pain (9/10), although less than they did for the pain of patients without such evidence. Further, a recent study echoed the latter findings in a hospital setting that involved more than 100 nurses and over 800 inpatients. In the presence of supporting medical information, nurses overestimated pain among patients reporting pain at low levels, but continued to underestimate pain among patients reporting high severity pain (Dekel et al., 2016).

In a vignette study with general practitioners and physiotherapists who were presented with videos of chronic low back pain patients, De Ruddere et al. (2014) found that health care practitioners were less inclined to help, felt less sympathy, disliked patients more, and suspected more deception when there was no clear medical explanation for the pain. Moreover, when patients presented with pain in the absence of tissue pathology, health care practitioners thought that the pain interfered less with daily activities and that pain medication would be less effective. Finally, the health care practitioners thought they were less able to treat the patients with medically unexplained pain.

In several studies that investigated the effect of absence versus presence of medical evidence upon observer responses, it is noteworthy that the robust effect of knowledge about medical evidence was not influenced by the levels of pain behavior that were displayed by patients (e.g., De Ruddere, Goubert, Stevens, et al., 2013;

De Ruddere, Goubert, Vervoort, et al., 2013). As noted previously, such behavior is a crucial cue for observers when estimating others' pain (Craig, Prkachin, & Grunau, 2001; Ferrell et al., 1991; Williams, 2002). The robust effect of medical evidence on observers' responses toward others' pain raises the question about its potential underlying mechanisms, such as observers' suspicions about deception and/or dislike of the patient. Pain in the absence of a clear medical explanation does not fit with common beliefs about pain, beliefs that reflect a strict biomedical model and that posit a direct connection between pain severity and the extent of tissue damage (Kent, Keating, & Taylor, 2009). Accordingly, skepticism may occur in individuals when confronted with patients whose pain complaints are not understood in terms of clear physiological damage. Unfortunately, an elaborated discussion of such mechanisms is not within the scope of this chapter. Instead, we refer the interested reader to a recent topical review regarding stigma and chronic pain (De Ruddere & Craig, 2016).

Presence of Psychological and/or Psychiatric Comorbidity
In clinical practice, patients with pain frequently present with psychological and/or psychiatric problems such as anxiety and mood disorders (Beesdo et al., 2010; Von Korff et al., 2005; Williams, Cox, & Enns, 2003), posttraumatic stress syndrome (Sharp & Harvey, 2001; Williams et al., 2003), substance use disorders (Morasco et al., 2011), severe sleep problems (Nicholson & Verma, 2004), and generally increased levels of daily stressors, both intrapersonal (e.g., feelings of insecurity) and interpersonal (e.g., lack of social recognition; Van Houdenhove et al., 2002). These comorbidities are sufficiently common that treatment guidelines recommend routine screening of patients for psychological distress (Airaksinen et al., 2006).

Despite the frequency with which such conditions co-occur in patients with chronic pain conditions, data suggest that patients who present with psychological comorbidities are vulnerable to having their symptoms discounted. For example, Zastrow et al. (2008) demonstrated that adult inpatients at internal medicine wards are at greater risk of pain underestimation when they suffered from depression and/or anxiety disorders. In an online experimental study, De Ruddere and colleagues found that both physiotherapists and general practitioners attributed less pain to patients when the patients presented with psychosocial stress factors, such as a depressed mood, anxiety, and relational or job problems (De Ruddere et al., 2014). Furthermore, in the presence of psychosocial stress factors in patients displaying high levels of pain behavior, health care practitioners gave lower disability ratings, felt less sympathy for the patient, and believed medication would be less effective. Moreover, they felt less likely to be effective in helping these patients.

In summary, the above findings suggest that observers take a patient's pain report less seriously when they know that psychosocial factors may influence the patient's pain experience. Such a pattern applies both to the lay public and to health care practitioners—the latter group reports greater concern regarding deception (De Ruddere et al., 2014) and greater dislike for patients when they present with elevated psychosocial stress (De Ruddere et al., 2014; Halfens, Evers, & Abu-Saad, 1990). However, research into the impact of psychological and/or psychiatric comorbidity upon observers' actual behavior toward pain patients is, to our knowledge, scarce.

Compensation/Litigation Status

Compensation and litigation status are considered jointly as both involve factors that reflect a person's involvement in a legally mediated situation. Whether involved in litigation or not, claimants who sustain a potentially compensable, pain-related injury share a similar stigma in the eyes of the medical profession, such that their symptoms often are viewed with skepticism (De Ruddere & Craig, 2016; Hadler, 1996; Merskey & Teasell, 2000).

The negative stereotypes behind such skepticism have some basis in fact: chronic pain patients involved in compensation proceedings consistently demonstrate poorer treatment outcomes than patients not involved in such proceedings (Rainville, Sobel, Hartigan, & Wright, 1997; Rohling, Binder, & Langhinrichsen-Rohling, 1995). More recent research, however, suggests that the issue may be more complex than simple legal involvement (Sullivan, Yakobov, Scott, & Tait, 2014). Further, research is quite mixed in regard to the effect of compensation involvement on symptom presentation: some studies have shown that such patients present with elevated symptom levels relative to patients not involved in compensation proceedings (Rohling et al., 1995; Turk & Okifuji, 1996), while other studies have not shown such a relationship (Mendelson, 1995).

Notwithstanding the complexities suggested above, the limited literature regarding the effects of litigation/compensation suggests that observers discount patients' pain-related symptoms. Results of a vignette study, conducted with undergraduates, showed that subjects in the latter condition discounted symptoms of pain, distress, and disability when the pain involved a person in an adversarial legal relationship (Tait & Chibnall, 1994). Another vignette study conducted with lay public participants yielded largely similar results (Chibnall & Tait, 1999): subjects perceived the symptoms to be magnified and lacking medical legitimacy.

Observer Features

Because pain, especially that of a chronic nature, often presents with biomedical, psychosocial, and sociocultural elements, it is not surprising that there is variability in its management. What is surprising, however, is the *level* of variability in the management of both chronic and acute conditions (Cottrell, Roddy, & Foster, 2010; Green & Wheeler, 2003; Green, Wheeler, Marchant, Laporte, & Guerrero, 2001). For example, Drayer, Henderson, and Reidenberg (1999) found that nurses and doctors differed substantially in the amount of pain that they attributed to hospitalized patients, reflected in a low correlation between nurses' and doctors' pain ratings

($r = 0.21$). In the case of chronic pain, there is evidence that physician approaches to treatment are virtually idiosyncratic, with little commonality in approach across providers (Chibnall, Dabney, & Tait, 2000). Such variability reflects the extreme ambiguity that characterizes pain-related decision-making, underscoring the importance of understanding the observer/provider factors that can influence such decisions. It also is important to consider factors that influence the judgments of non-providers, not only because those judgments typically reflect the cultural disposition of the lay public but because those factors can operate when family caregivers provide support to other family members who fall ill. Moreover, judgments of family caregivers often serve as a valued source of health information to health care providers.

Although the category of non-providers is large, research relevant to observer judgments of pain has focused on two primary groups. One group can generally be referenced as the lay public, as it includes students and people recruited from the nonmedical community. The other group that has received study involves those members of the lay community that have served as caregivers, typically for family members suffering from a chronic, often terminal condition such as cancer. The accuracy of proxy reports has been a focus of research for some years. Interestingly, much of that research has shown that proxy estimates of pain correlate less well with patient reports than with many other symptoms (Hilarius, Kloeg, Detmar, Muller, & Aaronson, 2007; Sneeuw, Sprangers, & Aaronson, 2002). Further, unlike pain estimates derived from the general public, proxies generally *over*estimate the patient's level of pain (Elliott, Elliott, Murray, Braun, & Johnson, 1996; Higginson & McCarthy, 1993; McPherson & Addington-Hall, 2003; McPherson, Wilson, Lobchuk, & Brajtman, 2008; Redinbaugh, Baum, Demoss, Fello, & Arnold, 2002; Sneeuw et al., 1999; Yeager, Miaskowski, Dibble, & Wallhagen, 1995). For each group, observer characteristics have been identified that can impact judgments of pain. The following sections review information for health care providers, members of the lay community, and family caregivers.

Experience

It would be natural to expect that providers, who have considerable experience in the treatment of patients in pain, would estimate a patient's pain more accurately than would the lay public. That expectation, however, would be disappointed, as the data show that providers consistently underestimate pain, generally to a greater degree than do non-providers (Cheng et al., 2007; Dekel et al., 2016; Kappesser et al., 2006; Lenburg, Glass, & Davitz, 1970; Prkachin, Solomon, Hwang, & Mercer, 2001; Tait et al., 2016) Moreover, those with greater experience underestimate a patient's pain to a greater degree than do those with less experience. The latter pattern has been found in such diverse groups and settings as student nurses (Halfens et al., 1990), nurses on a burn unit (Choinière, Melzack, Girard, Rondeau, & Paquin,

1990), physicians in an Emergency Department (Marquié et al., 2003), and physical/occupational therapists on a rehabilitation service (Prkachin et al., 2001).

While the prevalence of pain underestimation is well established among health providers, the mechanisms that drive it are less understood. There is some evidence that frequent exposures to patients in pain may desensitize providers to these complaints (Marquié et al., 2003; Prkachin, Mass, & Mercer, 2004; Prkachin & Rocha, 2010), possibly by re-calibrating comparison levels that they apply to a patient's reported experience (i.e., adapting different standards for "pain as bad as it can get"). This could explain differences in pain estimation found between surgeons, who deal with postoperative pain on a regular basis, and internists, whose exposure to patients in severe pain is less regular (Tait, Chibnall, Miller, & Werner, 2011) or between specialist and general nurses (Wilson & McSherry, 2006). Alternatively, high levels of cumulative experience could lead providers to attend selectively to information that supports their judgments, such that they rely on well-established heuristics (i.e., clinical intuition) at the expense of more effortful processes (Kahneman, 2003). Yet another explanation invokes negative affect toward a patient in pain: providers may develop a negative valence toward that general class of patients, making them indifferent toward patients who present with such symptoms (Epstein et al., 2006; Leclere, Beaulieu, Bordage, Sindon, & Couillard, 1990) or even predisposed to blame those with chronic pain for failing to respond more positively to treatment (Eccleston, Williams, Rogers, & Williams, 1997; Tait, Chibnall, Luebbert, & Sutter, 2005).

The finding that experience with others in pain is positively related to pain-underestimation is not unique to professional health care providers. In particular, Prkachin and colleagues (Prkachin et al., 2004; Prkachin & Rocha, 2010) demonstrated that even observers drawn from the lay public demonstrate more pronounced underestimation as their exposure increases to patients exhibiting severe pain. However, in these studies, only the mere exposure to facial pain expressions of strangers was manipulated, which may differ from responses to the pain of significant others. In fact, we might expect that observers who are familiar with and positively valenced toward others with chronic pain will display more sympathy than observers who are unfamiliar with or are negatively valenced. Indeed, there is limited research that suggests that lay observers with chronic pain in family members may discount pain to a lower degree than those without such a background (Prkachin et al., 2001). Interestingly, they still estimated pain at levels below the patient's ratings, so their pain history did not completely offset the underestimation effect described above.

Knowledge and Beliefs About Pain (Management)

As previously mentioned, both lay observers and health care providers still endorse a biomedical model of pain (Eccleston & Crombez, 2007; Kent et al., 2009). Of course, the adequacy of such a model in the treatment of patients who are at risk of developing chronic pain or who have developed such pain is problematic. Indeed, despite evidence described previously that documents the frequent psychosocial comorbidities associated with pain conditions, many health care practitioners have little knowledge about those risk factors in patients with pain and do not use tools and methods that can screen for these factors (Kent et al., 2009; Singla, Jones, Edwards, & Kumar, 2015). Hence, the application of a strict biomedical approach toward the management of chronic pain is likely to create "blind spots" to issues that might impede optimal adjustment to such conditions.

While the impact of adherence to a strict biomedical approach has not yet been the focus of substantial research, there is considerable research suggesting that bio-medically oriented observers react in a negative way to patients. As noted previously, a study of general practitioners and physiotherapists (De Ruddere et al., 2014) suggested that both lay observers and health care providers, in the absence of clear medical evidence, may take a patient's pain less seriously. Moreover, practitioners who doubt the credibility of a patient's pain complaints and/or associated pain behavior are likely to collaborate less effectively with patients than practitioners without such doubts (MacNeela, Gibbons, McGuire, & Murphy, 2010). Indeed, practitioner doubts may extend to the usefulness of treatment guidelines for patients with chronic pain: there is evidence that general practitioners are uncomfortable with recommendations that patients with chronic low back pain should stay active (Corbett, Foster, & Ong, 2009).

While the above findings relate to the impact of belief systems on attitudes of the lay public and providers, pain-specific beliefs also have been found to be important for family caregivers, especially parent–child dyads. In particular, several researchers have found that catastrophizing thoughts in parents are associated with higher parental estimates of a child's pain (Goubert, Vervoort, Cano, & Crombez, 2009), more parental distress (Caes et al., 2014), more parental attempts to control a child's pain (Caes, Vervoort, Eccleston, & Goubert, 2012), more protective behavior toward a child in pain (Caes et al., 2014), a higher tendency to restrict a child's activity (Caes, Vervoort, Eccleston, Vandenhende, & Goubert, 2011), and a higher inclination to engage in solicitous behaviors (Goubert, Vervoort, De Ruddere, & Crombez, 2012). Further, relative to cancer pain, caregivers who overestimate pain are vulnerable to more distress, themselves, because of the high levels of pain and distress that they perceive in the patients receiving care (Redinbaugh et al., 2002). Relatedly, people who describe caregiving as stressful and burdensome also are likely to overestimate symptoms (McPherson et al., 2008). Of course, it is likely that symptom overestimation is not one-way, but may be affected by a tendency on the part of patients to underreport symptoms as a means of reducing the burden on caregivers (McPherson & Addington-Hall, 2003). All of the above findings, whether related to providers, the lay public, or family members, raise questions about whether pain education or training might change the knowledge, attitudes and potentially the behaviors of individuals interacting with others in pain.

Training

The evidence is limited and mixed relative to the effectiveness of training as a means of improving provider judgments regarding the management of pain. Relative to assessment, training has been shown to improve the accuracy of pain estimation in physical therapists (Solomon, Prkachin, & Farewell, 1997). Relative to treatment, there is evidence that training in appropriate opioid management can improve the quality of pain care in a hypothetical patient with terminal cancer (Cleeland, Cleeland, Dar, & Rinehardt, 1986). Relative to the actual delivery of pain care, however, the data are less positive: an intensive training and feedback intervention employed in hospitalized, seriously ill patients with severe pain showed no effects on pain control relative to usual care (Desbiens et al., 1998). Similarly, the VA implemented an initiative that emphasized the importance of pain as a 5th vital sign; the initiative led to improved symptom recording, but no meaningful changes in care (Mularski et al., 2006).

While the abovementioned studies focused on practitioners' pain assessments and on reported pain relief, other studies have focused upon training aimed at change in provider beliefs, attitudes and knowledge with regard to pain. Several studies found support for training in a biopsychosocial model of pain: such training decreased physiotherapists' beliefs that pain alone contributes to impairment and disability (Domenech, Sánchez-Zuriaga, Segura-Ortí, Espejo-Tort, & Lisón, 2011), as well as increased knowledge about psychosocial prognostic factors (Overmeer, Boersma, Main, & Linton, 2009). Relative to the former study, the reduction in fear-avoidance and pain-impairment beliefs was associated with an increase in the activity and work recommendations made to patients, while training in a biomedical model occasioned more maladaptive beliefs that, in turn, were related to fewer activity recommendations (Domenech et al., 2011).

Notwithstanding the mixed results described above, the Department of Health and Human Services (DHHS) initiated a campaign to make case-based training in effective pain management broadly available to the US provider community. This is one of several DHHS strategies triggered by a recent study of pain care in the USA, which concluded, among other findings, that the health care provider community received inadequate training in pain management (Institute of Medicine (US) Committee on Advancing Pain Research Care and Education, 2011). In Europe, the European Federation of IASP Chapters recently developed a pain knowledge curriculum to support a multidisciplinary certification as a pain specialist (European Pain Federation (EFIC), 2016). Given these major undertakings, additional evidence regarding the effects of training on clinical judgment and practice is likely to emerge.

It is important to note that changing the knowledge and attitudes of lay observers might be of value, as well. For example, there is evidence that psychoeducational strategies can be effective in modifying beliefs of the lay public regarding the management of low back pain (George et al., 2009). Indeed, an Australian study in which such an intervention was conducted at a population level occasioned reductions in both low back claims and costs over a subsequent 2-year period (Buchbinder, Jolley, & Wyatt, 2001). Whether such education would be helpful in enhancing judgments of and responses to persons in pain (e.g., reducing levels of catastrophizing in family caregivers), however, has not been examined.

Empathy

There is some evidence that the prejudicial attitudes referenced above could be off-set by another provider characteristic, empathy. While empathy is the topic of another chapter, the limited research regarding the role of empathy in pain judgments deserves brief mention here. Both vignette-based (Chibnall, Tait, & Jovel, 2014) and applied clinical research (Chang, Lin, Chang, & Lin, 2005) show that providers characterized by higher levels of empathy, accessibility, and communicativeness are more likely to assess patients' levels of pain and disability accurately. Further, there is some evidence that providers that are higher in empathy are less likely to blame a patient for a failure to respond to treatment (Tait et al., 2005): relative to providers with lower levels of empathy, those with higher levels were less likely to blame a patient's psychological adjustment for bad outcomes. While there is more abundant evidence that patients of empathic providers will demonstrate higher adherence to treatment (Schneider, Kaplan, Greenfield, Li, & Wilson, 2004) and experience better outcomes (Stewart, 1996), a discussion of that literature is beyond the bounds of this chapter.

Conclusion

While this chapter provides an extensive overview of different "context" variables that are known to influence observer responses to others in pain, it does not provide the reader with an exhaustive list. Indeed, other factors, not discussed in this chapter, are of likely importance. For example, this chapter used a micro-level approach, leaving unaddressed macro-level issues, i.e., the impact of organizational or structural factors upon observer responses (e.g., the recent guidelines of the US Centers for Disease Control with regard to the prescription of opioid medication). Further, the work that we discussed mainly focused upon the interpersonal context of adults suffering from pain with relatively little attention to observer responses to children in pain. Although we examined the latter issue relatively little, we would argue that study of the interpersonal dynamics in parent–child dyads is important for both practical and theoretical reasons. Similarly, we did not address in any depth observer responses to individuals with some level of neurocognitive impairment, even though the evaluation and treatment of older adults with such impairments remains a challenging issue without a clear solution.

Despite these limitations, the studies reviewed in this chapter point to several obvious conclusions. First, the topic of observer responses to patients in pain is increasingly recognized as a fundamental contributor to the care of persons with (chronic) pain conditions and is of particular importance in trying to understand the variability associated with current approaches to that care. Second, while of increasing interest, mapping the impact of most contextual variables onto specific observer responses remains challenging. In part, this is due to the focus of most studies on the influence of particular variables, without the guidance that might be provided by a theoretical or heuristic framework. Future studies into the role of context variables upon observer responses would benefit from grounding in a clear theoretical approach, framing the variables under study within a general model that incorporates all variables of potential theoretical interest. Such an approach also would help to address a third factor that is evident in the literature, the high level of variability in methodologies across the studies that limits comparisons across research findings. Finally, we would be remiss if we did not call attention to the need for more study of links between observer responses to others in pain and the impact of those responses on treatment outcomes for patients in clinical or other caregiving contexts. Despite the increased understanding of and appreciation for the role of context in observer judgments, our knowledge of how context, judgment, and treatment outcomes interact remains sketchy and is in need of translational research. Such research is strongly recommended in order to build our understanding of how we can translate our current base of knowledge into improved assessment and treatment of patients in pain in clinical practice.

References

Airaksinen, O., Brox, J. I., Cedraschi, C., Hildebrandt, J., Klaber-Moffett, J., Kovacs, F., … Zanoli, G. (2006). Chapter 4. European guidelines for the management of chronic nonspecific low back pain. *European Spine Journal, 15*(S2), s192–s300. https://doi.org/10.1007/s00586-006-1072-1

Album, D., & Westin, S. (2008). Do diseases have a prestige hierarchy? A survey among physicians and medical students. *Social Science & Medicine, 66*, 182–188. https://doi.org/10.1016/j.socscimed.2007.07.003

Andersen, T., Christensen, F. B., Høy, K. W., Helmig, P., Niedermann, B., Hansen, E. S., & Bünger, C. (2010). The predictive value of pain drawings in lumbar spinal fusion surgery. *The Spine Journal, 10*, 372–379. https://doi.org/10.1016/j.spinee.2010.02.002

Bargh, J. A., Chaiken, S., Raymond, P., & Hymes, C. (1996). The automatic evaluation effect: Unconditional automatic attitude activation with a pronunciation task. *Journal of Experimental Social Psychology, 32*, 104–128.

Beesdo, K., Jacobi, F., Hoyer, J., Low, N. C. P., Höfler, M., & Wittchen, H.-U. (2010). Pain associated with specific anxiety and depressive disorders in a nationally representative population sample. *Social Psychiatry and Psychiatric Epidemiology, 45*(1), 89–104. https://doi.org/10.1007/s00127-009-0045-1

Bernardes, S. F., & Lima, M. L. (2011). A contextual approach on sex-related biases in pain judgements: The moderator effects of evidence of pathology and patients' distress cues on nurses' judgements of chronic low-back pain. *Psychology & Health, 26*(12), 1642–1658. https://doi.org/10.1080/08870446.2011.553680

Buchbinder, R., Jolley, D., & Wyatt, M. (2001). Population based intervention to change back pain beliefs and disability: Three part evaluation. *Bone, Muscle, & Joint, 322*, 1516–1520.

Butler, R. N. (1969). Age-ism: Another form of bigotry. *The Gerontologist, 9*, 243–246. https://doi.org/10.1093/geront/9.4_Part_1.243

Caes, L., Goubert, L., Devos, P., Verlooy, J., Benoit, Y., & Vervoort, T. (2014). The relationship between parental catastrophizing about child pain and distress in response to medical procedures in the context of childhood cancer treatment: A longitudinal analysis. *Journal of Pediatric Psychology, 39*(7), 677–686. https://doi.org/10.1093/jpepsy/jsu034

Caes, L., Vervoort, T., Devos, P., Verlooy, J., Benoit, Y., & Goubert, L. (2014). Parental distress and catastrophic thoughts about child pain: Implications for parental protective behavior in the context of child leukemia-related medical procedures. *The Clinical Journal of Pain, 30*(9), 787–799. https://doi.org/10.1097/AJP.0000000000000028

Caes, L., Vervoort, T., Eccleston, C., & Goubert, L. (2012). Parents who catastrophize about their child's pain prioritize attempts to control pain. *Pain, 153*(8), 1695–1701. https://doi.org/10.1016/j.pain.2012.04.028

Caes, L., Vervoort, T., Eccleston, C., Vandenhende, M., & Goubert, L. (2011). Parental catastrophizing about child's pain and its relationship with activity restriction: The mediating role of parental distress. *Pain, 152*(1), 212–222. https://doi.org/10.1016/j.pain.2010.10.037

Carnes, D., Ashby, D., & Underwood, M. (2006). A systematic review of pain drawing literature. *The Clinical Journal of Pain, 22*(5), 449–457. https://doi.org/10.1097/01.ajp.0000208245.41122.ac

Carron, H., & Rowlingson, J. (1981). Coordinated out-patient management of chronic pain at the University of Virginia Pain Clinic. *NIDA Research Monograph, 36*, 84–91.

Chang, Y., Lin, Y., Chang, H., & Lin, C. (2005). Cancer patient and staff ratings of caring behaviors: Relationship to level of pain intensity. *Cancer Nursing, 28*, 331–339.

Cheng, Y., Lin, C.-P., Liu, H.-L., Hsu, Y.-Y., Lim, K.-E., Hung, D., & Decety, J. (2007). Expertise modulates the perception of pain in others. *Current Biology, 17*(19), 1708–1713. https://doi.org/10.1016/j.cub.2007.09.020

Chibnall, J. T., Dabney, A., & Tait, R. C. (2000). Internist judgments of chronic low back pain. *Pain Medicine, 1*(3), 231–237. https://doi.org/10.1046/j.1526-4637.2000.00029.x

Chibnall, J. T., & Tait, R. C. (1995). Observer perceptions of low back pain—effects of pain report and other contextual factors. *Journal of Applied Social Psychology, 25*(5), 418–439.

Chibnall, J. T., & Tait, R. C. (1999). Social and medical influences on attributions and evaluations of chronic pain. *Psychology & Health, 14*(4), 719–729. https://doi.org/10.1080/08870449908410760

Chibnall, J. T., & Tait, R. C. (2001). Pain assessment in cognitively impaired and unimpaired older adults: A comparison of four scales. *Pain, 92*, 173–186.

Chibnall, J. T., Tait, R. C., & Jovel, A. (2014). Accountability and empathy effects on medical students' clinical judgments in a disability determination context for low back pain. *Journal of Pain, 15*(9), 915–924. https://doi.org/10.1016/j.jpain.2014.06.001

Chibnall, J. T., Tait, R. C., & Ross, L. R. (1997). The effects of medical evidence and pain intensity on medical student judgments of chronic pain patients. *Journal of Behavioral Medicine, 20*(3), 257–271. https://doi.org/10.1023/a:1025504827787

Choinière, M., Melzack, R., Girard, N., Rondeau, J., & Paquin, M.-J. (1990). Comparisons between patients' and nurses' assessment of pain and medication efficacy in severe burn injuries. *Pain, 40*, 143–152.

Cleeland, C. S. (1998). Undertreatment of cancer pain in elderly patients. *The Journal of the American Medical Association, 279*(23), 1914–1915.

Cleeland, C. S., Cleeland, L. M., Dar, R., & Rinehardt, L. C. (1986). Factors influencing physician management of cancer pain. *Cancer, 58*(3), 796–800. https://doi.org/10.1002/1097-0142(19860801)58:3<796::AID-CNCR2820580331>3.0.CO;2-#

Cleeland, C. S., Gonin, R., Hatfield, A. K., Edmonson, J. H., Blum, R. H., Stewart, J. A., & Pandya, K. J. (1994). Pain and its treatment in outpatients with metastatic cancer. *The New England Journal of Medicine, 330*(9), 592–596.

Corbett, M., Foster, N., & Ong, B. N. (2009). GP attitudes and self-reported behaviour in primary care consultations for low back pain. *Family Practice, 26*(5), 359–364. https://doi.org/10.1093/fampra/cmp042

Cottrell, E., Roddy, E., & Foster, N. E. (2010). The attitudes, beliefs and behaviours of GPs regarding exercise for chronic knee pain: A systematic review. *Family Practice, 11*, 4.

Craig, K. D., Prkachin, K. M., & Grunau, R. E. (2001). The facial expression of pain. In D. C. Turk & R. Melzack (Eds.), *Handbook of pain assessment* (2nd ed., pp. 153–169). New York, NY: The Guilford Press.

De Ruddere, L., Bosmans, M., Crombez, G., & Goubert, L. (2016). Patients are socially excluded when their pain has no medical explanation. *Journal of Pain, 17*(9), 1028–1035. https://doi.org/10.1016/j.jpain.2016.06.005

De Ruddere, L., & Craig, K. D. (2016). Understanding stigma and chronic pain: A state of the art review. *Pain, 157*(8), 1607–1610.

De Ruddere, L., Goubert, L., Prkachin, K. M., Louis Stevens, M. A., Van Ryckeghem, D. M. L., & Crombez, G. (2011). When you dislike patients, pain is taken less seriously. *Pain, 152*(10), 2342–2347. https://doi.org/10.1016/j.pain.2011.06.028

De Ruddere, L., Goubert, L., Stevens, M., Amanda, A. C., & Crombez, G. (2013). Discounting pain in the absence of medical evidence is explained by negative evaluation of the patient. *Pain, 154*(5), 669–676. https://doi.org/10.1016/j.pain.2012.12.018

De Ruddere, L., Goubert, L., Stevens, M. A. L., Deveugele, M., Craig, K. D., & Crombez, G. (2014). Health care professionals' reactions to patient pain: Impact of knowledge about medical evidence and psychosocial influences. *Journal of Pain, 15*(3), 262–270. https://doi.org/10.1016/j.jpain.2013.11.002

De Ruddere, L., Goubert, L., Vervoort, T., Kappesser, J., & Crombez, G. (2013). Impact of being primed with social deception upon observer responses to others' pain. *Pain, 154*(2), 221–226. https://doi.org/10.1016/j.pain.2012.10.002

De Ruddere, L., Goubert, L., Vervoort, T., Prkachin, K. M., & Crombez, G. (2012). We discount the pain of others when pain has no medical explanation. *Journal of Pain, 13*(12), 1198–1205. https://doi.org/10.1016/j.jpain.2012.09.002

Dekel, B. G. S., Gori, A., Vasarri, A., Sorella, M. C., Di Nino, G., & Melotti, R. M. (2016). Medical evidence influence on inpatients and nurses pain ratings agreement. *Pain Research and Management, 2016*, 1–11. https://doi.org/10.1155/2016/9267536

Desbiens, N. A., Wu, A. W., Yasui, Y., Lynn, J., Alzola, C., Wenger, N. S., … Fulkerson, W. (1998). Patient empowerment and feedback did not decrease pain in seriously ill hospitalized adults. *Pain, 75*, 237–246.

Dewar, A., White, M., Posade, S. T., & Dillon, W. (2003). Using nominal group technique to assess chronic pain, patients' perceived challenges and needs in a community health region. *Health Expectations, 6*, 44–52. https://doi.org/10.1046/j.1369-6513.2003.00208.x

Domenech, J., Sánchez-Zuriaga, D., Segura-Ortí, E., Espejo-Tort, B., & Lisón, J. F. (2011). Impact of biomedical and biopsychosocial training sessions on the attitudes, beliefs, and recommendations of health care providers about low back pain: A randomised clinical trial. *Pain, 152*(11), 2557–2563. https://doi.org/10.1016/j.pain.2011.07.023

Drayer, R. A., Henderson, J., & Reidenberg, M. (1999). Barriers to better pain control in hospitalized patients. *Journal of Pain and Symptom Management, 17*(6), 434–440. https://doi.org/10.1016/S0885-3924(99)00022-6

Eccleston, C., & Crombez, G. (2007). Worry and chronic pain: A misdirected problem solving model. *Pain, 132*(3), 233–236. https://doi.org/10.1016/j.pain.2007.09.014

Eccleston, C., Williams, A., Rogers, W., & Williams, A. C. (1997). Patient's and professionals understanding of the causes of chronic pain: Blame, responsibility and identity protection. *Social Science and Medicine, 45*(5), 699–709.

Elliott, B. A., Elliott, T. E., Murray, D. M., Braun, B. L., & Johnson, K. M. (1996). Patients and family members: The role of knowledge and attitudes in cancer pain. *Journal of Pain and Symptom Management, 12*, 209–220.

Epstein, R. M., Shields, C. G., Meldrum, S. C., Fiscella, K., Carroll, J., Carney, P. A., & Duberstein, P. R. (2006). Physicians' responses to patients' medically unexplained symptoms. *Psychosomatic Medicine, 68*(2), 269–276. https://doi.org/10.1097/01.psy.0000204652.27246.5b

European Pain Federation (EFIC). (2016). Diploma in Pain Medicine. Retrieved November 28, 2016, from http://www.europeanpainfederation.eu/core-curriculum/diploma-in-pain-medicine/

Ferrell, B. R., Eberts, M. R., McCaffery, M., & Grant, M. (1991). Clinical decision making and pain. *Cancer Nursing, 14*, 289–297.

George, S. Z., Teyhen, D. S., Wu, S. S., Wright, A. C., Dugan, J. L., … Childs, J. D. (2009). Psychosocial education improves low back pain beliefs: Results from a cluster randomized clinical trial (NCT00373009) in a primary prevention setting. *European Spine Journal, 18*, 1050–1058. https://doi.org/10.1007/s00586-009-1016-7

Gerhardt, A., Hartmann, M., Blumenstiel, K., Tesarz, J., & Eich, W. (2014). The prevalence rate and the role of the spatial extent of pain in nonspecific chronic back pain—a population-based study in the south-west of Germany. *Pain Medicine, 15*, 1200–1210.

Goubert, L., Craig, K. D., & Buysse, A. (2009). Perceiving others in pain: Experimental and clinical evidence on the role of empathy. In W. Ickes & J. Decety (Eds.), *The social neuroscience of empathy* (pp. 153–166). Cambridge, MA: MIT Press.

Goubert, L., Craig, K. D., Vervoort, T., Morley, S., Sullivan, M. J. L., Williams, A. C. d. C., … Crombez, G. (2005). Facing others in pain: The effects of empathy. *Pain, 118*(3), 285–288. https://doi.org/10.1016/j.pain.2005.10.025

Goubert, L., Vervoort, T., Cano, A., & Crombez, G. (2009). Catastrophizing about their children's pain is related to higher parent-child congruency in pain ratings: An experimental investigation. *European Journal of Pain, 13*(2), 196–201. https://doi.org/10.1016/j.ejpain.2008.03.009

Goubert, L., Vervoort, T., De Ruddere, L., & Crombez, G. (2012). The impact of parental gender, catastrophizing and situational threat upon parental behaviour to child pain: A vignette study. *European Journal of Pain, 16*(8), 1176–1184. https://doi.org/10.1002/j.1532-2149.2012.00116.x

Green, C. R., Anderson, K. O., Baker, T. A., Campbell, L. C., Decker, S., Fillingim, R. B., … Vallerand, A. H. (2003). The unequal burden of pain: Confronting racial and ethnic disparities in pain. *Pain Medicine, 4*(3), 277–295.

Green, C. R., & Wheeler, J. R. C. (2003). Physician variability in the management of acute postoperative and cancer pain: A quantitative analysis of the Michigan experience. *Pain Medicine, 4*(1), 8–20.

Green, C. R., Wheeler, J. R. C., Marchant, B., Laporte, F., & Guerrero, E. (2001). Analysis of the physician variable in pain management. *Pain Medicine, 2*(4), 317–327. https://doi.org/10.1046/j.1526-4637.2001.01045.x

Grossman, S. A., Sheidler, V. R., Swedeen, K., Mucenski, J., & Piantadosi, S. (1991). Correlation of patient and caregiver ratings of cancer pain. *Journal of Pain and Symptom Management, 6*(2), 53–57.

Hadjistavropoulos, H. D., Craig, K. D., Hadjistavropoulos, T., & Poole, G. D. (1996). Subjective judgments of deception in pain expression: Accuracy and errors. *Pain, 65*(2–3), 251–258. https://doi.org/10.1016/0304-3959(95)00218-9

Hadjistavropoulos, H. D., Ross, M. A., & Von Baeyer, C. L. (1990). Are physicians' ratings of pain affected by patients' physical attractiveness? *Social Science & Medicine, 31*, 69–72.

Hadjistavropoulos, T., Craig, K. D., Duck, S., Cano, A., Goubert, L., Jackson, P. L., … Fitzgerald, T. D. (2011). A biopsychosocial formulation of pain communication. *Psychological Bulletin, 137*(6), 910–939. https://doi.org/10.1037/a0023876

Hadjistavropoulos, T., LaChapelle, D., Hale, C. H., & MacLeod, F. K. (2000). Age-and appearance-related stereotypes about patients undergoing a painful medical procedure. *The Pain Clinic, 12*(1), 25–33.

Hadjistavropoulos, T., McMurtry, B., & Craig, K. D. (1996). Beautiful faces in pain: Biases and accuracy in the perception of pain. *Psychology and Health, 11*, 411–420.

Hadler, N. M. (1996). The disabled, the disallowed, the disaffected and the disavowed. *Journal of Occupational & Environmental Medicine, 38*(3), 247–251. https://doi.org/10.1097/00043764-199603000-00008

Halfens, R., Evers, G., & Abu-Saad, H. (1990). Determinants of pain assessment by nurses. *International Journal of Nursing Studies, 27*, 43–49. https://doi.org/10.1016/0020-7489(90)90022-B

Hayashi, K., Arai, Y. C. P., Morimoto, A., Aono, S., Yoshimoto, T., Nishihara, M., … Ushida, T. (2015). Associations between pain drawing and psychological characteristics of different body region pains. *Pain Practice, 15*(4), 300–307. https://doi.org/10.1111/papr.12173

Higginson, I. J., & McCarthy, M. (1993). Validity of the support team assessment schedule: Do staffs' ratings reflect those made by patients or their families? *Palliative Medicine, 7*(3), 219–228.

Hilarius, D. L., Kloeg, P. H. A. M., Detmar, S. B., Muller, M. J., & Aaronson, N. K. (2007). Level of agreement between patient self-report and observer ratings of health-related quality of life communication in oncology. *Patient Education and Counseling, 65*, 95–100. https://doi.org/10.1016/j.pec.2006.06.002

Hirsh, A. T., Hollingshead, N. A., Matthias, M. S., Bair, M. J., & Kroenke, K. (2014). The influence of patient sex, provider sex, and sexist attitudes on pain treatment decisions. *Journal of Pain, 15*(5), 551–559. https://doi.org/10.1016/j.jpain.2014.02.003

Holloway, I., Sofaer-Bennett, B., & Walker, J. (2007). The stigmatisation of people with chronic back pain. *Disability and Rehabilitation, 29*(18), 1456–1464. https://doi.org/10.1080/09638280601107260

Hooper, E. M., Comstock, L. M., Goodwin, J. M., & Goodwin, J. S. (1982). Patient characteristics that influence physician behavior. *Medical Care, 6*, 630–638.

Institute of Medicine (US) Committee on Advancing Pain Research Care and Education. (2011). *Relieving pain in America: A blueprint for transforming prevention, care, education, and research.* Washington, DC: National Academies Press.

International Association for the Study of Pain Task Force on Taxonomy. (1994). *Classification on chronic pain: Descriptions of chronic pain syndromes and definitions of pain terms* (2nd ed.). Seattle, WA: IASP Press.

Jones, M. R., Ehrhardt, K. P., Ripoll, J. G., Sharma, B., Padnos, I. W., Kaye, R. J., & Kaye, A. D. (2016). Pain in the elderly. *Current Pain and Headache Reports, 20*(4), 1–9. https://doi.org/10.1007/s11916-016-0551-2

Kahneman, D. (2003). A perspective on judgment and choice: Mapping bounded rationality. *American Psychologist, 58*(9), 697–720.

Kappesser, J., Williams, A. C. d. C., & Prkachin, K. M. (2006). Testing two accounts of pain underestimation. *Pain, 124*(1–2), 109–116. https://doi.org/10.1016/j.pain.2006.04.003

Kent, P. M., Keating, J. L., & Taylor, N. F. (2009). Primary care clinicians use variable methods to assess acute nonspecific low back pain and usually focus on impairments. *Manual Therapy, 14*(1), 88–100. https://doi.org/10.1016/j.math.2007.12.006

Leclere, H., Beaulieu, M.-D., Bordage, G., Sindon, A., & Couillard, M. (1990). Why are clinical problems difficult? General practitioners' opinions concerning 24 clinical problems. *Canadian Medical Association Journal, 143*, 1305–1315.

Lenburg, C. B., Glass, H. P., & Davitz, L. J. (1970). Inferences of physical pain and psychological distress. II. In relation to the stage of the patient's illness and occupation of the perceiver. *Nursing Research, 19*(5), 392–398.

Lord, B., Cui, J., & Kelly, A. M. (2009). The impact of patient sex on paramedic pain management in the prehospital setting. *The American Journal of Emergency Medicine, 27*(5), 525–529. https://doi.org/10.1016/j.ajem.2008.04.003

MacLeod, F. K., LaChapelle, D. L., & Hadjistavropoulos, T. (2001). The effect of disability claimants' coping styles on judgments of pain, disability, and compensation: A vignette study. *Rehabilitation Psychology, 46*(4), 417–435.

MacNeela, P., Gibbons, A., McGuire, B., & Murphy, A. (2010). "We need to get you focused": General practitioners' representations of chronic low back pain patients. *Qualitative Health Research, 20*(7), 977–986. https://doi.org/10.1177/1049732310364219

Marquié, L., Raufaste, E., Lauque, D., Mariné, C., Ecoiffier, M., & Sorum, P. (2003). Pain rating by patients and physicians: Evidence of systematic pain miscalibration. *Pain, 102,* 289–296.

Martel, M. O., Thibault, P., & Sullivan, M. J. L. (2011). Judgments about pain intensity and pain genuineness: The role of pain behavior and judgmental heuristics. *The Journal of Pain, 12,* 468–475. https://doi.org/10.1016/j.jpain.2010.10.010

McClure, M. J., Xu, J. H., Craw, J. P., Lane, S. P., Bolger, N., & Shrout, P. E. (2013). Understanding the costs of support transactions in daily life. *Journal of Personality, 82*(6), 563–574. https://doi.org/10.1111/jopy.12061

McPherson, C. J., & Addington-Hall, J. M. (2003). Judging the quality of care at the end of life: Can proxies provide reliable information? *Social Science & Medicine, 56,* 95–109.

McPherson, C. J., Wilson, K. G., Lobchuk, M. M., & Brajtman, S. (2008). Family caregivers' assessment of symptoms in patients with advanced cancer: Concordance with patients and factors affecting accuracy. *Journal of Pain and Symptom Management, 35*(1), 70–82. https://doi.org/10.1016/j.jpainsymman.2007.02.038

Melzack, R. (1975). The McGill Pain Questionnaire: Major properties and scoring methods. *Pain, 1,* 277–299.

Mendelson, G. (1995). "Compensation neurosis" revisited: Outcome studies of the effects of litigation. *Journal of Psychosomatic Research, 39*(6), 695–706.

Merskey, H., & Teasell, R. W. (2000). The disparagement of pain: Social influences on medical thinking. *Pain Research and Management, 5*(4), 259–270. https://doi.org/10.1155/2000/565309

Michael, G. E., Sporer, K. A., & Youngblood, G. M. (2007). Women are less likely than men to receive prehospital analgesia for isolated extremity injuries. *American Journal of Emergency Medicine, 25,* 901–906. https://doi.org/10.1016/j.ajem.2007.02.001

Monsivais, D. B. (2013). Decreasing the stigma burden of chronic pain. *Journal of the American Association of Nurse Practitioners, 25*(10), 551–556. https://doi.org/10.1111/1745-7599.12010

Morasco, B. J., Gritzner, S., Lewis, L., Oldham, R., Turk, D. C., & Dobscha, S. K. (2011). Systematic review of prevalence, correlates, and treatment outcomes for chronic non-cancer pain in patients with comorbid substance use disorder. *Pain, 152,* 488–497. https://doi.org/10.1016/j.pain.2010.10.009

Mularski, R. A., White-Chu, F., Overbay, D., Miller, L., Asch, S. M., & Ganzini, L. (2006). Measuring pain as the 5th vital sign does not improve quality of pain management. *Journal of General Internal Medicine, 21,* 607–612.

Nguyen, R. H. N., Turner, R. M., Rydell, S. A., MacLehose, R. F., & Harlow, B. L. (2013). Perceived stereotyping and seeking care for chronic vulvar pain. *Pain Medicine, 14*(10), 1461–1467. https://doi.org/10.1111/pme.12151

Nicholson, B., & Verma, S. (2004). Comorbidities in chronic neuropathic pain. *Pain Medicine, 5*(Suppl 1), S9–S27. https://doi.org/10.1111/j.1526-4637.2004.04019.x

Overmeer, T., Boersma, K., Main, C. J., & Linton, S. J. (2009). Do physical therapists change their beliefs, attitudes, knowledge, skills and behaviour after a biopsychosocially orientated university course? *Journal of Evaluation in Clinical Practice, 15*(4), 724–732. https://doi.org/10.1111/j.1365-2753.2008.01089.x

Prkachin, K. M., Mass, H., & Mercer, S. R. (2004). Effects of exposure on perception of pain expression. *Pain, 111*(1–2), 8–12. https://doi.org/10.1016/j.pain.2004.03.027

Prkachin, K. M., & Rocha, E. M. (2010). High levels of vicarious exposure bias pain judgments. *The Journal of Pain, 11*(9), 904–909. https://doi.org/10.1016/j.jpain.2009.12.015

Prkachin, K. M., Solomon, P., Hwang, T., & Mercer, S. R. (2001). Does experience influence judgements of pain behaviour? Evidence from relatives of pain patients and therapists. *Pain Research and Management, 6*(2), 105–112. https://doi.org/10.1155/2001/108098

Raftery, K. A., Smith-Coggins, R., & Chen, A. (1995). Gender-associated differences in emergency department pain management. *Annals of Emergency Medicine, 26*(4), 414–421.

Rainville, J., Sobel, J. B., Hartigan, C., & Wright, A. (1997). The effect of compensation involvement on the reporting of pain and disability by patients referred for rehabilitation of chronic low back pain. *Spine, 22*(17), 2016–2024.

Ransford, A. O., Douglas, C., & Mooney, V. (1976). The pain drawing as an aid to the psychologic evaluation of patients with low-back pain. *Spine, 1*(2), 1–127. https://doi.org/10.1097/01.brs.0000244674.99258.f9

Redinbaugh, E. M., Baum, A., DeMoss, C., Fello, M., & Arnold, R. (2002). Factors associated with the accuracy of family caregiver estimates of patient pain. *Journal of Pain and Symptom Management, 23*(1), 31–38.

Robinson, M. E., & Wise, E. A. (2003). Gender bias in the observation of experimental pain. *Pain, 104*(1–2), 259–264. https://doi.org/10.1016/S0304-3959(03)00014-9

Rohling, M. L., Binder, L. M., & Langhinrichsen-Rohling, J. (1995). Money matters: A meta-analytic review of the association between financial compensation and the experience and treatment of chronic pain. *Health Psychology, 14*(6), 537–547.

Safdar, B., Heins, A., Homel, P., Miner, J., Neighbor, M., Desandre, P., … Todd, K. H. (2009). Impact of physician and patient gender on pain management in the emergency department—a multicenter study. *Pain Medicine, 10*(2), 364–372. https://doi.org/10.1111/j.1526-4637.2008.00524.x

Salmon, P., & Manyande, A. (1996). Good patients cope with their pain: Postoperative analgesia and nurses' perceptions of their patients' pain. *Pain, 68*(1), 63–68. https://doi.org/10.1016/S0304-3959(96)03171-5

Scarry, E. (1985). *The body in pain*. New York, NY: Oxford University Press.

Schiavenato, M., & Craig, K. D. (2010). Pain assessment as a social transaction beyond the "gold standard". *The Clinical Journal of Pain, 26*, 667–676.

Schneider, J., Kaplan, S. H., Greenfield, S., Li, W., & Wilson, I. B. (2004). Better physician-patient relationships are associated with higher reported adherence to antiretroviral therapy in patients with HIV infection. *The Journal of General Internal Medicine, 19*, 1096–1103.

Sharp, T. J., & Harvey, A. G. (2001). Chronic pain and posttraumatic stress disorder: Mutual maintenance? *Clinical Psychology Review, 21*(6), 857–877.

Singla, M., Jones, M., Edwards, I., & Kumar, S. (2015). Physiotherapists' assessment of patients' psychosocial status: Are we standing on thin ice? A qualitative descriptive study. *Manual Therapy, 20*(2), 328–334. https://doi.org/10.1016/j.math.2014.10.004

Sjöström, B., Haljamäe, H., Dahlgren, L.-O., & Lindström, B. (1997). Assessment of postoperative pain: Impact of clinical experience and professional role. *Acta Anaesthesiologica Scandinavica, 41*(3), 339–344. https://doi.org/10.1111/j.1399-6576.1997.tb04695.x

Slade, S. C., Molloy, E., & Keating, J. L. (2009). Stigma experienced by people with nonspecific chronic low back pain: A qualitative study. *Pain Medicine, 10*(1), 143–154. https://doi.org/10.1111/j.1526-4637.2008.00540.x

Sneeuw, K. C. A., Aaronson, N. K., Sprangers, M. A. G., Detmar, S. B., Wever, L. D. V., & Schornagel, J. H. (1999). Evaluating the quality of life of cancer patients: Assessments by patients, significant others, physicians and nurses. *British Journal of Cancer, 81*(1), 87–94. https://doi.org/10.1038/sj.bjc.6690655

Sneeuw, K. C. A., Sprangers, M. A. G., & Aaronson, N. K. (2002). The role of health care providers and significant others in evaluating the quality of life of patients with chronic disease. *Journal of Clinical Epidemiology, 55*, 1130–1143.

Solomon, P. E., Prkachin, K. M., & Farewell, V. (1997). Enhancing sensitivity to facial expression of pain. *Pain, 71*(3), 279–284. https://doi.org/10.1016/S0304-3959(97)03377-0

Sommer, M., de Rijke, J. M., van Kleef, M., Kessels, A. G. H., Peters, M. L., Geurts, J. W. J. M., … Marcus, M. A. E. (2008). The prevalence of postoperative pain in a sample of 1490 surgical inpatients. *European Journal of Anaesthesiology, 25*(4), 267–274. https://doi.org/10.1017/S0265021507003031

Staton, L. J., Panda, M., Chen, I., Genao, I., Kurz, J., Pasanen, M., … Cykert, S. (2007). When race matters: Disagreement in pain perception between patients and their physicians in primary care. *Journal of the National Medical Association, 99*(5), 532–538.

Stewart, M. A. (1996). Effective physician-patient communication and health outcomes: A review. *Canadian Medical Association Journal, 152*, 1423–1433.

Sullivan, M. J. L., Martel, M. O., Tripp, D. A., Savard, A., & Crombez, G. (2006). Catastrophic thinking and heightened perception of pain in others. *Pain, 123*(1–2), 37–44. https://doi.org/10.1016/j.pain.2006.02.007

Sullivan, M. J. L., Thibault, P., Savard, A., Catchlove, R., Kozey, J., & Stanish, W. D. (2006). The influence of communication goals and physical demands on different dimensions of pain behavior. *Pain, 125*(3), 270–277. https://doi.org/10.1016/j.pain.2006.06.019

Sullivan, M. J. L., Yakobov, E., Scott, W., & Tait, R. (2014). Perceived injustice and adverse recovery outcomes. *Psychological Injury and Law, 7*(4), 325–324. https://doi.org/10.1007/s12207-014-9209-8

Tait, R. C. (1983). Psychological factors in chronic benign pain: Evaluation and treatment. *Current Concepts in Pain, 1*, 10–15.

Tait, R. C., & Chibnall, J. T. (1994). Observer perceptions of chronic low back pain. *Journal of Applied Social Psychology, 24*(5), 415–431.

Tait, R. C., & Chibnall, J. T. (1997). Physician judgments of chronic pain patients. *Social Science & Medicine, 45*(8), 1199–1205. https://doi.org/10.1016/S0277-9536(97)00033-6

Tait, R. C., Chibnall, J. T., House, K., & Biehl, J. (2016). Medical judgments across the range of reported pain severity: Clinician and lay perspectives. *Pain Medicine, 17*(7), 1269–1281. https://doi.org/10.1093/pm/pnv076

Tait, R. C., Chibnall, J. T., & Kalauokalani, D. (2009). Provider judgments of patients in pain: Seeking symptom certainty. *Pain Medicine (Malden, Mass.), 10*(1), 11–34. https://doi.org/10.1111/j.1526-4637.2008.00527.x

Tait, R. C., Chibnall, J. T., Luebbert, A., & Sutter, C. (2005). Effect of treatment success and empathy on surgeon attributions for back surgery outcomes. *Journal of Behavioral Medicine, 28*(4), 301–312. https://doi.org/10.1007/s10865-005-9007-6

Tait, R. C., Chibnall, J. T., & Margolis, R. B. (1990). Pain extent: Relations with psychological state, pain severity, pain history, and disability. *Pain, 41*(3), 295–301. https://doi.org/10.1016/0304-3959(90)90006-Y

Tait, R. C., Chibnall, J. T., Miller, L., & Werner, C. A. (2011). Judging pain and disability: Effects of pain severity and physician specialty. *Journal of Behavioral Medicine, 34*(3), 218–224. https://doi.org/10.1007/s10865-010-9302-8

Taylor, A. G., Skelton, J. A., & Butcher, J. (1984). Duration of pain condition and physical pathology as determinants of nurses' assessments of patients in pain. *Nursing Research, 33*, 4–8.

Teske, K., Daut, R. L., & Cleeland, C. S. (1983). Relationships between nurses' observations and patients' self-reports of pain. *Pain, 16*, 289–296. https://doi.org/10.1016/0304-3959(83)90117-3

Tesser, A., & Martin, L. (1996). The psychology of evaluation. In *Social psychology: Handbook of basic principles* (pp. 400–432). London, England: Guilford Press.

Todd, K. G., Samaroo, N., & Hoffman, J. R. (1993). Ethnicity as a risk factor for inadequate emergency department analgesia. *The Journal of the American Medical Association, 269*(3), 1537–1539. https://doi.org/10.1001/jama.269.12.1537

Toye, F., & Barker, K. (2010). "Could I be imagining this?"—the dialectic struggles of people with persistent unexplained back pain. *Disability and Rehabilitation, 32*(21), 1722–1732. https://doi.org/10.3109/09638281003657857

Toye, F., & Barker, K. (2012). Persistent non-specific low back pain and patients' experience of general practice: A qualitative study. *Primary Health Care Research & Development, 13*(1), 72–84. https://doi.org/10.1017/S1463423611000387

Turk, D. C., & Okifuji, A. (1996). Perception of traumatic onset, compensation status, and physical findings: Impact on pain severity, emotional distress, and disability in chronic pain patients. *Journal of Behavioral Medicine, 19*(5), 435–453. https://doi.org/10.1007/BF01857677

Turk, D. C., & Okifuji, A. (1999). Does sex make a difference in the prescription of treatments and the adaptation to chronic pain by cancer and non-cancer patients? *Pain, 82*(2), 139–148. https://doi.org/10.1016/S0304-3959(99)00041-X

Turk, D. C., & Okifuji, A. (2001). Pain terms and taxonomies. In D. Loeser, S. H. Butler, J. J. Chapman, & D. C. Turk (Eds.), *Bonica's management of pain* (3rd ed., pp. 18–25). Philadelphia, PA: Lippincott Williams & Wilkins.

Upshur, C. C., Bacigalupe, G., & Luckmann, R. (2010). "They don't want anything to do with you": Patient views of primary care management of chronic pain. *Pain Medicine, 11*(12), 1791–1798. https://doi.org/10.1111/j.1526-4637.2010.00960.x

Van Houdenhove, B., Neerinckx, E., Onghena, P., Vingerhoets, A., Lysens, R., & Vertommen, H. (2002). Daily hassles reported by chronic fatigue syndrome and fibromyalgia patients in tertiary care: A controlled quantitative and qualitative study. *Psychotherapy and Psychosomatics, 71*, 207–213.

Vervoort, T., Caes, L., Crombez, G., Koster, E., Van Damme, S., Dewitte, M., & Goubert, L. (2011). Parental catastrophizing about children's pain and selective attention to varying levels of facial expression of pain in children: A dot-probe study. *Pain, 152*(8), 1751–1757. https://doi.org/10.1016/j.pain.2011.03.015

Von Baeyer, C. L., Bergstrom, K. J., Brodwin, M. G., & Brodwin, S. K. (1983). Invalid use of pain drawings in psychological screening of back pain patients. *Pain, 16*(1), 103–107. https://doi.org/10.1016/0304-3959(83)90089-1

Von Korff, M., Crane, P., Lane, M., Miglioretti, D. L., Simon, G., Saunders, K., … Kessler, R. (2005). Chronic spinal pain and physical-mental comorbidity in the United States: Results from the national comorbidity survey replication. *Pain, 113*(3), 331–339. https://doi.org/10.1016/j.pain.2004.11.010

Weissman, D. E., & Haddox, J. D. (1989). Opioid pseudoaddiction—an iatrogenic syndrome. *Pain, 36*, 363–366.

Werner, A., & Malterud, K. (2003). It is hard work behaving as a credible patient: Encounters between women with chronic pain and their doctors. *Social Science & Medicine, 57*(8), 1409–1419. https://doi.org/10.1016/S0277-9536(02)00520-8

Williams, A. C. d. C. (2002). Facial expression of pain: An evolutionary account. *The Behavioral and Brain Sciences, 25*(4), 439–455. https://doi.org/10.1017/S0140525X02000080

Williams, A. C. d. C. (2004). Assessing chronic pain and its impact. In R. H. Dworkin & W. S. Breithart (Eds.), *Psychosocial aspects of pain: A handbook for health care providers* (pp. 97–115). Seattle, WA: IASP Press.

Williams, L. A., Cox, B. J., & Enns, M. W. (2003). Mood and anxiety disorders associated with chronic pain: An examination in a nationally representative sample. *Pain, 106*(1–2), 127–133. https://doi.org/10.1016/S0304-3959(03)00301-4

Wilson, B., & McSherry, W. (2006). A study of nurses' inferences of patients' physical pain. *Journal of Clinical Nursing, 15*(4), 459–468. https://doi.org/10.1111/j.1365-2702.2006.01358.x

Yeager, K. A., Miaskowski, C., Dibble, S. L., & Wallhagen, M. (1995). Differences in pain knowledge and perception of the pain experience between outpatients with cancer and their family caregivers. *Oncology Nursing Forum, 22*, 1235–1241.

Zastrow, A., Faude, V., Seyboth, F., Niehoff, D., Herzog, W., & Löwe, B. (2008). Risk factors of symptom underestimation by physicians. *Journal of Psychosomatic Research, 64*(5), 543–551. https://doi.org/10.1016/j.jpsychores.2007.11.010

Part V

Observer Responses to Others' Pain

Chapter 13
Beyond Operant Theory of Observer Reinforcement of Pain Behavior

Shannon M. Clark, Michelle T. Leonard, Annmarie Cano, and Bethany Pester

Abstract Operant theory has guided theoretical and empirical developments in the field of chronic pain for decades. This model has been the primary perspective from which behavioral interventions for chronic pain have been drawn. Recent evidence suggests that there is a need to expand upon the operant model with conceptual models found in the interpersonal, empathy, and pain communication literature. Although they each have a unique focus (e.g., communication, empathy), they each highlight the interpersonal dynamics that can impact the experience of pain for patients. Evidence is needed to know the extent to which treatment can intervene on these influential relationship variables and further, to elucidate the unique interplay between the communication of spouses in the context of pain and behavioral responses of close others. The theoretical models found in the interpersonal, empathy, and pain communication literature provide a way to view pain expressions in the context of the relationship and the deeper idiosyncratic meaning that these may have for an individual with chronic pain (ICP). These models provide a richer understanding of the motivations and antecedents that lead an observer to respond to a loved one's pain behaviors and the effects of different observer responses on an ICP's subjective rating of pain. Addressing communication, empathy, and intimacy correlates of observer responses to pain and gathering a better understanding of the communicative role of pain behaviors is necessary, as this is likely the direction that treatments for chronic pain are headed.

Keywords Partner responses · Reinforcement · Pain behavior · Emotional validation · Operant theory · Pain communication · Empathy

S. M. Clark · A. Cano · B. Pester
Wayne State University, Detroit, MI, USA

M. T. Leonard (✉)
University of Michigan–Dearborn, Dearborn, MI, USA
e-mail: acano@wayne.edu

© Springer International Publishing AG, part of Springer Nature 2018
T. Vervoort et al. (eds.), *Social and Interpersonal Dynamics in Pain*,
https://doi.org/10.1007/978-3-319-78340-6_13

Introduction

Operant theory has guided theoretical and empirical developments in the field of chronic pain for over four decades. In 1976, Fordyce published his seminal work, *Behavioral Methods for Chronic Pain and Illness* (Fordyce, 1976), which contextualized patient behavior in such a way that led to effective interventions that enlist the support of family members. Fordyce's operant model posits that reinforcement from close others influences another's experience of pain, including pain expressions and pain behaviors. This model has been the primary perspective from which behavioral interventions for chronic pain have drawn. Recent evidence, however, suggests that there is a need to expand upon the operant model with conceptual models found in the interpersonal, empathy, and pain communication literature. The purpose of this chapter is to provide an overview of the operant model of pain and to describe other perspectives that can be used to conceptualize the role of social responses to pain. Clinical recommendations based on these perspectives are also offered.

The Operant Theory of Pain

According to the operant theory, increased or prolonged pain severity or disability can be viewed as a function of learning and conditioning that occurs when one's environment directly or indirectly reinforces pain behaviors (Fordyce, 1976). Pain behaviors include but are not limited to facial expressions of pain, verbal and para-verbal expressions of pain, avoidance of painful activities, and bodily movements such as changes in gait, rubbing the affected area, and wincing. Close others, such as intimate partners or close family members, can be the most influential sources of reinforcement because of their frequent and close contact with individuals with chronic pain (ICPs). Loved ones may reinforce pain behavior in multiple ways. First, positive reinforcement of pain behaviors can increase the likelihood that an ICP expresses pain behaviors in the future. For instance, a loved one's attention in response to a verbal statement about pain (e.g., "I am in too much pain today") may increase the likelihood that an ICP will express that feeling again. Second, the removal of a difficult or painful task or activity can negatively reinforce pain behavior. For example, a loving spouse may wash the dishes for his/her partner when the partner engages in pain behaviors such as lying down, which in turn, may increase the likelihood that his partner will engage in this pain behavior the next time the dishes are dirty. Third, extinction may also play a role. For instance, not attending to pain behaviors is expected to result in a decrease of pain behaviors. Fourth, a lack of reinforcement of well behaviors, such as remaining active, eating a balanced diet, engaging in activity pacing, or using medications effectively to keep pain at a manageable level, may also occur. That is, a loved one may not notice or give attention to his partner in pain when the partner is taking steps to maintain wellness. Unfortunately, this pattern of not attending to well behaviors may lead to an extinction of well behaviors. Not only are ICPs' pain behaviors subject to reinforce-ment, but loved ones' responses may also be reinforced. Loved ones can be recipro-cally reinforced by ICPs' gratitude and/or feelings of caring that are elicited when assistance is provided. Operant theory, therefore, sets the stage for understanding couples' interaction patterns within the context of pain.

One frequent way in which these types of dynamics are studied quantitatively is through self-reported spouse responses. The Multidimensional Pain Inventory (MPI; Kerns, Turk, & Rudy, 1985) is among the most common measures used in the literature. Among other aspects of an ICP's pain experience, this measure provides scores on three different types of spouse or significant other responses to pain: solic-itous, punishing/negative, and distracting. Solicitous responses are best character-ized as attentive and concerned in nature (e.g., asking what he/she can do to help or taking over one's jobs/duties). Negative or punishing spouse responses represent actions that involve the direct expression of frustration or anger toward the ICP. Distracting spouse responses involve a close other attempting to divert an ICP's attention away from their pain by engaging in another activity (e.g., turning on the television or reading to their partner). In addition to the MPI, there are several other measures of spouse responding that have been used in the literature. For instance, the Spouse Response Inventory (Schwartz, Jensen, & Romano, 2005) was devel-oped to assess not only responses to pain behaviors but also responses to well behaviors.

Numerous research studies have shown support for the operant model of pain. A study utilizing healthy volunteers found that reinforcement increased the frequency of facial pain expressions to pain (Kunz, Rainville, & Lautenbacher, 2011). Moreover, this same study found that these reinforced facial responses were also associated with self-report pain ratings. This study is unique as much of the research on the operant model uses self-report measures like the ones mentioned above. For example, perceptions of an observing partner's responses to an ICP's pain behavior have been found to be associated with an ICP's pain severity, pain disability, and depressive symptoms (Stroud, Turner, Jensen, & Cardenas, 2006). Receiving nega-tive responses, as reported by ICPs, has also been found to be associated with depressive symptoms (Stroud et al., 2006). Additionally, perceived solicitous responses from loved ones appear to increase pain behaviors in ICPs as well. Block, Kremer, and Gaylor (1980) sampled 20 married patients with chronic pain and found that subjective numerical pain ratings increased in the presence of the spouse for those ICPs who reported that their partners were solicitous in responding to their pain. Further, pain decreased in the presence of the spouse when partners in pain reported that their spouses were non-solicitous in responding. In addition, partner anxiety has also been linked to perceived partner solicitous behavior and, in turn, increased reported pain by ICPs (Davis, Bergeron, Sadikaj, Corsini-Munt, & Steben, 2015). A complete review of the studies that rely on these self-report measures is not provided herein, as the use of self-report measures provides incomplete support from an operant perspective. That is, it is difficult to know whether a partner response reinforced behavior without also examining the consequences of the part-ner response. The MPI and SRI do not assess consequences. Another weakness of self-report surveys of partner responses is that they typically rely on retrospective reporting.

Thus, observational studies assessing the relationship between pain behaviors and observer responses as they occur in the moment have been conducted, which also support an operant theory of pain. A key breakthrough in this area comes from Romano et al. (1992), who observed couples while they engaged in routine household activities in a laboratory setting, such as sweeping a floor. Spouses of patients with pain, specifically with musculoskeletal pain, were more likely to respond to their partners' nonverbal pain behaviors (e.g., limping) with solicitous behavior (e.g., taking over a task) compared to spouses of healthy individuals. Additionally, ICPs were more likely to engage in nonverbal pain behaviors in response to spouse solicitous behaviors than their healthy counterparts. A second study using the same observational methodology and sample found that spouse solicitous responses to pain behaviors were related to greater observed patient pain behaviors and disability as assessed by the Sickness Impact Profile (Romano et al., 1995). Furthermore, spouse solicitous responses were related to physical dysfunction (e.g., mobility, body care) for only those patients who reported relatively greater depression. This suggests that solicitous behaviors may be especially reinforcing for individuals who report greater distress. Other studies utilizing behavioral observation similarly found that spouse solicitous responses were associated with increased pain behaviors in patients. Paulsen and Altmaier (1995) observed patients with chronic low back pain engage in routine daily activities such as walking up and down stairs. Consistent with the operant model, patients who reported greater frequency of spouse responses to displays of pain showed more pain behaviors compared to those who reported fewer solicitous responses.

However, there are notable limitations to the research supporting the operant model as a conceptual framework for chronic pain. As noted above, self-report measures relying on retrospective recall of interactions provide limited validity. Although the observational studies offer a more sophisticated approach, a limitation in this research is an apparent lack of attention to Fordyce's (1976) comments on ignoring pain behaviors. Fordyce placed less emphasis on ignoring (i.e., extinction of) pain behavior, and instead, highlighted the importance of reinforcing well behavior and adaptive coping skills. This is consistent with the behavioral literature that states that the reinforcement of alternative behavior is more effective than extinction (Petscher, Rey, & Bailey, 2009). However, researchers have not examined this idea in a chronic pain population and couple-based clinical interventions that offer support for an operant model tend to incorporate more than just behavioral techniques (e.g., psychoeducation) into the treatments, which could cloud the mechanism of action.

The utility of empirical studies supporting operant theory extends to the clinical literature on pain management as well. Because pain behavior is understood as a behavioral manifestation of pain sensations, as well as other factors including reinforcement history (Fordyce, 1976), an assumption underlying many individual treatments for pain has been that pain behavior and interference are symptoms that must be reduced or eliminated. Because of the presumptive link between pain severity and behaviors, it was assumed that pain severity would also decrease, as demonstrated by the many pain intervention studies that focused on pain severity as the primary outcome (Flor & Birbaumer, 1993; Keefe, Dunsmore, & Burnett, 1992; Sanders et al., 1989; Syrjala, Donaldson, Davis, Kippes, & Carr, 1995). Recently, however, intervention researchers have acknowledged that accompanying decreases in pain severity may not occur (McCracken, Gauntlett-Gilbert, & Vowles, 2007; McCracken, Vowles, & Eccleston, 2004, 2005). These researchers have acknowledged that while pain may not be alleviated by the interventions, the focus on pain behavior and interference with daily activities nevertheless has great clinical importance.

Outcomes for individual treatments based in behavioral methods that involve the reinforcement of more "healthy" behaviors have support from scholarly reviews on the operant model (Gatzounis, Schrooten, Crombez, & Vlaeyen, 2012; Turner & Chapman, 1982). More relevant to the scope of this chapter, however, is the work that incorporates romantic partners into these treatment paradigms. Keefe, Caldwell, Baucom, and Salley (1996) and Keefe et al. (1999) have shown that a couple-based intervention for the treatment of osteoarthritis (OA) that included an attention-based reinforcement by providing spousal pain coping skills training resulted in more decreased pain behavior and pain severity when compared to individual treatment. In a study comparing only an operant program to an operant program combined with cognitive coping skills training added to a wait list control group, Kole-Snijders et al. (1999) found that both treatment groups did better in terms of activity tolerance, pain behavior, and pain control post treatment. However, the treatment that included the cognitive skills component seemed to show more positive outcomes than the operant training program alone. More recent work with patients with OA and their spouses also seems to support an operant framework. Specifically, couples who participated in an education and support intervention showed decreased punishing responses post treatment (with a similar trend for distracting responses) and at a 6-month follow-up, an increase in supportive behavior (Martire, Schulz, Keefe, Rudy, & Starz, 2008).

Despite the support for the operant model, both clinically and empirically, not all research shows the proposed direct link between solicitous responses from spouses and loved ones reinforcing pain behaviors in ICPs. Although the operant model suggests that all verbal responses to pain, including empathic validation, should be considered reinforcing, the evidence from the observational studies, limitations standing, does not yet support this; thus, different ways of thinking about spouse responses are needed. Other theoretical perspectives may aid in understanding the role of a variety of observer responses to pain, such as empathic validation. These other perspectives look beyond the reinforcement of pain behavior and consider a broad variety of outcomes and meanings related to significant other responses, such as quality of life and relationship satisfaction for ICPs and their partners. Alternative models stemming from the literature on pain, empathy, and interpersonal relationships may provide additional perspectives and methods for investigating the role of spouse responses on ICPs.

Beyond Operant Theory: Alternative Theoretical Perspectives

There have been several alternative theoretical perspectives that have been put forth in the literature. Although they each have a unique focus (e.g., communication, empathy), they each highlight the interpersonal dynamics that can impact the experience of pain for patients. These models will be outlined below with supportive evidence from the literature.

Communal Coping Model

Pain catastrophizing has been described as a pattern of negative cognitions associated with the pain experience, with components of magnification, rumination, and helplessness. This construct has received a great deal of attention in the literature due to the association of pain catastrophizing with both pain and psychological distress (Sullivan et al., 2001). The communal coping model (Sullivan et al., 2001) was put forth to describe how an ICP's use of pain catastrophizing may serve to communicate an increased need of support from others. From this perspective, pain catastrophizing in both ICPs and their observing partners may influence the function of verbal pain expression. Pain catastrophizing may serve a social function and act to gain both positive and negative attention. From the viewpoint of the communal coping model, individuals engage in pain catastrophizing to elicit empathy, assistance, and social support from others. Receiving support may result in decreased pain, but more specifically, may validate that pain is difficult to cope with.

In support of this communicative hypothesis, Sullivan, Adams, and Sullivan (2004) found an interaction effect between the social environment and pain catastrophizing on the duration of emitted pain behaviors. People who underwent a painful task and reported higher levels of pain catastrophizing displayed facial and vocal expressions of pain for a longer duration when an observer was present during the task. However, individuals reporting lower levels of pain catastrophizing did not differ in the duration of pain expression when they were being observed or when they were alone. Keefe et al. (2003) found evidence for a communal model of pain catastrophizing in a sample of 70 patients with gastrointestinal cancers and their caregivers. Based on measures completed by patients and caregivers, caregivers of patients who engaged in catastrophizing perceived the patient as having more pain and pain behaviors, and the catastrophizing patient reported receiving more instrumental support. Similarly, Sullivan, Martel, Tripp, Savard, and Crombez (2006) found that pain catastrophizing impacts an observer's perception of pain severity. Forty participants were videotaped completing the cold pressor task, an acute pain task requiring participants to hold their hand in a basin of extremely cold water. Patients reporting higher levels of pain catastrophizing who underwent the cold pressor task reported more intense pain when being viewed by unknown observers versus when they were alone. Those who reported engaging in high pain catastrophizing were viewed as experiencing more intense pain from novel individuals watching them complete the cold pressor task. Additionally, the relationship between pain catastrophizing and inferred pain was mediated by the overt pain behavior displayed by the participant. Finally, Burns et al. (2015) also found support for the communal coping model in a sample of 105 couples. This study found that ICPs engaged in more pain catastrophizing when a partner was present. Moreover, the results from the study found that increases in pain catastrophizing were associated with increased spouse reports of ICP behavior. These same increases in pain catastrophizing were associated with patients' perceptions that their spouses were more supportive and engaged in fewer negative responses toward them. This provides evidence for the communal coping model and a social reinforcement component of pain behaviors, even in the presence of strangers.

In sum, the research literature seems to show support for the communal coping model of pain catastrophizing. This model has an element of more traditional models, in terms of how spouses respond to ICP pain catastrophizing; however, it provides a much more complex picture of the pain experience from an interpersonal sense. Although this model is supported, there are nonetheless limitations and directions for future research. Of note, most studies in this area utilize self-report measures of pain catastrophizing. Although the measures are well validated, using more observational methods in studies to understand how cognitive aspects of catastrophizing might specifically be communicated between partners would be fruitful (Cano, Leong, Williams, May, & Lutz, 2012). By understanding how specific elements of pain catastrophizing are communicated, more targeted interventions can be examined.

Sociocommunicative Models and Empathy

Hadjistavropoulos and Craig (2002) offer a sociocommunicative framework for understanding both self-reported and observed pain. From this model, pain is first processed internally by the individual experiencing it. This processing, however, is influenced by contextual factors that are specific to that individual. Next, the individual expresses pain, influenced by internal processes, to others around them (i.e., self-reported verbal and nonverbal expression). Observers then decode the verbal and nonverbal expressions provided by that individual in pain, which will in turn be influenced by the biases of the observer.

Goubert et al. (2005) built on this sociocommunications model to better understand the dyadic processes involved in the communication of chronic pain. The authors acknowledge that characteristics of the ICP and observer may influence the observer's sense of knowing about the ICP's experience. Observer responses to pain are shaped by several cognitive and environmental influences; both bottom-up (i.e., characteristics of the ICP) and top-down (i.e., characteristics of the observer) processes can alter the presence and type of responses provided by an observer witnessing a loved one in pain. Specific examples of these bottom-up factors could include pain history, expressed anticipatory distress, or pain behaviors. Top-down factors could include the observers' own experiences with pain, their level of perceived impact of the pain on their relationship, or the cues that they are detecting from their loved one who is expressing pain. Furthermore, social and developmental factors of both partners may influence their communication skills in general, and further, the expression and response to pain may serve an evolutionary function, informing both partners of danger or threat of actual injury (Craig, 2004).

These theoretical perspectives highlight the role that pain expression can play in terms of communication between couple members. This communication could serve to elicit instrumental or emotionally based support. Adding to the literature on the role of pain communication, cognitive factors have been thoroughly researched as both top-down and bottom-up characteristics of the ICP and observer that influence pain communication. One of these cognitive factors includes perceived threat (i.e., fear in the moment that pain is about to occur; Leeuw et al., 2007). Among ICPs, perceived threat has been linked to increased reported pain ratings. Among observers witnessing loved ones in pain, higher reported threat also increased the likelihood that one would have an avoidant response to pain (Vlaeyen & Linton, 2000). Pain beliefs (e.g., "My pain will be this bad forever"; Williams & Thorn, 1989) and pain rules are also cognitive variables that affect pain communication. Pain rules are rigid beliefs and generalizations that may not have been directly reinforced but are utilized when managing pain (e.g., "All exercise will put me at risk for increased pain and injury, because I assume something strenuous will lead to pain"; Main, Keefe, Jensen, Vlaeyen, & Vowles, 2015).

There has also been work on pain catastrophizing from a sociocommunications framework. Clark et al. (2016) found a significant interaction between pain catastrophizing in participants undergoing the cold pressor task and their observing partners. Couples in which both partners rated their pain anxiety as low or both high were more congruent on individual pain ratings of one partner's pain. That is, pain ratings of one partner's pain were more similar. This finding provides support that partners who report similar levels of pain catastrophizing are more attuned and have a greater "sense of knowing" about their loved one's pain (Goubert et al., 2005).

Batson, Fultz, and Schoenrade (1987) also offer a conceptualization to better understand pain communication and empathy by working backward from observer responses. Broadly, individuals may choose to help for reasons that serve themselves or for empathic reasons related to the person they are helping; these motivations are not mutually exclusive (Batson & Shaw, 1991). From this perspective, responses to distress in others can be divided into two categories: personal distress or empathy. Observers may be more likely to have empathic responses because their motivation to respond comes from their desire to reduce pain in others.

Empathic responses have emerged in the pain field as a point of great debate with researchers acknowledging the potentially positive and negative outcomes of empathic responses to pain such as emotional validation (Cano & Goubert, 2017; Cano & Williams, 2010; Edmond & Keefe, 2015; Linton, McCracken, & Vlaeyen, 2008). Based on work by Reis and Shaver (1988), Cano and colleagues have argued that emotional validation is a type of empathic response that conveys acceptance and attempted understanding of a person's pain-related emotional distress (Cano &

Goubert, 2017; Cano & Williams, 2010). Cano and Goubert (2017) state that emotional disclosures of pain-related distress such as anxiety, anger, or sadness about pain and its impact must be acknowledged in a validating way to promote health and well-being in the person with pain as well as intimacy and closeness with others. It has been suggested that empathic responses to pain can also reinforce pain behaviors (Edmond & Keefe, 2015). However, Cano and Goubert (2017) counter that the validation of emotional disclosures need not result in the reinforcement of other pain behaviors if a proper functional assessment including a range of behaviors and responses are closely investigated.

Regardless, instrumental help and/or emotional validation may increase feelings of well-being in the responding observer; they may find joy in knowing that they were a kind person. Alternatively, validating might also decrease distress or fear in the observer who feels uncomfortable until they have "done their part" (Batson, 1987). When one is not experiencing too much personal distress in response to another's pain, they may be more driven to respond in altruistic ways, focusing only on reducing the pain of others.

Viewing another in pain can also lead to excessive fear and worry in observing partners. Rather than trying to reduce pain in another, fearful and worried observing partners may instead be motivated to reduce stress and pain in themselves. Significant worry in an observer about the pain that their partner might experience (e.g., high pain catastrophizing), may lead to distress and avoidance; this, in turn, may interfere with their ability to perceive pain that is being communicated to them by their partner. Partners without pain may avoid and distance themselves physically and emotionally from their loved ones to decrease distress in themselves. Observers or romantic partners with significant anxiety may further underestimate their partner's pain severity. Underestimating pain may serve as a mechanism for decreasing pain catastrophizing and assist observers in distancing themselves from their partners' pain.

Discussed in Batson et al. (1987), Defensive Distancing Theory helps explain how observers may not respond with validation or support. Batson and colleagues note that in observing others in pain, individuals may feel empathy, which could result in validating the pain of others. However, if observing others in pain leads to psychological distress, individuals may create "distance" from the other in a form of self-protection. Batson et al. (1987) also support the idea that observers who experience distress when faced with a loved one in pain may have increased motivation to resolve their own distress instead of providing validation or support to that loved one (Jaremka, Bunyan, Collins, & Sherman, 2011; Pyszczynski et al., 1995). Distancing oneself from the pain of others may be influenced by low self-esteem that leads them to engage in self-doubt and self-protective behaviors (Jaremka et al., 2011). Observing partners may also attempt to distance themselves by trying to see themselves as different from those in pain. For example, observing partners who are distressed when seeing a loved one in pain may believe that they are inherently different, even on personality traits that are unrelated to illness susceptibility (e.g., cleanliness, wit, etc.; Pyszczynski et al., 1995). It is possible that low self-esteem, anxiety, and a desire to be unlike people who are ill causes some observing partners to struggle in taking the perspective of others and, in turn, have difficulties responding as a selfless and empathic partner. Hadjistavropoulos et al. (2011) support these additions to their original model by also suggesting that pain expression goes beyond a simple act of sharing an emotion and responding to that disclosure, but involves a partner's accurate interpretation of an ICP's pain expression.

The literature supports these top-down and bottom-up factors in regard to how pain messages are communicated, and by understanding these factors we may better predict what propels an observer to respond with validation or empathic concern versus a number of other behavioral responses to a loved one in pain (e.g., withdrawal, avoidance, or providing assistance). Leonard, Issner, Cano, and Williams (2013) gathered research evidence on how good spouses were at interpreting the cognitive/affective pain related communications relayed by patients with pain. Participants in this study were asked to discuss pain with their partners. Partners of ICPs were then asked to infer the feelings and thoughts of their loved one in pain and were assessed for empathic accuracy. Partners of ICPs who reported significant levels of pain catastrophizing about their loved ones' pain reported less empathic accuracy, and in fact, did a poorer job at inferring the feelings and thoughts of their partners in pain. Moreover, pain severity reported by ICPs was related to improved empathic accuracy from the observing partner. Both marital satisfaction and the observing partner's own pain experience served as moderators to these interactions.

In sum, the literature on validation and empathic responses to pain suggests that the outcomes of such responses are complex and may differ based on individual, interpersonal, and contextual differences. What is perceived as supportive by an ICP may result in increased distress for the observer and what is perceived by the observer as empathic, may function negatively for the ICP. Portions of this literature are theoretical in nature and need to be empirically tested to tease apart these caveats. Furthermore, the elements of pain specific instrumental support and emotional validation by one's partner are distinct couple dynamics. Continued research in this area is needed to understand the moderators that influence empathic communication between ICPs and their partners.

Interpersonal and Emotion Regulation Models

Other alternatives to the operant model come from the interpersonal relationships literature. From the perspective of the Intimacy Process Model (Reis & Shaver, 1988), intimacy is enhanced when two things happen: one person engages in emotional disclosure and the other is emotionally responsive to the disclosure. While this transaction assumes some sense of empathy in the observer, the focus is on behavior that conveys acceptance. From the perspective of this model, intimacy can be viewed as a transaction to gain an innate human need, achieved through mutual disclosure, emotional validation, and partner responsiveness. A similar view is taken by Dialectic Behavior Therapy researchers (Fruzzetti & Iverson, 2004, 2006). Emotionally validating responses are thought to increase the sense of intimacy within a couple whereas invalidating responses disturb healthy emotion regulation in the person who disclosed the emotion.

A biological perspective can also be integrated with this interpersonal framework to highlight the potential benefits for validation of an ICP's experience. Krahé, Springer, Weinman, and Fotopoulou (2013) conducted a systematic review of 26 experimental studies on pain that implies that intimacy and interpersonal closeness can modify biological responses to pain. They found that interpersonal interaction can have pain reducing effects, but are contingent on several variables, such as relationship history and individual differences. The authors further state that the effects of intimacy on pain relief are influenced by one's expectations about intimate interactions with others and whether one believes intimate interaction will lead to feelings of safety from threat. Validation may serve as a stress reducer and further decreases one's pain by soothing the emotional arousal that occurs with pain. In other words, responding to distress with acceptance and emotional validation may reinforce pain expression, but not reinforce distress. Validation may allow a person to regulate emotion at the neurological level and reduce stress. Research by Ditzen, Hoppmann, and Klumb (2008) supports that there are physical stress-reducing effects following intimate interaction, which they determined by measuring cortisol levels in participants' saliva. In contrast, reviews of studies on pain and validation reveal that responding with invalidation can result in increased levels of stress and negative affect for both ICPs and their significant others (Edmond & Keefe, 2015; Shenk & Fruzzetti, 2011).

Many empirically supported third generation psychotherapies (e.g., Acceptance and Commitment Therapy and Mindfulness-Based Stress Reduction) also support an intimacy process model and describe the role of validating responses in one's emotional experience. Specifically, these approaches note that validation is not necessarily agreeing with another's experience, but rather, acknowledges that one's feelings, emotions, and responses are legitimate, regardless of accuracy. In the context of significant others, this could be a form of radical acceptance of the other. In one particular study measuring verbalizations emitted by chronic pain patients, ICPs reported that they do not feel as if their suffering or pain is recognized or understood by their close others (Herbette & Rimé, 2004). The importance of feeling understood may be especially important in chronic pain due to the subjective nature of the illness. ICPs often encounter others who do not deem their symptoms to be genuine, and knowing that their experience is accepted and not judged by a close other is critical.

There also appears to be support for the intimacy process and emotion regulation models mentioned above when looking specifically at pain research. While completing an experimental manipulation of pain, the cold pressor task, in a laboratory setting, individuals in pain who disclosed more emotional and verbal expressions of pain were more likely to receive validation from their spouses (Leong, Cano, Wurm, Lumley, & Corley, 2015). Furthermore, in a study of couples in which one partner had chronic pain, it was found that validation from a spouse led to decreased negative affect and negative emotion for ICPs following validation training (Edlund, Carlsson, Linton, Fruzzetti, & Tillfors, 2015). Responses that are perceived by an ICP as invalidating are more closely related to receiving a punishing response from a spouse as opposed to a response of solicitous behavior, such as helping (Cano,

Barterian, & Heller, 2008). Moreover, invalidation from a spouse can result in negative effects for an ICP, and in turn, an ICP's response to that invalidation can exacerbate those negative effects. Cano and Williams (2010) also argued that validation of the emotional expression of pain by one's partner may lead to increased intimacy, more positive affect, and better functioning among individuals with chronic pain. Edmond and Keefe (2015) came to similar conclusions when they reported that validation was associated with increased disclosure of pain and decreased anger and frustration for ICPs. Moreover, they found that validation was not correlated with depression, anxiety, or increased pain in ICPs, but was associated with positive affect and decreased worry among a nonclinical population undergoing a painful task. That is, the consequences of an interchange between partners go beyond the response of one partner. Both the response of validation or invalidation, and the reaction that the ICP has to their partner's response, can alter the observing spouse's response to pain, which may result in positive or negative effects for the ICP. The gender of an ICP adds a complex variable to this interchange. Men and women with chronic pain respond differently when they receive validation or invalidation from their partners. Specifically, in couples where a male partner was struggling with pain, couple invalidation was associated with poorer pain outcomes, while validation was associated with both pain and marital satisfaction (Leong, Cano, & Johansen, 2011).

Further findings from Leonard et al. (2013), a study that looked at videotaped communication between ICPs and their partners, suggest that the observing partner's perceived empathic accuracy is not related to that partner's overt empathic behavior. The observer's perception of being empathic also did not relate to the overt empathic behaviors that were measured by blind observers. Although solicitousness and empathic responses were associated, marital satisfaction influenced this relationship. Among couples that reported higher levels of marital satisfaction, decreased solicitous behavior was related to greater empathic responding in observing partners. Among less satisfied couples, no significant relationship between solicitousness and empathic observer responses was found.

Validation from observers and loved ones plays an integral role in the pain experience of those suffering. It provides stress reduction, increased well-being, regulated affect, and improved intimacy beyond reducing one's subjective rating of pain. However, the perception of empathy determines whether validation provides positive or negative outcomes for ICPs. Given several personal and communicative variables, simply responding or attending to the pain of others may not function the same as validation that produces positive outcomes for ICPs.

Summary of Alternative Models

In sum, communication and interpersonal models, like operant models, hold that the social environment is highly influential in shaping pain behaviors, distress, and adjustment. One could argue that each of these models could be conceptualized as an operant model focusing on different behaviors and reinforcements. For instance, empathic responses could be conceptualized as reinforcing emotional disclosures. However, these other models provide additional avenues of exploration in terms of the mechanisms through which partner responses affect emotion regulation, relationship adjustment, and pain behaviors. Drawing from a larger pool of theoretical and conceptual work, communications, interpersonal, and empathy models offer an integrative way to examine the roles of thoughts, expectations, emotions, and relationship dynamics that can offer additional insights into intervention development. Researchers are beginning to tease apart just what it means for a behavior to be a pain behavior (Cano & Goubert, 2017; Papini et al., 2015), which is a critical preliminary step toward examining the effects of responses to those behaviors. Researchers are also exploring the extent to which a variety of responses may reinforce pain behaviors (Cano & Williams, 2010; Edmond & Keefe, 2015) as well as modulate pain more generally, without necessarily using an operant framework (Krahé et al., 2013).

Future Directions

Clearly understanding the interpersonal nature of pain is urgently important. Evidence is still needed to know the extent to which treatment can intervene on these influential relationship variables and further, to elucidate the unique interplay between the communication of spouses in the context of pain and behavioral responses of close others. Measuring only one partner's perception of validation and invalidation of emotional expression of pain may be too simple of a conceptualization to inform treatment approaches for ICPs and their spouses. Additionally, it is still unclear whether reducing stress and increasing intimacy outweigh the potential of reinforcing pain behaviors.

Nonetheless, partners can engage in a variety of responses to pain and there are numerous factors that influence these responses. Although the literature does seem to support the operant role of spouse responses, this process may be more complex than reinforcement alone. Spouses' responses may provide crucial emotion regulation and relationship enhancement functions. However, there are a great number of unanswered questions regarding spouse responses that must be addressed to develop more comprehensive models that can be used to develop effective interventions for pain.

First, questions remain regarding the operant model and treatment modalities that have branched from this theory. Most notably, the role of extinction of pain behaviors is still unclear and has not been sufficiently studied. Observational studies that measure in-moment pain behaviors followed immediately by a lack of observer response would be necessary to test the effects of planned ignoring on frequency of ICP pain behavior. Promising observational methods exist that can be used in this manner (Paulsen & Altmaier, 1995; Romano et al., 1992, 1995), where pain behaviors (either induced or recorded) are observed as they unfold and responses from close others are either manipulated or varied (e.g., validation, planned ignoring, solicitous helping, or punishing verbal remark). Measuring a spectrum of responses may lead to the development of more specific and effective interventions for ICPs and their loved ones that reduce pain behavior and increase well behaviors. If there is no direct correlation between pain behavior and pain ratings (Labus, Keefe, & Jensen, 2003), further research may continue to support the development of interventions that focus less on pain severity and more on behavior.

Such methodologies will also address questions that remain regarding the alternative theories mentioned above that are both competitive and compatible with the operant model. In this manner, researchers can better test whether emotional validation reinforces pain behaviors, and whether this is consistent in varied environments and with different observers responding. Further, researchers can examine the impact both partners' perceptions of intimacy, emotion regulation, distress, and well-being have on how close others respond. Such research may shed light on how observers can best respond to their partners in pain to maximize positive outcomes.

It is also necessary to integrate communal coping, sociocommunicative and empathy, and interpersonal models regarding observer responses to pain behaviors by assessing ICPs' and observers' perceptions of empathy and support. It is not enough to observe the overt behaviors and responses elicited by ICPs and observers, but researchers must also assess how behaviors are interpreted and how interpretations impact the pain experience. Indeed, in the social support literature, numerous studies have found that perceived support is more strongly associated with relationship satisfaction and well-being than is enacted support (Kaul & Lakey, 2003; Lemay, Clark, & Feeney, 2007; Qadir, Haqqani, Khalid, Huma, & Medhin, 2014). It may be that assessing the interpretation of behavior provided by both ICPs and their partners could provide invaluable insights into the couples' context of pain. For example, if an increase in an ICP's verbal expression of pain is observed, it is also possible to measure how the ICP perceived his/her partner's response. An observing loved one may respond with attention to another's pain; however, it is in the perception of the ICP whether he/she views that response as supportive, validating, or enabling disability. This knowledge is also necessary to inform research about the function of that observer's response in the current moment.

It should be stressed that to enrich research on the operant model of pain and integrate communicative, empathy, and interpersonal models, research must emphasize contemporaneous, in-moment data collection over that of retrospective measures that ask about pain behaviors and responses that have occurred in the past. It is possible that this direction of research will advance Fordyce's gold standard pain model and lead to a more comprehensive conceptualization of the social influences of pain.

Clinical Implications

Although research supports individual focused psychotherapy for ICPs, almost half of patients in a clinical population experiencing interpersonal distress will drop out of these interventions (Carmody, 2001). Furthermore, ICPs experiencing interpersonal distress, such as marital dissatisfaction, have poorer outcomes (Strategier, Chwalisz, Altmaier, Russell, & Lehmann, 1997; Turk, 2005; Turk, Okifuji, Sinclair, & Starz, 1998). This is likely because social stressors impede their ability to utilize the skills learned in their individual therapy (Baucom et al., 2009; Sullivan & Davila, 2010). Given that the operant model addresses a social component, a couple therapy approach focusing on the needs of both ICPs and their spouses would be a logical direction for future chronic pain interventions. Drawing from an operant model, observer behavioral training and education have been a longstanding staple for the treatment of chronic pain. Many treatment programs (as reviewed above) have been built around Fordyce's model (Anderson, Cole, Gullickson, Hudgens, & Roberts, 1977; Fordyce, 1976). Couple based approaches have been researched as a treatment modality for chronic pain and aim to treat the psychological well-being of both partners as this may be beneficial for the ICP's pain experience (Saarijarvi, 1991). There have been, however, alternative treatment approaches to chronic pain, and the evidence for these approaches is building.

Acceptance and commitment therapy has been strongly supported as a valid individual treatment for chronic pain (Hann & McCracken, 2014; Veehof, Oskam, Schreurs, & Bohlmeijer, 2011). While mindfulness-based stress reduction has been supported as an effective treatment component for chronic pain (Kabat-Zinn, 1982; Kabat-Zinn, Lipworth, & Burney, 1985; McCracken et al., 2007; Rosenzweig et al., 2010; Vowles & McCracken, 2008; Vowles, Wetherell, & Sorrell, 2009; Wicksell, Olsson, & Hayes, 2010; Zautra et al., 2008), there is evidence that mindfulness skills and psychological flexibility in the partners of ICPs can affect their own and their partners' pain and depressive symptoms (Cano, Johansen, & Franz, 2005; Cano, Miller, & Loree, 2009; Leonard & Cano, 2006). An increase in mindfulness skills among observing partners has also been shown to not only lead to higher relationship satisfaction but also an improved ability to respond in a constructive manner, perhaps by reducing the distress and fear that leads one to distance him or herself from a partner in pain (Barnes, Brown, Krusemark, Campbell, & Rogge, 2007). Research on couple therapy approaches to chronic pain has taken an acceptance approach using integrative behavioral couples therapy (IBCT) for chronic pain (Cano & Leonard, 2006; McCracken, Carson, Eccleston, & Keefe, 2004). In line with the alternative interpersonal and empathy models mentioned above, IBCT adds mindfulness and acceptance practices, emotional validation, understanding, and empathy to traditional couple communication techniques. Although repairing and building the communication and relationship satisfaction between partners may not be an intuitive treatment approach for chronic pain, research evidence suggests that there is a link between marital satisfaction, partner support, and partner responsiveness with a variety of pain variables (Leonard, Cano, & Johansen, 2006). Future couple-based treatment methods may utilize the best of traditional and integrative couple therapy and mindfulness-based stress reduction. An innovative intervention for couples with chronic pain does just this by teaching psychological and relational flexibility skills to both partners conjointly to promote psychological and relationship well-being in each partner as well as improved pain adjustment in positive relational context (Cano, Corley, Clark, & Martinez, 2017). Researchers are encouraged to continue to explore treatment approaches that target a variety of intrapersonal and interpersonal outcomes.

Conclusion

In sum, Fordyce's (1976) seminal work has led to significant applied and clinical research on the operant model of pain and its associated processes. Further, this work has been informative to treatment modalities centered on manipulating the contingencies of pain behaviors to reduce pain severity among individuals with chronic pain. Although research supporting the operant model holds merit today, there are limitations and nuances that are better accounted for by integrating communicative, empathy, and interpersonal models into the understanding of the function of pain behaviors. Furthermore, the literature suggests that a straightforward operant approach toward intervention may not be the most fruitful approach to dyadic interventions as many of the effect sizes, albeit significant, are small in nature. It has been suggested that other targets to treatment including spousal communication, cognitive aspects of pain (e.g., worry or fear), or even focusing on the quality of the relationship as an important moderator for outcomes (Keefe, Somers, & Martire, 2008; Martire, Schulz, Helgeson, Small, & Saghafi, 2010). These potential targets are consistent with the other theoretical perspectives presented above, and given the role of the observing loved one in responding contingently to pain behaviors, it is vital to integrate these processes into current operant conceptualizations of couple's interactions in the context of pain.

The theoretical models outlined in this chapter provide a way to view pain expressions (whether verbal or behavioral) in the context of the relationship and the deeper idiosyncratic meaning that these may have for IPCs. Furthermore, they provide a richer understanding of the motivations and antecedents that lead an observer to respond to a loved one's pain behaviors and the effects of different observer responses on an ICP's subjective rating of pain. Addressing communication, empathy and intimacy correlates of observer responses to pain and gathering a better understanding of the communicative role of pain behaviors is necessary, as this is likely the direction that treatments for chronic pain are headed.

References

Anderson, T. P., Cole, T. M., Gullickson, G., Hudgens, A., & Roberts, A. H. (1977). Behavior modification of chronic pain: A treatment program by a multidisciplinary team. *Clinical Orthopaedics and Related Research, 129*, 96–100.

Barnes, S., Brown, K. W., Krusemark, E., Campbell, W. K., & Rogge, R. D. (2007). The role of mindfulness in romantic relationship satisfaction and responses to relationship stress. *Journal of Marital and Family Therapy, 33*(4), 482–500.

Batson, C. D. (1987). Prosocial motivation: Is it ever truly altruistic? *Advances in Experimental Social Psychology, 20*, 65–122.

Batson, C. D., Fultz, J., & Schoenrade, P. A. (1987). Distress and empathy: Two qualitatively distinct vicarious emotions with different motivational consequences. *Journal of Personality, 55*(1), 19–39.

Batson, C. D., & Shaw, L. L. (1991). Evidence for altruism: Toward a pluralism of prosocial motives. *Psychological Inquiry, 2*(2), 107–122.

Baucom, D. H., Porter, L. S., Kirby, J. S., Gremore, T. M., Wiesenthal, N., Aldridge, W., … Keefe, F. J. (2009). A couple-based intervention for female breast cancer. *Psycho-Oncology, 18*(3), 276–283. https://doi.org/10.1002/pon.1395

Block, A. R., Kremer, E. F., & Gaylor, M. (1980). Behavioral treatment of chronic pain: The spouse as a discriminative cue for pain behavior. *Pain, 9*(2), 243–252.

Burns, J. W., Gerhart, J. I., Post, K. M., Smith, D. A., Porter, L. S., Schuster, E., … Keefe, F. J. (2015). The communal coping model of pain catastrophizing in daily life: A within-couples daily diary study. *The Journal of Pain, 16*(11), 1163–1175.

Cano, A., Barterian, J. A., & Heller, J. B. (2008). Empathic and nonempathic interaction in chronic pain couples. *Clinical Journal of Pain, 24*(8), 678–684. https://doi.org/10.1097/AJP. 0b013e31816753d8

Cano, A., Corley, A. M., Clark, S. M., & Martinez, S. C. (2017). A couple-based psychological treatment for chronic pain and relationship distress. *Cognitive and Behavioral Practice*.

Cano, A., & Goubert, L. (2017). What's in a name? The case of emotional disclosure of pain-related distress. *The Journal of Pain, 18*(8), 881–888. https://doi.org/10.1016/j.jpain.2017.01.008

Cano, A., Johansen, A. B., & Franz, A. (2005). Multilevel analysis of couple congruence on pain, interference, and disability. *Pain, 118*(3), 369–379. https://doi.org/10.1016/j.pain.2005.09.003

Cano, A., & Leonard, M. T. (2006). Integrative behavioral couple therapy for chronic pain: Promoting behavior change and emotional acceptance. *Journal of Clinical Psychology: In Session, 62*, 1409–1418. https://doi.org/10.1002/jclp.20320

Cano, A., Leong, L. E., Williams, A. M., May, D. K., & Lutz, J. R. (2012). Correlates and consequences of the disclosure of pain-related distress to one's spouse. *Pain, 153*(12), 2441–2447.

Cano, A., Miller, L. R., & Loree, A. (2009). Spouse beliefs about partner chronic pain. *The Journal of Pain, 10*(5), 486–492. https://doi.org/10.1016/j.jpain.2008.11.005

Cano, A., & Williams, A. C. d. C. (2010). Social interaction in pain: Reinforcing pain behaviors or building intimacy? *Pain, 149*, 9–11. https://doi.org/10.1016/j.pain.2009.10.010

Carmody, T. P. (2001). Psychosocial subgroups, coping, and chronic low-back pain. *Journal of Clinical Psychology in Medical Settings, 8*, 137–148.

Clark, S. M., Cano, A., Goubert, L., Vlaeyen, J. W. S., Wurm, L. H., & Corley, A. M. (2016). Pain anxiety and its association with pain congruence trajectories during the cold pressor task. *The Journal of Pain, 18*(4), 396–404.

Craig, K. D. (2004). Social communication of pain enhances protective functions: A comment on Deyo, Prkachin and Mercer (2004). *Pain, 107*(1–2), 5–6.

Davis, S. N., Bergeron, S., Sadikaj, G., Corsini-Munt, S., & Steben, M. (2015). Partner behavioral responses to pain mediate the relationship between partner pain cognitions and pain outcomes in women with provoked vestibulodynia. *Journal of Pain, 16*(6), 549–557. https://doi.org/10.1016/j.jpain.2015.03.002

Ditzen, B., Hoppmann, C., & Klumb, P. (2008). Positive couple interactions and daily cortisol: On the stress-protecting role of intimacy. *Psychosomatic Medicine, 70*(8), 883–889. https://doi.org/10.1097/PSY.0b013e318185c4fc

Edlund, S. M., Carlsson, M. L., Linton, S. J., Fruzzetti, A. E., & Tillfors, M. (2015). I see you're in pain—the effects of partner validation on emotions in people with chronic pain. *Scandinavian Journal of Pain, 6*, 16–21.

Edmond, S., & Keefe, F. J. (2015). Validating pain communication: Current state of the science. *Pain, 156*(2), 215–219.

Flor, H., & Birbaumer, N. (1993). Comparison of the efficacy of electromyographic biofeedback, cognitive-behavioral therapy, and conservative medical interventions in the treatment of chronic musculoskeletal pain. *Journal of Consulting and Clinical Psychology, 61*(4), 653.

Fordyce, W. E. (Ed.). (1976). *Behavioral methods for chronic pain and illness.* St. Louis, MO: C. V. Mosby.

Fruzzetti, A. E., & Iverson, K. M. (2004). Mindfulness, acceptance, validation, and "individual" psychopathology in couples. In S. C. Hayes, V. M. Follette, & M. M. Linehan (Eds.), *Mindfulness and acceptance: Expanding the cognitive-behavioral tradition* (pp. 168–191). New York, NY: Guilford Press.

Fruzzetti, A. E., & Iverson, K. M. (2006). Intervening with couples and families to treat emotion dysregulation and psychopathology. In D. K. Snyder, J. Simpson, & J. N. Hughes (Eds.), *Emotion regulation in couples and families: Pathways to dysfunction and health* (pp. 249–267). Washington, DC: American Psychological Association.

Gatzounis, R., Schrooten, M. G., Crombez, G., & Vlaeyen, J. W. (2012). Operant learning theory in pain and chronic pain rehabilitation. *Current Pain and Headache Reports, 16*(2), 117–126.

Goubert, L., Craig, K., Vervoort, T., Morley, S., Sullivan, M., Williams, A., … Crombez, G. (2005). Facing others in pain: The effects of empathy. *Pain, 118*(3), 285–288. https://doi.org/10.1016/j.pain.2005.10.025

Hadjistavropoulos, T., & Craig, K. (2002). A theoretical framework for understanding self-report and observational measures of pain: A communications model. *Behaviour Research and Therapy, 40*(5), 551–570.

Hadjistavropoulos, T., Craig, K. D., Duck, S., Cano, A., Goubert, L., Jackson, P., … Dever Fitzgerald, T. (2011). A biopsychosocial formulation of pain communication. *Psychological Bulletin, 137*(6), 910–939. https://doi.org/10.1037/a0023876

Hann, K. E., & McCracken, L. M. (2014). A systematic review of randomized controlled trials of acceptance and commitment therapy for adults with chronic pain: Outcome domains, design quality, and efficacy. *Journal of Contextual Behavioral Science, 3*(4), 217–227.

Herbette, G., & Rimé, B. (2004). Verbalization of emotion in chronic pain patients and their psychological adjustment. *Journal of Health Psychology, 9*(5), 661–676.

Jaremka, L. M., Bunyan, D. P., Collins, N. L., & Sherman, D. K. (2011). Reducing defensive distancing: Self-affirmation and risk regulation in response to relationship threats. *Journal of Experimental Social Psychology, 47*(1), 264–268. https://doi.org/10.1016/j.jesp.2010.08.015

Kabat-Zinn, J. (1982). An outpatient program in behavioral medicine for chronic pain patients based on the practice of mindfulness meditation: Theoretical considerations and preliminary results. *General Hospital Psychiatry, 4*, 33–47. https://doi.org/10.1016/0163-8343(82)90026-3

Kabat-Zinn, J., Lipworth, L., & Burney, R. (1985). The clinical use of mindfulness meditation for the self-regulation of chronic pain. *Journal of Behavioral Medicine, 8*(2), 163–190.

Kaul, M., & Lakey, B. (2003). Where is the support in perceived support? The role of generic relationship satisfaction and enacted support in perceived support's relation to low distress. *Journal of Social and Clinical Psychology, 22*(1), 59–78.

Keefe, F. J., Caldwell, D. S., Baucom, D., & Salley, A. (1996). Spouse-assisted coping skills training in the management of osteoarthritic knee pain. *Arthritis Care & Research, 9*(4), 279–291. https://doi.org/10.1002/1529-0131(199608)9:4<279::AID-ANR1790090413>3.0.CO;2-6

Keefe, F. J., Caldwell, D. S., Baucom, D., Salley, A., Robinson, E., Timmons, K., … Helms, M. (1999). Spouse-assisted coping skills training in the management of knee pain in osteoarthritis: Long-term followup results. *Arthritis Care & Research, 12*(2), 101–111. https://doi.org/10.1002/1529-0131(199904)12:2<101::AID-ART5>3.0.CO;2-9

Keefe, F. J., Dunsmore, J., & Burnett, R. (1992). Behavioral and cognitive-behavioral approaches to chronic pain: Recent advances and future directions. *Journal of Consulting and Clinical Psychology, 60*(4), 528.

Keefe, F. J., Lipkus, I., Lefebvre, J. C., Hurwitz, H., Clipp, E., Smith, J., & Porter, L. (2003). The social context of gastrointestinal cancer pain: A preliminary study examining the relation of patient pain catastrophizing to patient perceptions of social support and caregiver stress and negative responses. *Pain, 103*(1–2), 151–156. https://doi.org/10.1016/S0304-3959(02)00447-5

Keefe, F. J., Somers, T. J., & Martire, L. M. (2008). Psychologic interventions and lifestyle modifications for arthritis pain management. *Rheumatic Disease Clinics of North America, 34*(2), 351–368.

Kerns, R. D., Turk, D. C., & Rudy, T. E. (1985). The West Haven-Yale Multidimensional Pain Inventory (WHYMPI). *Pain, 23*(4), 345–356. https://doi.org/10.1016/0304-3959(85)90004-1

Kole-Snijders, A. M., Vlaeyen, J. W., Goossens, M. E., Rutten-van Mölken, M. P., Heuts, P. H., van Breukelen, G., & van Eek, H. (1999). Chronic low-back pain: What does cognitive coping skills training add to operant behavioral treatment? Results of a randomized clinical trial. *Journal of Consulting and Clinical Psychology, 67*(6), 931.

Krahé, C., Springer, A., Weinman, J. A., & Fotopoulou, A. (2013). The social modulation of pain: Others as predictive signals of salience—a systematic review. *Frontiers in Human Neuroscience, 7*, 386.

Kunz, M., Rainville, P., & Lautenbacher, S. (2011). Operant conditioning of facial displays of pain. *Psychosomatic Medicine, 73*(5), 422–431.

Labus, J. S., Keefe, F. J., & Jensen, M. P. (2003). Self-reports of pain intensity and direct observations of pain behavior: When are they correlated? *Pain, 102*(1), 109–124.

Leeuw, M., Houben, R., Severeijns, R., Picavet, H. S. J., Schouten, E. G., & Vlaeyen, J. W. (2007). Pain-Related fear in low back pain: A prospective study in the general population. *European Journal of Pain, 11*(3), 256–266.

Lemay, E. P., Clark, M. S., & Feeney, B. C. (2007). Projection of responsiveness to needs and the construction of satisfying communal relationships. *Journal of Personality and Social Psychology, 92*(5), 834.

Leonard, M. T., & Cano, A. (2006). Pain affects spouses too: Personal experience with pain and catastrophizing as correlates of spouse distress. *Pain, 126*, 139–146. https://doi.org/10.1016/j.pain.2006.06.022

Leonard, M. T., Cano, A., & Johansen, A. B. (2006). Chronic pain in a couples context: A review and integration of theoretical models and empirical evidence. *The Journal of Pain, 7*(6), 377–390. https://doi.org/10.1016/j.jpain.2006.01.442

Leonard, M. T., Issner, J. B., Cano, A., & Williams, A. M. (2013). Correlates of spousal empathic accuracy for pain-related thoughts and feelings. *Clinical Journal of Pain, 29*, 324–333. https://doi.org/10.1097/AJP.0b013e3182527bfd

Leong, L., Cano, A., & Johansen, A. B. (2011). Sequential and base rate analysis of emotional validation and invalidation in chronic pain couples: Patient gender matters. *Journal of Pain, 12*(11), 1140–1148. https://doi.org/10.1016/j.jpain.2011.04.004

Leong, L., Cano, A., Wurm, L. H., Lumley, M. A., & Corley, A. M. (2015). A perspective taking manipulation leads to greater empathy and less pain during the cold pressor task. *The Journal of Pain, 16*(11), 1176–1185.

Linton, S. J., McCracken, L. M., & Vlaeyen, J. W. (2008). Reassurance: Help or hinder in the treatment of pain. *Pain, 134*(1–2), 5–8.

Main, C. J., Keefe, F. J., Jensen, M. P., Vlaeyen, J. W., & Vowles, K. E. (Eds.). (2015). *Fordyce's behavioral methods for chronic pain and illness: Republished with invited commentaries.* Philadelphia, PA: Wolters Kluwer Health.

Martire, L. M., Schulz, R., Helgeson, V. S., Small, B. J., & Saghafi, E. M. (2010). Review and meta-analysis of couple-oriented interventions for chronic illness. *Annals of Behavioral Medicine, 40*(3), 325–342. https://doi.org/10.1007/s12160-010-9216-2

Martire, L. M., Schulz, R., Keefe, F. J., Rudy, T. E., & Starz, T. W. (2008). Couple-oriented education and support intervention for osteoarthritis: Effects on spouses' support and responses to patient pain. *Families, Systems, & Health, 26*(2), 185.

McCracken, L. M., Carson, J. W., Eccleston, C., & Keefe, F. J. (2004). Acceptance and change in the context of chronic pain. *Pain, 109*(1–2), 4–7. https://doi.org/10.1016/j.pain.2004.02.006

McCracken, L. M., Gauntlett-Gilbert, J., & Vowles, K. E. (2007). The role of mindfulness in a contextual cognitive-behavioral analysis of chronic pain-related suffering and disability. *Pain, 131*(1–2), 63–69. https://doi.org/10.1016/j.pain.2006.12.013

McCracken, L. M., Vowles, K. E., & Eccleston, C. (2004). Acceptance of chronic pain: Component analysis and a revised assessment method. *Pain, 107*(1), 159–166.

McCracken, L. M., Vowles, K. E., & Eccleston, C. (2005). Acceptance-based treatment for persons with complex, long standing chronic pain: A preliminary analysis of treatment outcome in comparison to a waiting phase. *Behaviour Research and Therapy, 43*(10), 1335–1346.

Paulsen, J. S., & Altmaier, E. M. (1995). The effects of perceived versus enacted social support on the discriminative cue function of spouses for pain behaviors. *Pain, 60,* 103–110. https://doi.org/10.1016/0304-3959(94)00096-W

Papini, M. R., Fuchs, P. N., & Torres, C. (2015). Behavioral neuroscience of psychological pain. *Neuroscience & Biobehavioral Reviews, 48,* 53–69.

Petscher, E. S., Rey, C., & Bailey, J. S. (2009). A review of empirical support for differential reinforcement of alternative behavior. *Research in Developmental Disabilities, 30*(3), 409–425. https://doi.org/10.1016/j.ridd.2008.08.008

Pyszczynski, T., Greenberg, J., Solomon, S., Cather, C., Gat, I., & Sideris, J. (1995). Defensive distancing from victims of serious illness: The role of delay. *Personality & Social Psychology Bulletin, 21,* 13–20. https://doi.org/10.1177/0146167295211003

Qadir, F., Haqqani, S., Khalid, A., Huma, Z., & Medhin, G. (2014). A pilot study of depression among older people in Rawalpindi, Pakistan. *BMC Research Notes, 7*(1), 1.

Reis, H. T., & Shaver, P. (1988). Intimacy as an interpersonal process. In S. Duck (Ed.), *Handbook of interpersonal relationships* (pp. 367–389). Chichester, England: Wiley.

Romano, J. M., Turner, J. A., Friedman, L. S., Bulcroft, R. A., Jensen, M. P., Hops, H., & Wright, S. F. (1992). Sequential analysis of chronic pain behaviors and spouse responses. *Journal of Consulting and Clinical Psychology, 60,* 777–782. https://doi.org/10.1037/0022-006X.60.5.777

Romano, J. M., Turner, J. A., Jensen, M. P., Friedman, L. S., Bulcroft, R. A., Hops, H., & Wright, S. F. (1995). Chronic pain patient-spouse behavioral interactions predict patient disability. *Pain, 63*(3), 353–360. https://doi.org/10.1016/0304-3959(95)00062-3

Rosenzweig, S., Greeson, J. M., Reibel, D. K., Green, J. S., Jasser, S. A., & Beasley, D. (2010). Mindfulness-based stress reduction for chronic pain conditions: Variation in treatment outcomes and role of home meditation practice. *Journal of Psychosomatic Research, 68*(1), 29–36. https://doi.org/10.1016/j.jpsychores.2009.03.010

Saarijarvi, S. (1991). A controlled study of couple therapy in chronic low back pain patients: Effects on marital satisfaction, psychological distress and health attitudes. *Journal of Psychosomatic Research, 35,* 265–272. https://doi.org/10.1016/0022-3999(91)90080-8

Sanders, M. R., Rebgetz, M., Morrison, M., Bor, W., Gordon, A., Dadds, M., & Shepherd, R. (1989). Cognitive-behavioral treatment of recurrent nonspecific abdominal pain in children: An analysis of generalization, maintenance, and side effects. *Journal of Consulting and Clinical Psychology, 57*(2), 294–300.

Schwartz, L., Jensen, M. P., & Romano, J. M. (2005). The development and psychometric evaluation of an instrument to assess spouse responses to pain and well behavior in patients with chronic pain: The spouse response inventory. *The Journal of Pain, 6*(4), 243–252. https://doi.org/10.1016/j.jpain.2004.12.010

Shenk, C. E., & Fruzzetti, A. E. (2011). The impact of validating and invalidating responses on emotional reactivity. *Journal of Social and Clinical Psychology, 30*(2), 163–183.

Strategier, L. D., Chwalisz, K., Altmaier, E. M., Russell, D. W., & Lehmann, T. R. (1997). Multidimensional assessment of chronic low back pain: Predicting treatment outcomes. *Journal of Clinical Psychology in Medical Settings, 4,* 91–110.

Stroud, M. W., Turner, J. A., Jensen, M. P., & Cardenas, D. D. (2006). Partner responses to pain behaviors are associated with depression and activity interference among persons with chronic pain and spinal cord injury. *The Journal of Pain, 7*(2), 91–99. https://doi.org/10.1016/j.jpain.2005.08.006

Sullivan, K. T., & Davila, J. (Eds.). (2010). *Support processes in intimate relationships*. New York, NY: Oxford University Press.

Sullivan, M. J. L., Adams, H., & Sullivan, M. E. (2004). Communicative dimensions of pain catastrophizing: Social cueing effects on pain behaviour and coping. *Pain, 107*(3), 220–226. https://doi.org/10.1016/j.pain.2003.11.003

Sullivan, M. J. L., Martel, M. O., Tripp, D., Savard, A., & Crombez, G. (2006). The relation between catastrophizing and the communication of pain experience. *Pain, 122*, 282–288. https://doi.org/10.1016/j.pain.2006.02.001

Sullivan, M. J. L., Thorn, B., Haythornthwaite, J. A., Keefe, F., Martin, M. Y., Bradley, L. A., & Lefebvre, J. C. (2001). Theoretical perspectives on the relation between catastrophizing and pain. *Clinical Journal of Pain, 17*, 52–64. https://doi.org/10.1097/00002508-200103000-00008

Syrjala, K. L., Donaldson, G. W., Davis, M. W., Kippes, M. E., & Carr, J. E. (1995). Relaxation and imagery and cognitive-behavioral training reduce pain during cancer treatment: A controlled clinical trial. *Pain, 63*(2), 189–198.

Turk, D. C. (2005). The potential of treatment matching for subgroups of patients with chronic pain. *Clinical Journal of Pain, 21*, 44–55. https://doi.org/10.1097/00002508-200501000-00006

Turk, D. C., Okifuji, A., Sinclair, J. D., & Starz, T. W. (1998). Differential responses by psychosocial subgroups of fibromyalgia syndrome patients to an interdisciplinary treatment. *Arthritis Care and Research, 11*, 397–404. https://doi.org/10.1002/art.1790110511

Turner, J. A., & Chapman, C. R. (1982). Psychological interventions for chronic pain: A critical review. II. Operant conditioning, hypnosis, and cognitive-behavioral therapy. *Pain, 12*(1), 23–46.

Veehof, M. M., Oskam, M.-J., Schreurs, K. M., & Bohlmeijer, E. T. (2011). Acceptance-based interventions for the treatment of chronic pain: A systematic review and meta-analysis. *Pain, 152*(3), 533–542.

Vlaeyen, J. W., & Linton, S. J. (2000). Fear-avoidance and its consequences in chronic musculoskeletal pain: A state of the art. *Pain, 85*(3), 317–332.

Vowles, K. E., & McCracken, L. M. (2008). Acceptance and values-based action in chronic pain: A study of treatment effectiveness and process. *Journal of Consulting and Clinical Psychology, 76*(3), 397–407. https://doi.org/10.1037/0022-006X.76.3.397

Vowles, K. E., Wetherell, J. L., & Sorrell, J. T. (2009). Targeting acceptance, mindfulness, and values-based action in chronic pain: Findings of two preliminary trials of an outpatient group-based intervention. *Cognitive and Behavioral Practice, 16*, 49–58. https://doi.org/10.1016/j.cbpra.2008.08.001

Wicksell, R. K., Olsson, G. L., & Hayes, S. C. (2010). Psychological flexibility as a mediator of improvement in acceptance and commitment therapy for patients with chronic pain following whiplash. *European Journal of Pain, 14*(10), e1–e11.

Williams, D. A., & Thorn, B. E. (1989). An empirical assessment of pain beliefs. *Pain, 36*(3), 351–358.

Zautra, A. J., Davis, M. C., Reich, J. W., Nicassio, P., Tennen, H., Finan, P., … Irwin, M. R. (2008). Comparison of cognitive-behavioral and mindfulness meditation interventions on adaptation to rheumatoid arthritis for patients with and without history of recurrent depression. *Journal of Consulting and Clinical Psychology, 76*(3), 408–421. https://doi.org/10.1037/0022-006X.76.3.408

Chapter 14
The Role of Nonverbal Features of Caregiving Behavior

Kaytlin Constantin, Rachel L. Moline, and C. Meghan McMurtry

Abstract Pain experience and expression are complex and multiply determined by numerous biological, psychological, and social factors. However, the interpersonal context in which pain occurs has been largely understudied compared to intrapersonal factors. This chapter aims to review existing literature on nonverbal features of caregiving behavior occurring during transactions in pain contexts. Thus, we are shifting the spotlight to the *observer* of the individual in pain in considering the observer's expressive behaviors, in addition to physiological responses which may influence observable actions. The nonverbal features of caregiving behavior reviewed include: vocal paralanguage and linguistics, kinesics and haptics, proxemics, and physiological activity. For each nonverbal feature, a review of the existing literature is provided by summarizing illustrative work first in the context of acute pain followed by chronic pain, during spousal interactions and parent–child interactions. Concrete recommendations for future research are provided in the concluding section.

Keywords Pain · Spousal interactions · Parent–child interactions · Nonverbal communication · Vocal paralanguage · Linguistics · Kinesics · Haptics · Proxemics · Physiological responses

K. Constantin · R. L. Moline
Department of Psychology, University of Guelph, Guelph, ON, Canada

C. M. McMurtry (✉)
Department of Psychology, University of Guelph, Guelph, ON, Canada

Pediatric Chronic Pain Program, McMaster Children's Hospital, Hamilton, ON, Canada

Children's Health Research Institute, London, ON, Canada

Department of Paediatrics, Schulich School of Medicine & Dentistry, Western University, London, ON, Canada
e-mail: cmcmurtr@uoguelph.ca

© Springer International Publishing AG, part of Springer Nature 2018
T. Vervoort et al. (eds.), *Social and Interpersonal Dynamics in Pain*,
https://doi.org/10.1007/978-3-319-78340-6_14

Introduction

Overview: Pain and Nonverbal Communication

An individual's pain experience (internal) and pain expression (external, observable) are complex and multiply determined by a host of biological, psychological, and social factors. The social factors within this biopsychosocial conceptualization of pain have been under-studied compared to intrapersonal factors (Craig, 2009; Craig et al., 2010; Hadjistavropoulos et al., 2011). However, the interpersonal context is critical to an individual's experience of pain. For example, the behavior of caregivers, such as parents and spouses, plays an important role in the experience and expression of acute and chronic pain (e.g., Chambers, Craig, & Bennett, 2002; Coan, Schaefer, & Davidson, 2006; Dahlquist, Power, & Carlson, 1995; Dunford, Thompson, & Gauntlett-Gilbert, 2014; Johansen & Cano, 2007; Smith, Keefe, Caldwell, Romano, & Baucom, 2004). The effects of these caregiver behaviors are thought to extend beyond the immediate temporal context to long-term pain experience, expression, and functioning (e.g., via social learning: Bandura, 1977; operant conditioning: Craig, 1986; Fordyce, 1986; Hadjistavropoulos et al., 2011; and intimacy models of interaction: Cano & Williams, 2010). Consistent with each of the aforementioned models, emotions communicated by caregivers may be particularly important when conceptualizing possible mechanisms behind the impact of caregiving behaviors on child and spousal pain outcomes.

Two models which are consistent with the biopsychosocial conceptualization of pain are critical to understanding the role of non-verbal features of caregiving behavior: the social communication model of pain (Craig, 1986, 2009) and the pain empathy model (Goubert et al., 2005). The social context of pain is emphasized in the social communication model of pain (Craig, 1986, 2009), which draws attention to the intra and interpersonal factors that can shape an individual's pain experience and expression such as context and relationship with observers. The pain empathy model proposed by Goubert et al. (2005) posits that both bottom-up (e.g., behavior by the person in pain) and top-down (e.g., observer's pain catastrophizing) variables influence an observer's affective and behavioral response to another's pain.

If the social context of pain has been neglected, the nonverbal features of communication in the context of pain as exhibited by *caregivers* have been almost ignored. The majority of the research examining caregiver behavior in pain contexts has focused on verbal content (what caregivers say) which neglects numerous other cues or "*actions*" (messages sent from sender to receiver; Duck & McMahan, 2015). Consider the following *interactions* (messages exchanged between individuals; Duck & McMahan, 2015):

> Example 1:
>> *Child about to receive a needle:*   I'm scared! It's going to hurt.
>> *Mother:*   Shhhh.

Example 2:
Adult with chronic low back pain: [reaching to remove a heavy dish from the dishwasher]
Spouse: No… allow me.
Example 3:
Child falls down and skins knee: Daddy! Look at this.
Father: Oh! Let's see.

How do we understand what is happening in these examples? Is the mother showing an angry facial expression and saying "shhh" sharply and loudly (i.e., telling her child to be quiet)? Or does she have a concerned look on her face and is she saying "shhhh" in a soft and soothing voice? Is the spouse offering to help (e.g., moving to pick up the dish, speaking in a falling tone) or perhaps being sarcastic and critical (e.g., standing back with his/her hands on hips and laughing)? Finally, is the father curious or alarmed?[1] A description of the non-verbal cues/features is needed to guide interpretation of these actions and associated interactions.

Communication occurs through a variety of channels including verbal (*what* is said), vocal paralanguage (*how* something is said), kinesics (facial expression, gestures, limb and body movements), haptics (touch), and proxemics (interpersonal distance; Heath & Bryant, 2000). Each of these observable features is also likely connected to the person's internal physiologic arousal. To understand these communications as *transactions*, we would need to understand individuals' "construction of shared meanings or understandings" (Duck & McMahan, 2015, p. 16). Furthermore, the constitutive approach to communication holds that not only is communication integral to the social nature of our species, but that communication itself is a creator (e.g., of relationships; Duck & McMahan, 2015). For example, non-verbal cues may be critical to whether the communication is perceived as empathic and validating or invalidating. These non-verbal cues may also be particularly important for children who are attuned to this form of communication and rely on adults for emotion regulation (Vannorsdall, Dahlquist, Pendley, & Power, 2004). Non-verbal behaviors are believed to be more involuntary, automatic, and thus more reliable indicators of one's experience/response/state compared to verbal behaviors (Craig et al. 2010).

Objectives

In this chapter we aim to review the existing literature on non-verbal features of caregiving behavior occurring during transactions in pain contexts. Thus, we are shifting the spotlight to the *observer* of the individual in pain in considering the observer's expressive behaviors and, to a lesser extent, physiological responses which may influence observable actions. First, Table 14.1 provides a summary of specific non-verbal features of caregiving behavior [i.e., vocal paralanguage and

---

[1] And not the focus of this chapter but is the child in pain and distressed, or interested in the appearance of a skinned knee?

Table 14.1 Terminology, capture/measurement, and coding

Category of behavior	Term	Definition	Typical capture/measurement and coding	Comments and example caregiver pain-related citations
Vocal paralanguage and linguistic features				
	Tone	Voice or vocal tone includes intonation, emphasis, pitch, and amplitude of speech and involves characteristics of spoken communication apart from words (DiMatteo et al., 1993)	*Capture:* audio recording *Sign-based coding via software:* phonetics programs (e.g., Praat; Boersma & Weenink, www.praat.org) can measure different acoustic properties, and can yield, among other parameters, pitch contours which coders can use to identify rising versus falling tonal contours from digital audio *Judgment-based manual coding:* individuals are asked to provide typically holistic "judgments" about the tone of voice heard during a particular utterance or exchange. Verbal content may be removed or not. Most frequently used when coding for emotion (Elfenbein & Ambady, 2002)	Several behavioral coding schemes include references to vocal tone (e.g., Reid et al., 2005), relying on judgment-based coding in which an operational definition was not clearly reported McMurtry et al. (2010)
	Pitch	*Pitch:* Cyclic, repetitive nature of the vibrations that comprise sound. Fundamental frequency (F_0) refers to the rate at which the vocal folds open and close around the glottis (Von Bismarck, 1974) *Pitch contour:* Sequence of F_0 values across utterance, changes in pitch (Harrigan & Rosenthal, 2008)	*Capture:* audio recording *Sign-based coding via software:* output indicates F_0 for pitch and the proportion of rising to falling F_0 contours in a sentence for pitch contour *Judgment-based manual coding:* assessing for pitch by listening and providing "judgments" about the pitch, typically classifying pitch according to qualitative descriptors (e.g., high or low; Andrews & Madeira, 1977)	Has not been studied in pain contexts

Voice quality	*High-frequency energy*: How "sharp" and "soft" a voice is. Relative proportion of total acoustic energy above, versus below, a cut-off frequency (Harrigan & Rosenthal, 2008)	*Capture*: audio recording *Sign-based coding via software*: obtained by measuring the long-term average spectrum (LTAS), or the distribution of energy over a range of frequencies, averaged over an extended period of time (Harrigan & Rosenthal, 2008)	Has not been studied in pain contexts
Temporal aspects	*Segmental reduction*: Articulatory short-cuts, typically in fast-speech to keep a constant speech rate. Reduction of utterance length *Speech rate*: speed of speech (Harrigan & Rosenthal, 2008)	*Capture*: audio recording *Sign-based manual coding*: segmental reduction being measured in terms of number of phonetic syllables per utterance (Engstrand & Krull, 2001); speech rate measured in terms of number of words per minute (Harrigan & Rosenthal, 2008)	Has not been studied in pain contexts
Intensity	How "loud" or "soft" the sound is. Totalled number of auditory nerve stimulations over short cyclic time periods, most likely over the duration of theta wave cycles (Harrigan & Rosenthal, 2008)	*Capture*: audio recording *Sign-based coding via software*: output indicates loudness in decibels (dB)	Greenbaum, Turner, Cook, and Melamed (1990) (dentists and patients)
Structure and function	*Structure*: Verbal delivery of a verbalization in terms of phrasing meanings behind sentences and *Speech function*: Refers to verbalizations such as "statement," "question," or "command." Speech function is associated with grammatical features of clauses, such as the order of subject and verb and clause finiteness	*Capture*: audio recording and transcription *Judgment-based manual coding*: assessing for content and grammatical features (e.g., presence of tense for statements and questions but absence of tense for command)	McMurtry et al. (2007) and Dahlquist et al. (2001)

(continued)

Table 14.1 (continued)

Category of behavior	Term	Definition	Typical capture/measurement and coding	Comments and example caregiver pain-related citations
Kinesics and haptics				
	Facial expression	Changes in facial muscles, blood flow, skin temperature, coloring. Emphasis on movements	*Capture:* video recording *Sign-based manual coding or coding via software:* coding of changes/movements in muscles of the face, often using facial action units *Judgment-based manual coding:* individuals are asked to provide typically holistic judgments about the "message" of what was observed such as emotion conveyed	Two approaches are considered complementary (Cohn & Ekman, 2008) Sign-based coding: Horton and Pillai Riddell (2010) (infants) Judgment-based coding: in pain literature often collapses across caregiver nonverbal features (e.g., Romano et al., 1991)
	Solicitous behaviors	Physical assistance or taking over a task	*Capture:* video recording *Combination of sign-based and judgment-based manual coding:* often focus on physically assisting or taking over a task *Questionnaires:* person in pain (child, adult) is asked to report on caregiver's (e.g., parent, spouse) behaviors. Caregiver report may also be elicited	Observed behavior frequently coded using the modified version of the Living in Family Environments (LIFE) coding scheme which collapses over several nonverbal features: Romano et al. (1991, 1992, 2000) These behaviors could arguably fall within several other categories (e.g., attending, supportive, task-related)
	Touch behaviors	Tactile contact that is either instrumental or supportive in nature	*Capture:* video recording *Sign-based manual coding:* although coding is frequently sign-based, categorization of touch may also rely on judgment-based coding by trained researchers	Various coding schemes have been used including: Child Behavior Coding System, Postanesthesia Care Unit (CBCS-P; as seen in Rancourt et al., 2015); Modified versions of the Child-Adult Medical Procedure Interaction Scale (as seen in Chorney et al., 2009; Dahlquist et al., 1995; Pedro et al., 2010), and a coding method developed by Peterson et al. (2007)

Supportive or empathic touch	Any form of physical contact initiated by an adult that either serves to communicate reassurance or is supportive or neutral in nature	*Capture:* video recording *Sign-based manual coding:* often includes slow patting, rubbing, hand-holding, rocking, and giving hugs or kisses	Thompson et al. (2016)
Instrumental or task-related touch	Touch that serves a function or purpose; task-oriented	*Capture:* video recording *Sign-based manual coding:* may include forceful restraint, touch to an area that may cause pain, or positioning the individual for a procedure	Rancourt et al. (2015)
Attending behavior	Behaviors that focus attention to the pain or distress the individual in pain is experiencing	*Capture:* video recording *Sign-based manual coding:* may include looking at the individual in pain, rubbing or massaging muscles, completing exercise with the individual. Coding may involve a combination of sign- and judgment-based manual coding	Reid et al. (2005)
Proxemics			
Interpersonal distance	How far apart individuals are from one another physically	*Capture:* video recording *Sign-based manual coding:* based on approximations of space between caregiver and the individual's head (e.g., intimate distance as less than 30 cm, personal distance as 30–90 cm, etc.)	Peterson et al. (2007)
Physiology			
Heart rate (HR)	Speed of the heart contractions	*Capture:* electrocardiogram (ECG; most common) *Sign-based coding via software:* beats per minute	Provides a measure of stress or physiological arousal (Smith et al. 2007)

(continued)

Table 14.1 (continued)

Category of behavior	Term	Definition	Typical capture/measurement and coding	Comments and example caregiver pain-related citations
	Heart rate variability (HRV)	Fluctuations in the length between consecutive heartbeats A distinction is typically made between: *Resting or tonic HRV*: heart rate variability under resting or normal conditions *Reactive or phasic HRV*: change in HRV from baseline to a stimulus or event	*Capture*: electrocardiogram is used to collect the data and software is used to analyze the data, which can be done using various *sign-based coding via software* techniques, including: *Time domain methods*: the interval between successive QRS complexes (called the normal-to-normal or NN interval) in an ECG wave are determined and statistical methods are used to calculate the variations in heart rate. Most common methods are: the root mean square of the successive differences between NN intervals (RMSSD); and the number of interval differences of successive NN intervals greater than 50 ms (NN50) *Frequency domain methods*: examines how power (variance) is distributed as a function of frequency using power spectral density analyses. This can be accomplished with the Fast Fourier Transform (FFT) or autoregressive methods. Two spectral components are typically identified: low frequency and high frequency (HF) components HF-HRV (spectral analysis), RMSSD (statistical analysis)	These two methods are highly correlated, although time domain methods are computationally straightforward compared to frequency domain methods (Goedhart, van der Sluis, Houtveen, Willemsen, & de Geus, 2007) *Resting HRV*: stable, individual differences in the capacity for emotion regulation. Although not examined in the observer, has been explored in relation to pain adaptation (e.g., Nahman-Averbuch et al., 2016) *Reactive HRV*: ongoing self-regulatory efforts and emotional experience (Vervoort et al., 2014)
	Electrodermal activity	Activity of eccrine sweat gland secretions, controlled by the sympathetic nervous system	*Capture*: ambulatory physiologic data recorder *Sign-based coding via software*: skin conductance level, transformed as a percentage	Index of emotional arousal. Kain et al. (2003)

Mean arterial pressure	Average blood pressure	*Capture*: blood pressure cuff *Sign-based coding via software*: mean arterial pressure is calculated using the following equation: [(Diastolic blood pressure × 2) + systolic blood pressure]/3	Smith et al. (2007)
Diastolic blood pressure (DBP)	Measures the pressure in the blood vessels between heart beats	*Capture*: blood pressure cuff *Sign-based coding via software*: measured in units of millimeters of mercury (mmHg). Two measures: Mean diastolic blood pressure Diastolic blood pressure reactivity: changes in diastolic blood pressure from resting state to a stressful event	Kain et al. (2003)
Systolic blood pressure (SBP)	Measures the pressure in the blood vessels during heart beats	*Capture*: blood pressure cuff *Sign-based coding via software*: measured in units of millimeters of mercury (mmHg). Two measures: Mean systolic blood pressure Systolic blood pressure reactivity: changes in systolic blood pressure from resting state to a stressful event	Kain et al. (2003)

Note: In determining the approach to capture and describe the nonverbal features of interest, a number of decisions will need to be made (Chorney, McMurtry, Chambers, & Bakeman, 2015): (1) *granularity or specificity desired* (e.g., micro vs. macro coding, exhaustive vs. selective); (2) *when* to measure and describe the feature (e.g., continuously, a portion of an interaction tied to an event, by intervals); (3) *how* to score the feature (e.g., nominal codes, ordinal scores) including whether duration, frequency, or timing matter; (4) *presenting the results* (e.g., proportions, rates, averages, ranges). To highlight various coding methods, we have distinguished sign-based vs. judgment-based coding. Admittedly, the distinction is not uniformly clear. However, we intend sign-based coding to indicate the measurement and reporting of specific features/actions/movements that are based on discrete, operationalized qualities (e.g., range of pitch in Hz, hand-holding, eyebrow raise). In contrast, judgment-based coding is based on more holistic determinations related to the nonverbal feature in question and may include interpretations of the intended *meaning* or *message* (e.g., a fearful vocal tone, an aggressive facial expression, comforting touch). Although the individuals providing the "judgments" could be "experts," they are typically trained observers linguistics, kinesics, haptics, and proxemics]; we also review caregiver internal physiology as, although not "visible" in and of itself, it relates to an individual's emotional experience and regulation, and observable behaviors (Appelhans & Luecken, 2006; Porges, 2007). The bulk of the chapter is organized by non-verbal feature. For each non-verbal feature, we will review the existing literature by summarizing illustrative work first in the context of acute pain followed by chronic pain. The concluding section will provide concrete recommendations for future research.

Each of these non-verbal features typically exists within an interactive, and ultimately transactive process (Duck & McMahan, 2015). However, our focus is on the "actions" and responses of caregivers in the context of another's pain whether intentional or not (Duck & McMahan, 2015; Hadjistavropoulos et al., 2011; Heath & Bryant, 2000). When possible, we will explore the exchange of actions with the individual in pain ("interaction"), and relations between these individual actions/features with outcome for the person in pain.[2] We will review data for parents of children (>2 years of age) and spouses of adults who are experiencing either chronic or acute pain. Given the non-verbal caregiving behaviors for infants are likely to be qualitatively different (e.g., skin-to-skin/kangaroo care), studies focusing solely on infants will not be reviewed. Parents and spouses are often longitudinal partners in these interactions and are the focus of this chapter. Although the nonverbal behavior of medical professionals as they interact with individuals in pain is also important, they will not be covered.

In summary, the following empirically informed premises are important to our starting point: (1) the social context of pain is important; (2) pain experience and expression are impacted by others' behavior, both immediately and over time; (3) the behaviors of caregivers (e.g., parents, spouses) in long-term relationships with individuals in pain who are likely to be present in day-to-day pain contexts may be particularly important; (4) communicative behavior goes beyond verbal content—it has been argued that "the non-verbal content of messages often *is* the message" (Burgoon & Hoobler, 2002, p. 241); and (5) the (eventual) integration of verbal and non-verbal features of communication is paramount to a full understanding.

Vocal Paralanguage and Linguistic Features

Vocal paralanguage and linguistic cues offer important information about speaker state, as emotion and meaning are expressed by both *what* is being said in addition to *how* it is being said (Scherer, 2003). Prosody consists of the elements of speech that contribute to vocal paralanguage functions including intensity, pitch, and length, associated with rhythm and intonation in a language (Frick, 1985). Acoustic features of prosody reflect the underlying emotional state of the speaker, and are linked to the expression of emotions that are apparent to others (Frick, 1985;

---

[2] Please note that in the majority of cases, results pertaining to specific nonverbal features and pain outcome are not available.

Scherer, 2003). For example, if the statement "I'm so proud of you!" is made by a mother congratulating her child after scoring at a soccer game, her voice will reflect a state of joy and happiness and exhibit distinctive vocal cues (e.g., high pitch) which, in turn, will precipitate the listener's attribution of a happy emotional state to the mother.

Acute Pain

Parent–Child Interactions Infants and young children appear to be sensitive to prosodic features in speech, and by early childhood are typically able to identify emotion from acoustic cues (Morton & Trehub, 2001; Mumme, Fernald, & Herrera, 1996; Sauter, Panattoni, & Happé, 2013; Vaish & Striano, 2004). For example, 4–10-year-olds are able to identify joy or sadness from prosody, with accuracy increasing with age (Morton & Trehub, 2001), and children as young as 5 years are able to accurately interpret negative and positive emotions from vocal cues (Sauter et al., 2013). To date, parental vocal tone (McMurtry, Chambers, McGrath, & Asp, 2010; McMurtry, McGrath, Asp, & Chambers, 2007), speech structure (Dahlquist et al., 2001), and speech function (McMurtry et al., 2007) have been studied in the pediatric acute pain context.

A study by McMurtry et al. (2007) investigated the role of speech function and tone during the provision of parental reassurance in the context of pediatric immunizations with 5-year-old children. Speech function of parent verbalizations were classified as statement, question, command, or minor clause. Additionally, using descriptions of Halliday's (1970) primary tones, and the computer software Praat (Boersma & Weenink, 2016), vocal tone of parental reassurance was analyzed. This novel methodology provided a basic acoustic description of reassurance, and identified that half of the instances of reassurance were said with a falling tone, which corresponds with speaker protectiveness and certainty (McMurtry et al., 2007). Importantly, this linguistic description is the only attempt to define a "reassuring" tone, often cited in the literature, using an operationalized methodology.

In a subsequent study investigating 5–10-year-old children's perception of caregiver emotion, McMurtry et al. (2010) used video vignettes to systematically manipulate the verbal content (informative, uninformative), facial expression (happy, fearful), and vocal tone (falling, rising) of reassurance; distraction was used as a comparison (McMurtry et al., 2010). The actor portrayed instances of reassurance with either a rising tone, intended to indicate uncertainty or vulnerability, or verbalizations spoken with a falling tone, to indicate certainty or protectiveness (McMurtry et al., 2010). Children endorsed greatest adult fear intensity when reassurance was portrayed using a rising tone in combination with a fearful facial expression (McMurtry et al., 2010). During distraction, children rated adults as being more fearful when using a falling tone, but only in the presence of a fearful facial expression. Thus, vocal tone appears to impact children's perceptions of the caregiver's emotion during instances of reassurance and distraction, although facial cues and verbal content also play important roles.

Dahlquist et al. (2001) studied parental command structure in relation to 5–15-year-old children's distress during invasive cancer procedures (intra-muscular injections, lumbar punctures). Command structure, or the way in which a command is phrased, was coded using the Command Structure subscale of the Pediatric Medical Interaction Scale (PMIS; Dahlquist, Pendley, Power, Landthrip, & Jones, 1994). Specific direct requests (e.g., "Get up on the table") were associated with lower child distress, and vague commands, or commands phrased as questions (e.g., "Do you want to get up on the table?") were associated with increased child distress (Dahlquist et al., 2001).

Other studies involving parent–child interactions during acute painful procedures have made reference to considering vocal tones in their coding methodology (Blount, Landolf-Fritsche, Powers, & Sturges, 1991; Blount, Sturges, & Powers, 1990; Kleiber & McCarthy, 1999; Svendsen, Moen, Pedersen, & Bjørk, 2016; Taylor, Sellick, & Greenwood, 2011). However, these studies did not have a clear operationalization of vocal tone and a coding scheme was not systematically applied (e.g., Blount et al., 1990). Rather, judgment-based, qualitative descriptors of vocal tone to code parent verbalizations were described, such as a "harshness in tone" (Blount et al., 1991). Qualitative descriptions of vocal tone in an observational study included reference to a "commanding voice" or a "light, powerful, enthusiastic voice" (Svendsen et al., 2016). Though informative, qualitative descriptors provide different information than clearly operationalized measures of vocal properties.

Spousal Interactions To the best of our knowledge, there have been no studies examining linguistic cues in spousal interactions in an acute pain context.

Chronic Pain

Parent–Child Interactions Two studies have mentioned vocal tone in the context of parent interactions with children diagnosed with chronic pain within a potentially acutely painful context (Dunford et al., 2014; Reid, McGrath, & Lang, 2005). Reid et al. (2005) investigated parent–child interactions during a painful exercise task involving children aged 11–17 years old with a diagnosis of fibromyalgia or juvenile rheumatoid arthritis, and pain-free controls and their parents. Parent verbalizations were categorized as discouraging coping, encouraging coping, or other. Reference to vocal tone was included in the discouraging coping category, as "... said with tone of voice that sympathizes with child's pain". A specific example was 'Remember it's up to you. If it hurts you can stop' or 'You okay?', said in a sympathetic voice (Reid et al., 2005). Dunford et al. (2014) studied adolescents with chronic pain undergoing a physical exercise session and their primary caregiver. Parent verbal and nonverbal behaviors were coded, and were categorized as "monitoring," "protecting," "encouraging," or "instructing." In the qualitative description of the 'instructing category', the authors described parent voices as sometimes having a "critical tone" as determined by global judgment coding (Dunford et al., 2014). Both studies provided judgment-based descriptions of parent vocal tone, without describing a specific method of operationalization. Furthermore, vocal tone was conceptualized as an illustrative example or component of a particular coding category; thus, it is unclear whether the vocal tone was actually present when the code was applied.

Spousal Interactions To date, several studies have used the Living in Family Environments coding scheme (LIFE; Hops, Davis, & Longoria, 1995; Romano et al., 1991, 1992; Romano, Jensen, Turner, Good, & Hops, 2000) to assess interactions of patients with chronic pain and their spouses during completion of household tasks. The modified coding system assesses behaviors (i.e., non-verbal pain, verbal pain, solicitous, negative) using 22 verbal content codes and eight non-verbal affect codes; the latter are dependent upon vocal tone, facial expressions, gestures, and body posture. For example, reference to vocal tone was made in the category of aggressive affect, and later coded in the aversive affect category, defined as "irritated, angry, or sarcastic facial expression or voice tone". A reduction in non-verbal pain behaviors (e.g., wincing, facial expression of pain) in response to aggressive spousal behavior was observed in the chronic pain group relative to the healthy control group (Romano et al., 1992). However, due to the criteria of "Aggressive" behavior, distinguishing if vocal tone was utilized to code the behavior, in addition to or instead of facial expression, was not possible. No descriptive information regarding observed vocal tone was provided (e.g., frequency). This use of general, and broad descriptors of categories (e.g., not identifying which cue was observed, such as facial expression or vocal tone) is a common issue found throughout the reviewed literature.

Johansen and Cano (2007) investigated spousal interactions for dyads that included one partner with chronic pain. The Specific Affect Coding System (SPAFF; Gottman, McCoy, Coan, & Collier, 1995) considers context, vocal tone, facial expressions, body movement as well as cultural specific data. Participants and their spouses engaged in a 15-min discussion about a topic of disagreement of their choosing which was then coded using the SPAFF. Prior to coding, the coders were trained using audiotapes that accompanied the SPAFF manual to learn differentiation of vocal tone, however, no more detail regarding this methodology was provided. Overall, marital satisfaction was related to their expressions of humor, and sadness in one spouse was negatively related to marital satisfaction (Johansen & Cano, 2007). However, as vocal tone was not a specific criterion in the coding system, nor were descriptive results regarding vocal tone provided, there are no relevant results pertaining this non-verbal feature.

Summary: Vocal Paralanguage and Linguistic Features

There is very little literature on vocal paralanguage and linguistic features in pain contexts, particularly work that isolates these features from other caregiving features to enable specific conclusions. During painful procedures caregiver vocal tone and speech function appear relevant to pain outcomes (Dahlquist et al., 2001; McMurtry et al., 2007). Parental procedural reassurance is often said with a falling tone, as consistent with speaker protectiveness and certainty; however, parent facial expressions play an important role in how children interpret parent emotion during specific utterances (McMurtry et al., 2007). Use of direct, and specific commands may be most helpful during pediatric procedures (vs. vague commands; Dahlquist et al., 2001). No research has examined vocal paralanguage and linguistic features in pediatric chronic pain. No conclusions can be reached for spousal behavior in the acute or chronic pain context.

Future research should include quantifiable and/or replicable operationalizations of vocal tone; the relations between judgment-based coding and objective, quantitative measures should be explored. Capturing the level of confidence that coders endorse and reliability observed with regard to providing judgment-based coding of vocal tone in the absence of instruction beyond an adjective (e.g., sympathetic voice) would help address limitations of existing literature. There are also numerous aspects of vocal paralanguage and linguistics (e.g., pitch, loudness) deserving of examination in pain contexts as they are likely important to communication and pain outcomes.

Kinesics and Haptics

Facial Expressions

The importance of the face as a signal of the expresser's emotion has long been recognized (Darwin, 1998). Facial expressions are a salient cue in social interactions and have been argued to be the "most commanding and complicated" non-verbal behavior (Cohn & Ekman, 2008, p. 9). The basic perceptual abilities for perceiving and recognizing facial expressions of emotion appear early in life (Ekman & Oster, 1979; Walker-Andrews, 1997). Although facial expressions of the individual who is in pain have received attention (Prkachin, 2009), little is known regarding caregivers' facial expressions in these contexts.

Acute Pain

Parent–Child Interactions   In a study on the effects of social modeling on *subsequent* pain response, Goodman and McGrath (2003) assigned mothers whose 10–14-year-old children were about to complete the cold pressor task to one of three groups: (a) *exaggerate*, in which they were asked to show exaggerated pain behavior, particularly through their face; (b) *minimize*, in which they were asked to mask any pain behavior; and (c) a *control* group, in which they were given no particular instructions for pain behavior (Goodman & McGrath, 2003). Children watched their mothers complete the cold pressor and then completed the task themselves. Consistent with social learning, children of mothers in the *exaggerate* condition showed a lower pain threshold when completing the task themselves.

As reviewed in the vocal paralanguage section, McMurtry et al.' (2010) experimental manipulation of caregivers' facial expressions (happy, fearful) when engaging in reassurance or distraction impacted children's perceptions of emotion. Although verbal content and vocal tone were also found to be important, the largest effect sizes were found for facial expressions, particularly happy facial expressions, clearly demonstrating the salience of this cue. Other work (Schinkel, Chambers, Caes, & Moon, 2016; Svendsen et al., 2016) has included reference to facial expressions within more general codes or analyses but as the codes did not require facial expressions specifically, there are no data to report. For example, in Schinkel et al.' (2016) novel study comparing father and mother non-verbal behaviors during children's acute pain (via the cold pressor task), facial expressions were referenced in the codes for humor ("funny face"), facial and behavioral sympathy ("parent makes a sympathetic expression"), and criticism ("parent gives a disapproving facial expression"; p. 4). The authors found no significant associations between child pain outcomes and frequency of these behavioral constellations by mothers or fathers (Schinkel et al., 2016).

Spousal Interactions   To the best of our knowledge, there have been no studies examining spousal facial expressions in the context of acute pain.

Chronic Pain

Parent–Child Interactions   To the best of our knowledge, there have been no published reports of parental facial expressions in the context of pediatric chronic pain. Although Reid et al. (2005) originally included facial expressions as cues within their affective coding scheme, all affect codes were eventually dropped. Facial expressions were also referenced within other codes (e.g., an example of the "attend" code is "parent smiles at child") but as they were not required components of the code, there are no data to report (Reid et al., 2005).

Spousal Interactions   As reviewed in the vocal paralanguage and linguistics section, several studies have included spousal facial expressions within the LIFE coding system (Romano et al., 1991, 1992, 2000) and the SPAFF coding system (Johansen & Cano, 2007). However, as facial expressions were incorporated as one affective cue for the codes in question, there are no data to report specific to observed spousal facial expressions.

Gestures, Bodily Movements, and Touch

These behaviors include movement of the hands, face, or other parts of the body and have been frequently examined in the pain context, particularly touch behaviors (see Table 14.1). Caregiver touch behaviors can be divided into supportive or empathic touch and instrumental touch (Peterson et al., 2007). Supportive touch involves bodily contact to soothe or reassure a child, while instrumental touch is task-oriented (e.g., moving the individual for medical procedures; Peterson et al., 2007; Rancourt, Chorney, & Kain, 2015). In parent–child contexts, the touch of an adult may help children feel more secure, comforted, and cared for, which may reduce children's distress during painful medical procedures (Vannorsdall et al., 2004). Parent touch is important for social and emotional development, and has positive physiological effects including reducing heart rate, blood pressure, cortisol, and increasing oxytocin in both parent–child and spousal interactions (see Field, 2010 for a review). Touch may convey a sense of validation and enhance intimacy in spousal interactions and relationships. Sensory stimulation (e.g., rubbing, massaging) may also activate sensory nerve fibers and interfere with the transmission of incoming pain signals (Melzack & Wall, 1965; Vannorsdall et al., 2004). Further, touch may distract the individual from the pain and associated negative emotions (Vannorsdall et al., 2004). Alternatively, caregiver supportive touch behavior may increase experienced distress because it focuses the individual's attention on the distressing events (Peterson et al., 2007).

Acute Pain

Parent–Child Interactions Acute pain literature suggests that instrumental touch is typically associated with child (from 2 to 12 years old) fear and distress, although this has been hypothesized to occur in response to a child who is already distressed (e.g., in use of restraint; Peterson et al., 2007; Rancourt et al., 2015). The findings on supportive touch are mixed. Parent empathic touch and physical comfort (e.g., hand-holding) are common during painful medical procedures (e.g., anesthesia induction, bone marrow aspirations, lumbar punctures; Chorney et al., 2009; Dahlquist et al., 1995; Rancourt et al., 2015) and have been linked to higher levels of pain intensity and distress behavior in children ranging from 2 to 13 years old (Chorney et al., 2009; Dahlquist et al., 1995; Schinkel et al., 2016). Other investigators have found that empathic touch was related to children's distress following port starts and lumbar punctures, suggesting parents may use empathic touch in response to children's distress, particularly in younger children (Peterson et al., 2007). Sequential analyses revealed that mothers were more likely to use supportive touch in response to child (2–11 years old) distress (Rancourt et al., 2015); in contrast, greater distress in 3–6-year-old children was related to lower provision of physical comfort by the parent during anesthesia induction (Wright, Stewart, Finley, & Raazi, 2014).

Alternatively, other research suggests parent supportive touch and physical comfort may be unrelated to children's distress behaviors (Pedro, Barros, & Moleiro, 2010; Peterson et al., 2007; Thompson, Ayers, Pervilhac, Mahoney, & Seddon, 2016; Vannorsdall et al., 2004). This has been found in various age ranges (3–15 years of age) and contexts (immunizations, port starts, lumbar punctures, venipunctures; Pedro et al., 2010; Peterson et al., 2007; Thompson et al., 2016; Vannorsdall et al., 2004). Similarly, caregiver supportive gestures (e.g., gives child thumbs up, "high-5") have also been found to be unrelated to child pain (Schinkel et al., 2016). Although a relation is not always found between caregiver touch, bodily movements, and child pain outcomes, caregiver close physical proximity and holding or cuddling their child (1–11 years old) has been linked to lower parent ratings of child fear, pain intensity, and pain behaviors (Cavender, Goff, Hollon, & Guzzetta, 2004; Kankkunen, Vehviläinen-Julkunen, Pietilä, & Halonen, 2003). Not only might children be accustomed to their parents physically soothing them while they are distressed, but it appears these behaviors may have positive effects on parents' experience and ratings of their child's pain (Kankkunen et al., 2003; Vannorsdall et al., 2004).

Spousal Interactions This literature is sparse, although relatively consistent in suggesting potential benefits of social touch, specifically hand-holding, in alleviating acute pain. Spousal hand-holding, compared to holding a stranger's hand, has been shown to effectively reduce anxiety associated with anticipated pain (i.e., threat of electric shock; Coan et al., 2006). Similarly, in experimental laboratory studies, women who held their partner's hand, provided lower ratings of thermal pain (Goldstein, Shamay-Tsoory, Yellinek, & Weissman-Fogel, 2016; Master et al., 2009).

Chronic Pain

Parent–Child Interactions In the study by Reid et al. (2005), parent physical contact (e.g., massaging or rubbing muscles) was also included in the "attend" code, which was defined as behaviors that direct attention to the child. The attend code was found to be unrelated to children's task compliance (i.e., rate of engagement in the exercise, ranging from the required rate to not being engaged at all) and children's self-reported coping with general pain. However, other forms of parent physical comfort (e.g., supportive touch, hugs) that may not occur during experimental exercise tasks may be important (Reid et al., 2005). A recent qualitative observational study of parents and adolescents (mean age 14) seeking chronic pain treatment identified categories of parent behaviors during a physical exercise session (Dunford et al., 2014). Parental unprompted assisting, exercise modelling, and modifying behavior (e.g., parent physically moving adolescent's body parts to complete the exercise) were observed, although further research is needed to examine how these behaviors influence/are related to children and adolescents' pain coping (Dunford et al., 2014).

Spousal Interactions As noted in the vocal paralanguage and linguistic section, several studies have examined spousal gestures and bodily movements (e.g., physical assistance, taking over a task) within the LIFE coding system (Romano et al., 1991, 1992, 2000; Smith et al., 2004). Spousal solicitous behavior during household chores, including physical assistance or taking over a task, are common (Romano et al., 1991) and are associated with, or lead to, higher rates of verbal and non-verbal pain behaviors and physical disability in patients with chronic back pain and musculoskeletal pain (Romano et al., 1992, 1995, 2000). However, as gestures were incorporated as one cue within the solicitous behaviors code, there are no data to report specific to observed spousal bodily movements or gestures.

Summary: Kinesics and Haptics

Literature extant to pain would suggest that facial expressions of caregivers are critical to social communication (Ekman & Oster, 1979) and the little research that has been conducted examining parents' facial expressions during pediatric pain supports this contention. The current pediatric evidence-base suggests that parents should avoid fearful facial expressions in the acute pain context[3] and that the use of a happy facial expression may supersede the processing of other non-verbal cues by the person in pain. No literature has examined the impact of spousal facial expression in acute or chronic pain or parental facial expression in pediatric chronic pain.

The majority of research examining kinesics and haptics in the acute pain context has focused on parent–child interactions and results are mixed; one potential explanation for this is that procedure-related touch behaviors are frequently examined in combination with other parent verbal and nonverbal behaviors (e.g., reassurance, empathy, apologizing; Chorney et al., 2009). Differences in the behavioral measures used, study design and pain context (e.g., venipuncture, anesthesia induction), and age range may also account for the variability in child pain outcomes. Based on existing research, particular forms of instrumental touch (e.g., restraint)

---

[3] Of note, however, Horton and Pillai Riddell (2010) examined mothers' facial expressions immediately prior to their infants' immunizations and found that mothers whose infants looked at their faces prior to the needle expressed more facial fear than mothers of infants who did not look at their faces. Surprisingly, these facial expressions of fear by the mothers were associated with less infant pain (as measured by facial action) in the 10 s following the injection. These results were interpreted within a maternal sensitivity framework, such that mothers who, over time, have typically displayed congruent affect with their infants' emotions have infants who are more able to cope with pain and regulate their distress (Horton & Pillai Riddell, 2010).

are typically linked to higher levels of distress and should be minimized or avoided (cf. Taddio et al., 2015). A small literature has demonstrated benefits for spousal hand-holding (e.g., Master et al., 2009). It remains unclear how caregiver gestures and bodily movements are related to pain outcomes in children and spouses with chronic pain. Further research is needed to describe the topography of naturalistic kinesic (including facial expressions) and haptic cues and clarify how these non-verbal features affect pain in children and spouses. Understanding whether parental behaviors are reactive (i.e., in response to child behaviors) or proactive (i.e., occurring prior to child behaviors) will be helpful in clarifying the causal nature of the relation between parent touch and child pain outcomes.

Proxemics

Interpersonal distance (see Table 14.1) has been explored (Schinkel et al., 2016), and can range from intimate, personal, social, and public distance (Peterson et al., 2007). As outlined by Peterson et al. (2007), intimate distance occurs when the caregiver is less than 12 inches from the individual in pain, and is the distance within which physical contact is likely to occur. Personal distance occurs when the caregiver is 1–3 ft. from the individual in pain, a distance where the caregiver is within reach. Social distance is characterized by more than 3 and less than 6 ft. of distance, and is typical during formal conversations, whereas clinical distance occurs when the caregiver is more than 6 ft. from the child (Peterson et al., 2007). Interpersonal distance behaviors can be examined in the context of immediacy behaviors serving to communicate availability, involvement, warmth, and decrease physical and psychological distance (Andersen & Andersen, 2005; Peterson et al., 2007). For example, a forward lean towards a spouse or child, minimal interpersonal distance (i.e., intimate or personal distance), appropriate use of touch, and eye gaze communicate emotional support (Andersen & Andersen, 2005; Peterson et al., 2007).

Acute Pain

Parent–Child Interactions   Caregivers typically spend most of their time within intimate or personal distances (Peterson et al., 2007; Thompson et al., 2016), and this appears to be stable across all phases (i.e., preprocedure, procedure, postprocedure) of a medical procedure (Peterson et al., 2007). It has been recommended that parents remain physically close to their child in order to facilitate interactions and decrease child distress (Naber, Halstead, Broome, & Rehwaldt, 1995); however, physical distance during or following certain painful procedures may help to avoid stimulating a child when they are required to rest or be still (Cline et al., 2006).

Caregiver intimate distance has been linked to 7–16-year-olds' distress during venipunctures, suggesting parents may sit closer to their child when they are distressed, although it may also be due to prearranged seating and staff directing caregivers to a seat (Thompson et al., 2016). Similarly, use of a close distance was positively related to parent and nurses' ratings of child distress prior to, and during, port starts and lumbar punctures in 3–12-year-old children (Peterson et al., 2007). However, Schinkel et al. (2016) found that paternal and maternal proximity were unrelated to child pain outcomes during the cold pressor task.

Spousal Interactions To the best of our knowledge, there have been no studies to examine proxemics during spousal interactions during acute pain.

Chronic Pain

Parent–Child Interactions To the best of our knowledge, there have been no studies to examine proxemics during parent–child interactions in the chronic pain context.

Spousal Interactions To the best of our knowledge, there have been no studies to examine proxemics during spousal interactions in the chronic pain context.

Summary: Proxemics Existing knowledge on caregivers' interpersonal distance during acute pain is limited, and nonexistent in chronic pain contexts. Parents are typically at a close distance to their child during medical procedures, and this closeness has been related to higher child distress (e.g., Thompson et al., 2016). However, it is unclear if this behavior is proactive or reactive; it is recommended younger children undergoing vaccinations sit on their parents' lap to maximize comfort (Taddio et al., 2015). It may be beneficial for some parents to remain at a distance during or following certain medical procedures to avoid stimulating child movement (e.g., lumbar punctures in pediatric oncology; Cline et al., 2006), which highlights the need to examine this behavior in different contexts. Also, caregiver distance may be governed by how the room is set-up, the type of procedure, and whether staff direct caregiver seating. Future experimental research could control for these factors, and may help clarify the effects of caregiver distance on child pain by assigning parents to different distances. Investigations are also needed to understand caregiver proxemics during spousal interactions, and in chronic pain contexts.

Physiological Activity

The autonomic nervous system (ANS) plays an important role in homeostatic regulation in response to internal and external demands and stressors (Brummelte, Oberlander, & Craig, 2013; Kreibig, 2010). The ANS consists of the sympathetic nervous system (dominates under conditions of stress) and the parasympathetic nervous system (dominates under states of rest and safety) and these two systems work to balance responses to changing environments. The majority of the physiological and psychophysiological investigations in the pain context to date have focused on the individual in pain (Brummelte et al., 2013; Kyle & McNeil, 2014). However, witnessing a spouse or child in pain can be a stressful event and distressing to caregivers (Goubert et al., 2005), and they may experience increased physiological arousal in these situations (e.g., Smith, Shah, Goldman, & Taddio, 2007). Caregivers must manage their own emotional experience in order to effectively attend to and support their child's or spouse's needs in the pain context (Constantin, McMurtry, & Bailey, 2016; Goubert et al., 2005).

Indices of autonomic functioning (e.g., electrodermal activity, blood pressure [BP], heart rate [HR], heart rate variability [HRV]) can be used to inform emotional experience and regulation (see Table 14.1; Appelhans & Luecken, 2006; Berna, Ott, & Nandrino, 2014; Kreibig, 2010). Moreover, HRV is posited to index the activity of the vagus (10th cranial) nerve, which receives input from cortical circuits involved in cognitive, autonomic, and emotion regulation (Porges, 2007; Thayer & Lane, 2000). HRV may more distally index the functioning of these systems (Thayer, Åhs, Fredrikson, Sollers, & Wager, 2012; Thayer & Lane, 2000); high HRV has been linked to greater capacity to flexibly respond to environmental demands (e.g., context-appropriate emotions), with decreases in HRV posited to occur in response to high stress situations (Park, Vasey, Van Bavel, & Thayer, 2014; Thayer et al., 2012; Thayer & Lane, 2000). Therefore, exploring physiological activity in caregivers can be informative in understanding caregiver emotional arousal, regulation, and observable behaviors. Research has only recently started to investigate the physiological response in caregivers.

Acute Pain

Parent–Child Interactions Parent–child interactions during anesthesia induction (via mask) and a venipuncture procedure in the emergency department have been examined in children ranging from 1 month to 18 years of age (Kain et al., 2003; Smith et al., 2007). Parents experienced increases in sympathetic activity (HR, mean arterial pressure, systolic BP, skin conductance) during the venipuncture and leading up to the anesthesia induction (particularly in parents who were present during the induction vs. in the waiting room; Kain et al., 2003; Smith et al., 2007). Further, parents' HR was linked to children's pain outcomes, with higher parental HR associated with children's preoperative anxiety during induction of anesthesia (Kain et al., 2003) and distress following a venipuncture (Smith et al., 2007). These variables may be involved in a positive feedback loop: child pain/distress leads to caregiver anxiety, elevated stress (HR, BP), and distress-promoting verbalizations, which in turn contribute to child pain and distress, and then the cycle repeats (Smith et al., 2007).

In a lab-based experimental investigation, parent HR and HRV were examined before and after an attention manipulation and viewing task (Vervoort, Trost, Sütterlin, Caes, & Moors, 2014). Parents viewed pictures of other people's children, who had previously completed the CPT, exhibiting varying levels of pain facial expression. They were instructed to either focus their eyes on the pain face (i.e., "attend to pain" group), or to focus on the neutral face (i.e., "avoid pain" group). This task interacted with parents' state level of anxiety to affect HR. Specifically, parents reporting low levels of anxiety experienced greater distress (i.e., high HR) when required to attend to child pain, while parents reporting high levels of anxiety experienced greater distress (i.e., high HR) when required to focus attention away from child pain (Vervoort et al., 2014). HRV, included as a measure of parent emotion regulation, decreased significantly from the pre- to post-viewing task, indicating increases in emotional distress (Vervoort et al., 2014). Although not focused on caregiver responses, related research has examined adult physiological activity towards the threat of pain in others (i.e., strangers; Caes et al., 2012). When anticipating pain, observers experienced increases in corrugator activity (i.e., muscle responsible for frowning of the eyebrow) and fear-potentiated startle response (Caes et al., 2012); it is likely these responses would be magnified when observing a loved one in pain.

Spousal Interactions To the best of our knowledge, there have been no studies to examine physiological activity during spousal interactions in the acute pain context.

Chronic Pain

Parent–Child Interactions To the best of our knowledge, there have been no studies examining caregiver physiological activity in the chronic pain context.

Spousal Interactions Block (1981) examined spouses' skin conductance and HR activity while watching videos of painful and neutral facial expressions by: their spouses who experience chronic pain, unfamiliar patients with chronic pain, or performers. Painful facial expressions were associated with higher skin conductance levels, and it was particularly high when viewing painful expressions from spouses with high levels of marital satisfaction. A similar but nonsignificant pattern was found with HR (Block, 1981). Viewing spouses with osteoarthritis complete a painful task and having their partner discuss this experience following the task was associated with increases in BP and HR in caregivers (Monin et al., 2010). In spouses of individuals with musculoskeletal pain, recalling and describing their partners' suffering (e.g., physical discomfort or pain, feeling psychologically distressed) was associated with higher systolic BP reactivity (Mitchell, Levy, Keene, & Monin, 2015).

Summary: Physiology

Anticipating, witnessing, and recalling a child or spouse in pain is distressing for caregivers and associated with higher sympathetic activity, which has been linked to child distress. This suggests that caregivers of individuals with chronic pain may be at a heightened risk for cardiovascular disease given the frequent sympathetic activation and distress associated with viewing a loved one in pain (Monin et al., 2010). Therefore, understanding how caregivers are internally regulating their experienced distress has implications regarding their behavioral responses as well as their own cardiovascular health. These findings also highlight the importance of effective pain management and the implications this has not only for those experiencing pain, but also for caregivers. Future research is needed to clarify the relation(s) between caregivers' physiological responding, particularly the role of parasympathetic activity (e.g., HRV), in the pain context and their observable behaviors. Understanding caregiver physiology can inform how an observer is emotionally processing their spouse or child's pain, which may add context to their behavioral responses to another's pain experience. Research is needed to enhance our understanding of how caregivers respond physiologically to their child's chronic pain, and how spouses respond physiologically to their partner's acute pain.

Overall Summary and Future Research Directions

Due to the historical foci on (a) intrapersonal factors, (b) expressive communication by the individual in pain (e.g., pain behaviors such as grimacing, guarding, crying), (c) and verbal communication by caregivers, the understanding of nonverbal features of caregiving behavior in pain contexts has been largely overlooked. The small body of literature examining caregiver nonverbal behaviors including haptics, body movements, facial expression, and vocal paralanguage, typically combines these various indices together. This emphasizes a grouped, "functional" approach; without complementary detailed topography, valuable information may be missing (Cano & Williams, 2010). Furthermore, the "function" of a behavior is often presumed by researchers (e.g., physical *reassurance*, *solicitous* behaviors) rather than elicited from the person in pain who may have a different perspective (Cano & Williams, 2010). Beyond considering/assuming a gestalt of nonverbal features, these cues are also frequently grouped together with verbal behaviors to form general codes. This is logical in the sense that we typically communicate via multiple channels simultaneously; yet, it negates identification and description of which specific behaviors occurred and their relations with pain-related outcomes.

Future research should measure the full spectrum of naturalistic communication between caregivers and individuals in pain so that the relations among various nonverbal features as well as verbal content are examined (Burgoon & Hoobler, 2002). The individual measurement and eventual integration of these channels are perhaps daunting tasks but will undoubtedly yield rich information which can be used to drive theory and models of pain, assessment, as well as interventions in both acute and chronic pain. A consideration of interactions in pain contexts from multiple interpretative models/perspectives including social communication, pain empathy, intimacy, operant, and cognitive behavioral models is an area ripe for future work. A major challenge for researchers is the longitudinal nature of communication as each interaction builds on historical ones (Heath & Bryant, 2000). The importance of the (preexisting) relationship between communicative partners (here the caregiver and the person in pain) is widely acknowledged (Hadjistavropoulos et al., 2011; Heath & Bryant, 2000); thus, differences are expected in the nature of the interactions and nonverbal features depending on the relationship of the caregiver to the person in pain and these differences should be explored.

As noted above, capturing and clearly describing the naturalistic topography of these features is imperative; this should occur first on a feature-by-feature basis and be well contextualized (e.g., considering the painful context, demographic variables such as age, sex, and culture as well as the relationship between interacting people). Incorporating physiological measures will also contribute to understanding the complex interactions that occur in the pain context. Next, relations among the various nonverbal features and physiology can be considered in a similar manner. This includes the timing of various features within a given interaction which can be gleaned from the use of sequential analyses. Investigating the relations among the nonverbal features and observable pain expression, self-report of pain experience, caregiver perception of the pain experience, and self-report of both intended message (by caregiver) and perceived "message" (by person in pain) will all be important to study. In particular, incorporating an individual's perceptions of discrete caregiver behaviors may help drive the field forward; use of methodology like video-mediated recall tasks as in McMurtry et al. (2010) may be helpful. An important factor to consider is also the degree of automaticity versus controlled acts for the various nonverbal caregiving behaviors (Hadjistavropoulos & Craig, 2002; Heath & Bryant, 2000). As in Schinkel et al. (2016), examination of sex differences in nonverbal features (expression, interpretation) would also be an informative avenue as would consideration of the role of culture. These descriptive studies can then inform experimental methodologies systematically manipulating nonverbal and contextual features of interest to clarify their effect on pain experience and expression.

In conclusion, it is evident that a more robust understanding of pain can emerge from a deeper exploration of nonverbal caregiving behaviors in acute and chronic pain contexts. Research to date has focused almost exclusively on caregiver verbal behavior, which, though important, comprises only a fraction of the related social interaction and transaction, and therefore translates to a limited understanding of the pain experience. The study of nonverbal features of caregiving behavior in both acute and chronic pain contexts offers numerous opportunities for novel and important future work. We urge pain researchers to consider nonverbal features in their work on interactions in the context of pain which will contribute to existing frameworks of pain communication and look forward to contributions in this area.

References

Andersen, P. A., & Andersen, J. F. (2005). Measurements of perceived nonverbal immediacy. In V. L. Manusov (Ed.), *The sourcebook of nonverbal measures* (pp. 113–126). Mahwah, NJ: Lawrence Erlbaum Associates.

Andrews, M. L., & Madeira, S. S. (1977). The assessment of pitch discrimination ability in young children. *Journal of Speech and Hearing Disorders, 42*(2), 279–286.

Appelhans, B. M., & Luecken, L. J. (2006). Heart rate variability as an index of regulated emotional responding. *Review of General Psychology, 10*, 229–240. https://doi.org/10.1037/1089-2680.10.3.229

Bandura, A. (1977). *Social learning theory*. Englewood Cliffs, NJ: Prentice-Hall.

Berna, G., Ott, L., & Nandrino, J. (2014). Effects of emotion regulation difficulties on the tonic and phasic cardiac autonomic response. *PLoS One, 9*(7), e102971. https://doi.org/10.1371/journal.pone.0102971

Block, A. R. (1981). An investigation of the response of the spouse to chronic pain behavior. *Psychosomatic Medicine, 43*(5), 415–422.

Blount, R. L., Landolf-Fritsche, B., Powers, S. W., & Sturges, J. W. (1991). Differences between high and low coping children and between parent and staff behaviors during painful medical procedures. *Journal of Pediatric Psychology, 16*(6), 795–809. https://doi.org/10.1093/JPEPSY/16.6.795

Blount, R. L., Sturges, J. W., & Powers, S. W. (1990). Analysis of child and adult behavioral variations by phase of medical procedure. *Behavior Therapy, 21*(1), 33–48. https://doi.org/10.1016/S0005-7894(05)80187-X

Boersma, P., & Weenink, D. (2016). *Praat: Doing phonetics by computer [computer program]*. http://www.praat.org/

Brummelte, S., Oberlander, T. F., & Craig, K. D. (2013). Biomarkers of pain: Physiological indices of pain reactivity in infants and children. In P. J. McGrath, B. J. Stevens, S. M. Walker, & W. T. Zempsky (Eds.), *Oxford textbook of paediatric pain* (pp. 391–398). Oxford, England: Oxford University Press.

Burgoon, J. K., & Hoobler, G. D. (2002). Non-verbal signals. In M. L. Knapp & J. A. Daly (Eds.), *Handbook of interpersonal communication* (pp. 240–299). London, England: Sage.

Caes, L., Uzieblo, K., Crombez, G., De Ruddere, L., Vervoort, T., & Goubert, L. (2012). Negative emotional responses elicited by the anticipation of pain in others: Psychophysiological evidence. *The Journal of Pain, 13*, 467–476. https://doi.org/10.1016/j.jpain.2012.02.003

Cano, A., & Williams, A. C. d. C. (2010). Social interaction in pain: Reinforcing pain behaviors or building intimacy? *Pain, 149*, 9–11. https://doi.org/10.1016/jpain.2009.10.010

Cavender, K., Goff, M., Hollon, E. C., & Guzzetta, C. E. (2004). Parents' positioning and distracting children during venipuncture. *Journal of Holistic Nursing, 22*(1), 32–56. https://doi.org/10.1177/0898010104263306

Chambers, C. T., Craig, K. D., & Bennett, S. M. (2002). The impact of maternal behavior on children's pain experiences: An experimental analysis. *Journal of Pediatric Psychology, 27*(3), 293–301. Retrieved from http://www.ncbi.nlm.nih.gov/pubmed/11909936

Chorney, J. M., McMurtry, C. M., Chambers, C. T., & Bakeman, R. (2015). Developing and modifying behavioral coding schemes in pediatric psychology: A practical guide. *Journal of Pediatric Psychology, 40*, 154–164. https://doi.org/10.1093/jpepsy/jsu099

Chorney, J. M., Torrey, C., Blount, R., McLaren, C. E., Chen, W., & Kain, Z. N. (2009). Healthcare provider and parent behavior and children's coping and distress at anesthesia induction. *Anesthesiology, 111*(6), 1290–1296. https://doi.org/10.1097/ALN.0b013e3181c14be5

Cline, R. J. W., Harper, F. W. K., Penner, L. A., Peterson, A. M., Taub, J. W., & Albrecht, T. L. (2006). Parent communication and child pain and distress during painful pediatric cancer treatments. *Social Science & Medicine, 63*(4), 883–898. https://doi.org/10.1016/j.socscimed.2006.03.007

Coan, J. A., Schaefer, H. S., & Davidson, R. J. (2006). Lending a hand: Social regulation of the neural response to threat. *Psychological Science, 17*(12), 1032–1039. https://doi.org/10.1111/j.1467-9280.2006.01832.x

Cohn, J. F., & Ekman, P. (2008). Measuring facial action. In J. A. Harrigan, R. Rosenthal, & K. R. Scherer (Eds.), *The new handbook of methods in non-verbal behavior research* (pp. 9–64). Oxford, England: Oxford University Press.

Constantin, K., McMurtry, C. M., & Bailey, H. N. (2016). Parental cardiac response in the context of pediatric acute pain: Current knowledge and future directions. *Pain Management, 7*(2), 81–87. https://doi.org/10.2217/pmt-2016-0033

Craig, K. D. (1986). Social modeling influences: Pain in context. In R. A. Sternbach (Ed.), *The psychology of pain* (2nd ed., pp. 67–95). New York, NY: Raven Press.

Craig, K. D. (2009). The social communication model of pain. *Canadian Psychology, 50*, 22–32. https://doi.org/10.1037/a0014772

Craig, K. D., Versloot, J., Goubert, L., Vervoort, T., & Crombez, G. (2010). Perceiving pain in others: Automatic and controlled mechanisms. *The Journal of Pain, 11*(2), 101–108. https://doi.org/10.1016/j.jpain.2009.08.008

Dahlquist, L. M., Pendley, J. S., Power, T. G., Landthrip, D. S., Jones, C. L., & Steuber, C. P. (2001). Adult command structure and children's distress during the anticipatory phase of invasive cancer procedures. *Children's Health Care, 30*(2), 151–167. https://doi.org/10.1207/S15326888CHC3002_5

Dahlquist, L. M., Pendley, J. S., Power, T. G., Landthrip, D. S., & Jones, C. M. (1994). *The pediatric medical interaction scale.* (Unpublished manuscript). Baltimore, MD: University of Maryland, Baltimore County.

Dahlquist, L. M., Power, T. G., & Carlson, L. (1995). Physician and parent behavior during invasive pediatric cancer procedures: Relationships to child behavioral distress. *Journal of Pediatric Psychology, 20*(4), 477–490. https://doi.org/10.1093/jpepsy/20.4.477

Darwin, C. (1998). *The expression of the emotions in man and animals* (3rd ed.). London, England: Harper Collins. (Original work published 1872).

DiMatteo, M. R., Sherbourne, C. D., Hays, R. D., Ordway, L., Kravitz, R. L., McGlynn, E. A., … Rogers, W. H. (1993). Physicians' characteristics influence patients' adherence to medical treatment: Results from the medical outcomes study. *Health Psychology, 12*(2), 93. Retrieved from https://www.ncbi.nlm.nih.gov/pubmed/8500445

Duck, S. W., & McMahan, D. T. (2015). *Communication in everyday life: The basic course edition with public speaking.* Thousand Oaks, CA: Sage.

Dunford, E., Thompson, M., & Gauntlett-Gilbert, J. (2014). Parental behavior in paediatric chronic pain: A qualitative observational study. *Clinical Child Psychology and Psychiatry, 19*(4), 561–575. https://doi.org/10.1177/1359104513492347

Ekman, P., & Oster, H. (1979). Facial expressions of emotion. *Annual Review of Psychology, 30*, 527–554.

Elfenbein, H. A., & Ambady, N. (2002). On the universality and cultural specificity of emotion recognition: A meta-analysis. *Psychological Bulletin, 128*(2), 203–235. https://doi.org/10.1037//0033-2909.128.2.203

Engstrand, O., & Krull, D. (2001). Simplification of phonotactic structures in unscripted Swedish. *Journal of the International Phonetic Association, 31*(1), 41–50. https://doi.org/10.1017/S0025100301001049

Field, T. (2010). Touch for socioemotional and physical well-being: A review. *Developmental Review, 30*(4), 367–383. https://doi.org/10.1016/j.dr.2011.01.001

Fordyce, W. E. (1986). Learning processes in pain. In R. A. Sternbach (Ed.), *The psychology of pain* (2nd ed., pp. 49–65). New York, NY: Raven Press.

Frick, R. W. (1985). Communicating emotion: The role of prosodic features. *Psychological Bulletin, 97*(3), 412–429.

Goedhart, A. D., van der Sluis, S., Houtveen, J. H., Willemsen, G., & de Geus, E. J. C. (2007). Comparison of time and frequency domain measures of RSA in ambulatory recordings. *Psychophysiology, 44*(2), 203–215. https://doi.org/10.1111/j.1469-8986.2006.00490.x

Goldstein, P., Shamay-Tsoory, S., Yellinek, S., & Weissman-Fogel, I. (2016). Empathy predicts an experimental pain reduction during touch. *The Journal of Pain, 17*(10), 1049–1057. https://doi.org/10.1016/j.jpain.2016.06.007

Goodman, J. E., & McGrath, P. J. (2003). Mothers' modeling influences children's pain during a cold pressor task. *Pain, 104*, 559–565. https://doi.org/10.1016/S0304-3959(03)00090-3

Gottman, J. M., McCoy, K., Coan, J., & Collier, H. (1995). *The Specific Affect Coding System (SPAFF) for observing emotional communication in marital and family interaction.* Mahwah, NJ: Lawrence Erlbaum Associates.

Goubert, L., Craig, K. D., Vervoort, T., Morley, S., Sullivan, M. J. L., Williams, A. C., … Crombez, G. (2005). Facing others in pain: The effects of empathy. *Pain, 118*, 285–288. https://doi.org/10.1016/j.pain.2005.10.025

Greenbaum, P. E., Turner, C., Cook, E. W., & Melamed, B. G. (1990). Dentists' voice control: Effects on children's disruptive and affective behavior. *Health Psychology, 9*(5), 546–558. https://doi.org/10.1037/0278-6133.9.5.546

Hadjistavropoulos, T., & Craig, K.D. (2002). A theoretical framework for understanding self-report and observational measures of pain: a communications model. *Behaviour Research and Therapy, 40*(5), 551–570.

Hadjistavropoulos, T., Craig, K. D., Duck, S., Cano, A., Goubert, L., Jackson, P. L., … Fitzgerald, T. D. (2011). A biopsychosocial formulation of pain communication. *Psychological Bulletin, 137*, 910–939. https://doi.org/10.1037/a0023876

Halliday, M. A. (1970). Functional diversity in language as seen from a consideration of modality and mood in English. *Foundations of Language, 6*(3), 322–361. Retrieved from http://www.jstor.org/stable/25000463

Harrigan, J., & Rosenthal, R. (2008). *New handbook of methods in nonverbal behavior research.* Oxford, England: Oxford University Press.

Heath, R. L., & Bryant, J. (2000). *Human communication theory and research: Concepts, contexts, and challenges* (2nd ed.). Mahwah, NJ: Lawrence Erlbaum Associates.

Hops, H., Davis, B., & Longoria, N. (1995). Methodological issues in direct observation: Illustrations with the living in familial environments (LIFE) coding system. *Journal of Clinical Child Psychology, 24*(2), 193–203. https://doi.org/10.1207/s15374424jccp2402_7

Horton, R. E., & Pillai Riddell, R. R. (2010). Mothers' facial expressions of pain and fear and infants' pain response during immunization. *Infant Mental Health Journal, 31*, 397–411. https://doi.org/10.1002/imhj.20262

Johansen, A. B., & Cano, A. (2007). A preliminary investigation of affective interaction in chronic pain couples. *Pain, 132*, S86–S95. https://doi.org/10.1016/j.pain.2007.04.016

Kain, Z. N., Caldwell-Andrews, A. A., Mayes, L. C., Wang, S. M., Krivutza, D. M., & LoDolce, M. E. (2003). Parental presence during induction of anesthesia: Physiological effects on parents. *Anesthesiology, 98*, 58–64. Retrieved from http://www.ncbi.nlm.nih.gov/pubmed/12502980

Kankkunen, P., Vehviläinen-Julkunen, K., Pietilä, A. M., & Halonen, P. (2003). Parents' use of nonpharmacological methods to alleviate children's postoperative pain at home. *Journal of Advanced Nursing, 41*(4), 367–375. https://doi.org/10.1046/j.1365-2648.2003.02536.x

Kleiber, C., & McCarthy, A. M. (1999). Parent behavior and child distress during urethral catheterization. *Journal of the Society of Pediatric Nurses: JSPN, 4*(3), 95–104. Retrieved from http://www.ncbi.nlm.nih.gov/pubmed/10472541

Kreibig, S. D. (2010). Autonomic nervous system activity in emotion: A review. *Biological Psychology, 84*(3), 394–421. https://doi.org/10.1016/j.biopsycho.2010.03.010

Kyle, B. N., & McNeil, D. W. (2014). Autonomic arousal and experimentally induced pain: A critical review of the literature. *Pain Research & Management, 19*(3), 159–167. https://doi.org/10.1155/2014/536859

Master, S. L., Eisenberger, N. I., Taylor, S. E., Naliboff, B. D., Shirinyan, D., & Lieberman, M. D. (2009). A picture's worth: Partner photographs reduce experimentally induced pain. *Psychological Science, 20*(11), 1316–1318. https://doi.org/10.1111/j.1467-9280.2009.02444.x

McMurtry, C. M., Chambers, C. T., McGrath, P. J., & Asp, E. (2010). When "don't worry" communicates fear: Children's perceptions of parental reassurance and distraction during a painful medical procedure. *Pain, 150*(1), 52–58. https://doi.org/10.1016/j.pain.2010.02.021

McMurtry, C. M., McGrath, P. J., Asp, E., & Chambers, C. T. (2007). Parental reassurance and pediatric procedural pain: A linguistic description. *The Journal of Pain, 8*(2), 95–101. https://doi.org/10.1016/j.jpain.2006.05.015

Melzack, R., & Wall, P. (1965). Pain mechanisms: A new theory. *Science, 150*, 971–978.

Mitchell, H., Levy, B. R., Keene, D. E., & Monin, J. K. (2015). Reactivity to a spouse's interpersonal suffering in late life marriage: A mixed-methods approach. *Journal of Aging and Health, 27*(6), 939–961. https://doi.org/10.1177/0898264315569456

Monin, J. K., Schulz, R., Martire, L. M., Jennings, J. R., Lingler, J. H., & Greenberg, M. S. (2010). Spouses' cardiovascular reactivity to their partners' suffering. *The Journals of Gerontology Series B, Psychological Sciences and Social Sciences, 65*((2), 195–201. https://doi.org/10.1093/geronb/gbp133

Morton, J. B., & Trehub, S. E. (2001). Children's understanding of emotion in speech. *Child Development, 72*(3), 834–843. Retrieved from http://www.ncbi.nlm.nih.gov/pubmed/11405585

Mumme, D. L., Fernald, A., & Herrera, C. (1996). Infants' responses to facial and vocal emotional signals in a social referencing paradigm. *Child Development, 67*(6), 3219–3237. https://doi.org/10.1111/j.1467-8624.1996.tb01910.x

Naber, S. J., Halstead, L. K., Broome, M. E., & Rehwaldt, M. (1995). Communication and control: Parent, child, and health care professional interactions during painful procedures. *Issues in Comprehensive Pediatric Nursing, 18*(2), 79–90.

Nahman-Averbuch, H., Dayan, L., Sprecher, E., Hochberg, U., Brill, S., Yarnitsky, D., & Jacob, G. (2016). Sex differences in the relationships between parasympathetic activity and pain modulation. *Physiology & Behavior, 154*, 40–48.

Park, G., Vasey, M. W., Van Bavel, J. J., & Thayer, J. F. (2014). When tonic cardiac vagal tone predicts changes in phasic vagal tone: The role of fear and perceptual load. *Psychophysiology, 51*, 419–426. https://doi.org/10.1111/psyp.12186

Pedro, H., Barros, L., & Moleiro, C. (2010). Brief report: Parents and nurses' behaviors associated with child distress during routine immunization in a Portuguese population. *Journal of Pediatric Psychology, 35*(6), 602–610. https://doi.org/10.1093/jpepsy/jsp062

Peterson, A. M., Cline, R. J. W., Foster, T. S., Penner, L. A., Parrott, R. L., Keller, C. M., . . . Albrecht, T. L. (2007). Parents' interpersonal distance and touch behavior and child pain and distress during painful pediatric oncology procedures. Journal of Nonverbal Behavior, 31(2), 79–97. doi:https://doi.org/10.1007/s10919-007-0023-9

Porges, S. W. (2007). The polyvagal perspective. *Biological Psychology, 74*, 116–143. https://doi.org/10.1016/j.biopsycho.2006.06.009

Prkachin, K. M. (2009). Assessing pain by facial expression: Facial expression as nexus. *Pain Research & Management, 14*, 53–58. https://doi.org/10.1155/2009/542964

Rancourt, K. M., Chorney, J. M., & Kain, Z. (2015). Children's immediate postoperative distress and mothers' and fathers' touch behaviors. *Journal of Pediatric Psychology, 40*(10), 1115–1123. https://doi.org/10.1093/jpepsy/jsv069

Reid, G. J., McGrath, P. J., & Lang, B. A. (2005). Parent–child interactions among children with juvenile fibromyalgia, arthritis, and healthy controls. *Pain, 113*(1), 201–210. https://doi.org/10.1016/j.pain.2004.10.018

Romano, J. M., Jensen, M. P., Turner, J. A., Good, A. B., & Hops, H. (2000). Chronic pain patient-partner interactions: Further support for a behavioral model of chronic pain. *Behavior Therapy, 31*(3), 415–440. https://doi.org/10.1016/S0005-7894(00)80023-4

Romano, J. M., Turner, J. A., Friedman, L. S., Bulcroft, R. A., Jensen, M. P., & Hops, H. (1991). Observational assessment of chronic pain patient-spouse behavioral interactions. *Behavior Therapy, 22*(4), 549–567. https://doi.org/10.1016/S0005-7894(05)80345-4

Romano, J. M., Turner, J. A., Friedman, L. S., Bulcroft, R. A., Jensen, M. P., Hops, H., & Wright, S. F. (1992). Sequential analysis of chronic pain behaviors and spouse responses. *Journal of Consulting and Clinical Psychology, 60*(5), 777–782. https://doi.org/10.1037/0022-006X.60.5.777

Romano, J. M., Turner, J. A., Jensen, M. P., Friedman, L. S., Bulcroft, R. A., Hops, H., & Wright, S. F. (1995). Chronic pain patient–spouse behavioral interactions predict patient disability. *Pain, 63*(3), 353–360.

Sauter, D. A., Panattoni, C., & Happé, F. (2013). Children's recognition of emotions from vocal cues. *The British Journal of Developmental Psychology, 31*(1), 97–113. https://doi.org/10.1111/j.2044-835X.2012.02081.x

Scherer, K. (2003). Vocal communication of emotion: A review of research paradigms. *Speech Communication, 40*(1–2), 227–256. https://doi.org/10.1016/S0167-6393(02)00084-5

Schinkel, M. G., Chambers, C. T., Caes, L., & Moon, E. (2016). A comparison of maternal versus paternal non-verbal behavior during child pain. *Pain Practice*. https://doi.org/10.1111/papr.12415

Smith, R., Shah, V., Goldman, R., & Taddio, A. (2007). Caregivers' responses to pain in their children in the emergency department. *Archives of Pediatrics & Adolescent Medicine, 161*, 578–582. Retrieved from http://www.ncbi.nlm.nih.gov/pubmed/17548763

Smith, S. J., Keefe, F. J., Caldwell, D. S., Romano, J., & Baucom, D. (2004). Gender differences in patient–spouse interactions: A sequential analysis of behavioral interactions in patients having osteoarthritic knee pain. *Pain, 112*(1), 183–187. https://doi.org/10.1016/j.pain.2004.08.019

Svendsen, E. J., Moen, A., Pedersen, R., & Bjørk, I. T. (2016). Parent-healthcare provider interaction during peripheral vein cannulation with resistive preschool children. *Journal of Advanced Nursing, 72*(3), 620–630. https://doi.org/10.1111/jan.12852

Taddio, A., McMurtry, C. M., Shah, V., Pillai Riddell, R., Chambers, C. T., Noel, M., & the HELPinKids&Adults Team. (2015). Reducing pain during vaccine injections: Clinical practice guideline (summary). *Canadian Medical Association Journal, 187*(13), 975–982. https://doi.org/10.1503/cmaj.150391

Taylor, C., Sellick, K., & Greenwood, K. (2011). The influence of adult behaviors on child coping during venipuncture: A sequential analysis. *Research in Nursing & Health, 34*(2), 116–131. https://doi.org/10.1002/nur.20424

Thayer, J. F., Åhs, F., Fredrikson, M., Sollers, J. J., & Wager, T. D. (2012). A meta-analysis of heart rate variability and neuroimaging studies: Implications for heart rate variability as a marker of stress and health. *Neuroscience and Biobehavioral Reviews, 36*, 747–756. https://doi.org/10.1016/j.neubiorev.2011.11.009

Thayer, J. F., & Lane, R. D. (2000). A model of neurovisceral integration in emotion regulation and dysregulation. *Journal of Affective Disorders, 61*, 201–216. https://doi.org/10.1016/S0165-0327(00)00338-4

Thompson, S., Ayers, S., Pervilhac, C., Mahoney, L., & Seddon, P. (2016). The association of children's distress during venepuncture with parent and staff behaviors. *Journal of Child Health Care, 20*(3), 267–276. https://doi.org/10.1177/1367493515598643

Vaish, A., & Striano, T. (2004). Is visual reference necessary? Contributions of facial versus vocal cues in 12-month-olds' social referencing behavior. *Developmental Science, 7*(3), 261–269. https://doi.org/10.1111/j.1467-7687.2004.00344.x

Vannorsdall, T., Dahlquist, L., Pendley, J. S., & Power, T. (2004). The relation between nonessential touch and children's distress during lumbar punctures. *Children's Health Care, 33*(4), 299–315. https://doi.org/10.1207/s15326888chc3304_4

Vervoort, T., Trost, Z., Sütterlin, S., Caes, L., & Moors, A. (2014). Emotion regulatory function of parent attention to child pain and associated implications for parental pain control behavior. *Pain, 155*(8), 1453–1463. https://doi.org/10.1016/j.pain.2014.04.015

von Bismarck, G. (1974). Sharpness as an attribute of the timbre of steady sounds. Acta Acustica united with Acustica, *30*(3), 159–172.

Walker-Andrews, A. S. (1997). Infants' perception of expressive behaviors: Differentiation of multimodal information. *Psychological Bulletin, 121*, 437–456.

Wright, K. D., Stewart, S. H., Finley, G. A., & Raazi, M. (2014). A sequential examination of parent-child interactions at anesthetic induction. *Journal of Clinical Psychology in Medical Settings, 21*(4), 374–385. https://doi.org/10.1007/s10880-014-9413-4

Chapter 15
Interpersonal Pain Dynamics in Couples: Interactions Between Spouses' Physical Health Predict Caregiver Outcomes

Julie K. Cremeans-Smith

Abstract Pain is a private experience which patients may express through verbal or behavioral means. The communication of such suffering can result in the individual's pain potentially becoming a social stressor. Patients' verbal or nonverbal pain behaviors may elicit social support from others, frequently including their spouse. In high quality marriages, spouses engage in shared efforts to cope with the stress of one partner's painful condition. However, prior research on the interpersonal dynamics of pain among couples has focused on the impact of one partner's health condition while ignoring the potential that both spouses may be coping with a chronic health condition. Congruence frequently occurs between marital partners in respect to health behaviors and diagnoses. Herein, the interactions between the physical health of 101 older women with osteoarthritis and their caregiving husbands are considered. Results illustrate significant interactions between spouses' physical health, which predict the behavior and mental health of the caregiving spouse. Further, husbands' provision of emotional support and depressive symptoms are influenced by actor effects, while provision of instrumental support and life satisfaction are associated with partner effects. Therefore, future research on interpersonal dynamics of pain within married couples should consider the health status of both spouses.

Keywords Chronic pain · Couples · Caregiver stress · Dyadic coping · Marital satisfaction · Emotional support · Congruence · Physical health

Satisfying marriages are associated with a variety of mental and physical health benefits (Kiecolt-Glaser & Newton, 2001). Marriage may exert these positive effects by enhancing emotion regulation, increasing the practice of healthy behaviors, and buffering individuals from the physiological consequences of stress (Robles, Slatcher, Trombello, & McGinn, 2014). The intimate nature of marriage, as well as

J. K. Cremeans-Smith (✉)
Department of Psychological Sciences, Kent State University at Stark,
North Canton, OH, USA
e-mail: jcremean@kent.edu

© Springer International Publishing AG, part of Springer Nature 2018
T. Vervoort et al. (eds.), *Social and Interpersonal Dynamics in Pain*,
https://doi.org/10.1007/978-3-319-78340-6_15

the sharing of space, time, and resources on a daily basis, differentiates this type of relationship from other dyadic interactions (i.e., family members, friends; Robles et al., 2014). The marital context provides individuals with an important source of support, as the spouse is often reported to be a primary provider of social support (Phillipson, 1997). Therefore, the interpersonal dynamics that occur between married partners have the potential to significantly impact the psychological and physical well-being of patients coping with chronic pain. It is important to recognize that such effects are bidirectional. A systems perspective would suggest that the illness of one spouse alters the structure of the relationship and impacts the psychological and physical well-being of the other partner (Burman & Margolin, 1992). This chapter will review research demonstrating that chronic pain is a social phenomenon, the stress of which impacts both marital partners and prompts shared coping efforts. Relationship variables (e.g., marital satisfaction), as well as individual factors (e.g., personal experience with pain) that may influence the support provision and psychological adjustment of spouses will also be considered.

Chronic pain conditions, such as arthritis, low back pain, and fibromyalgia, pose a significant burden. Estimates suggest that 11.2% of the US population experienced chronic pain during the past 3 months (Nahin, 2015). Further, individuals coping with chronic, severe pain are also likely to be impacted by experiences of fatigue, depression, anxiety, and disability, compared to healthy individuals (Nahin, 2015). Pain is fundamentally a private experience, which must be made known to others through the verbal or nonverbal expression of distress (Turk, Kerns, & Rosenberg, 1992). However, behavioral displays may not accurately reflect an individual's pain experience. For example, structured interviews with chronic pain patients revealed that the vast majority (90%) had tried to hide their pain from others (Morley, Doyle, & Beese, 2000). A history of negative interactions with support providers may encourage patients to be cautious in future communications and to minimize outward expressions of pain. Such interactions are frequent. More than 60% of patients interviewed by Morley et al. (2000) had experienced negative reactions (lack of sympathy, distrust, etc.) from support providers after talking about their pain. However, the use of verbal disclosure and nonverbal pain behaviors by patients is essential for communicating suffering to others and eliciting their support (Craig, Prkachin, & Grunau, 2001). The extensive interdependence between married partners may increase the saliency of these pain behaviors and likelihood of a response by the caregiving spouse (Preston & de Waal, 2002). Spouses' empathic responses to patients' pain behaviors are determined by multiple factors, including the frequency of these expressions and an evaluation of whether such communication is typical for the patient (Wilson et al., 2013). Although the communication of distress and suffering is beneficial to patients, outward expressions of pain are associated with greater depressive symptoms among caregiving spouses (Stephens, Martire, Cremeans-Smith, Druley, & Wojno, 2006).

The Impact of Spousal Support on Patient Outcomes

The provision of emotional and/or instrumental support by a spouse can enhance patients' psychological and physical well-being. For example, women with rheumatoid arthritis whose spouses were highly supportive reported lower levels of anxiety and depression during times of stress (Zautra et al., 1998). Further, patients whose marital relationships were characterized by frequent positive interactions (e.g., affection, emotional closeness, physical intimacy) exhibited lower levels of disease activity (Zautra et al., 1998). Similarly, patients recovering from knee arthroplasty feel more efficacious to manage their pain and adhere to medical recommendations when their spouses are emotionally supportive. Three months following surgery, these patients are characterized by better physical and mental health outcomes (Khan et al., 2009). In addition to benefitting the patient, adequate support that matches patients' need can positively influence couple-level outcomes such as trust and relationship satisfaction (Rafaeli & Gleason, 2009). The provision of emotional support, in particular, has the potential to enhance intimacy as it communicates to the patient that their spouse is attentive and responsive to their needs (Revenson, Schiaffino, Majerovitz, & Gibofsky, 1991).

Not all support is beneficial, however. In some instances, spouses' attempts to be helpful are miscarried or interpreted negatively by the patient (Revenson et al., 1991). Patients who highly value their independence are more likely to react negatively (i.e., greater depressive symptoms and lower self-efficacy) to support attempts by their spouse (Martire, Stephens, & Schulz, 2011). Further, caregiver behaviors which communicate to patients that they are incapable of coping without the provider's assistance may undermine patients' self-efficacy or autonomy (Rafaeli & Gleason, 2009). Additionally, when support turns into control (e.g., persuasion or pressure to induce behavioral change), there are negative consequences for both the patient (e.g., poor adherence) as well as the spouse (e.g., distress; Franks, Wehrspann, August, Rook, & Stephens, 2016). Researchers have suggested various mechanisms through which spouses' problematic support may negatively impact patients' psychological and physical health, such as failing to meet patients' needs (Fekete, Stephens, Druley, & Greene, 2007; Revenson et al., 1991) and creating a sense of indebtedness to their partner (Rafaeli & Gleason, 2009).

Operant models have proposed that spousal support or attention to pain behaviors may positively reinforce such expressions (Turk et al., 1992). Laboratory studies with chronic back pain patients support the operant model, finding reduced pain threshold and tolerance on cold pressor (Flor, Breitenstein, Birbaumer, & Furst, 1995) and less time spent walking on a treadmill in the presence of solicitous spouses (i.e., overly attentive to or concerned about the patient's pain; Lousberg, Schmidt, & Groenman, 1992). Among clinical samples, spousal solicitousness is associated with greater disability and more pain behaviors on the part of the patient (Schwartz, Jensen, & Romano, 2005). Patients may employ fewer active coping methods or be reluctant to accept pain when spouses engage in solicitous behaviors, the result of which is an increase in patients' distress and disability (McCracken,

2005). A more thorough review of this topic may be found in Chap. 5 of this volume.

Solicitous spousal behaviors are not always reinforcing, however. In fact, such behaviors are rated less positively by chronic pain patients than spousal promotion of cognitive-behavioral strategies for pain management (e.g., encouragement of task persistence or problem solving; Newton-John & Williams, 2006). Conversely, intimacy models suggest that spousal responses that have been previously labelled as solicitous may play an important role in promoting relationship quality and satisfaction (Cano & Williams, 2010). For instance, when a spouse responds with empathy and validation to a patient's disclosure of pain-related thoughts or feelings, both partners are likely to experience an increased sense of closeness and intimacy (Cano & Williams, 2010; Rime, 2009). Therefore, the experience and expression of pain by one individual has the potential to significantly impact the dynamics of the marital relationship.

Dyadic Coping with Chronic Pain

A growing body of research has focused on dyadic coping, examining couples' interactions and shared efforts to adapt to the painful condition of one partner. Bodenmann (2005), for example, suggests that researchers "cannot examine one partner's stress appraisals or coping efforts without considering the effects on the other partner and the marriage" (p. 36). Couples who are confronted with persistent, health-related stressors engage in a transactional process of coping that evolves over time (Berg & Upchurch, 2007). Therefore, threat appraisals and coping efforts occur not only at the individual level (e.g., actor or partner effects), but also at the level of the couple (joint effects). When dyadic efforts are engaged to cope with patients' chronic pain, the combined resources of both partners are utilized to manage the stressor (Bodenmann, 1997). Conceptualizing stress and coping efforts at the level of the dyad, however, introduces the potential for relationship variables such as marital satisfaction to significantly impact the situation. Couples with high levels of marital satisfaction may be more likely to engage in shared appraisal or communal coping, which further enhances their relationship (Berg & Upchurch, 2007). In contrast, conflicts within a marriage may increase the propensity of caregiving spouses to respond negatively (i.e., with unsupportive responses to or criticism) to patients' expressions of pain (Manne & Zautra, 1989).

High quality marriages are characterized by high levels of relationship satisfaction, positive attitudes towards one's partner, and low frequency of hostile or negative behaviors (Robles et al., 2014). Partners in such relationships typically interpret each other's behaviors as motivated by altruism, empathy, and compassion, creating a self-reinforcing cycle that further enhances their relationship satisfaction (Clark & Stephens, 1996). Further, the needs of both partners may be fulfilled within the context of the marriage when spouses provide equitable levels of emotional support and disclosure (Berg & Upchurch, 2007). High levels of marital satisfaction encourage spouses to engage in pro-relationship rather than self-serving behaviors, illustrating a transformation of motivation (Lewis et al., 2006). When the couple is then confronted with the stress of one's chronic pain, such a relationship offers a significant resource for both partners. High marital satisfaction has been shown to mutually buffer partners in the aforementioned scenario: patients demonstrated enhanced illness management and both spouses experience better psychosocial adjustment (Berg & Upchurch, 2007). One important caveat is that marital satisfaction may increase the value that patients place on attention from their spouse, potentially enhancing the risks associated with solicitous responses (Turk et al., 1992). A significant limitation of research with couples is the lack of information regarding the quality of their relationship prior to the onset of one partner's chronic pain condition (Burman & Margolin, 1992). Therefore, it is difficult to know whether negative interactions result from the stress of coping with chronic pain or reflect preexisting communication patterns (Burman & Margolin, 1992). Although research has acknowledged the stress associated with caregiving, studies typically focus on the support needs of the patient without recognizing the needs of the spouse (Berg & Upchurch, 2007; Rafaeli & Gleason, 2009). Reciprocated and equitable support within the relationship is known to enhance marital satisfaction and psychological well-being of both partners (Acitelli & Antonucci, 1994). In contrast, inequity between the amount of support that is received versus that which is provided to a partner may produce emotional distress (e.g., guilt, resentment; Walster, Walster, & Berscheid, 1978). Patients coping with a chronically painful condition may be less able to provide support to their partner (Burman & Margolin, 1992). For example, differences in physical health status encourage the healthy spouse to take on more household responsibilities. Such a situation may result in the patient over-benefiting from the relationship and introduce the potential for negative reactions to this inequity by both partners (Yorgason & Choi, 2016). However, it is likely that both partners have been diagnosed with a chronic health condition. Thus, there may not be a clear distinction between patients and caregivers during late adulthood (Berg & Upchurch, 2007). This raises the possibility that an interaction between spouses' physical health status may influence the provision of supportive behaviors and occurrence of psychological distress within the couple. Although models of communal coping encourage the appraisal of the patient's diagnosis as "ours" (e.g., Lyons, Michelson, Sullivan, & Coyne, 1998), such research typically focuses on the health of only one spouse without taking into consideration potential interactions.

The Role of Couple Congruence

The concept of congruence was initially examined in regard to emotional expression and indicators of mental health between spouses. Emotions are suggested to be contagious among social partners, as one mimics and synchronizes expressions, vocalizations, and postures with another (Hatfield, Cacioppo, & Rapson, 1993). Among married couples, the sharing of social space and the intimacy of the relationship may increase the likelihood of emotional contagion (Bookwala & Schulz, 1996; Rime, 2009). Congruence between spouses is evident in moment-to-moment emotions, as well as on indicators of mental well-being, including depressive symptoms, life satisfaction, and purpose in life (Hoppmann & Gerstorf, 2009). Such congruence appears to be domain specific; depressive symptoms in one spouse are significantly related to those symptoms in the other, but not to other indicators of well-being (i.e., life satisfaction, purpose in life; Bookwala & Schulz, 1996). Shared negative emotions frequently occur among couples in which one partner is coping with chronic pain (Druley, Stephens, Martire, Ennis, & Wojno, 2003). Further, congruence in these negative emotions is more likely to occur when the patient frequently expresses their pain and suffering (i.e., pain behaviors; Druley et al., 2003). As marital quality is known to impact the well-being of caregiving spouses (e.g., Goodman & Shippy, 2002), it may also influence the degree of emotional contagion between partners.

More recently, studies have revealed that congruence also occurs in partners' physical health. Health behaviors (e.g., physical activity, diet, substance use), as well as indicators of physical health (e.g., blood pressure, cholesterol, triglycerides, and blood glucose), are often highly similar between spouses (Meyler, Stimpson, & Peek, 2007). Support for congruence in such measures is evident between patients with chronic pain and their caregiving spouses. For example, daily activity (e.g., duration of moderate-intensity exercise, number of steps) among patients with osteoarthritis of the knee is higher on days when their spouses are also more active (Martire et al., 2013). Spousal effects on physical activity are evident even after controlling for demographic characteristics, physical health comorbidities, and relationship quality (Martire et al., 2013). Congruence between married partners is also evident in specific health diagnoses, including arthritis, hypertension, and cancer (Stimpson & Peek, 2005). After controlling for demographics and health behaviors, individuals who have a spouse with arthritis are 200% more likely to be diagnosed with the same condition, compared to those with a healthy partner (Stimpson & Peek, 2005). However, it is possible that congruence in physical health diagnoses reflects differences in medical consultations or screening. For instance, Campbell, Sharim, Jordan, and Dunn (2016) found that wives were more likely to have a consultation for a musculoskeletal pain condition, if their husband had previously sought medical treatment for a similar condition. Although this study controlled for the effects of emotional contagion, socioeconomic status, and age, Campbell et al. (2016) did not include measures of health behaviors (diet, obesity, physical fitness, etc.) that may confer shared vulnerability.

Several theories have been suggested to account for emotional and physical health congruence among married couples. For instance, individuals may seek out spouses who are similar in emotional or physical characteristics. Research supports assortative mating on the basis of health behaviors, including smoking, alcohol use, and exercise (Ask, Rognmo, Torvik, Roysamb, & Tambs, 2012). In contrast, congruence may develop over time as common risks that exist within the shared social environment translate into congruence in physical health (Stimpson & Peek, 2005).

Others have suggested that participation in social activities, which are highly correlated among elderly spouses, is a key variable in understanding congruence (Hoppmann, Gerstorf, & Luszcz, 2008).

Among couples coping with chronic pain, congruence, or lack thereof, between partners' assessments of patients' pain severity may influence expressions of empathy and provision of support. When spouses are discordant in their ratings of patients' pain, there is a greater likelihood that the person in pain will feel misunderstood or receive inadequate care (see Goubert et al., 2005). For example, spousal underestimation of patients' pain severity is associated with more depressive symptoms, less positive affect, and less self-efficacy to manage chronic pain among these patients (compared to congruent couples; Cremeans-Smith et al., 2003). In addition, spousal overestimation of pain is also associated with greater depressive symptoms among patients—suggesting that lack of congruence, regardless of type, has negative implications for patient well-being (Cremeans-Smith et al., 2003). Spouses who hold similar beliefs about the nature of chronic pain (i.e., controllability, cyclic nature) may be better able to offer support that matches patients' needs (Sterba et al., 2008). Leonard, Issner, Cano, and Williams (2013) suggest that marital satisfaction is an important piece of this puzzle, moderating the relationship between spouses' ratings of patients' pain severity and their provision of empathy. Specifically, spouses with high levels of marital satisfaction who rated their partner's pain as intense showed greater accuracy in understanding their partner's feelings (Leonard et al., 2013).

The Role of Partner Personal Experience

Spouses who have personal experiences with health conditions, such as chronic pain, may display greater empathy or provide more appropriate support to the patient. Empathy is characterized by a deep understanding of the experiences of another, which results in affective and behavioral responses in the observer (Goubert et al., 2005). When caregivers perceive the suffering of another (e.g., pain behaviors, verbal expression) cognitive representations of personal experiences associated with that behavior are activated, according to the Perception-Action Model of empathy (Preston & de Waal, 2002). Spouses who have personal experiences with pain may have a greater wealth of cognitive resources (i.e., memory, appraisal, coping) that become activated when observing pain expressions by their partner, compared to a spouse who has not experienced similar health-related stressors. Such resources may encourage spouses with a personal history of health-related stressors to appraise the patient's pain as a significant threat to the couple, thereby increasing the likelihood of communal coping (Lewis et al., 2006). Previous findings, however, are mixed as whether personal history of pain impacts one's responses to the suffering of others. For example, nursing professionals with personal experience of intense pain tended to be more sympathetic to patients' pain and resulting distress (Holm, Cohen, Dudas, Medema, & Allen, 1989). When interpreting their results, Holm et al. (1989) suggested that nurses remember their own emotional suffering in reaction to intensely painful experiences, which is then reflected in their assessment of the patient. In contrast, spouses who have been diagnosed with a chronic musculoskeletal condition were significantly less validating of their partners' pain, compared to healthy partners (Issner, Cano, Leonard, & Williams, 2012). Further, Leonard et al. (2013) reported that spouses afflicted with chronic pain are no more accurate in assessing the emotional state of the patient than are healthy spouses. Such findings may reflect the degree to which spouses are successfully coping with their own painful condition. Issner et al. (2012) suggest that spouses who are focused on their own pain may not be sensitive to patient needs, while spouses who are successfully coping may not understand a patient who is struggling to do so. Further, the discrepant findings within the literature may reflect different levels of intimacy with the patient (i.e., health professionals versus spouses) or the assessment of personal experience (i.e., self-report of prior severe pain versus medical diagnosis). Given the frequency with which older adults experience chronic pain and rely on spousal caregivers, further insight into the role that physical health plays in an individual's ability and willingness to provide support is clearly needed.

Although prior studies have revealed a significant degree of congruence between married partners' mental and physical health, much of the social support literature has failed to consider the potential impact of spousal health. For instance, research examining the impact of caregiving on spouses' mental health has not controlled for the spouse's general physical health or specific diagnoses (e.g., Baanders & Heijmans, 2007; Brouwer et al., 2004; Druley et al., 2003; Lee, Brennan, & Daly, 2001). Further, studies of spousal support provision have not controlled for spouses' physical health (e.g., Iida, Stephens, Rook, Franks, & Salem, 2010; Khan et al., 2009). In fact, the social support literature routinely ignores spouses' general health and physical comorbidities, while acknowledging that such factors could impact the quality of couples' interactions (e.g., Khan et al., 2009). Further, spousal health conditions or symptoms (e.g., arthritis pain of moderate or greater intensity) are often used as exclusion criteria in such studies (e.g., Manne & Zautra, 1989; Martire et al., 2013). There are, however, notable exceptions (e.g., Issner et al., 2012; Leonard et al., 2013). For instance, nearly half of the couples (47.4%) surveyed by Issner et al. (2012) reported that both partners experienced chronic pain. In sum, prior research has typically focused on the impact of one partner's health condition on either the patient's or spouse's psychological well-being. Such efforts concentrate on actor and partner effects, while ignoring potential joint effects. Interdependence theory defines joint effects as the interaction between actor and partner effects (Rusbult & Van Lange, 2003), such that factors of the wife and husband may interact to impact husbands' outcomes (Lewis et al., 2006).

An Illustrative Example of Couples Coping with Chronic Pain

In response to the above described gap in the existing literature, let us turn our attention to the possibility that interactions between partners' health may impact the provision of support and mental well-being of caregiving spouses. As prior research has suggested that individuals with personal experience with severe pain are more empathetic to other's suffering (e.g., Holm et al., 1989), one might expect that spouses with greater physical health burden would provide greater levels of support when patients were also in poorer health and consequently in greater need of support. Further, poor spousal physical health may function as an additive risk factor (in combination with poor patient health) for spouses' mental health (i.e., greater depressive symptoms, lower life satisfaction).

For this example, we will consider an existing dataset, consisting of 101 older women with a primary diagnosis of osteoarthritis and their caregiving spouses (details regarding the recruitment strategy and sample may be found in Martire, Stephens, Druley, & Wojno, 2002). Briefly, eligibility criteria for patients included age of at least 60 years, married, and living with their spouse. In addition, patients must have experienced pain during the past month, experienced difficulty carrying out personal care or instrumental activities of daily living, received assistance from her spouse with at least one activity, and the spouse was the individual who had provided the most assistance with daily activities. Both patients and spouses were screened for intact cognitive function with the Short Portable Mental Status Questionnaire (SPMSQ, Pfeiffer, 1975). In contrast to much of the existing research on interpersonal pain dynamics within couples, no health or activity restriction on the part of the spouse was used for eligibility screening.

On average, patients were 69.3 years of age (SD = 5.9; range 61–90), and spouses were 71.3 years (SD = 6.7; range 52–92). Most of the sample was Caucasian (97%, 3% African American). The couples had been married for an average of 42.2 years (SD = 13.5; range 1–69). The patients reported having arthritis for 19.7 years on average (SD = 14.9; range 1–66) and typically reported having arthritis in five joints or sets of joints (e.g., knees). The most common sites of arthritis were knees (70% of participants), back (69%), and hands (67%). The average level of pain experienced over the past month was 17.2 (SD = 4.4; range 7–25) using the pain subscale of the Arthritis Impact Measurement Scale, which has a potential range of 5–25 (AIMS2; Meenan, Mason, Anderson, Guccione, & Kazis, 1992). Participants reported having at least some difficulty with an average of 2.9 out of six personal care activities (e.g., bathing, dressing) (SD = 1.9; range = 0–6) and at least some difficulty with an average of 2.2 out of four instrumental activities of daily living (e.g., shopping, household tasks) (SD = 1.2; range = 0–4).

Data were collected using in-person interviews conducted in couples' homes and partners were interviewed separately. During these interviews, both patients and spouses responded to items assessing their general physical health (House, 1986). Self-rated general health is thought to accurately reflect individuals' health burden (e.g., Mantyselka, Turunen, Ahonen, & Kumpusalo, 2003; Siedlecki, 2006), although this data was not confirmed via medical records. Caregiving husbands also provided information regarding their provision of support over the past month. Emotional support items reflected husbands' supportive communication and empathic understanding regarding wives' pain (e.g., "listened to your wife talk about how she was feeling" and "tried to put yourself in your situation"; adapted from Stephens & Clark, 1997). Instrumental support items assessed husbands' assistance with activities (e.g., household tasks, opening things) and personal care (e.g., bathing, dressing; based on Clark and Stephens (1996). Husbands' mental well-being was assessed on the basis of depressive symptoms (The Center for Epidemiologic Studies—Depression scale [CES-D]; Radloff, 1977) and life satisfaction (House, 1986; Neugarten, Havighurst, & Tobin, 1961).

As prior research has suggested that spouses who provide care for partners with more severe pain experience greater emotional distress (e.g., Schwartz, Slater, Birchler, & Atkinson, 1991), patient's pain severity was controlled in regression analyses. Husbands' completed the pain subscale of the AIMS2 (Meenan et al., 1992) based on perceptions of their wives' pain severity. Additionally, marital satisfaction has also been shown to impact emotional distress (e.g., Cutrona, 1996) and partners' insight into the emotional experience of each other (Leonard et al., 2013). Therefore, husbands' marital satisfaction was assessed using the Quality of Marriage Index (QMI; Norton, 1983).

Interactions Between Spouses' Health Predict Caregivers' Behaviors and Mental Health

Descriptive statistics and bivariate correlations between study variables are presented in Table 15.1. Wives' general health was significantly correlated with husbands' provision of instrumental support, as well as husbands' life satisfaction. In contrast, husbands' general health was significantly correlated with their depressive

Table 15.1 Descriptive statistics and bivariate correlations between study variables

	Mean	(SD)	Range	1	2	3	4	5	6
1. Wives' physical health	7.614	(2.063)	3–12	–	0.094	−0.035	−0.436**	−0.137	0.310**
2. Husbands' physical health	10.178	(2.326)	5–15	–	–	−0.186[a]	−0.032	−0.434**	0.222*
3. Empathy	19.970	(4.260)	9–28	–	–	–	0.157	−0.092	0.173
4. Instrumental support	25.564	(8.164)	10–44	–	–	–	–	0.004	−0.244*
5. Depressive symptoms	7.835	(5.807)	0–28	–	–	–	–	–	−0.174
6. Life satisfaction	15.005	(2.396)	9–21	–	–	–	–	–	–

$*p < 0.05$, $**p < 0.01$, $^a p < 0.065$

symptoms and life satisfaction, as well as marginally related to their provision of emotional support.

Hierarchical multiple regression was used to examine the potential interactions between spouses' general health and outcomes of interest. All analyses controlled for husbands' ratings of their marital satisfaction and patient pain severity in step one, wives' and husbands' self-reported general health was entered in step two, and centered interaction terms in step three. Table 15.2 displays the results of these regression analyses. Husbands' levels of emotional and instrumental support are displayed in the top half of the table, while indices of husbands' psychological well-being are presented in the bottom half.

Consistent with expectations, a significant main effect was evident between husbands' general health and their provision of empathy ($\Delta R^2 = 0.077$, $p = 0.016$). Husbands with poorer health ($\beta = -0.247$, $p = 0.012$) provided greater emotional support to their wives. In contrast, wives' general health was not predictive of husbands' empathy ($\beta = -0.125$, $p = 0.224$). A significant interaction was evident between spouses' physical health in relation to husbands' emotional support ($\Delta R^2 = 0.047$, $p = 0.022$). Decomposition analyses revealed the slope of husbands' general health on emotional support to be significant when wives' general health was poor ($t[97] = -3.553$, $p < 0.01$). As displayed in Fig. 15.1, husbands provided greater levels of emotional support when both spouses indicated their physical health to be poor.

In contrast to the above findings for empathy, husbands' provision of instrumental support was determined by patients' general health ($\Delta R^2 = 0.116$, $p = 0.002$). Husbands provided greater instrumental support when wives were in poorer health ($\beta = -0.366$, $p < 0.001$). Neither the main effect for husbands' general health nor the interaction of spouses' health were significant predictors of husbands' instrumental support (ps > 0.10).

Spouses' physical health was also examined in relation to husbands' psychological well-being. Regression analyses revealed a significant main effect of husbands' physical health on their depressive symptoms ($\Delta R^2 = 0.172$, $p < 0.001$). Husbands reported more frequent depressive symptoms when their own health was poor ($\beta = -0.418$, $p < 0.001$), but showed no relationship to patients' physical ($\beta = -0.013$, $p = 0.893$). In addition, there was a significant interaction between spouses' general health in predicting husbands' depressive symptoms ($\Delta R^2 = 0.035$, $p = 0.039$). Decomposition analyses revealed the slope of husbands' general health on depressive symptoms to be significant when wives' general health was poor ($t[97] = -4.681$, $p < 0.01$). Similar to the pattern of findings for empathy, Fig. 15.2 illustrates that husbands suffer more depressive symptoms when both spouses report poor general health.

Lastly, the relationship between spouses' physical health and husbands' life satisfaction was examined. Results revealed wives' physical health to be a significant predictor of husbands' life satisfaction ($\Delta R^2 = 0.079$, $p = 0.018$). When wives reported better physical health, husbands experienced greater life satisfaction ($\beta = 0.216$, $p = 0.041$). Neither husbands' physical heath (at the individual level) nor

Table 15.2 Regression analyses predicting husbands' support and well-being from spouses' physical health

Step no.	Variables	Husbands' empathy					Husbands' instrumental support				
		B	SE	β	ΔR^2	F of ΔR^2	B	SE	β	ΔR^2	F of ΔR^2
1.	Marital satisfaction	0.650	0.182	0.354**	0.124	6.412**	−0.355	0.345	−0.102	0.118	6.110**
	Wives' pain severity	0.080	0.101	0.078			0.606	0.191	0.315**		
2.	Wives' physical health	−0.262	0.214	−0.125	0.077	4.304*	−1.445	0.394	−0.366**	0.116	6.763**
	Husbands' physical health	−0.453	0.176	−0.247*			0.193	0.326	0.056		
3.	Wife X husband health	0.234	0.100	0.224*	0.047	5.448*	−0.082	0.190	−0.042	0.002	0.186

Step no.	Variables	Husbands' depressive symptoms					Husbands' life satisfaction				
		B	SE	β	ΔR^2	F of ΔR^2	B	SE	β	ΔR^2	F of ΔR^2
1.	Marital satisfaction	−0.729	0.255	−0.289**	0.086	4.282*	0.280	0.103	0.276**	0.083	4.094*
	Wives' pain severity	0.031	0.142	0.022			−0.027	0.057	−0.049		
2.	Wives' physical health	−0.038	0.282	−0.013	0.172	10.331**	0.250	0.120	0.216*	0.079	4.177*
	Husbands' physical health	−1.053	0.233	−0.418**			0.184	0.099	0.182		
3.	Wife X husband health	0.279	0.133	0.195*	0.035	4.391*	0.022	0.058	0.038	0.001	0.139

*$p < 0.05$; **$p < 0.01$

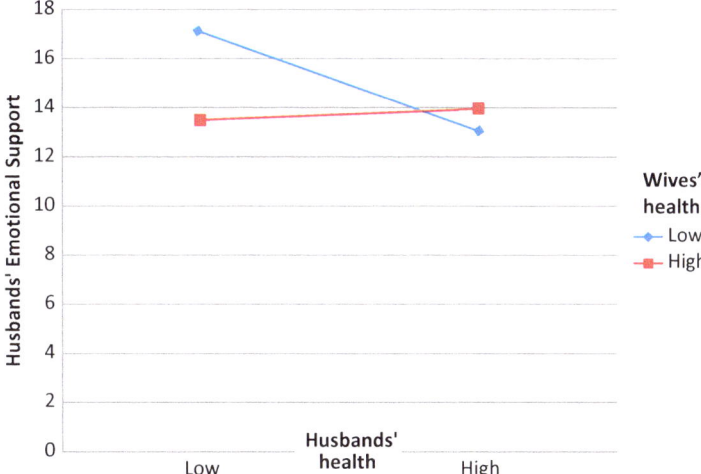

Fig. 15.1 The interaction between spouses' physical health predicting husbands' levels of emotional support

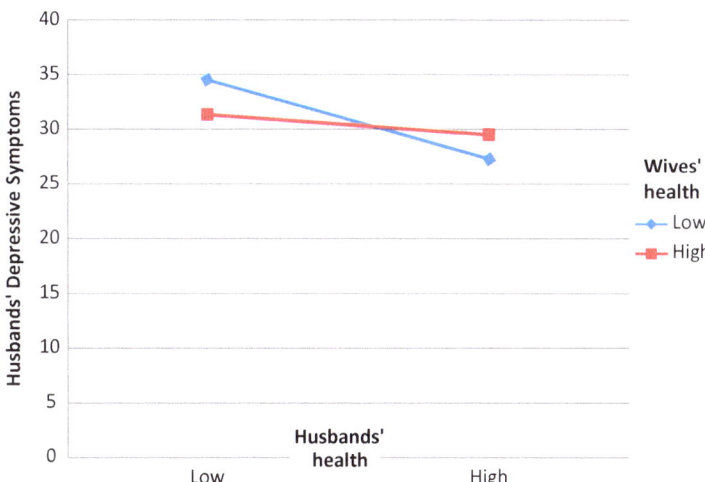

Fig. 15.2 The interaction between spouses' physical health predicting husbands' depressive symptoms

the interaction between spouses' health were significant predictors of husbands' life satisfaction (ps > 0.65).

The literature reviewed herein as well as the present findings lend further support to the social dynamics of physical health conditions, which impact both members of the marital dyad. Prior research on the interpersonal dynamics of pain among couples typically assumes one spouse to be the "patient" in need of support. However, an estimated 88% of older adults have at least one chronic health condition, increasing the likelihood that both partners are coping with pain or other chronic health conditions (Berg & Upchurch, 2007). The current findings reveal the presence of significant interactions between spouses' physical health, which predict the behavior and mental health of the caregiving spouse. That is, when both spouses report poor physical health, caregiving husbands express greater empathy but experience more depressive symptoms. These findings support the joint effects as specified by interdependence theory (Rusbult & Van Lange, 2003). Further, main effects revealed that husbands' provision of emotional support and depressive symptoms are under actor influence, while provision of instrumental support and life satisfaction are associated with partner effects.

Explaining Effects on Caregivers' Provision of Support

Husbands' levels of instrumental support in the present example were associated with wives' health, in agreement with prior research. Patients coping with chronic pain (e.g., osteoarthritis, rheumatoid arthritis) frequently depend on spouses for assistance with daily tasks. In such cases, spouses typically assume responsibility for household tasks (meal prep, house cleaning, grocery shopping, etc.; Brouwer et al., 2004). Patients' physical symptoms and pain behaviors may elicit the provision of support by the spouse (e.g., Craig et al., 2001; Iida et al., 2010). Wives in poor health may display more frequent or salient cues, which influence the degree of instrumental support provided by their husband. As husbands' health did not predict levels of instrumental support, this finding suggests their health may not have restricted their ability to provide support to the patient.

Main effects revealed that husbands' provision of emotional support in the present study was related to their own health. This finding stands in contrast to prior research. For instance, Leonard et al. (2013) found no difference in empathic accuracy between spouses with and without a painful condition. Further, Issner et al. (2012) reported that spouses coping with a painful condition are less validating of their partner's pain. Spouses in these studies were classified on the basis of diagnosis with a painful condition, while data regarding their efficacy in managing that condition was absent. In contrast, the present study examined the self-rated health of marital partners, rather than simply diagnostic label. Self-rated health is useful in assessing health-related burdens and is an accurate predictor of mortality, even after controlling for factors such as functional status, depression, and comorbidity (DeSalvo, Bloser, Reynolds, He, & Muntner, 2005). Perhaps indices of self-rated health provide more insight into individuals' perceptions and experiences than a diagnostic label. For example, prior research has demonstrated that poor self-rated health is associated with suffering daily or chronic pain (Mantyselka et al., 2003), as well as greater disability, depression, and powerlessness (Siedlecki, 2006).

Explaining Effects on Caregivers' Mental Health

Among couples in which both partners reported poor physical health, husbands engaged in more emotional support but experienced greater depressive symptoms. While these findings may seem to contradict one another, there are several possible explanations for this effect. For instance, individuals high in empathy are likely to experience greater stress in response to the suffering of others due to their heightened awareness or sensitivity (Schieman & Turner, 2001). Therefore, high empathy may increase vulnerability to depressive symptoms in response to partners' poor health. Another possibility lies with the affective responses to suffering. When witnessing the distress of another, an observer may respond with affect that is self-oriented (e.g., distress), other-oriented (e.g., sympathy), or a combination of the two (Batson, 1991, cited in Goubert et al., 2005). Perhaps husbands in the present example were more apt to experience combined affective responding (i.e., displaying sympathy and distress) when they are confronted with poor health of both self and partner.

The present example suggests that effects on spouses' psychological well-being depend on the characteristic in question. That is, main effects revealed that husbands' depressive symptoms were related to their own general health, while life satisfaction was predicted by wives' physical health. Although prior research has assumed that the stress and burden associated with caregiving negatively impacts spouses (e.g., Adelman, Tmanova, Delgado, Dion, & Lachs, 2014; Baanders & Heijmans, 2007), the present findings reveal the importance of considering the caregiver's own physical health. In agreement with Manne and Zautra (1990), the present results suggest that spousal distress is better understood as a product of their own physical health rather than a result of caregiving. Additionally, cognitive characteristics (e.g., pain catastrophizing) may moderate the level of distress experienced by spousal caregivers. Notably, this is the case among spouses who experience chronic pain (in addition to the patient) and not among pain-free caregiving spouses (Leonard & Cano, 2006). Therefore, future research concerning partners' health status and outcomes will need to consider cognitive-emotional characteristics that influence the coping of the actor and partner, as well as the dyad.

The current findings stand in contrast to the assertion that caregiver depression may reflect distress about the patient's disability (e.g., Capistrant, Berkman, & Glymour, 2014). Husbands' depressive symptoms in the present study were *not* predicted by wives' self-reported health. In fact, decomposition analyses revealed that husbands reported the fewest depressive symptoms when wives' health was poor but their own health was good. This finding is in agreement with Lee et al. (2001), who reported that caregivers' depression was not related to patients' functional limitations, but instead was correlated with their own physical health. Notably, the participants surveyed by Lee et al. (2001) differed substantially from the present study: only 55% of caregivers were spouses, the majority of whom were caring for a patient with Alzheimer's disease. As the present example focused on older women with osteoarthritis and their caregiving husbands it is unclear whether the current findings generalize to caregivers of both genders. Significant gender differences are known to exist within the context of marriage relative to perceived social support (Acitelli & Antonucci, 1994), as well as caregiver burden and psychological well-being (Lin, Fee, & Wu, 2012). Therefore, gender differences within the context of chronic pain and caregiving may provide a fruitful area for future study.

The women in the present sample reported that they had been coping with the chronic pain of arthritis for an average of nearly 15 years. Perhaps husbands who have been providing support for such an extended period of time come to accept their wife's declining health, thereby reducing its impact on their mental health. When confronted with an unresolvable problem, such as providing care for a partner with dementia, research suggests that adopting an acceptance style of coping may reduce caregiver burden (Kneebone & Martin, 2003). Additionally, it is possible that husbands' declining health is a relatively new phenomenon, evoking worries about the future independence of the couple. For instance, Manne and Zautra (1990) found that the psychological well-being of caregiving husbands was predicted by their own perceived vulnerability to illness, rather than aspects of their wife's rheumatoid arthritis. These findings may indicate that caregiving spouses who anticipate their own health decline become distressed at the prospect of the couple losing their independence and increasing their reliance on others (e.g., family members, nursing facility; Manne & Zautra, 1990). Unfortunately, the present data set does not contain information pertaining to duration of various diagnoses or long-term fluctuations in husbands' physical health. The collection of such information in future studies could provide valuable insights into the present findings.

As expected, there was a significant interaction between spouses' physical health in predicting the depressive symptoms of caregiving husbands. Specifically, husbands experience greater depressive symptoms when both spouses rate their general health as poor. This finding suggests a synergistic risk, such that caregiving may be particularly detrimental to psychological well-being when the spouse is also coping with their own declining health. The stress associated with such a situation may overwhelm the coping resources of the spouse, increasing their vulnerability to depression. Prior research suggests that spouses are more likely to experience caregiving burden (e.g., interference, strain, and burnout) when they rate their own health as poor (Lin et al., 2012). However, Lin et al. (2012) did not control for influence of pain severity or marital satisfaction on caregiver outcomes. Additionally, patients in the present study with poorer self-rated health may engage in more frequent expressions of their suffering, which in turn takes a negative toll on their spouse. For instance, Stephens et al. (2006) found that high levels of verbal pain disclosure by women who are experiencing severe arthritis pain predicted a significant increase in husbands' depressive symptoms over a 6 month period.

When wives report better physical health, spouses experience greater life satisfaction. Although analyses controlled for patients' pain severity, perhaps wives who perceive their physical health in a favorable light rely less on their husbands for support or have enhanced self-efficacy in their ability to manage pain. Prior research has revealed that patients with greater self-efficacy to manage arthritis-related pain and disability have caregivers who are less burdened and show more optimism (Beckham,

Burker, Rice, & Talton, 1995). Further, caregivers are likely to appraise the situation as less stressful or threatening when patients are in better health or demonstrate fewer impairments, resulting in better life satisfaction (Lee et al., 2001). In contrast, when patients exhibit greater impairments in physical, mental, or social domains, spousal caregivers experience personal strain and poorer social relations (Baanders & Heijmans, 2007). Better physical health may enable patients to participate in shared activities and hobbies with their spouse, which may enhance the quality of their communication and marital relationship (Orthner & Mancini, 1990).

Conclusions and Future Research

Existing research on the interpersonal dynamics of chronic pain supports the need for interventions, treatments, and educational efforts to include the spouse. Psychosocial interventions have been shown to be effective in reducing the depression, anxiety, and burden experienced by caregivers (Martire, Lustig, Schulz, Miller, & Helgeson, 2004). Further, interventions are particularly beneficial to the well-being of both patients and spouses when they focus on aspects of their relationship (Martire et al., 2004). Such benefits are also evident in studies that have focused specifically on patients coping with painful conditions. For instance, Keefe et al. (2004) report that subjecting spouses in pain to a coping skills training and exercise intervention yielded greater improvements in patients' self-efficacy, physical fitness, and muscle strength. Couple-oriented interventions can be beneficial for the spouse as well as patient, but the efficacy of such programs depend on levels of marital satisfaction (Martire, Schulz, Keefe, Rudy, & Starz, 2007). As marital satisfaction may fluctuate over time, longitudinal studies are needed to examine the changing dynamic within couples impacted by chronic pain.

Much of the research on couples coping with chronic pain has focused on those in long-term marriages. Couples in the present example, for instance, had been married for an average of approximately 42 years. However, demographic trends suggest that individuals are increasingly likely to divorce (Berg & Upchurch, 2007). This trend poses a number of interesting topics for future research, including the impact of divorce on pain expression and support, as well as efforts by individuals to replace supportive resources lost via divorce. Additionally, intervention efforts that were couple-oriented may need to consider the efficacy of incorporating other types of supportive relationships (e.g., family members, friends). Following divorce, there are significant gender differences in the likelihood to remarry. That is, men are more likely to remarry, while women are at an increased risk for aging alone (Phillipson, 1997). These gender differences will impact individuals' adjustment following divorce and the availability of supportive resources. As a result, older individuals (women in particular) may increasingly look to other relationships for support and assistance when confronted with declining physical health. Chronic pain is a social phenomenon, impacting social networks and dyads outside of the marital relationship.

Acknowledgments   The author expresses sincere gratitude to Mary Ann Stephens, PhD for grant-ing permission to analyze the data described herein: Couples Coping with Arthritis Pain. In addi-tion, the author thanks Courtney L. Fleisher and Melissa A. Berthoff for their assistance with recruitment and data collection.

References

Acitelli, L. K., & Antonucci, T. C. (1994). Gender differences in the link between marital support and satisfaction in older couples. *Journal of Personality and Social Psychology, 67*, 688–698.

Adelman, R. D., Tmanova, L. L., Delgado, D., Dion, S., & Lachs, M. S. (2014). Caregiver burden: A clinical review. *Journal of the American Medical Association, 311*, 1052–1059.

Ask, H., Rognmo, K., Torvik, F. A., Roysamb, E., & Tambs, K. (2012). Non-random mating and convergence over time for alcohol consumption, smoking, and exercise: The Nord-Trondelag Health Study. *Behavioral Genetics, 42*, 354–365.

Baanders, A. N., & Heijmans, M. J. W. M. (2007). The impact of chronic diseases: The partner's perspective. *Family and Community Health, 30*, 305–317.

Beckham, J. C., Burker, E. J., Rice, J. R., & Talton, S. L. (1995). Patient predictors of caregiver burden, optimism, and pessimism in rheumatoid arthritis. *Behavioral Medicine, 20*, 171–178.

Berg, C. A., & Upchurch, R. (2007). A developmental-contextual model of couples coping with chronic illness across the adult life span. *Psychological Bulletin, 133*, 920–954.

Bodenmann, G. (1997). Dyadic coping: A systemic-transactional view of stress and coping among couples: Theory and empirical findings. *Revue Europenne de Psychologie Appliquee, 47*, 137–140.

Bodenmann, G. (2005). Dyadic coping and its significance for marital functioning. In T. Revenson, K. Kayser, & G. Bodenmann (Eds.), *Couples coping with stress: Emerging perspectives on dyadic coping* (pp. 33–50). Washington, DC: American Psychological Association.

Bookwala, J., & Schulz, R. (1996). Spousal similarity in subjective Well-being: The cardiovascular health study. *Psychology and Aging, 11*, 582–590.

Brouwer, W. B. F., van Exel, J. A., van de Berg, B., Dinant, H. J., Koopmanschap, M. A., & van den Bos, G. A. M. (2004). Burden of caregiving: Evidence of objective burden, subjective burden, and quality of life impacts on informal caregivers of patients with rheumatoid arthritis. *Arthritis and Rheumatism, 51*, 570–577.

Burman, B., & Margolin, G. (1992). Analysis of the association between marital relationships and health problems: An interactional perspective. *Psychological Bulletin, 112*, 39–63.

Campbell, P., Sharim, M., Jordan, K. P., & Dunn, K. M. (2016). In sickness and in health: A cross-sectional analysis of concordance for musculoskeletal pain in 13, 507 couples. *European Journal of Pain, 20*, 438–446.

Cano, A., & Williams, A. C. d. C. (2010). Social interaction in pain: Reinforcing pain behaviors of building intimacy? *Pain, 149*, 9–11.

Capistrant, B. D., Berkman, L. F., & Glymour, M. M. (2014). Does duration of spousal caregiving affect risk of depression onset? Evidence from the Health and Retirement Study. *American Journal of Geriatric Psychiatry, 22*, 766–770.

Clark, S. L., & Stephens, M. A. P. (1996). Stroke patients' well-being as a function of caregiving spouses' helpful and unhelpful actions. *Personal Relationships, 3*, 171–184.

Craig, K. D., Prkachin, K., & Grunau, R. E. (2001). The facial expression of pain. In D. Turk & R. Melzack (Eds.), *Handbook of pain assessment* (pp. 153–169). New York, NY: Guilford Press.

Cremeans-Smith, J. K., Stephens, M. A. P., Franks, M. M., Druley, J. A., Martire, L. M., & Wojno, W. C. (2003). Spouses' and physicians' perceptions of pain severity in older women with osteoarthritis: Dyadic agreement and patients' well-being. *Pain, 106*, 27–34.

Cutrona, C. (1996). *Social support in couples: Marriage as a resource in times of stress*. Thousand Oaks, CA: Sage.

DeSalvo, K. B., Bloser, N., Reynolds, K., He, J., & Muntner, P. (2005). Mortality prediction with a single general self-rated health question: A meta-analysis. *Journal of General Internal Medicine, 20*, 267–275.

Druley, J. A., Stephens, M. A. P., Martire, L. M., Ennis, N., & Wojno, W. C. (2003). Emotional congruence in older couples coping with wives' osteoarthritis: Exacerbating effects of pain behavior. *Psychology and Aging, 18*, 406–414.

Fekete, E. M., Stephens, M. A. P., Druley, J. A., & Greene, K. A. (2007). Couples' support provision during illness: The role of perceived emotional responsiveness. *Families, Systems, and Health, 25*, 204–217.

Flor, H., Breitenstein, C., Birbaumer, N., & Furst, M. (1995). A psychophysiological analysis of spouse solicitousness towards pain behaviors, spouse interaction, and pain perception. *Behavior Therapy, 26*, 255–272.

Franks, M. M., Wehrspann, E., August, K. J., Rook, K. S., & Stephens, M. A. P. (2016). Chronic disease management in older couples: Spousal support versus control strategies. In J. Bookwala (Ed.), *Couple relationships in the middle and later years: Their nature, complexity, and role in health and illness* (pp. 303–323). Washington, DC: American Psychological Association.

Goodman, C. R., & Shippy, R. A. (2002). Is it contagious? Affect similarity among spouses. *Aging and Mental Health, 6*, 266–274.

Goubert, L., Craig, K. D., Vervoort, T., Morley, S., Sullivan, M. J., Williams, C. A. d. C., … Crombez, G. (2005). Facing other in pain: The effects of empathy. *Pain, 118*, 285–288.

Hatfield, E., Cacioppo, J. T., & Rapson, R. L. (1993). Emotional contagion. *Current Directions in Psychological Science, 2*, 96–99.

Holm, K., Cohen, F., Dudas, S., Medema, P. G., & Allen, B. L. (1989). Effect of personal pain experience on pain assessment. *Journal of Nursing Scholarship, 21*, 72–75.

Hoppmann, C., & Gerstorf, D. (2009). Spousal interrelations in old age—a mini-review. *Gerontology, 55*, 449–459.

Hoppmann, C. A., Gerstorf, D., & Luszcz, M. (2008). Spousal social activity trajectories in the Australian longitudinal study of ageing in the context of cognitive, physical, and affective resources. *Journal of Gerontology: Psychological Sciences, 63B*, P41–P50.

House, J. S. (1986). *America's changing lives: Wave 1 (survey study report)*. Ann Arbor, MI: Survey Research Center, University of Michigan (Producer)/Inter-University Consortium for Political and Social Research.

Iida, M., Stephens, M. A. P., Rook, K. S., Franks, M. M., & Salem, J. K. (2010). When the going gets tough, does support get going? Determinants of spousal support provision to type 2 diabetic patients. *Personality and Social Psychology Bulletin, 36*, 780–791.

Issner, J. B., Cano, A., Leonard, M. T., & Williams, A. M. (2012). How do I empathize with you? Let me count the ways: Relations between facets of pain-related empathy. *The Journal of Pain, 13*, 167–175.

Keefe, F. J., Blumenthal, J., Bausom, D., Affleck, G., Waugh, R., Caldwell, D. S., … Lefebvre, J. (2004). Effects of spouse-assisted coping skills training and exercise training in patients with osteoarthritic knee pain: A randomized controlled study. *Pain, 110*, 539–549.

Khan, C. M., Iida, M., Stephens, M. A. P., Fekete, E. M., Druley, J. A., & Greene, K. A. (2009). Spousal support following knee surgery: Roles of self-efficacy and perceived emotional responsiveness. *Rehabilitation Psychology, 54*, 28–32.

Kiecolt-Glaser, J. K., & Newton, T. L. (2001). Marriage and health: His and hers. *Psychological Bulletin, 127*, 472–503.

Kneebone, I. I., & Martin, P. R. (2003). Coping and caregivers of people with dementia. *British Journal of Health Psychology, 8*, 1–17.

Lee, H. S., Brennan, P. F., & Daly, B. J. (2001). Relationship of empathy to appraisal, depression, life satisfaction, and physical health in informal caregivers of older adults. *Research in Nursing and Health, 24*, 44–56.

Leonard, M. T., & Cano, A. (2006). Pain affects spouses too: Personal experience with pain and catastrophizing as correlates of spouse distress. *Pain, 126*, 139–146.

Leonard, M. T., Issner, J. H., Cano, A., & Williams, A. M. (2013). Correlates of spousal empathic accuracy for pain-related thoughts and feelings. *Clinical Journal of Pain, 29*, 324–333.

Lewis, M. A., McBride, C. M., Pollak, K. I., Puleo, E., Butterfield, R. M., & Emmons, K. M. (2006). Understanding health behavior change among couples: An interdependence and communal coping approach. *Social Science and Medicine, 62*, 1369–1380.

Lin, I. F., Fee, H. R., & Wu, H. S. (2012). Negative and positive caregiving experiences: A closer look at the intersection of gender and relationship. *Family Relations, 61*, 343–358.

Lousberg, R., Schmidt, A. J. M., & Groenman, N. H. (1992). The relationship between spouse solicitousness and pain behavior: Searching for more experimental evidence. *Pain, 51*, 75–79.

Lyons, R. F., Michelson, K. D., Sullivan, M. J., & Coyne, J. C. (1998). Coping as a communal process. *Journal of Personal and Social Relationships, 15*, 579–605.

Manne, S. L., & Zautra, A. J. (1989). Spouse criticism and support: Their association with coping and psychological adjustment among women with rheumatoid arthritis. *Journal of Personality and Social Psychology, 56*, 607–617.

Manne, S. L., & Zautra, A. J. (1990). Couples coping with chronic illness: Women with rheumatoid arthritis and their healthy husbands. *Journal of Behavioral Medicine, 13*, 327–342.

Mantyselka, P. T., Turunen, J. H. O., Ahonen, R. S., & Kumpusalo, E. A. (2003). Chronic pain and poor self-rated health. *Journal of the American Medical Association, 290*, 2435–2442.

Martire, L. M., Lustig, A. O., Schulz, R., Miller, G. E., & Helgeson, V. S. (2004). Is it beneficial to involve a family member? A meta-analysis of psychosocial interventions for chronic illness. *Health Psychology, 23*, 599–611.

Martire, L. M., Schulz, R., Keefe, F. J., Rudy, T. E., & Starz, T. W. (2007). Couple-oriented education and support intervention: Effects on individuals with osteoarthritis and their spouses. *Rehabilitation Psychology, 52*, 121–132.

Martire, L. M., Stephens, M. A. P., Druley, J. A., & Wojno, W. (2002). Negative reactions to received spousal care: Predictors and consequences of miscarried support. *Health Psychology, 21*, 167–176.

Martire, L. M., Stephens, M. A. P., Mogle, J., Schulz, R., Brach, J., & Keefe, F. (2013). Daily spousal influence on physical activity in knee osteoarthritis. *Annals of Behavioral Medicine, 45*, 213–223.

Martire, L. M., Stephens, M. A. P., & Schulz, R. (2011). Independence centrality as a moderator of the effects of spousal support on patient well-being and physical functioning. *Health Psychology, 30*, 651–655.

McCracken, L. M. (2005). Social context and acceptance of chronic pain: The role of solicitous and punishing responses. *Pain, 113*, 155–159.

Meenan, R. F., Mason, J. H., Anderson, J. J., Guccione, A. A., & Kazis, L. E. (1992). AIMS2: The content and properties of a revised and expanded Arthritis Impact Measurement Scales health status questionnaire. *Arthritis and Rheumatism, 35*, 1–10.

Meyler, D., Stimpson, J. P., & Peek, M. K. (2007). Health concordance within couples: A systematic review. *Social Science and Medicine, 64*, 2297–2310.

Morley, S., Doyle, K., & Beese, A. (2000). Talking to others about pain: Suffering in silence. *Proceedings of the Ninth World Congress on Pain, Progress in Pain Research and Management, 16*, 1123–1129.

Nahin, R. L. (2015). Estimates of pain prevalence and severity in adults: United States, 2012. *Journal of Pain, 16*, 769–780.

Neugarten, B. L., Havighurst, R. J., & Tobin, S. S. (1961). The measurement of life satisfaction. *Journal of Gerontology, 16*, 134–143.

Newton-John, T. R., & Williams, A. C. d. C. (2006). Chronic pain couples: Perceived marital interactions and pain behaviors. *Pain, 123*, 53–63.

Norton, R. (1983). Measuring marital quality: A critical look at the dependent variable. *Journal of Marriage and the Family, 45*, 141–151.

Orthner, D. K., & Mancini, V. A. (1990). Leisure impacts on family interaction and cohesion. *Journal of Leisure Research, 22*, 125–137.

Pfeiffer, E. (1975). A short portable mental status questionnaire for the assessment of organic brain deficit in elderly patients. *Journal of the American Geriatrics Society, 23*, 433–441.

Phillipson, C. (1997). Social relationships in later life: A review of the research literature. *International Journal of Geriatric Psychiatry, 12*, 505–512.

Preston, S. D., & de Waal, F. B. M. (2002). Empathy: Its ultimate and proximate bases. *Behavioral and Brain Sciences, 25*, 1–72.

Radloff, L. S. (1977). The CES-D scale: A self-report depression scale for research in the general population. *Applied Psychological Measurement, 1*, 385–401.

Rafaeli, E., & Gleason, M. E. J. (2009). Skilled support within intimate relationships. *Journal of Family Theory and Review, 1*, 20–37.

Revenson, T. A., Schiaffino, K. M., Majerovitz, D., & Gibofsky, A. (1991). Social support as a double-edged sword: The relation of positive and problematic support to depression among rheumatoid arthritis patients. *Social Science and Medicine, 33*, 807–813.

Rime, B. (2009). Emotion elicits the social sharing of emotion: Theory and empirical review. *Emotion Review, 1*, 60–85.

Robles, T. F., Slatcher, R. B., Trombello, J. M., & McGinn, M. M. (2014). Marital quality and health: A meta-analytic review. *Psychological Bulletin, 140*, 140–187.

Rusbult, C. E., & Van Lange, P. A. M. (2003). Interdependence, interaction, and relationships. *Annual Review of Psychology, 54*, 351–375.

Schieman, S., & Turner, H. A. (2001). "When feeling other people's pain hurts": The influence of psychosocial resources on the association between self-reported empathy and depressive symptoms. *Social Psychology Quarterly, 64*, 376–389.

Schwartz, L., Jensen, M. P., & Romano, J. M. (2005). The development and psychometric evaluation of an instrument to assess spouse responses to pain and well behavior in patients with chronic pain: The spouse response inventory. *The Journal of Pain, 6*, 243–252.

Schwartz, L., Slater, M. A., Birchler, G. R., & Atkinson, J. H. (1991). Depression in spouses of chronic pain patients: The role of patient pain and anger, and marital satisfaction. *Pain, 44*, 61–67.

Siedlecki, S. L. (2006). Predictors of self-rated health in patients with chronic nonmalignant pain. *Pain Management Nursing, 7*, 109–116.

Stephens, M. A. P., & Clark, S. L. (1997). Reciprocity in the expression of emotional support among later-life couples coping with stroke. In B. H. Gottlieb (Ed.), *Coping with chronic stress* (pp. 221–242). New York, NY: Plenum.

Stephens, M. A. P., Martire, L. M., Cremeans-Smith, J. K., Druley, J. A., & Wojno, W. C. (2006). Older women with osteoarthritis and their caregiving husbands: Effects of pain and pain expression on husbands' well-being and support. *Rehabilitation Psychology, 51*, 3–12.

Sterba, K. R., DeVellis, R. F., Lewis, M. A., DeVellis, B. M., Jordan, J. M., & Baucom, D. H. (2008). Effect of couple illness perception congruence on psychological adjustment in women with rheumatoid arthritis. *Health Psychology, 27*, 221–229.

Stimpson, J. P., & Peek, K. (2005). Concordance of chronic conditions in older Mexican American couples. *Preventing Chronic Disease: Public Health Research, Practice, and Policy, 2*, 1–7.

Turk, D. C., Kerns, R. D., & Rosenberg, R. (1992). Effects of marital interaction on chronic pain and disability: Examining the down side of social support. *Rehabilitation Psychology, 37*, 259–274.

Walster, E., Walster, G. W., & Berscheid, E. (1978). *Equity: Theory and research*. Boston, MA: Allyn and Bacon.

Wilson, S. J., Martire, L. M., Keefe, F. J., Mogle, J. A., Stephens, M. A. P., & Schulz, R. (2013). Daily verbal and nonverbal expression of osteoarthritis pain and spouse responses. *Pain, 154*, 2045–2053.

Yorgason, J. B., & Choi, H. (2016). Health contributions to marital quality: Expected and unexpected links. In J. Bookwala (Ed.), *Couple relationships in the middle and later years: Their nature, complexity, and role in health and illness* (pp. 177–196). Washington, DC: American Psychological Association.

Zautra, A. J., Hoffman, J. M., Matt, K. S., Yocum, D., Potter, P. T., Castro, W. L., & Roth, S. (1998). An examination of individual differences in the relationship between interpersonal stress and disease activity among women with rheumatoid arthritis. *Arthritis and Rheumatology, 11*, 271–279.

Chapter 16
Caregiving Impact upon Sufferers' Cognitive Functioning

Lauren C. Heathcote, Tine Vervoort, and Melanie Noel

Abstract Pain by its evolutionary nature demands attention, warrants interpretation, and often etches itself into our lifelong memories. These cognitive processes of attending, interpreting, and remembering are central components of the pain experience and guide our approach and avoidance of future pain-related experiences. In this chapter, we discuss how cognitive processes influence and are influenced by our experience of pain, and the role of caregivers in the development and malleability of pain-related cognition. We focus on the parent–child relationship, as this is where most research has been conducted. We present evidence suggesting that the experience of chronic pain, or maladaptive pain behaviors, is often associated with distortions in cognitive processes—known as *cognitive biases*. Biases in attention, interpretation, and memory may help maintain pain over time, and contribute to distress and disability. Evidence for the influence of parents in children's pain memory development is growing. However, little research has investigated the role of parents and caregivers in attention and interpretation biases specifically. Here, we draw from research in anxiety disorders and depression indicating that caregivers may play a role in triggering, strengthening, and reducing threat-related cognitive biases. Indeed, threat-related cognitive biases appear to pass down through generations. Experimental studies in particular reveal that these biases can be influenced by parents' verbal information, emotion, and behaviors, indicating potential mechanisms for this intergenerational transmission of cognitive bias. We suggest ways in which we can draw from these studies in anxiety and depression to design novel studies for understanding the role of caregivers in the experience of pain-related cognition. Targeting pain-related cognitive biases in caregivers and patients may provide novel therapeutic targets for individuals suffering from pain.

L. C. Heathcote (✉)
Stanford University, Stanford, CA, USA
e-mail: lcheath@stanford.edu

T. Vervoort
Department of Experimental-Clinical and Health Psychology, Ghent University,
Ghent, Belgium

M. Noel
University of Calgary, Calgary, AB, Canada

T. Vervoort et al. (eds.), *Social and Interpersonal Dynamics in Pain*,
https://doi.org/10.1007/978-3-319-78340-6_16

347

Keywords Cognition · Cognitive bias · Attention · Interpretation · Memory · Parents and caregivers · Children and adolescents · Development

Introduction

As an evolutionary threat, pain by its very nature demands attention, warrants interpretation, and propels action to either approach or avoid. Pain is also not limited to the present moment. Rather, pain experiences are remembered and these memories guide subsequent pain behaviors. Therefore, pain engages cognitive processes of attention, interpretation, and memory, which motivate behavior and influence how pain is experienced in the future. Cognition is integral to the pain experience itself. Indeed, cognitive components have been incorporated into recent proposals for an updated definition of pain (Williams & Craig, 2016). What's more, cognitive biases have been implicated in the development and maintenance of chronic pain (Aldrich, Eccleston, & Crombez, 2000; Eccleston & Crombez, 2007; Pincus & Morley, 2001; Todd et al., 2015).

At the core of the pain experience is its command of one's attention. The intrinsic threat value of pain serves adaptive functions by capturing one's attention and motivating action to escape, reduce, or avoid tissue damage (Eccleston & Crombez, 1999). However, when pain is perceived as excessively severe or harmful, individuals may selectively attend to pain and pain-related cues over other important, competing demands (Crombez, Eccleston, Baeyens, & Eelen, 1998; Helzer, Connor-Smith, & Reed, 2009; Karsdorp, Ranson, Schrooten, & Vlaeyen, 2012; Van Damme, Crombez, & Eccleston, 2004; Verhoeven et al., 2010). This is often referred to as *attention bias*. Consequently, these individuals may experience increased attentional capture and interruption by pain. Indeed, some have argued that the experience of chronic pain should be redefined as "chronic interruption" (Eccleston & Crombez, 1999).

Once pain-related information is attended to, it is interpreted. Pain can be ambiguous and demand interpretation in terms of its meaning (is there something wrong with my body?), threat value (how much danger is there to my body?), and longevity (how long will it take to heal?). Other ambiguous somatic cues can also contribute to our interpretations of impending pain (does this funny feeling in my stomach mean that I am getting cramps?). Cues from our external environment may also indicate an upcoming pain experience (is that angry person going to hit me?). The way we make sense of this pain-related ambiguity—our *interpretations* of ambiguity—guide and shape our experiences of pain and the extent of our suffering (Todd et al., 2015). In particular, the habitual tendency to interpret ambiguous bodily information in a pain-related, threatening way—often referred to as *interpretation bias*—is likely to substantially impact pain experiences across the life span.

Long after the present pain experience, pain is remembered. Memories of pain are by their very nature susceptible to distortion. Individuals can remember pain accurately (i.e., no difference in recalled and initial pain) or in positively or negatively biased ways (i.e., recalled pain is less or greater than the initial pain report).

The nature of these memory distortions—often referred to as *memory bias*—plays a powerful role in shaping future pain response. Individuals who remember pain in a negatively biased way are at higher risk for developing greater distress, pain, and fear at future pain experiences. Conversely, accurate and positively framed memories are linked to adaptive pain outcomes (Chen, Zeltzer, Craske, & Katz, 2000; Noel, Chambers, McGrath, Klein, & Stewart, 2012).

Research is beginning to reveal that biases in attention, interpretation, and memory for pain and pain-related information are influenced and shaped by caregivers. Indeed, given that caregivers are likely to have profound influences on children's perceptions and appraisals of the world around them, they are also likely to provide salient models of children's pain-related cognitive processing. In this chapter we review and summarize research to date on the impact of caregivers upon the cognitive functioning of those in pain, particularly focusing on attention, interpretation, and memory biases. Given the infancy of this research area, we also review other relevant literatures that provide evidence of caregiver impact on threat-related cognitive biases, and highlight where these studies can be applied to the study of pain. Caregiver influences on pain and pain-related cognitive functioning are likely present and salient throughout the life span. However, this chapter focuses on the pediatric period (i.e., ages 0–18 years). The reasons for this are twofold: (1) Biases in cognitive processes (attention, interpretation, memory) for pain are particularly malleable in childhood (Jaaniste, Noel, & von Baeyer, 2016), opening up important avenues for intervention and, we argue, prevention of pain problems; (2) The impact of caregivers (parents) on individuals is particularly salient during these developmental periods (Noel, Palermo, Chambers, Taddio, & Hermann, 2015).

Attention Bias to Pain: State of the Art

Biased attention to pain has been linked to increased levels of pain severity, chronicity, and disability (e.g., Chapman & Martin, 2011; Sharpe, Haggman, Nicholas, Dear, & Refshauge, 2014). Van Ryckeghem and colleagues (2013) also demonstrated that elevated levels of attention bias to pain strengthened the relationship between daily pain severity and distractibility from ongoing daily activity. Attention bias has thus been shown to play a critical role in pain outcomes. However, evidence is not unequivocal; some studies do not identify expected associations between attention, avoidance, and pain-related psychological factors (Huber, Kunz, Artelt, & Lautenbacher, 2010; Roelofs, Peters, van der Zijden, Thielen, & Vlaeyen, 2003; Van Ryckeghem, Crombez, Van Hulle, & Van Damme, 2012), or find evidence counter to expectations (Boston & Sharpe, 2005; Vervoort, Caes, Crombez, et al., 2011; Vervoort, Caes, Trost, Notebaert, & Goubert, 2012). To date, the pediatric literature is limited, yet it is likewise marked by inconclusiveness. For example, biased attention to pain-related stimuli was observed among a sample of children with recurrent abdominal pain (Beck et al., 2011), but the reverse pattern (attentional avoidance) was found in a seperate sample of children with recurrent abdominal pain (Boyer et al., 2006). Furthermore, Vervoort, Trost, and Van Ryckeghem (2013) indicated the association between child catastrophizing, attention bias, and avoidance behavior was counter to expectations. Specifically, they observed increased attention *away* from pain faces (i.e., attentional avoidance) among children who magnified the consequences of pain.

Discrepant or inconsistent findings may owe to methodological limitations of existing attention bias research. Attention bias to pain is typically assessed using a computeised manual response task (most often the dot-probe task) using pain words as stimuli. When using the dot-probe task, participants are briefly shown a pair of stimuli at two different spatial locations on a computer screen. One of the stimuli is threatening (e.g., a word related to pain) while the other is neutral (e.g., a neutral word like 'table'). When these stimuli disappear from the screen, a small probe (often a dot) emerges at the location of either the threatening or neutral stimulus ("congruent" vs. "incongruent" trials, respectively). Selective attention to pain is inferred when responding (i.e., pressing a key) is faster to probes on congruent trials than to probes on incongruent trials. Conversely, faster responding to probes on incongruent trials is considered indicative of threat avoidance. A first central methodological limitation of these often used tasks may be the use of word stimuli (see Crombez, Van Ryckeghem, Eccleston, & Van Damme, 2013), that may have low ecological validity and are only indirectly related to pain (Heathcote, Lau, et al., 2016). More ecologically valid stimuli, such as facial expression of pain, may constitute a significant advance in the study of attention to pain, particularly when these facial pain stimuli relate to personally salient impending pain (Heathcote, Lau, et al., 2016; Vervoort et al., 2013). What's more, the dot-probe measures attention indirectly via manual response latencies. In addition, current methodology does not allow a continuous assessment of attention and thus does not permit distinguishing between initial attentional allocation and subsequent maintenance (e.g., sustaining) of attention. This distinction is theoretically and clinically important as literature supports the conclusion that, particularly among individuals who report high catastrophizing thoughts about pain, attentional disruption by pain stems mainly from difficulties in attentional disengagement (and thus increased attentional maintenance to pain) rather than initial attentional allocation (Liossi, Schoth, Bradley, & Mogg, 2009; Sharpe, Dear, & Schrieber, 2009; Van Damme et al., 2004). Recently, eye-tracking technology using pictures that relate to an impending personal pain experience has been introduced into pain-related attention bias research, thereby representing a significant advance in the study of attentional processing of another's pain, as this provides a more ecologically valid approach and a direct window onto behavioral dynamics as they unfold over time (see for example Heathcote, Lau, et al., 2016; Vervoort et al., 2013, further discussed below).

However, discrepant or inconsistent findings also imply that the nature of attention bias is not trait-like, and that the motivational qualities of biased pain-related attention are not intrinsic to attention. That is, selective attention to pain may not—in and of itself—lead to avoidance behavior. Similarly, attentional avoidance of pain may not always contribute to pain persistence, but may also motivate escape or avoidance behaviors. Instead, the nature of pain-related attention bias as well as the relationship between attention bias to pain, psychological variables such as pain catastrophizing and pain-related outcomes may be modulated by other variables. These may, as outlined below, include individual differences, such as one's attention control ability, but, may also include *how caregivers respond to their own as well as their child's pain.*

Individual Differences in Attention Bias to Pain

Attention control, which is defined as the ability to focus effortfully in the face of distraction and flexibly shift attention, has been suggested to be important in understanding the variable relationship between pain catastrophizing, pain attending, and pain-related outcomes such as avoidance behavior (Heathcote et al., 2015; Heathcote, Koopmans, et al., 2016; Heathcote, Lau, et al., 2016). This suggestion draws on dual process models of information processing—which have been mostly invoked in the context of anxiety disorders (e.g., Derryberry & Reed, 2002). Specifically, according to dual process models, anxiety is framed as a consequence of an imbalance between a fast, impulsive responding system, and a regulatory control system. Attention control, in turn, is proposed as a key variable buffering (i.e., moderating) the association between anxiety and attention bias to threat (Derryberry & Reed, 2002; Helzer et al., 2009; Mathews & Mackintosh, 1998; Mathews & MacLeod, 2005; Susa, Pitică, Benga, & Miclea, 2012). Studies have indeed revealed that only anxious participants with low levels of attention control demonstrate an attention bias towards threat (see for example Derryberry & Reed, 2002; Susa et al., 2012). Recently, these findings have been extended to pain contexts. Specifically, Heathcote and colleagues (2015) observed, using a dot-probe task with pain faces as stimuli, that adolescents who catastrophize about pain, and report *low* attention control, show high vigilance to facial expressions of pain. No such pattern was observed for adolescents reporting high attention control. Another study by Heathcote, Lau, and colleagues (2016), using eye tracking and personally relevant pain faces as stimuli, further attested to the buffering and potentially protective role of attention control. In particular, findings indicated that attention control again fulfilled a buffering role on self-reported pain intensity and behavioral avoidance (i.e., pain tolerance). Specifically, high anxious children who reported *low* levels of attention control anticipated more pain prior to experimental pain induction (i.e., cold pressor pain) and showed lower pain tolerance. While preliminary, these findings attest to the important role of individual differences in understanding both the nature and impact of biased attention to pain. Yet, not only individual characteristics matter. A growing body of research has shown that how others respond to our pain influences our adaptation to pain.

The Influence of Caregiver Responses on Attention Biases to Pain

Considerable research is available demonstrating that parent responses to their child's pain may directly impact the child's pain experience and functioning (see for example Caes, Vervoort, Eccleston, & Goubert, 2012; Caes, Vervoort, Eccleston, Vandenhende, & Goubert, 2011; Langer, Romano, Levy, Walker, & Whitehead, 2009). Further, how parents respond to the child's pain may also, through observational learning processes, indirectly affect adaptation to pain for that child (Goubert, Vlaeyen, Crombez, & Craig, 2011; Palermo & Chambers, 2005; Wilson, Moss, Palermo, & Fales, 2014). Below, we review the small number of studies in this area to date, and highlight how parent responses may, *indirectly or directly*, be particularly relevant in understanding both the nature and impact of children's attentional processing of pain.

Indirect Pathways: The Role of Observational Learning

Pain problems tend to run in families (Stone & Wilson, 2016). While various factors may account for this observation, learning processes emerging via observing another person in pain may be critically important. Indeed, findings in adults indicate that fear-avoidance beliefs, and associated behaviors, can be acquired in healthy adults after watching videos of others displaying painful expressions (Helsen, Goubert, Peters, & Vlaeyen, 2011). In pediatric populations, there is also preliminary evidence for the role of observational learning on children's pain experiences. For example, Goodman and McGrath (2003) demonstrated that pain behaviors in children increased after observing their mother expressing pain. Underlying mechanisms accounting for these findings remain unclear. Yet, it is reasonable to assume that observational learning will occur when individuals selectively encode and dwell upon pain-related information; hence, *biased attentional processing of pain-related information in the other* is likely key. Indirectly supporting this notion are findings from Horton and Riddell (2010) in the context of routine needle injections for immunization purposes. They demonstrated that infants were more likely to attend to their mother's face if the mother had expressed greater fear prior to a needle. Mothers who expressed greater fear, in turn, had infants who expressed greater facial displays of distress in response to the needle.

While attending towards pain in the other is likely to contribute to increased learning, the reverse, attentional avoidance, may also contribute to learning. For example, attentional avoidance of those who previously expressed pain may hamper extinction of what was previously learned and likewise contribute to deleterious outcomes. In one relevant study, Vervoort and colleagues (2013) examined the impact of child and parental catastrophizing (magnification, rumination, helplessness) about their own pain on the child's attentional processing of pain. They also examined the impact on the child's behavioral avoidance of pain. Findings revealed that children showed greater attentional avoidance of pain-related information (personally relevant pain facial expressions) in the context of high levels of parental rumination and helplessness about their own pain. Children who magnified the consequences of their pain also showed attentional avoidance of the same pain-related information. In turn, this attentional avoidance was related to increased child avoidance behavior. Not surprisingly, child pain magnification was significantly correlated with both parental rumination and helplessness. This association is consistent with a social learning perspective, which posits that parents indirectly affect their children's pain responses by means of observational learning (Chambers, 2003; Goodman & McGrath, 2003; Goubert et al., 2011). Specifically, children attending towards parental pain, fear, and avoidant behaviors in the context of potentially pain-inducing activities may adjust their interpretation of such activities and their consequences to match the parent behaviors (Chambers, Craig, & Bennett, 2002). Drawing on previous research showing that adult pain catastrophizing is associated with increased pain expressiveness (Sullivan, Adams, & Sullivan, 2004; Sullivan, Martel, Tripp, Savard, & Crombez, 2006) and behavioral pain avoidance (Karsdorp et al., 2012; Vlaeyen, Kole-Snijders, Boeren, & van Eek, 1995), it is likely that these behaviors will, in turn, be communicated to an observer. Hence, observational learning and attentional biases for pain are likely intrinsically linked.

Direct Pathways: The Role of Caregiving Behavior

Not only how others respond to their own pain, but also how others respond to the sufferer's pain, may impact the sufferer's pain-related attention. In the pediatric literature, parent responses to their child's pain are often broadly categorized as "pain-control'" versus "non-pain-control" behaviors. Pain-control behaviors, encompassing behaviors such as comforting, reassuring, or restricting child activities, are considered behaviors that direct the child's attention toward pain. Hence, these could be considered *pain-attending behaviors.* Conversely, non-pain-control behaviors, encompassing behaviors such as the use of humor, distraction, or encouraging activity, are considered behaviors that direct the child's attention away from pain. Hence, these could be considered *non-pain-attending behaviors* (Caes et al., 2014; Vervoort, Caes, Trost, et al., 2011; Walker et al., 2006). While pain-attending behaviors may protect the child from further harm or pain, such efforts may, in the context of long-term or inescapable pain, become maladaptive. That is, pain-attending behaviors may decrease engagement in valued daily activities, thereby fostering disability and maintaining or exacerbating pain problems. Indeed, studies have shown that whereas parental pain-attending behaviors are associated with increased child pain and distress, non-pain-attending behaviors are associated with increased child coping (Blount et al., 1997; Caes et al., 2014; Walker et al., 2006). However, the impact of parent pain-attending and non-pain-attending behaviors on the child's pain-related attention remains to be examined. Since parental pain-attending behaviors are thought to increasingly draw the child's attention to pain, they may also prime children towards biased attention to pain. Research in children with functional abdominal pain indicates that the impact of parental pain-attending behaviors upon child disability is mediated by child pain catastrophizing (Cunningham et al., 2014). Pain catastrophizing, in turn, has previously been found to impact biased attentional processing of pain (i.e., increased attentional avoidance; Vervoort et al., 2013), hence suggesting that parental pain-attending behaviors and child pain-related attention bias may indeed be linked.

Parent behaviors may also buffer or strengthen the impact of the child's cognitive factors upon pain-related outcomes. For instance, Vervoort, Huguet, Verhoeven, and Goubert (2011) demonstrated that the negative effect of child pain catastrophizing on disability was less pronounced when parents promoted child coping behavior (e.g., encourage using distraction). These behaviors can be subsumed under the umbrella of non-pain-attending behaviors. Accordingly, it is also likely that parental pain-attending behavior *moderates* the relationship between child attention bias and deleterious pain-related outcomes such as increased disability or distress. Indeed, children may become increasingly vulnerable for the hypothesized negative impact of pain-related attention bias when exposed to high levels of parental pain-attending behaviors. However, there has yet to be systematic empirical inquiry into *whether* parental pain-attending behavior impacts the child's attention bias for pain, and *how* such impact occurs; by moderating (i.e., strengthening) the impact of a child's pain-related attention bias and/or by priming the child's attention towards or away from pain. Indeed, future research is needed to propel forward this line of inquiry.

Interpretation Bias for Pain and Bodily Threat: State of the Art

The way we appraise and interpret pain plays a central role in almost all psychological models of chronic pain (e.g., Aldrich et al., 2000; Eccleston & Crombez, 1999; Van Damme, Legrain, Vogt, & Crombez, 2010; Vlaeyen & Linton, 2000). Thus, it is not surprising that the tendency to habitually interpret ambiguous information in a pain-related way—interpretation bias—has received much attention in the last decade. To examine interpretation bias, studies typically use self-report measures where participants are presented with ambiguous stimuli that could be appraised in a pain-related or a non-pain-related (e.g., benign or neutral) manner. For example, participants may be presented with homophones, which are words that sound the same yet have different spellings and meanings (e.g., pain/pane) or homographs, which are words that have identical spellings yet distinct meanings (e.g., terminal; causing death/airport building) (Pincus, Pearce, McClelland, Farley, & Vogel, 1994; Pincus, Pearce, & Perrott, 1996). Studies have also used word-stem completion tasks (e.g., ten___; could be completed as "tender" or "tennis") (Edwards & Pearce,

1994). In these paradigms, ambiguous stimuli have at least one pain-related or bodily-threat meaning and one benign meaning. Other studies employ "ambiguous situation tasks" in which participants are presented with vignettes of real-life situations which have plausible pain-related as well as benign interpretations (Keogh & Cochrane, 2002; Keogh, Hamid, Hamid, & Ellery, 2004; Vancleef, Hanssen, & Peters, 2016; Vancleef & Peters, 2008). Participants are then asked to generate their own interpretations, or to report whether experimenter-generated interpretations match their own interpretations. More recently, studies have also used computerized cognitive tasks that can measure more spontaneous (on-line) interpretations, for example through measurement of manual response times (Khatibi, Schrooten, Vancleef, & Vlaeyen, 2014; Khatibi, Sharpe, Jafari, Gholami, & Dehghani, 2015).

Most studies to date have investigated interpretation biases in adult pain populations, and all within an *intra*personal context. Indeed, no studies have investigated pain-related interpretation biases within an *inter*personal context. Schoth and Liossi (2016) pooled available data from adult chronic pain populations, performing meta-analyses to investigate whether or not adults with chronic pain display an interpretation bias for pain-related information. The meta-analyses revealed that adult chronic pain patients demonstrate significantly more pain-related interpretations of ambiguous stimuli relative to individuals without chronic pain, and that this bias may exist even outside of self-report (Khatibi et al., 2015). Interestingly, there is also evidence that negative interpretations of ambiguous pain-related and bodily-threat information characterize healthy individuals who score highly on measures of pain-related fear and catastrophizing (Heathcote, Koopmans, et al., 2016; Vancleef & Peters, 2008; Vancleef, Peters, & De Jong, 2009). Taken together, data suggests that pain-related interpretation biases are relevant for the experience of chronic pain, and may also be a pain-related vulnerability factor that exists in populations without chronic pain.

Only two studies to date have examined the role of pain-related interpretation biases in young people, once again within an *intra*personal context. In a first study, Heathcote, Koopmans, and colleagues (2016) developed a new measure to investigate interpretations of ambiguous pain and bodily-threat information in youth: the Adolescent Interpretations of Bodily Threat (AIBT) task. Results indicated that the tendency to endorse negative interpretations and to reject benign interpretations of ambiguous pain-related vignettes was associated with higher pain catastrophizing and recently experienced pain. This interpretation pattern was not specific for situations regarding pain and bodily threat, but generalized across ambiguous social situations. This lack of specificity may be because the sample was unselected, and the authors suggested we may expect more specific interpretation biases for pain and bodily threat information in clinical pain samples. To examine this, Heathcote, Jacobs, Eccleston, Fox, and Lau (2017) conducted a second study in which the AIBT task was administered to adolescent patients with chronic pain. As predicted, adolescents with chronic pain were less likely to endorse benign (i.e., non-threatening) interpretations of ambiguous bodily situations, than adolescents without chronic pain. This was particularly the case when reporting on the strength of belief in those interpretations being true. These differences between patients and controls in interpretational style were not evident for social situations, and not explained by differences in anxious or depressive symptoms. Weaker endorsement of benign interpretations was also associated with more functional disability even after controlling for chronic pain severity and pain catastrophizing. These results suggest that pain-related interpretations differ for adolescents with and without chronic pain, and may be clinically relevant for understanding levels of functioning among adolescent pain patients.

No published studies have examined the role of caregivers on interpretation biases. Yet, there are good reasons to believe that caregivers may have a profound impact on interpretations of pain and pain-related information for those they care for. These reasons are fourfold. (1) There is evidence from both the pain literature and from the psychopathology literature that interpretation biases are malleable and can be learned. (2) There is evidence from studies on pediatric anxiety that parent interpretation biases extend to the child's environment, and anxious parents expect their child to have negative interpretation biases. (3) Studies on pediatric anxiety show that threat-related interpretation biases can be learned vicariously from experimenters, peers, and, most importantly, parents. (4) Parents are a salient influence on child pain appraisals and beliefs. These points will now be discussed in turn.

The Malleability of Interpretation Biases to Pain

If caregivers influence pain-related interpretation biases in those they care for, interpretation biases must be malleable and subject to learning. Since negative interpretation biases have been identified as a potential driver of psychopathology such as anxiety and depression, studies have examined whether these biases can be modified through training. That is, whether they can be learned and unlearned. Cognitive Bias Modification of Interpretations (CBM-I) is one computerized training approach that is designed to change biases and, in turn, reduce psychopathological symptoms (MacLeod, 2012). During training participants are repeatedly presented with incomplete ambiguous scenarios, which can only be completed by endorsing a benign interpretation (in positive training) or a negative interpretation (in threat training) of the scenario (Lau, Pettit, & Creswell, 2013). Over time, these benign interpretations, which can be reinforced by feedback, are supposed to become automatic, and are argued to extend to the participant's own environment. Only one study to date has employed CBM-I within the context of pain. Jones and Sharpe (2014) randomly allocated 106 undergraduate students to receive computerized CBM-I that encouraged more threatening or more benign interpretations of ambiguous pain-related situations. As predicted, participants in the threat-training group endorsed more threatening interpretations of ambiguous pain-related information at a post-training test phase, and they hesitated more before immersing their hand in a cold pressor container. Most importantly, interpretive bias mediated the relationship between training condition and hesitance time, supporting a causal role of interpretation biases for pain avoidance behaviors. Outside of the pain context, studies have also investigated the use of CBM-I for anxiety populations, including for children and young people. While evidence for the efficacy of CBM-I in reducing anxiety symptoms is mixed, studies have typically shown that CBM-I is efficacious in changing interpretation biases (see MacLeod & Mathews, 2012). Thus, there is evidence that both pain-related and threat-related interpretation biases are malleable and can be (un)learned, including in youth.

While CBM-I data can tell us if interpretation biases are malleable, they do not inform us about caregiver influence on this malleability. Other studies within the field of pediatric anxiety have, however, examined the influence of parents on children's interpretation biases. This literature is highly relevant for our understanding of pain experiences because (1) chronic pain, like anxiety, runs in families (Stone & Wilson, 2016); (2) there is high comorbidity between anxiety disorders and chronic pain (Tsang et al., 2008), including in pediatric populations (Dorn et al., 2003). This indicates that a transdiagnostic approach to studying etiology, as well as intervention, may be beneficial; (3) there is a clear unifying construct across models of interpretation bias in pain and anxiety; the perception of threat. Although there may be differences in the content of the threat; for example, whether it is external to the individual (e.g., negative social cues in the case of social anxiety disorder), or internal to the individual (e.g., physiological sensations such as respiration in the case of panic disorder, and painful sensations in the case of chronic pain), the processes that facilitate and enhance threat perception may be similar across disorders. Thus, studies on parental influence on broad child threat interpretations will be an important source to draw on for understanding potential caregiver effects on interpretation biases in pain. These studies will now be briefly discussed.

The Influence of Caregivers on Threat-Related Interpretation Bias

In a seminal study, Barrett, Rapee, Dadds, and Ryan (1996) revealed that family discussions of ambiguous scenarios enhanced anxious children's avoidant plans of actions for those scenarios. Thus, early findings indicated family enhancement of cognitive style in anxious children. In a later series of studies, Creswell and colleagues demonstrated that mother and child threat interpretations of ambiguous situations were correlated (Creswell, Schniering, & Rapee, 2005), and that mothers who make threatening interpretations of their own environment also expect their child to make threatening interpretations (Orchard, Cooper, & Creswell, 2015). Lester and colleagues (Lester, Field, & Cartwright-Hatton, 2012; Lester, Field, Oliver, & Cartwright-Hatton, 2009) further showed that greater parental anxiety was associated with interpreting both self-referent and child-referent ambiguous situations in a more threatening way. The degree of self-referent interpretation bias also mediated the relation between parental anxiety and the tendency to interpret child-related ambiguous situations in a threatening manner (Lester et al., 2009), suggesting that parents' own interpretation biases are the driving force on their interpretations of the child's environment. Critically, Lester, Seal, Nightingale, and Field (2010) subsequently showed that children who made threat interpretations of ambiguous situations also anticipated that their mother would disambiguate situations for them in a threatening way. Taken together, there is strong evidence that parents' own threat-related interpretation biases may be a powerful predictor of the child's own bias.

A 2008 study on pediatric anxiety provides more direct relevance for understanding parent influences on child interpretation biases within potentially painful environments. Price-Evans and Field (2008) gave 6–10-year-old children threatening, positive, or no verbal information about three novel animals before asking the children to place their hands in the boxes they believed these animals inhabited. The threatening information may have indicated potential pain-related threat in terms of animal aggression, for example scratching or biting the child's hand. Results suggested that a neglectful maternal parenting style mediated the effect that verbal threat information had on the child's physiological responses to the potentially painful consequence of placing their hand in the box. Interestingly, a punitive maternal parenting style, maternal warmth, and overprotection were not found to have a significant effect, suggesting that certain parenting styles may be more important than others within this context. This study thus provides some of the first evidence that parenting style may be relevant for understanding child responses to ambiguous pain-related environments. In particular, maternal parenting style may be particularly relevant for understanding child avoidance behavior in the face of pain-related threat. Given that avoidance behavior is proposed as a key driving factor in pain chronicity in children (Asmundson, Noel, Petter, & Parkerson, 2012), parenting styles are likely an important factor for understanding child pain chronicity. Interestingly, studies have indeed revealed effects of parent factors on the child's experience of experimentally induced pain, thus mimicking findings from the pediatric anxiety literature. For instance, a 2003 study found that children's responses to the cold pressor test (CPT) were related to their mothers' style of responding, such that children who viewed their mother exaggerating displays of pain had lower pain thresholds than did children whose mothers were not given instructions on how to respond (Goodman & McGrath, 2003). An important next step will be to investigate whether the child's negative interpretations and thus expectations of the CPT mediate the associations between maternal responding and child response to the CPT.

Although there is a lack of research examining caregiver influences on children's pain-related interpretation biases, there is substantial evidence that child and parental pain experiences are closely linked. Family history of pain frequently emerges as a strong predictor of child pain functioning in chronic pain and acute experimental settings (see Evans et al., 2008). For example, in one study, family history of pain was related to increased pain episodes and sensitivity to an experimental thermal pain stimulus, although this was only in females (Fillingim, Edwards, & Powell, 2000). In another study, the number of family members with pain was related to greater daily pain, although counterintuitively, it was also associated with decreased

CPT pain intensity (Zeichner, Widner, Loftin, Panopoulos, & Allen, 1999). Of more direct relevance here, child catastrophizing, an interpretational style that focuses on catastrophic consequences of pain, has been shown to correlate with parent catastrophizing about their own pain (Lynch-Jordan, Kashikar-Zuck, Szabova, & Goldschneider, 2013). From a social-learning perspective, this intergenerational transmission of pain-related behaviors, beliefs, and expectations may be driven by vicarious learning, modelling, and reinforcement (Evans et al., 2008).

Memory Biases for Pain: State of the Art

Explicit (i.e., declarative, available to consciousness) and implicit (i.e., nonconscious, beyond conscious awareness) memory biases for pain have been implicated in the development and maintenance of ongoing pain problems (Flor, 2012) and fears and avoidance of medical care into adulthood (McMurtry et al., 2016). Given the powerful role of memories in shaping future pain experiences, and the particularly high malleability of pain memories in childhood, research attention has increasingly been paid to the pediatric period. Children's memories for pain are multidimensional, characterized by sensory, affective, and contextual aspects of the experience (Ornstein, Manning, & Pelphrey, 1999); however, traditionally, research has emphasized children's recall of pain's sensory aspects. Research on children's pain memories has employed a variety of methodologies ranging from open ended free recall interviews, prompted recall of contextual aspects of the pain experience, and readministration of single-item pain scales following the painful event. Important insights have been gained across studies taking different methodological approaches and common discoveries, such as the powerful role of pain memories on subsequent pain experience, have been made across a variety of populations and contexts, attesting to the robustness of these effects.

Memory Biases for Pain: Individual Differences

Early research on pain memory biases sought to address whether or not pain could be accurately recalled. Across a variety of pain contexts, data converged to suggest that the majority of children are indeed capable of accurately recalling their past pain experiences. However, a sizeable minority of children either under- or overestimate their pain, leading to positive and negative memory biases, respectively. In a seminal paper, Lander, Hodgins, and Fowler-Kerry (1992) examined children (5–17 years) undergoing venipuncture and assessed their pain, state anxiety, and recalled pain ratings 2 months later. Recall for the affective aspects of pain was found to be more accurate than recall for sensory pain (75% versus 43% recalled within ±1 face on a faces pain scale). The majority (74/138) of children recalled equivalent levels of pain as compared to their experienced pain reports. Relatively fewer children developed negative memory biases, with recalled pain being higher than experienced pain. However, positive memory biases were found among the smallest (12/138) group of youth. Among youth with cancer undergoing repeated lumbar punctures, Chen and colleagues (2000) similarly demonstrated that the majority of children accurately recalled details of their procedure; however, more positive than negative factual details were recalled. Even after a year, the majority of children and their parents remember children's acutely painful experiences in an accurate way (Badali, Riddell, Craig, Giesbrecht, & Chambers, 2000; Merritt, Ornstein, & Spicker, 1994; Rocha, Marche, & von Baeyer, 2009; Zonneveld, McGrath, Reid, & Sorbi, 1997).

Although research has demonstrated that while children *can* accurately recall their past pain experiences, these memories are also highly susceptible to distortion and biases (e.g., through provision of post-event feedback/processing), and this is particularly so in childhood (Jaaniste et al., 2016; Noel, Rabbitts, Tai, & Palermo, 2015). Moreover, remembering is dynamic. Just the act of retrieving the pain memory can serve to destabilize it, and negative memory biases are an established risk factor for worse pain outcomes (Chen et al., 2000; Noel, Chambers, McGrath, et al., 2012). All children do not remember pain in the same way; some children will remember pain accurately or even positively, whereas others will remember it in an increasingly distressing way over time. Therefore, research efforts in this area have shifted from demonstrating the overall accuracy of children's pain memories to identifying individual difference factors that predict which children will go on to develop negative biases in recall. Several intrapersonal factors have emerged as important in predicting pain memory biases including age, child sex, emotional distress (e.g., anxiety), pain, post-event information, and language used by observers. Across a variety of pain contexts, age has been shown to be a strong predictor of pain memory accuracy: younger children have been shown to have poorer recall accuracy than older children in the context of procedural (Burgwyn-Bailes, Baker-Ward, Gordon, & Ornstein, 2001; Chen et al., 2000; Goodman, Quas, Batterman-Faunce, Riddlesberger, & Kuhn, 1994; Salmon, Price, & Pereira, 2002; Zonneveld et al., 1997) and chronic pain (Chogle et al., 2012).

Despite the mounting evidence for sex differences in children's pain (Boerner, Birnie, Caes, Schinkel, & Chambers, 2014; Boerner, Schinkel, & Chambers, 2015) that appear to emerge around the time of puberty (and consequently, the onset of most types of pediatric chronic pain; King et al., 2011), few studies have examined sex as an individual risk factor for negative memory biases. In a notable exception, Hechler and colleagues (2009) examined the pain memories of a sample of adolescents with cancer using a single item numerical rating scale. Findings revealed that girls were more likely than boys to recall higher levels of pain intensity in the past 1 and 4 weeks, despite similar diagnosis and disease status.

Anxiety is critical to consider in understanding the development of pain memory biases. Highly anxious individuals have been shown to better recall their expectancies of a painful event than their actual experience of pain (Arntz, van Eck, & Heijmans, 1990). Anxiety is also central in several broader theoretical models of cognitive, and specifically, memory biases (Beck & Clark, 1997; Eysenck, Derakshan, Santos, & Calvo, 2007). Anxiety serves to interrupt information processing and favor the processing, encoding, and retrieval of threatening information. Experimental research has shown that children with higher state and trait anxiety, as well as anxiety sensitivity, tend to develop more negatively biased memories of pain (Noel, Chambers, McGrath, et al., 2012). Once these memories develop they become more powerful predictors of future pain response than the initial experience of pain itself (Noel, et al., 2012). Similar findings have been shown in the context of dental pain. Rocha and colleagues (2009) found that 5–12-year-old children with higher levels of trait anxiety tended to recall higher levels of pain over time than children with lower trait anxiety. A particularly relevant anxiety-related construct that has been implicated in the development of memory and other cognitive biases is pain catastrophizing. In the first study to examine this in youth, Noel, Rabbitts, and colleagues (2015) prospectively examined adolescents undergoing major surgeries (spinal fusion and pectus repair surgeries) and their parents. Parents and youth who reported more catastrophic thinking prior to surgery subsequently developed more distressing memories of pain 2–4 months later. Interestingly, parents' catastrophic thinking about pain (rumination, magnification) was a more important, direct and robust predictor of negative memory biases than children's own pain catastrophizing. The authors suggested that this catastrophizing-memory relationship could be mediated by post-event processing and language based interactions that parents and youth have about pain; however, such hypotheses have not yet been empirically tested. Beyond anxiety, more distressing emotions such as embarrassment (Goodman et al., 1994), depressed mood (Van Den Brink, Bandell-Hoekstra, & Huijer Abu-Saad, 2001), and fear (Merritt et al., 1994) have been linked to less accurate pain memories.

Research on children's pain memories has shown them to be strongly related to pain experienced at the time of the event. Just as pain predicts pain, pain also predicts biases in pain memories. This is a consistent and robust finding across populations, age groups, and settings. Among children with and without chronic illnesses undergoing venipuncture (Noel, McMurtry, Chambers, & McGrath, 2010), healthy children undergoing experimental (cold pressor) pain (Noel, Chambers, McGrath, et al., 2012; Noel, Chambers, Petter, et al., 2012; Noel, et al., 2012; Noel, Taylor, Quinlan, & Stewart, 2012), adolescents undergoing major surgery (Noel, Rabbitts, et al., 2015), children undergoing dental procedures (Rocha et al., 2009), and children with cancer experiencing lumbar punctures (Chen et al., 2000), those children and adolescents experiencing higher levels of experienced pain developed more negatively biased pain memories.

Conceptual Models of Children's Pain Memories: Accounting for the Role of Caregivers

In 2012, Noel and colleagues (Noel, Chambers, Petter, et al., 2012) proposed a model of acute pain memory development in childhood to account for the intrapersonal and interpersonal factors implicated in the process of pain memory formation and subsequent pain experience. This model began to integrate attention and memory. The model posits that children with higher levels of general and pain-specific anxiety tendencies are more likely to selectively attend to threatening and pain-related information in their environments. This attention then amplifies the pain experience and influences the aspects of the experience and environment that are encoded in memory. Enhanced attentional tendencies toward or away from threat are more likely to lead to negative biases in memory which then become a powerful predictor of subsequent pain, distress, and fear, thereby serving to fuel a cycle of increased cognitive biases, fear, and avoidance. Importantly, the model was the first to begin to account, albeit in a nondirectional way, for the role of parent cognitions and behaviors in shaping children's pain experiences and pain memories. The role of parents and parent–child language-based interactions as an important intervention target in memory reframing and pain management interventions was emphasized. A subsequent framework put forth by Noel, Palermo, and colleagues (2015) reiterated the importance of parent factors, particularly in the period of early childhood, when children's memories are most malleable and social influences of parents are strongest.

Caregiver Influences on Children's Memories for Pain

Similar to caregiver influences on attention and interpretation, such influences on children's pain memory development have been relatively understudied. There are a few notable exceptions, the majority of which are drawn from the field of developmental psychology. For several decades, it has been demonstrated and known that the manner in which parents talk to children about past events (including those that involve pain, e.g., injuries requiring emergency room treatment), plays a powerful role in shaping children's recall of those events (Peterson, Ross, & Charlene Tucker, 2002; Sales, Fivush, & Peterson, 2003). The influence of post-event information and parent–child narratives were traditionally examined to elucidate whether children could be reliable eye-witnesses in forensic settings and to inform how to harness parent–child narratives about pain in interventions to maximize cognitive-developmental outcomes (language and autobiographical memory). Nevertheless, we argue that this work is highly relevant to the study of children's pain memories and offer a valuable lens through which to understand this aspect of pain phenomenonology.

In an early investigation of memory accuracy among young children (aged 3–10 years) undergoing a painful procedure involving catheterization (voiding cystourethrogram; VCUG), Goodman and colleagues (1994) revealed an important influence of caregivers on children's recall. Maternal support predicted children's recall accuracy: mothers who did not physically comfort children (e.g., hug) or did not talk to them sympathetically had children who provided significantly more incorrect information during the recall interview. In addition, children of mothers who did not discuss or explain the VCUG to them were found to be more suggestible (i.e., making more errors of omission to misleading questions) than children whose mothers discussed the procedure with them after the fact. Taken together, the findings revealed that parent–child post-event discussion following an invasive painful procedure may buffer against the development of biases in recall. Nevertheless, post-procedural discussions in this study were measured using a self-report questionnaire and specific aspects of parental language that are particularly adaptive or maladaptive to children's recall accuracy were not captured.

Although research on memory-reframing interventions for children's pain management has not yet utilized parents as intervention agents, this work is relevant for understanding the influence of post-event language of adults on children's pain memory development. To date, there have been three trials of pain memory reframing interventions in children (Bruck, Ceci, Francoeur, & Barr, 1995; Chen, Zeltzer, Craske, & Katz, 1999; Pickrell et al., 2007). While the pain stimulus under investigation has consistently been needles (lumbar punctures, vaccine injections, dental anesthetic injections), study populations have included a wide age range (3–18 years) spanning several developmental periods and both youth with and without chronic illnesses (healthy children, pediatric oncology sample). Interventions were brief— ranging from a few sentences (e.g., telling children that they were brave and they did not cry; Bruck et al., 1995) to interactions lasting several minutes (e.g., using more cognitive-restructuring techniques and increasing children's sense of self-efficacy; Chen et al., 1999)—and all aimed to have adults talk to children in ways to reframe children's memories of pain to be more accurate and/or more positive. Findings across studies suggest that these types of interventions that manipulate adult-child conversations about painful events in the aftermath of those events do serve to modify children's pain memories to be less negatively biased. Moreover, some studies revealed that modifications in pain memories led to reductions in children's distress (Chen et al., 2000) and pain-related fear (Pickrell et al., 2007) at subsequent pain experiences. Beyond *remembering*, adult-led language based interventions have been targeted in interventions aimed at facilitating children's *forgetting* of pain memories. Marche, Briere, and von Baeyer (2016) used a retrieval induced forgetting task wherein researchers had children rehearse positive details of a past pain memory which then led to enhanced forgetting of its negative aspects. Although the task was not implemented as a pain management intervention, children who had a greater ability to forget negative aspects of their pain memory reported less anticipatory anxiety during an experimental pain task (e.g., cold pressor task). Taken together, this work suggests that children's memory biases for pain can be altered through language based interventions led by adults.

In the broader field of child development, parent–child language-based interactions about past events (e.g., vacations, injuries, and medical procedures), have been shown to strongly influence the retrieval and reframing of their autobiographical memories of those events (Salmon & Reese, 2015). Parent–child narrative style has also been shown to impact children's coping and psychological functioning (Salmon & Reese, 2015). Young children whose parents are topic-extending and elaborative (e.g., who ask open-ended questions to pull for richer, more detailed accounts of the past) and who use emotional language when they talk about past events, including those involving pain (e.g., lacerations, stitches, X-rays, casting, burns, and bruises) have children who are more accurate and detailed in recalling their pasts (Reese, Haden, & Fivush, 1993; Sales et al., 2003). Furthermore, parental reminiscing style is modifiable in interventions: young children of mothers who were taught to talk more elaborately about positive events subsequently provided richer memories of those events (Boland, Haden, & Ornstein, 2003; Reese & Newcombe, 2007).

Beyond *post*-event processing, through parent–child language based interactions, research has also examined *present*-event processing at the time of the painful event. Noel and colleagues (2010) sought to examine the influence of parent and staff behaviors during outpatient venipuncture on children's subsequent memories of pain and fear. Parent and staff verbal utterances during venipuncture were coded as either coping-promoting or distress-promoting using a validated observational coding system (CAMPIS-R; Blount et al., 1997). Children rated their pain and fear at the time of venipuncture and then again two weeks later, but this time based on their memories of the event. Recall accuracy for contextual details (who, what, when, where) was also assessed. Although parent behaviors were linked to children's anxiety and distress during venipuncture, they were not related to children's pain memories. Nevertheless, greater use of staff coping-promoting behaviors was predictive of children's recall accuracy of contextual details of the procedure. Given that distraction is encompassed within coping-promoting behaviors, the authors suggested that this finding could reflect greater attention toward contextual details. However, other researchers have shown that non-procedural talk/distraction during VCUG was related to deterioration of memory accuracy (Salmon et al., 2002). Discrepant findings across studies could be due to the heterogeneity in the methods used to assess memory (e.g., recalled levels of pain using single item measures, number of contextual details recalled).

Recent research suggests that parents' style of thinking about child pain prior to painful events may be particularly important in children's pain memory development. Noel, Rabbitts, and colleagues (2015) examined a cohort of adolescents undergoing major surgery (e.g., pectus repair, spinal fusion). Parents and youth completed measures of catastrophic thinking about child pain at baseline and their pain was assessed at baseline in the acute recovery phase (i.e., initial weeks following surgery). Children and parents then completed a memory interview at 2–4 months post-surgery during which time their memories of child pain were elicited using the same single-item pain measures administered previously. Findings revealed that parental catastrophic thinking about child pain was the most direct and robust predictor of children's and parents' pain memories. Specifically, children of parents who tended to magnify the threat value of their child's pain more frequently developed more negatively biased affective memories of pain. In addition, parents who tended to perseverate more frequently on the threatening aspects of their child's pain prior to surgery, went on to develop more negatively biased sensory memories of pain themselves. The authors of this study as well as other authors (Simons & Sieberg, 2015) suggested that these findings may reflect the influence of pain catastrophizing on verbally based interactions that parents and children have following surgery (e.g., narratives characterized by more threatening details). However, this hypothesis requires empirical testing.

Future Research

Cognition is fundamental to the pain experience and pain is, in large part, a social phenomenon (Williams & Craig, 2016). Cognitive processes of attending, interpreting, and remembering influence, and are influenced by, pain. Moreover, they are dynamic and malleable, making them fruitful targets for interventions (Crombez, Heathcote, & Fox, 2015). To date, investigations into the various cognitive biases for pain have proceeded in isolation, despite the fact that the mechanisms underlying attention, interpretation, and memory are invariably linked. Indeed, cognitive and attention theories of psychopathology hold that attention biases are integral in the development of memory biases. Specifically, these theories posit that memory biases develop because anxious individuals selectively encode, dwell upon, and retrieve threatening information (Beck & Clark, 1997). Moreover, close linkages between attention biases toward threatening information and negative memory biases (i.e., enhanced recall of threatening information and/or reduced forgetting) have been demonstrated among anxious and dysphoric individuals (Everaert & Koster, 2015; Noel, Taylor, Quinlan, & Stewart, 2012). More specific to pain, conceptual models of children's pain memory development posit that the child's attending to pain, and parental influences, are key in shaping biases in children's remembering. Shared parental mechanisms of action underlying attention and memory biases are also supported by empirical findings demonstrating that negative biases in children's attention and memory are most salient when parents perceive their child's pain as threatening (e.g., they think in catastrophic ways about their child's pain) (Noel, Palermo, et al., 2015; Vervoort et al., 2013). Interpretation is also closely tied to attention and memory; however, interpretation biases have received relatively less attention in the field of pediatric pain to date. Conceptual frameworks that integrate attention, interpretation, and memory biases specifically for pain in an affective-motivational context are needed and will serve to propel forward research in this area. With the introduction of new methods and measures to assess cognitive biases (Heathcote, Koopmans, et al., 2016; Heathcote, Lau, et al., 2016) in the context of pediatric pain, we expect this line of inquiry to rapidly grow.

While there is growing evidence of caregiver influence on child pain memories (Noel et al., 2010; Noel, Palermo, et al., 2015), examinations of the interpersonal factors influencing children's pain-related attention and interpretation biases are particularly limited. It remains to be tested whether child–family associations can be explained in part by the child's learning from their parent's cognitive biases, and if so, how this learning takes place. It will first be useful to examine whether child and parent pain-related cognitive biases are correlated. Moreover, expert consensus on how biases should be defined and measured will be important. Novel experimental methods have been used in the context of attention biases for anxiety that could be applied to similar investigations in pediatric pain. Following Rapee and colleagues (Barrett et al., 1996), it would be interesting to examine whether family discussions of ambiguous pain-related scenarios change children's interpretations of and plans of action for those scenarios, and whether these changes are different for parents and children with and without chronic pain. Validated tools that measure pain-related interpretation biases, such as the AIBT task (Heathcote, Koopmans, et al., 2016) could be adapted for these studies. Alternatively, studies on pediatric anxiety described above offer potential experimental tools that could be adapted for pain populations. For example, Field and Storksen-Coulson (2007) developed a powerful paradigm in which children are presented with novel, unfamiliar animals, for which mothers provide either threatening or non-threatening information. Children subsequently complete a measure of fear beliefs/interpretations, and are asked to put their hand into different boxes to feel each animal. A behavioral avoidance index is calculated to reflect how long it takes for children to put their hand in each box. A similar design could be implemented within the context of the CPT, in which threatening and non-threatening information could be provided by parents about different cold pressor containers, and a similar behavioral avoidance index could be calculated for how long it takes the child to immerse their hand in each water tank. Attention and memory biases for cold pressor pain could also be assessed in this context, and would be expected to be impacted given the strong influence of pre- and post-event processing on altering child attention and memory for painful information. Tasks are also needed to examine the transmission of parent cognitive style through verbal information as well as behaviors that can be directly modelled. A toolbox of experimental and clinical protocols must be developed to truly understand the "whens, whys, and hows" of caregiver influence on child attention, interpretation, and memory biases within the context of pain.

This area of inquiry has important clinical implications and could inform research and practice in acute and chronic pediatric pain management. Given that caregivers are likely to influence child pain-related cognition, and many cognitive-behavioral interventions for pediatric chronic (Fisher et al., 2014; Law, Beals-Erickson, Noel, Claar, & Palermo, 2015) and acute (Uman et al., 2013) pain target parental processes, research is needed to examine whether these interventions impact child pain-related outcomes through parent biases and their reactions to child biases. At the heart of cognitive behavioral interventions for pain are attempts to change children's cognitions about pain to be less threatening and instigate behavioral change strategies to confront pain and cope with it more adaptively. Conversely, the parent aspects of these interventions seem much more heavily weighted on changing parent behaviors (without focus on parental cognitions). We argue that to improve treatment efficacy, interventions will likely need to target antecedents of parent responses to child pain and not solely emphasize behavior change. Enhanced understanding of why parents engage in certain behavioral responses and how these behaviors become maintained over time is needed. Parents' own cognitive biases may be a key intervention target. Indeed, research is pointing to the powerful role of parents' own cognitions and biases in influencing children's pain and pain cognitions (e.g., pain memories). For example, research suggests that parent catastrophic thinking about child pain is a better predictor of pain persistence (Rabbitts, Groenewald, Tai, & Palermo, 2015) and children's pain memories (Noel, Rabbitts, et al., 2015) than the child's own pain and cognitions. Therefore, interventions may shift to incorporating more cognitive techniques with parents, particularly as they relate to their tendencies to think in catastrophic ways about their child's pain.

In addition to parental catastrophic thinking about child pain, adult language is a robust factor influencing children's pain and pain cognitions and is also directly targeted in interventions to modify children's cognitive biases. More nuanced examinations are needed to tease apart the specific aspects of parent–child language-based interactions that are important in shaping cognitive biases. Assessment of content (to include pain as well as other aspects of the experience), affective tone, and interaction style, is important to consider (e.g., moving beyond dichotomizing language-based interactions solely in relation to their focus on pain. Understanding how caregivers shape cognitions for pain in comparison (or contrast) to other kinds of emotional events (i.e., those involving sadness, distress) is also important to inform intervention efforts in this area. Moreover, many of the studies considered herein have considered how caregivers *negatively* impact child cognitive processing of pain. There is emerging evidence to suggest that parents and observers can *positively* impact child cognitive processing of pain. In a recent study by Marche and colleagues (2016), adult researcher-led discussions, wherein positive aspects of children's past pain experience were rehearsed with the children, led to enhanced forgetting of its negative aspects. Investigating which caregiver behaviors lead to positive child cognitive processing of pain will be important to develop interventions that aim to boost positive child pain outcomes.

Future research is needed to examine the influence of caregivers on pain-related cognitive biases across the life span. The relative influence of caregivers on children's cognitions (both general and pain-specific) is thought to be relatively stronger early in child development, with importance shifting to peer influences throughout adolescence (Noel, Palermo, et al., 2015) and then likely romantic partner influences into adulthood. However, research has not examined developmental trajectories of caregiver influences on cognitive biases. It is possible that mechanisms underlying caregiver influences on pain cognitions may be different across different caregiver and observer models. For example, vicarious learning about pain might be most salient among children and caregivers; however, research is needed to test this hypothesis. In addition, almost all studies described in this chapter were conducted within, or interpreted within, the assumption that caregiver influence is behaviorally transmitted. Indeed, experimental studies in which parent behavior is manipulated and shown to have a direct impact on child pain perception and reporting (e.g., Chambers et al., 2002), suggesting that caregiver behaviors influence how children perceive and think about pain. However, many researchers contend that the link between parent and child cognitive biases could also be explained by shared genes. Indeed, there is growing interest in the familial transmission of cognitive biases through shared genetic vulnerability (Fox & Beevers, 2016). This shared vulnerability may again be reinforced through caregiver behaviors. Although not a goal of this chapter, a future direction for the field is to consider both hereditary as well as environmental explanations for caregiver influence (caregivers can influence children's cognitions through their behaviors and genetic transmission).

In summary, cognitive biases for pain span attention, interpretation, and memory, and are thought to play a critical role in both the development and maintenance of pain problems. Pain cognitions are intricately shaped by emotional factors and threat perception and are thought to unfold within an interpersonal context. Particularly during the pediatric period, caregivers play a critical role in influencing the salience, interpretation, and processing of pain. Nevertheless, little research has examined the role of caregivers in the development of children's pain-related cognitive biases. In this chapter, we put forth a research agenda to guide future work in this area. Given the fundamental role that cognition plays in the pain experience, its plasticity, and role in intervention, this line of inquiry will inform theoretical and empirical advances to improve pain management and prevention across the life span.

References

Aldrich, S., Eccleston, C., & Crombez, G. (2000). Worrying about chronic pain: Vigilance to threat and misdirected problem solving. *Behavior Research and Therapy, 38*(5), 457–470. https://doi.org/10.1016/S0005-7967(99)00062-5

Arntz, A., van Eck, M., & Heijmans, M. (1990). Predictions of dental pain: The fear of any expected evil, is worse than the evil itself. *Behavior Research and Therapy, 28*(1), 29–41. https://doi.org/10.1016/0005-7967(90)90052-K

Asmundson, G. J. G., Noel, M., Petter, M., & Parkerson, H. A. (2012). Pediatric fear-avoidance model of chronic pain: Foundation, application and future directions. *Pain Research and Management, 17*, 397–405.

Badali, M. A., Riddell, R. P., Craig, K. D., Giesbrecht, K., & Chambers, C. T. (2000). Accuracy of Children's and parents' memory for a novel painful experience. *Pediatric Pain Management, 5*(2), 161–168.

Barrett, P. M., Rapee, R. M., Dadds, M. M., & Ryan, S. M. (1996). Family enhancement of cognitive style in anxious and aggressive children. *Journal of Abnormal Child Psychology, 24*(2), 187–203. https://doi.org/10.1007/BF01441484

Beck, A. T., & Clark, D. A. (1997). An information processing model of anxiety: Automatic and strategic processes. *Behavior Research and Therapy, 35*(1), 49–58. https://doi.org/10.1016/S0005-7967(96)00069-1

Beck, J. E., Lipani, T. A., Baber, K. F., Dufton, L., Garber, J., Smith, C. A., & Walker, L. S. (2011). Attentional bias to pain and social threat in pediatric patients with functional abdominal pain and pain-free youth before and after performance evaluation. *Pain, 152*(5), 1061–1067. https://doi.org/10.1016/j.pain.2011.01.029

Blount, R. L., Cohen, L. L., Frank, N. C., Bachanas, P. J., Smith, A. J., Manimala, M. R., & Pate, J. T. (1997). The child-adult medical procedure interaction scale-revised: An assessment of validity. *Journal of Pediatric Psychology, 22*(1), 73–88. https://doi.org/10.1093/jpepsy/22.1.73

Boerner, K. E., Birnie, K. A., Caes, L., Schinkel, M., & Chambers, C. T. (2014). Sex differences in experimental pain among healthy children: A systematic review and meta-analysis. *Pain, 155*(5), 983–993. https://doi.org/10.1016/j.pain.2014.01.031

Boerner, K. E., Schinkel, M., & Chambers, C. T. (2015). It is not as simple as boys versus girls: The role of sex differences in pain across the lifespan. *Pain Management, 5*(1), 1–4.

Boland, A., Haden, C., & Ornstein, P. (2003). Boosting children's memory by training mothers in the use of an elaborative conversational style as an event unfolds. *Journal of Cognition and Development, 4*(1), 39–65. https://doi.org/10.1207/S15327647JCD4,1-02

Boston, A., & Sharpe, L. (2005). The role of threat-expectancy in acute pain: Effects on attentional bias, coping strategy effectiveness and response to pain. *Pain, 119*(1–3), 168–175. https://doi.org/10.1016/j.pain.2005.09.032

Boyer, M. C., Compas, B. E., Stanger, C., Colletti, R. B., Konik, B. S., Morrow, S. B., & Thomsen, A. H. (2006). Attentional biases to pain and social threat in children with recurrent abdominal pain. *Journal of Pediatric Psychology, 31*(2), 209–220. https://doi.org/10.1093/jpepsy/jsj015

Bruck, M., Ceci, S. J., Francoeur, E., & Barr, R. (1995). "I hardly cried when I got my shot!" influencing children's reports about a visit to their pediatrician. *Child Development, 66*, 193–208. https://doi.org/10.2307/1131200

Burgwyn-Bailes, E., Baker-Ward, L., Gordon, B. N., & Ornstein, P. A. (2001). Children's memory for emergency medical treatment after one year: The impact of individual difference variables on recall and suggestibility. *Applied Cognitive Psychology, 15*(7 spec. iss). https://doi.org/10.1002/acp.833

Caes, L., Vervoort, T., Devos, P., Verlooy, J., Benoit, Y., & Goubert, L. (2014). Parental distress and catastrophic thoughts about child pain: Implications for parental protective behavior in the context of child leukemia-related medical procedures. *The Clinical Journal of Pain, 30*(9), 787–799. https://doi.org/10.1097/AJP.0000000000000028

Caes, L., Vervoort, T., Eccleston, C., & Goubert, L. (2012). Parents who catastrophize about their child's pain prioritize attempts to control pain. *Pain, 153*(8), 1695–1701. https://doi.org/10.1016/j.pain.2012.04.028

Caes, L., Vervoort, T., Eccleston, C., Vandenhende, M., & Goubert, L. (2011). Parental catastrophizing about child's pain and its relationship with activity restriction: The mediating role of parental distress. *Pain, 152*(1), 212–222. https://doi.org/10.1016/j.pain.2010.10.037

Chambers, C. T. (2003). The role of family factors in pediatric pain. In P. J. McGrath & G. A. Finley (Eds.), *Context of pediatric pain: Biology, family, culture* (pp. 99–130). Seattle, WA: IASP Press.

Chambers, C. T., Craig, K. D., & Bennett, S. M. (2002). The impact of maternal behaviour on children's pain experiences: An experimental analysis. *Journal of Pediatric Psychology, 27*, 293–301.

Chapman, S., & Martin, M. (2011). Attention to pain words in irritable bowel syndrome: Increased orienting and speeded engagement. *British Journal of Health Psychology, 16*, 47–60. https://doi.org/10.1348/135910710X505887

Chen, E., Zeltzer, L. K., Craske, M. G., & Katz, E. R. (1999). Alteration of memory in the reduction of children's distress during repeated aversive medical procedures. *Journal of Consulting and Clinical Psychology, 67*(4), 481–490.

Chen, E., Zeltzer, L. K., Craske, M. G., & Katz, E. R. (2000). Children's memories for painful cancer treatment procedures: Implications for distress. *Child Development, 71*(4), 933–947. https://doi.org/10.2307/1132335

Chogle, A., Sztainberg, M., Bass, L., Youssef, N. N., Miranda, A., Nurko, S., … Saps, M. (2012). Accuracy of pain recall in children. *Journal of Pediatric Gastroenterology and Nutrition, 55*(3), 288–291.

Creswell, C., Schniering, C. A., & Rapee, R. M. (2005). Threat interpretation in anxious children and their mothers: Comparison with nonclinical children and the effects of treatment. *Behavior Research and Therapy, 43*(10), 1375–1381. https://doi.org/10.1016/j.brat.2004.10.009

Crombez, G., Eccleston, C., Baeyens, F., & Eelen, P. (1998). When somatic information threatens, catastrophic thinking enhances attentional interference. *Pain, 75*(2–3), 187–198. https://doi.org/10.1016/S0304-3959(97)00219-4

Crombez, G., Heathcote, L. C., & Fox, E. (2015). The puzzle of attentional bias to pain: Beyond attention. *Pain, 156*(9), 1581–1582.

Crombez, G., Van Ryckeghem, D. M. L., Eccleston, C., & Van Damme, S. (2013). Attentional bias to pain-related information: A meta-analysis. *Pain, 4*, 497–510. https://doi.org/10.1016/j.pain.2012.11.013

Cunningham, N. R., Lynch-Jordan, A., Barnett, K., Peugh, J., Sil, S., Goldschneider, K., & Kashikar-Zuck, S. (2014). Child pain catastrophizing mediates the relation between parent responses to pain and disability in youth with functional abdominal pain. *Journal of Pediatric Gastroenterology and Nutrition, 59*(6), 732–738. https://doi.org/10.1097/MPG.0000000000000529

Derryberry, D., & Reed, M. A. (2002). Anxiety-related attentional biases and their regulation by attentional control. *Journal of Abnormal Psychology, 111*(2), 225–236. https://doi.org/10.1037//0021-843x.111.2.225

Dorn, L. D., Campo, J. C., Thato, S., Dahl, R. E., Lewin, D., Chandra, R., & Di Lorenzo, C. (2003). Psychological comorbidity and stress reactivity in children and adolescents with recurrent abdominal pain and anxiety disorders. *Journal of the American Academy of Child & Adolescent Psychiatry, 42*(1), 66–75. https://doi.org/10.1097/01.CHI.0000024897.60748.43

Eccleston, C., & Crombez, G. (1999). Pain demands attention: A cognitive-affective model of the interruptive function of pain. *Psychological Bulletin, 125*(3), 356–366. https://doi.org/10.1037/0033-2909.125.3.356

Eccleston, C., & Crombez, G. (2007). Worry and chronic pain: A misdirected problem solving model. *Pain, 132,* 233–236.

Edwards, L. C., & Pearce, S. A. (1994). Word completion in chronic pain: Evidence for schematic representation of pain? *Journal of Abnormal Psychology, 103*(2), 379–382. https://doi.org/10.1037/0021-843X.103.2.379

Evans, S., Tsao, J. C. I., Lu, Q., Myers, C., Suresh, J., & Zeltzer, L. K. (2008). Parent-child pain relationships from a psychosocial perspective: A review of the literature. *Journal of Pain Management, 1*(3), 237–246.

Everaert, J., & Koster, E. H. W. (2015). Interactions among emotional attention, encoding, and retrieval of ambiguous information: An eye-tracking study. *Emotion, 15*(5), 539–543. https://doi.org/10.1037/emo0000063

Eysenck, M. W., Derakshan, N., Santos, R., & Calvo, M. G. (2007). Anxiety and cognitive performance: Attentional control theory. *Emotion, 7*(2), 336–353. https://doi.org/10.1037/1528-3542.7.2.336

Field, A. P., & Storksen-Coulson, H. (2007). The interaction of pathways to fear in childhood anxiety: A preliminary study. *Behaviour Research & Therapy, 45*(12), 3051–3059.

Fillingim, R. B., Edwards, R. R., & Powell, T. (2000). Sex-dependent effects of reported familial pain history on recent pain complaints and experimental pain responses. *Pain, 86*(1–2), 87–94. https://doi.org/10.1016/S0304-3959(00)00239-6

Fisher, E., Heathcote, L. C., Palermo, T. M., de C Williams, A. C., Lau, J., & Eccleston, C. (2014). Systematic review and meta-analysis: Psychological therapies for children with chronic pain. *Journal of Pediatric Psychology, 39*(8), 763–782. https://doi.org/10.1093/jpepsy/jsu008

Flor, H. (2012). New developments in the understanding and management of persistent pain. *Current Opinion in Psychiatry, 25*(2), 109–113. https://doi.org/10.1097/YCO.0b013e3283503510

Fox, E., & Beevers, C. G. (2016). Differential sensitivity to the environment: contribution of cognitive biases and genes to psychological wellbeing. *Molecular Psychiatry, 21,* 1657–1662. https://doi.org/10.1038/mp.2016.114

Goodman, G. S., Quas, J. A., Batterman-Faunce, J. M., Riddlesberger, M. M., & Kuhn, J. (1994). Predictors of accurate and inaccurate memories of traumatic events experienced in childhood. *Consciousness and Cognition, 3–4,* 269–294. https://doi.org/10.1006/ccog.1994.1016

Goodman, J. E., & McGrath, P. J. (2003). Mothers' modeling influences children's pain during a cold pressor task. *Pain, 104*(3), 559–565. https://doi.org/10.1016/S0304-3959(03)00090-3

Goubert, L., Vlaeyen, J. W. S., Crombez, G., & Craig, K. D. (2011). Learning about pain from others: An observational learning account. *Journal of Pain, 12*(2), 167–174. https://doi.org/10.1016/j.jpain.2010.10.001

Heathcote, L. C., Jacobs, K., Eccleston, C., Fox, E., & Lau, J. Y. (2017). Biased interpretations of ambiguous bodily threat information in adolescents with chronic pain. *Pain, 158*(3), 471–478.

Heathcote, L. C., Koopmans, M., Eccleston, C., Fox, E., Jacobs, K., Wilkinson, N., & Lau, J. Y. F. (2016). Negative interpretation bias and the experience of pain in adolescents. *The Journal of Pain, 17*(9), 972–981. https://doi.org/10.1016/j.jpain.2016.05.009

Heathcote, L. C., Lau, J. Y. F., Mueller, S. C., Eccleston, C., Fox, E., Bosmans, M., & Vervoort, T. (2016). Child attention to pain and pain tolerance are dependent upon anxiety and attention control: An eye-tracking study. *European Journal of Pain, 21*(2), 250–263. https://doi.org/10.1002/ejp.920

Heathcote, L. C., Vervoort, T., Eccleston, C., Fox, E., Jacobs, K., Van Ryckeghem, D. M. L., & Lau, J. Y. F. (2015). The relationship between adolescents' pain catastrophizing and attention bias to pain faces is moderated by attention control. *Pain, 156*(7), 1334–1341. https://doi.org/10.1097/j.pain.0000000000000174

Hechler, T., Chalkiadis, G. A., Hasan, C., Kosfelder, J., Meyerhoff, U., Vocks, S., & Zernikow, B. (2009). Sex differences in pain intensity in adolescents suffering from cancer: Differences in pain memories? *Journal of Pain, 10*(6), 586–593. https://doi.org/10.1016/j.jpain.2008.11.011

Helsen, K., Goubert, L., Peters, M. L., & Vlaeyen, J. W. S. (2011). Observational learning and pain-related fear: An experimental study with colored cold pressor tasks. *Journal of Pain, 12*(12), 1230–1239. https://doi.org/10.1016/j.jpain.2011.07.002

Helzer, E. G., Connor-Smith, J. K., & Reed, M. A. (2009). Traits, states, and attentional gates: Temperament and threat relevance as predictors of attentional bias to social threat. *Anxiety, Stress, and Coping, 22*(1), 57–76. https://doi.org/10.1080/10615800802272244

Horton, R. E., & Riddell, R. R. P. (2010). Mothers' facial expressions of pain and fear and infants' pain response during immunization. *Infant Mental Health Journal, 31*(4), 397–411. https://doi.org/10.1002/imhj.20262

Huber, C., Kunz, M., Artelt, C., & Lautenbacher, S. (2010). Attentional and emotional mechanisms of pain processing and their related factors: A structural equations approach. *Pain Research and Management, 15*(4), 229–237.

Jaaniste, T., Noel, M., & von Baeyer, C. L. (2016). Young children's ability to report on past, future and hypothetical pain states: A cognitive developmental perspective. *Pain, 157*(11), 2399–2409. https://doi.org/10.1097/j.pain.0000000000000666

Jones, E. B., & Sharpe, L. (2014). The effect of cognitive bias modification for interpretation on avoidance of pain during an acute experimental pain task. *Pain, 155*(8), 1569–1576. https://doi.org/10.1016/j.jpain.2014.05.003

Karsdorp, P. A., Ranson, S., Schrooten, M. G. S., & Vlaeyen, J. W. S. (2012). Pain catastrophizing, threat, and the informational value of mood: Task persistence during a painful finger pressing task. *Pain, 153*(7), 1410–1417. https://doi.org/10.1016/j.jpain.2012.02.026

Keogh, E., & Cochrane, M. (2002). Anxiety sensitivity, cognitive biases, and the experience of pain. *The Journal of Pain, 3*(4), 320–329. https://doi.org/10.1054/jpai.2002.125182

Keogh, E., Hamid, R., Hamid, S., & Ellery, D. (2004). Investigating the effect of anxiety sensitivity, gender and negative interpretative bias on the perception of chest pain. *Pain, 111*(1–2), 209–217. https://doi.org/10.1016/j.pain.2004.06.017

Khatibi, A., Schrooten, M. G. S., Vancleef, L. M. G., & Vlaeyen, J. W. S. (2014). An experimental examination of catastrophizing-related interpretation bias for ambiguous facial expressions of pain using an incidental learning task. *Frontiers in Psychology, 5*, 1–10. https://doi.org/10.3389/fpsyg.2014.01002

Khatibi, A., Sharpe, L., Jafari, H., Gholami, S., & Dehghani, M. (2015). Interpretation biases in chronic pain patients: An incidental learning task. *European Journal of Pain, 19*, 1139–1147.

King, S., Chambers, C. T., Huguet, A., MacNevin, R. C., McGrath, P. J., Parker, L., & MacDonald, A. J. (2011). The epidemiology of chronic pain in children and adolescents revisited: A systematic review. *Pain, 152*(12), 2729–2738. https://doi.org/10.1016/j.pain.2011.07.016

Lander, J., Hodgins, M., & Fowler-Kerry, S. (1992). Children's pain predictions and memories. *Behavior Research and Therapy, 30*(2), 117–124. https://doi.org/10.1016/0005-7967(92)90134-3

Langer, S. L., Romano, J. M., Levy, R. L., Walker, L. S., & Whitehead, W. E. (2009). Catastrophizing and parental response to child symptom complaints. *Children's Health Care, 38*(3), 169–184. https://doi.org/10.1080/02739610903038750

Lau, J. Y. F., Pettit, E., & Creswell, C. (2013). Reducing children's social anxiety symptoms: Exploring a novel parent-administered cognitive bias modification training intervention. *Behavior Research and Therapy, 51*(7), 333–337. https://doi.org/10.1016/j.brat.2013.03.008

Law, E. F., Beals-Erickson, S. E., Noel, M., Claar, R., & Palermo, T. M. (2015). Pilot randomized controlled trial of internet-delivered cognitive-behavioral treatment for pediatric headache. *Headache, 55*(10), 1410–1425. https://doi.org/10.1111/head.12635

Lester, K. J., Field, A. P., & Cartwright-Hatton, S. (2012). Maternal anxiety and cognitive biases towards threat in their own and their child's environment. *Journal of Family Psychology, 26*(5), 756–766. https://doi.org/10.1037/a0029711

Lester, K. J., Field, A. P., Oliver, S., & Cartwright-Hatton, S. (2009). Do anxious parents interpretive biases towards threat extend into their child's environment? *Behavior Research and Therapy, 47*(2), 170–174. https://doi.org/10.1016/j.brat.2008.11.005

Lester, K. J., Seal, K., Nightingale, Z. C., & Field, A. P. (2010). Are children's own interpretations of ambiguous situations based on how they perceive their mothers have interpreted ambiguous situations for them in the past? *Journal of Anxiety Disorders, 24*(1), 102–108. https://doi.org/10.1016/j.janxdis.2009.09.004

Liossi, C., Schoth, D. E., Bradley, B. P., & Mogg, K. (2009). Time-course of attentional bias for pain-related cues in chronic daily headache sufferers. *European Journal of Pain, 13*(9), 963–969. https://doi.org/10.1016/j.ejpain.2008.11.007

Lynch-Jordan, A. M., Kashikar-Zuck, S., Szabova, A., & Goldschneider, K. R. (2013). The interplay of parent and adolescent catastrophizing and its impact on adolescents' pain, functioning, and pain behavior. *The Clinical Journal of Pain, 29*(8), 681–688. https://doi.org/10.1097/AJP.0b013e3182757720

MacLeod, C. (2012). Cognitive bias modification procedures in the management of mental disorders. *Current Opinion in Psychiatry, 25*(2), 114–120. https://doi.org/10.1097/YCO.0b013e32834fda4a

MacLeod, C., & Mathews, A. (2012). Cognitive bias modification approaches to anxiety. *Annual Review of Clinical Psychology, 8*(1), 189–217. https://doi.org/10.1146/annurev-clinpsy-032511-143052

Marche, T. A., Briere, J. L., & von Baeyer, C. L. (2016). Children's forgetting of pain-related memories. *Journal of Pediatric Psychology, 41*(2), 220–231. https://doi.org/10.1093/jpepsy/jsv111

Mathews, A., & Mackintosh, B. (1998). A cognitive model of selective processing in anxiety. *Cognitive Therapy and Research, 22*(6), 539–556. https://doi.org/10.1023/A:1018738019346

Mathews, A., & MacLeod, C. (2005). Cognitive vulnerability to emotional disorders. *Annual Review of Clinical Psychology, 1*, 167–195. https://doi.org/10.1146/annurev.clinpsy.1.102803.143916

McMurtry, C. M., Taddio, A., Noel, M., Antony, M. M., Chambers, C. T., Asmundson, G. J. G., … Scott, J. (2016). Exposure-based interventions for the management of individuals with high levels of needle fear across the lifespan: A clinical practice guideline and call for further research. *Cognitive Behavior Therapy, 45*(3), 217–235. https://doi.org/10.1080/16506073.2016.1157204

Merritt, K. A., Ornstein, P. A., & Spicker, B. (1994). Children's memory for a salient medical procedure: Implications for testimony. *Pediatrics, 94*(1), 17.

Noel, M., Chambers, C. T., McGrath, P. J., Klein, R. M., & Stewart, S. H. (2012). The influence of children's pain memories on subsequent pain experience. *Pain, 153*(8), 1563–1572. https://doi.org/10.1016/j.pain.2012.02.020

Noel, M., Chambers, C. T., Petter, M., McGrath, P. J., Klein, R. M., & Stewart, S. H. (2012). Pain is not over when the needle ends: A review and preliminary model of acute pain memory development in childhood. *Pain Management, 2*(5), 487–497. https://doi.org/10.2217/pmt.12.41

Noel, M., McMurtry, C. M., Chambers, C. T., & McGrath, P. J. (2010). Children's memory for painful procedures: The relationship of pain intensity, anxiety, and adult behaviors to subsequent recall. *Journal of Pediatric Psychology, 35*(6), 626–636. https://doi.org/10.1093/jpepsy/jsp096

Noel, M., Chambers, C. T., McGrath, P. J., Klein, R. M., & Stewart, S. H. (2012). The role of state anxiety in children's memories for pain. *Journal of Pediatric Psychology, 37*(5), 567–579.

Noel, M., Palermo, T. M., Chambers, C. T., Taddio, A., & Hermann, C. (2015). Remembering the pain of childhood: Applying a developmental perspective to the study of pain memories. *Pain, 156*(1), 31–34.

Noel, M., Rabbitts, J. A., Tai, G. G., & Palermo, T. M. (2015). Remembering pain after surgery: A longitudinal examination of the role of pain catastrophizing in children's and parents' recall. *Pain, 156*(5), 800–808. https://doi.org/10.1097/j.pain.0000000000000102

Noel, M., Taylor, T. L., Quinlan, C. K., & Stewart, S. H. (2012). The impact of attention style on directed forgetting among high anxiety sensitive individuals. *Cognitive Therapy and Research, 36*(4), 375–389. https://doi.org/10.1007/s10608-011-9366-y

Orchard, F., Cooper, P. J., & Creswell, C. (2015). Interpretation and expectations among mothers of children with anxiety disorders: Associations with maternal anxiety disorder. *Depression and Anxiety, 32*(2), 99–107. https://doi.org/10.1002/da.22211

Ornstein, P. A., Manning, E. L., & Pelphrey, K. A. (1999). Children's memory for pain. *Journal of Developmental and Behavioral Pediatrics, 20*(4), 262–277.

Palermo, T. M., & Chambers, C. T. (2005). Parent and family factors in pediatric chronic pain and disability: An integrative approach. *Pain, 119*(1–3), 1–4. https://doi.org/10.1016/j.pain.2005.10.027

Peterson, C., Ross, A., & Charlene Tucker, V. (2002). Hospital emergency rooms and children's health care attitudes. *Journal of Pediatric Psychology, 27*(3), 281–291. https://doi.org/10.1093/jpepsy/27.3.281

Pickrell, J. E., Heima, M., Weinstein, P., Coolidge, T., Coldwell, S. E., Skaret, E., … Milgrom, P. (2007). Using memory restructuring strategy to enhance dental behavior. *International Journal of Paediatric Dentistry, 17*(6), 439–448. https://doi.org/10.1111/j.1365-263X.2007.00873.x

Pincus, T., & Morley, S. (2001). Cognitive-processing bias in chronic pain: A review and integration. *Psychological Bulletin, 127*(5), 599–617. https://doi.org/10.1037//0033-2909.127.5.599

Pincus, T., Pearce, S., McClelland, A., Farley, S., & Vogel, S. (1994). Interpretation bias in responses to ambiguous cues in pain patients. *Journal of Psychosomatic Research, 38*(4), 347–353. https://doi.org/10.1016/0022-3999(94)90039-6

Pincus, T., Pearce, S., & Perrott, A. (1996). Pain patients' bias in the interpretation of ambiguous homophones. *The British Journal of Medical Psychology, 69*, 259–266. https://doi.org/10.1111/j.2044-8341.1996.tb01868.x

Price-Evans, K., & Field, A. P. (2008). A neglectful parenting style moderates the effect of the verbal threat information pathway on children's heart rate responses to novel animals. *Behavioral and Cognitive Psychotherapy, 36*(4), 473–482.

Rabbitts, J. A., Groenewald, C. B., Tai, G. G., & Palermo, T. M. (2015). Presurgical psychosocial predictors of acute postsurgical pain and quality of life in children undergoing major surgery. *The Journal of Pain, 16*, 226–234. https://doi.org/10.1016/j.jpain.2014.11.015

Reese, E., Haden, C. A., & Fivush, R. (1993). Mother-child conversations about the past: Relationships of style and memory over time. *Cognitive Development, 8*, 403–430. https://doi.org/10.1016/S0885-2014(05)80002-4

Reese, E., & Newcombe, R. (2007). Training mothers in elaborative reminiscing enhances children's autobiographical memory and narrative. *Child Development, 78*(4), 1153–1170. https://doi.org/10.1111/j.1467-8624.2007.01058.x

Rocha, E. M., Marche, T. A., & von Baeyer, C. L. (2009). Anxiety influences children's memory for procedural pain. *Pain Research & Management, 14*(3), 233–237.

Roelofs, J., Peters, M. L., van der Zijden, M., Thielen, F. G. J. M., & Vlaeyen, J. W. S. (2003). Selective attention and avoidance of pain-related stimuli: A dot-probe evaluation in a pain-free population. *The Journal of Pain, 4*(6), 322–328. https://doi.org/10.1016/S1526-5900(03)00634-5

Sales, J. M., Fivush, R., & Peterson, C. (2003). Parental reminiscing about positive and negative events. *Journal of Cognition and Development, 4*(2), 185–209. https://doi.org/10.1207/S15327647JCD0402_03

Salmon, K., Price, M., & Pereira, J. K. (2002). Factors associated with young children's long-term recall of an invasive medical procedure: A preliminary investigation. *Journal of Developmental and Behavioral Pediatrics, 23*(5), 347–352.

Salmon, K., & Reese, E. (2015). Talking (or not talking) about the past: The influence of parent-child conversation about negative experiences on children's memories. *Applied Cognitive Psychology, 29*(6), 791–801. https://doi.org/10.1002/acp.3186

Schoth, D. E., & Liossi, C. (2016). Biased interpretation of ambiguous information in patients with chronic pain: A systematic review and meta-analysis of current studies. *Health Psychology, 35*(9), 944–956. https://doi.org/10.1037/hea0000342

Sharpe, L., Dear, B. F., & Schrieber, L. (2009). Attentional biases in chronic pain associated with rheumatoid arthritis: Hypervigilance or difficulties disengaging? *The Journal of Pain, 10*(3), 329–335. https://doi.org/10.1016/j.jpain.2008.10.005

Sharpe, L., Haggman, S., Nicholas, M., Dear, B. F., & Refshauge, K. (2014). Avoidance of affective pain stimuli predicts chronicity in patients with acute low back pain. *Pain, 155*(1), 45–52. https://doi.org/10.1016/j.pain.2013.09.004

Simons, L. E., & Sieberg, C. B. (2015). Parents—to help or hinder pain memories in children. *Pain, 156*(5), 761–762. https://doi.org/10.1097/j.pain.0000000000000127

Stone, A. L., & Wilson, A. C. (2016). Transmission of risk from parents with chronic pain to offspring: An integrative conceptual model. *Pain, 157*, 2628–2639. https://doi.org/10.1097/j.pain.0000000000000637

Sullivan, M. J. L., Adams, H., & Sullivan, M. E. (2004). Communicative dimensions of pain catastrophizing: Social cueing effects on pain behavior and coping. *Pain, 107*(3), 220–226. https://doi.org/10.1016/j.pain.2003.11.003

Sullivan, M. J. L., Martel, M. O., Tripp, D., Savard, A., & Crombez, G. (2006). The relation between catastrophizing and the communication of pain experience. *Pain, 122*(3), 282–288. https://doi.org/10.1016/j.pain.2006.02.001

Susa, G., Pitică, I., Benga, O., & Miclea, M. (2012). The self regulatory effect of attentional control in modulating the relationship between attentional biases toward threat and anxiety symptoms in children. *Cognition & Emotion, 26*(6), 1069–1083. https://doi.org/10.1080/02699931.2011.638910

Todd, J., Sharpe, L., Johnson, A., Nicholson, K., Colagiuri, B., & Dear, B. F. (2015). Towards a new model of attentional biases in the development, maintenance, and management of pain. *Pain, 156*(9), 1589–1600. https://doi.org/10.1097/j.pain.0000000000000214

Tsang, A., Von Korff, M., Lee, S., Alonso, J., Karam, E., Angermeyer, M. C., … Watanabe, M. (2008). Common chronic pain conditions in developed and developing countries: Gender and age differences and comorbidity with depression-anxiety disorders. *Journal of Pain, 9*(10), 883–891. https://doi.org/10.1016/j.jpain.2008.05.005

Uman, L. S., Birnie, K. A., Noel, M., Parker, J. A., Chambers, C. T., McGrath, P. J., & Kisely, S. R. (2013). Psychological interventions for needle-related procedural pain and distress in children and adolescents. *The Cochrane Database of Systematic Reviews, 10*, CD005179. https://doi.org/10.1002/14651858.CD005179.pub3

Van Damme, S., Crombez, G., & Eccleston, C. (2004). Disengagement from pain: The role of catastrophic thinking about pain. *Pain, 107*(1–2), 70–76. https://doi.org/10.1016/j.pain.2003.09.023

Van Damme, S., Legrain, V., Vogt, J., & Crombez, G. (2010). Keeping pain in mind: A motivational account of attention to pain. *Neuroscience and Biobehavioral Reviews, 34*(2), 204–213. https://doi.org/10.1016/j.neubiorev.2009.01.005

Van Den Brink, M., Bandell-Hoekstra, E. N. G., & Huijer Abu-Saad, H. (2001). The occurrence of recall bias in pediatric headache: A comparison of questionnaire and diary data. *Headache, 41*(1), 11–20. https://doi.org/10.1046/j.1526-4610.2001.111006011.x

Van Ryckeghem, D. M. L., Crombez, G., Goubert, L., De Houwer, J., Onraedt, T., & Van Damme, S. (2013). The predictive value of attentional bias towards pain-related information in chronic pain patients: A diary study. *Pain, 154*(3), 468–475. https://doi.org/10.1016/j.pain.2012.12.008

Van Ryckeghem, D. M. L., Crombez, G., Van Hulle, L., & Van Damme, S. (2012). Attentional bias towards pain-related information diminishes the efficacy of distraction. *Pain, 153*(12), 2345–2351. https://doi.org/10.1016/j.pain.2012.07.032

Vancleef, L. M. G., Hanssen, M. M., & Peters, M. L. (2016). Are individual levels of pain anxiety related to negative interpretation bias? An examination using an ambiguous word priming task. *European Journal of Pain, 20*(5), 833–841. https://doi.org/10.1002/ejp.809

Vancleef, L. M. G., & Peters, M. L. (2008). Examining content specificity of negative interpretation biases with the Body Sensations Interpretation Questionnaire (BSIQ). *Journal of Anxiety Disorders, 22*(3), 401–415. https://doi.org/10.1016/j.janxdis.2007.05.006

Vancleef, L. M. G., Peters, M. L., & De Jong, P. J. (2009). Interpreting ambiguous health and bodily threat: Are individual differences in pain-related vulnerability constructs associated with an on-line negative interpretation bias? *Journal of Behavior Therapy and Experimental Psychiatry, 40*(1), 59–69. https://doi.org/10.1016/j.jbtep.2008.03.004

Verhoeven, K., Crombez, G., Eccleston, C., Van Ryckeghem, D. M. L., Morley, S., & Van Damme, S. (2010). The role of motivation in distracting attention away from pain: An experimental study. *Pain, 149*(2), 229–234. https://doi.org/10.1016/j.pain.2010.01.019

Vervoort, T., Caes, L., Crombez, G., Koster, E., Van Damme, S., Dewitte, M., & Goubert, L. (2011). Parental catastrophizing about children's pain and selective attention to varying levels of facial expression of pain in children: A dot-probe study. *Pain, 152*(8), 1751–1757. https://doi.org/10.1016/j.pain.2011.03.015

Vervoort, T., Caes, L., Trost, Z., Notebaert, L., & Goubert, L. (2012). Parental attention to their child's pain is modulated by threat-value of pain. *Health Psychology, 31*(5), 623–31. https://doi.org/10.1037/a0029292

Vervoort, T., Caes, L., Trost, Z., Sullivan, M., Vangronsveld, K., & Goubert, L. (2011). Social modulation of facial pain display in high-catastrophizing children: An observational study in schoolchildren and their parents. *Pain, 152*(7), 1591–1599. https://doi.org/10.1016/j.pain.2011.02.048

Vervoort, T., Huguet, A., Verhoeven, K., & Goubert, L. (2011). Mothers' and fathers' responses to their child's pain moderate the relationship between the child's pain catastrophizing and disability. *Pain, 152*(4), 786–793. https://doi.org/10.1016/j.pain.2010.12.010

Vervoort, T., Trost, Z., & Van Ryckeghem, D. M. L. (2013). Children's selective attention to pain and avoidance behavior: The role of child and parental catastrophizing about pain. *Pain, 154*(10), 1979–1988. https://doi.org/10.1016/j.pain.2013.05.052

Vlaeyen, J. W. S., Kole-Snijders, A. M. J., Boeren, R. G. B., & van Eek, H. (1995). Fear of movement/(re)injury in chronic low back pain and its relation to behavioral performance. *Pain, 62*(3), 363–372. https://doi.org/10.1016/0304-3959(94)00279-N

Vlaeyen, J. W. S., & Linton, S. J. (2000). Fear-avoidance and its consequences in chronic musculoskeletal pain: A state of the art. *Pain, 85*(3), 317–32. https://doi.org/10.1016/S0304-3959(99)00242-0

Walker, L. S., Williams, S. E., Smith, C. A., Garber, J., Van Slyke, D. A., & Lipani, T. A. (2006). Parent attention versus distraction: Impact on symptom complaints by children with and without chronic functional abdominal pain. *Pain, 122*(1–2), 43–52. https://doi.org/10.1016/j.pain.2005.12.020

Williams, A. C. de C., & Craig, K. D. (2016). Updating the definition of pain. *Pain, 157*(11), 2420–2423.

Wilson, A. C., Moss, A., Palermo, T. M., & Fales, J. L. (2014). Parent pain and catastrophizing are associated with pain, somatic symptoms, and pain-related disability among early adolescents. *Journal of Pediatric Psychology, 39*(4), 418–426. https://doi.org/10.1093/jpepsy/jst094

Zeichner, A., Widner, S., Loftin, M., Panopoulos, G., & Allen, J. (1999). Effects of familial pain models on daily pain indices and performance during the cold pressor task. *Psychological Reports, 84*, 955–960.

Zonneveld, L. N. L., McGrath, P. J., Reid, G. J., & Sorbi, M. J. (1997). Accuracy of children's pain memories. *Pain, 71*(3), 297–302. https://doi.org/10.1016/S0304-3959(97)03379-4

Part VI
Across the Lifespan

Chapter 17
Pain in Infancy: The Primacy of the Social Context

Hannah Gennis and Rebecca Pillai Riddell

Abstract With rare exception, pain is a universal personal experience. As with all sensations and their perceptions, physical pain can be seen as the end product of process that transduces the physical world into a subjective experience using physiological, cognitive, and emotional perspectives that are formed and experienced in a social context. Due to their unique developmental stage, infant pain is much more dependent on the social context, specifically the caregiver, than at any other stage in the life span. This chapter reviews evidence to suggest that Attachment Theory is an important lens in which to understand infant pain behavior. Attachment Theory demands a dyadic approach to understanding both pained infants and their caregivers. Assessing and managing infant pain through an attachment lens also acknowledges that infants are in a critical period of development in terms of developing core schemas about pain/distress and their own ability to regulate pain-related distress.

Keywords Infant pain · Caregiver · Parent · Mother · Attachment · Social · Soothing · Pain management · Pain assessment

In the dead of night, a newborn infant feels pain while lying in their crib. Despite being just days post-birth, she was born knowing how to signal her distress. One can envision, given knowledge of basic infant development, she would spend little cognitive resource on targeting this nocturnal signal to any particular caregiver or tailoring the signal to a particular cause (e.g., hunger versus lonliness versus pain). Rather the newborn reflexively mounts nonspecific behaviors to draw caregivers close. Under normative circumstances, a sleep-deprived mother or father, will approach the infant. They will make decisions about how to read and respond to the infants

H. Gennis
Department of Psychology, York University, Toronto, ON, Canada

R. Pillai Riddell (✉)
Department of Psychology, York University, Toronto, ON, Canada

Department of Psychiatry, Hospital for Sick Children, Toronto, ON, Canada

Department of Psychiatry, University of Toronto, Toronto, ON, Canada
e-mail: rpr@yorku.ca

© Springer International Publishing AG, part of Springer Nature 2018   379
T. Vervoort et al. (eds.), *Social and Interpersonal Dynamics in Pain*,
https://doi.org/10.1007/978-3-319-78340-6_17

distress signals. Day and night, this cycle of infant signal and adult response will occur thousands of times over the first year of life.

Unlike any other stage in the life span, these repeated mundane interactions between caregiver and the distressed infant, contribute to actually defining how a child (and the adult they will become) expresses and experiences pain. Beyond simply expressing a signal directly commensurate with a pain stimulus, an infant learns over time how to express pain within the context of the caregiving they receive. Using Attachment Theory (Bowlby, 1969/1982) and research conducted examining healthy infants and adults in an acute pain context, this chapter explores the social context of the infant in pain.

The Social Context of the Infant in Pain

Pain can be considered a universal personal experience. As with all sensations and their perceptions, physical pain can be seen as the end product of process that transduces the physical world into a subjective experience—the nuances of which can only truly be known by the individual experiencing the pain. Moreover, fundamental to its study is an acceptance of its biological, emotional, cognitive, and social dimensions (Williams & Craig, 2016). This complexity ensures that the same noxious physical stimulus will not be perceived in the same way between individuals because of the differing intraindividual balance of the biological, emotional, cognitive, and social dimensions factors working in concert to create a cognitive representation of the noxious stimulus and the resultant behavioral response. However, unlike the sensory, cognitive, and emotional components of pain, the social context does not reside solely within the individual. Akin to the pain experience itself, it is an external phenomenon that must be transduced into a subjective experience. While all four dimensions interrelate, the social context could be operationalized as impacting a person's' entire experience of pain by setting the foundation in which pain's biological, cognitive, and emotional sensations can occur. In children, parents are a critical factor to understanding a child's experience of pain. It will be argued that in early childhood, across the first years of life, parents are the most important factor within the social dimension of pain.

Early childhood is unique because it is a sensitive time for building schemas relating to how one perceives pain across the life span. Parents' interactions with infants in pain have not only shown to be critical to how a child processes painful experiences during a painful medical appointment but also to impact pain-related distress years later into preschool (Racine et al., 2016). Moreover, at no other stage in the healthy life span are humans as dependent on another to discern and manage pain as they are in infancy. This dependency actually forces a young child's pain experiences to be subject to the social, biological, cognitive, and emotional pain framework of another person for detection (assessment) and for action (management). Accordingly, without self-report, what is acknowledged as an infant's pain experience will actually differ according to which caregiver is perceiving the child's overt behaviors. Moreover, unlike other stages in the life span, the social context of a young child in pain is critical for building their core schemas of pain, distress, and their beliefs about their own agency over both.

As will be described below, an infant's early experiences with pain and distress coupled with their primary caregiver's responses to their distress forges a lasting schema that often relates to how an individual will process pain and distress throughout the life span (Bowlby, 1969/1982). This makes early childhood and the social dimensions of pain during this time different than any other stage in the life span. We assert that without an understanding of the caregiver and the young child's relationship pattern to the caregiver, clinicians and researchers will ultimately come to a flawed synthesis of a young child's pain experience.

Using work in our laboratory over the past decade as evidence, we will argue that because of the developmental stage of the young child, their perception of threats such as pain, are centred on how they have been socialized to experience distress by their primary caregiver (Bowlby, 1969/1982). This primary social relationship actually defines the young child's perception and understanding of pain unlike other stages in the life span because of the limited cognitive ability of infants and young children to bring in other factors to shape their pain experience (e.g., past pain experiences, knowledge of the duration of the pain experience, temporal considerations outside the present moment). Early in life, pain has been shown to trigger instinctive social behavior—the young infant enacts behaviors that will increase proximity to a caregiver when in distress. While this need for closeness to parents also occurs in older children, physical and cognitive development allows the possibility for older children to enact behaviors that reflect processing of the larger context of the painful stimulus beyond the caregiver (e.g., trying to rub the area that is in pain; walking away from a painful stimulus; remembering that the pain will go away). For the healthy infant, there is no ability to draw upon context beyond their parent's immediate behaviors.

These postulates about the young child in pain find their root in Bowlby's Attachment Theory (Bowlby, 1969/1982) which is fundamentally a theory of how the infant learns over the first year of life to use their primary caregivers to regulate distress (known as the attachment relationship). The early attachment relationship between the distressed infant and the primary caregiver forges a cognitive framework that is seen to relate to how humans perceive and react to distress throughout the lifetime. The goal of the infant's attachment system is to bring the caregiver close. While dimensional approaches have been taken, building on classic Bowlbian theory, there are four basic attachment categorizations (Ainsworth, Blehar, Waters, & Wall, 1978; Main & Solomon, 1990) that have been acknowledged—secure, resistant, avoidant, and disorganized. They all represent stable ways infants have been socialized to react to distress based on how their parents have responded to their distress. Secure infants express high distress and regulate when in presence of their caregiver because they have learned their caregiver will soothe them. Resistant infants express high distress and have trouble regulating despite the presence of their caregiver because of inconsistent patterns of parental soothing and proximity. Avoidant infants learn to mute their distress response outwardly in the presence of their caregiver because they have learned this is an organized strategy that will keep caregiver closer (caregivers of avoidant children have a tendency to not encourage expressions of emotion in others). Disorganized infants, as the category name implies, have behaviors that do not have an organized strategy to bring the caregiver close. This is often the result when the parent often reacts to the child's distress in frightening or distress-exacerbating ways.

Pain is considered a classic trigger of the infant's attachment system (Bowlby, 1969/1982). Critical to this is to understand that when this attachment relationship begins to show stability (i.e., the pattern in which the child uses the caregiver to regulate from distress stabilizes around 1 year of age), who the caregiver is when the infant or young child undergoes the painful experience will change the very nature of the pain experience and expression for that child. An infant or young child could experience and express pain differently based on whether it is a mother, a father, or a strange medical professional is holding them.

Broadly speaking, this chapter will focus on the primacy of the social dimension on a young child's perceptions of pain as discerned through work examining young children's behavioral responses to acute pain. Based on our research with the OUCH Cohort (http://bit.ly/2oLXbUq), a longitudinal study that followed children through vaccinations and psychological assessments over early childhood, we will examine the social context of pain responses during infancy (roughly the first year of life). We will first turn towards a more detailed discussion of the attachment context and then review research in the vaccination context presented through an attachment lens.

The Attachment Relationship as the Primary Social Context for Pain in Young Children

The stage prior to a child's first birthday is often referred to as "attachment in the making" by attachment theorists. During this stage, children are not only responding to pain and distress by signalling their caregiver as a primary goal, they are also concurrently in the process of building lasting schemas regarding their expression of distress and parent's response to that distress. These schemas are dependent on caregiver responses to their distress.

Infants are heavily reliant on their caregiver(s). Apart from meeting the basic needs of the infant (e.g., feeding), caregivers are important for helping the infant develop more complex skills required throughout the life span, such as their ability to regulate distress (Kopp, 1982; Pillai Riddell & Racine, 2009). An infant has not yet had enough experience, nor has not fully developed the cognitive ability to understand or remember that the pain will end. In fact, an infant's perception of pain is entirely constructed in the immediate moment (Craig, Korol, & Pillai, 2002). While a sophisticated combination of past, present, and future will develop throughout the life span to idiosyncratically influence a person's pain perception, this ability is outside of an infant's ability. Moreover, they lack the physical ability to independently enact self-regulation enhancing strategies (e.g., deep breathing, changing position) and are completely dependent on the support from individuals surrounding them (i.e., parents, other caregivers, or health professionals) to better cope with the painful experience. From an early age, over many distressing experiences, infants learn that specific types of signalling behaviors instigates proximity from their caregiver (Pillai Riddell & Racine, 2009). This process can be understood as the building of the attachment relationship.

Attachment theory (Bowlby, 1969/1982) is a prominent developmental theory to understand the socioemotional bond and expectations between the distressed infant and primary caregiver. As John Bowlby described it, the goal of the attachment system within the infant is to gain and maintain close proximity to the caregiver when security is threatened (Bowlby, 1969/1982; Marvin & Britner, 1999). The infant is said to have an "attachment behavioral control system" that works akin to a thermostat. When threat or distress is low, the attachment thermostat is off and this facilitates a child's exploration away from the caregiver. When threat or distress is high, the attachment thermostat turn on and a child focuses their energy on enacting behaviors devoted to bringing the caregiver close. Bowlby's theory of instinctive behavior is particularly relevant as it focuses on behaviors that are used to bring the caregiver closer during pain, such as cry, facial expressions, and body movement (Pillai Riddell & Chambers, 2007). The goal of the infant's signalling in that moment is that the caregiver will attend to these cues, and will make attempts to reduce the infant's pain/distress. The attachment system in the infant (which works with a reciprocal system in the caregiver—the caregiving system) has been postulated as one of human being's primary survival mechanisms in early life (Cassidy, 1994). Thus, although human infants and young children are born unable to meet any basic need without support, their brains are hardwired to signal adults to garner support when they are distressed.

Taking this one step further, if one accepts that early infant pain behaviors are innately determined survival reactions, then the initial behavioral signalling by the pained young infant could be seen as more accurately reflecting an infant's primary biological experience of pain than the pain expressions at any other stage of the life span. Infant's first signalling behavior is not yet a fully integrated expression of pain formulated as the result of weighing cognitive, emotional, sensory, and social factors. Thus, around the time the attachment bond is newly established (approximately 12 months of age), the responses may represent a more pure reflection of the social context of their painful experience than any other stage in the life span. Attachment theory provides a clear theoretical framework outlining why an infant's pain experience and expression are more heavily intertwined and more heavily weighted towards the social context (i.e., primary caregivers such as parents) than at any other stage in the life span.

How Do Attachment Categorizations Relate to Parent and Infant Behaviors in the Pain Context

We have attempted to understand if parent–infant dyads from varying attachment classifications act differently in the vaccination context. Hillgrove-Stuart, Pillai Riddell, Flora, Greenberg, and Garfield (2015) examined how caregiver behaviors during vaccination across four different ages in infancy (2, 4, 6, and 12 months), as well as at different time points within a vaccination appointment, were related to formal attachment classifications that were assessed using the Strange Situation Procedure (SSP; Ainsworth et al., 1978). The SSP involves a series of separations (intended to cause infant distress) and reunions with the parent to see how the infant uses the caregiver to regulate from the separation distress.

It was found that at 12 months, when the attachment relationship begins to be reliably measured, greater levels of parental proximal soothing (e.g., holding the infant close, rocking, rubbing; soothing that requires proximity) was related to infants' organized attachment classification (i.e., clear and consistent responding to signal distress upon separation and regulate from distress upon reunion), and caregivers who proximally soothed for a longer duration following the needle, had infants with organized, secure attachment styles. Findings also showed that steeper decreases in proximal soothing throughout vaccinations over the first year (engaging in less and less proximal soothing as the infant ages), was related to infant disorganized attachment (Hillgrove-Stuart et al., 2015). As would have been predicted by Attachment Theory, more proximal soothing within a painful medical appointment and over painful medical appointments over the first year of life were linked to secure attachment categorizations.

Using only the 12-month wave of the OUCH cohort and the attachment data, two accompanying papers (Horton, Pillai Riddell, Flora, Moran, & Pederson, 2015; Horton, Pillai Riddell, Moran, & Lisi, 2016) elucidated the relationships between infant attachment and infant pain behaviors. Infants with avoidant attachment classifications tended to show less distress compared to securely attached infants prior to the needle. However, after the needle there was a significant interaction with having a fearful or inhibited temperament (loosely defined as an infant's tendency to be withdrawn or slow to adapt in novel situations). In the conditions of a low fear temperament, avoidant infants regulated their pain-related distress much more quickly than secure infants (as would be expected). However, in higher fearful temperaments, avoidant infants regulated their pain related-distress more slowly. The interpretation of this result posited that the pain context is extra stressful on avoidant children who have a more fearful temperament such that their organized strategy to bring their parent close (i.e., muting their pain response) is overwhelmed; thus, triggering greater distress responding overall. This shows a clear example that the social context of the infant (i.e., the attachment relationship categorization of the infant that was developed by how the primary caregiver soothed their infant over the first year of life) actually may vary according to the child's personality.

Finally, given the interest in how the infant signals distress during vaccination and how that may vary according to caregiver soothing behavior patterns, analyses were also conducted to whether infant behaviors during the vaccination could predict their attachment classification. Suggesting a clear link to the attachment system and pain-related distress, no behaviors pre-vaccination were linked to attachment classifications (i.e., when there was no to little distress in our sample). However, after vaccination, it was found that "snuggling in" to the parent when distressed was significantly related. "Snuggling in" could be considered a classic proximity seeking behavior. Specifically, the greater the proportion of time after the vaccination needle that was spent snuggling into the caregiver, the greater the likelihood of a secure attachment classification. Securely attached infants used more proximity seeking during the vaccination compared to those infants classified as disorganized, or who were more avoidant of their parents during the SSP.

These novel analyses validate Bowlby's initial proposition that his theory relates to infants in pain and has relevance to the acute pain context. Stable patterns of caregiver and infant behavior during vaccination directly link to the attachment relationship categorizations. Thus, an exploration of the social context that caregivers create for the infant in pain through their behaviors will be reviewed after a brief discussion of a pain-specific model that takes into account attachment theory.

The Relationship Between Caregiver Behaviors on Infant Pain

The Development of Infant Acute Pain Responding (DIAPR) model was developed (Pillai Riddell, Racine, Craig, & Campbell, 2013; see Fig. 17.1) to depict how infant pain reactivity and infant pain regulation develops over the first year of life. Infant pain reactivity is seen as distinct to infant pain regulation, in part due to the attachment relationship. As aforementioned, attachment is a stable categorization of how an infant uses their caregiver to regulate distress. By this definition, there is a distinction between a child's immediate response to the pain stimulus and the responses that are distal to the pain stimulus as the child tries to re-attain homeostasis or a non-pained state. Thus, caregiver behaviors are postulated to directly impact pain regulation—how the infant calms down after the peak response and indirectly impact pain reactivity (as the impact would accrue over time as the caregiver behavioral responses to the child's distress shape the child's responses to pain).

Importantly, larger social/societal influences such as cultural beliefs about pain expression, gender biases about pain, availability of pain medications are seen to only influence the infant in pain through the caregiver. This is another distinction about the social context of the pained infant—larger spheres of influence outside of the immediate soother—are seen to only indirectly relate to infant pain responding (rather than having a direct impact as in older children and adults). Interestingly, despite the links between infant and caregiver behaviors during the vaccinations and attachment, the reader will note below that the relationships between caregiver behaviors and infant pain expression are not as strong as one would expect over the first year of life.

In a study by Lisi, Campbell, Pillai Riddell, Garfield, and Greenberg (2013), researchers aimed to assess descriptively what parents of healthy infants in the OUCH cohort spontaneously did to manage their infant's pain, without receiving information or coaching from researchers or their physician. Health professional behaviors were not controlled as it was a naturalistic observational methodology. Researchers found that the three most frequent behaviors used by parents were

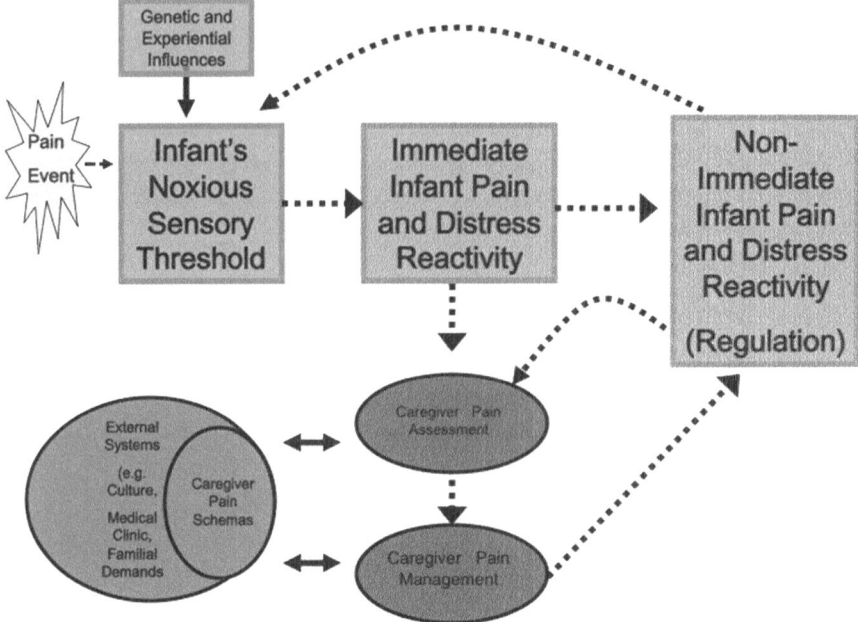

Fig. 17.1 The DIAPR model (Pillai Riddell et al., 2013)

physical comfort (e.g., bringing the baby close), rocking, and verbal reassurance (e.g., making statements such as, "you're ok"), occurring between 18 and 47% of the time. Notably, only physical comfort and rocking changed in frequency among the different ages. In particular, there was a clinically significant decrease in use of physical comfort (~10% decrease) between 2 and 12 months in the minutes following the vaccination, as well as rocking. Further, there was an increase in parents' use of distraction. This change in behaviors may be due to the increasing cognitive maturity of the infant at 12 months, and the ability for parents to engage their infant in distraction. Further, parents may be responding to the increased mobility of their infant at 12 months, and the child's desire to react to the needle in a less confined space.

The next phase of this study was to assess whether these parent behaviors actually reduced infant pain-related distress. It was found that at 4 and 12 months, frequency of these behaviors was not related to infant pain-related distress behaviors (cry, facial activity, body movements) post-needle. Parent behaviors only accounted for a maximum of 2.8% of the variance in infant pain scores at 2 months, and at most 10.2% of variance at 6 months following the needle. Specifically, use of a pacifier (a form of non-nutritive sucking) and distraction were related to decreased pain-related distress post-needle at these two ages. Perhaps one of the most interesting findings of this study is that with the exception of pacifying and distraction at two and 6 months, all behaviors had *positive* relationships with infant pain scores suggesting an actual *increase* in pain-related distress. This is contrary to what one might expect, but given this is a correlational study, it is likely that the distress signals (pain expression) are so intense, that this leads parents to embark on a greater frequency of soothing behaviors (pain management). It may be that the pain response is predicting more parent behavior, as opposed to the parent behavior predicting the infant pain response (Lisi et al., 2013).

Further research on the OUCH cohort assessing proximal soothing in particular found that minimal to no variance in infant pain behavior at all 2-, 4-, 6-, and 12-month vaccinations was accounted for by caregiver proximal soothing immediately following the needle or in the minutes following the needle (Campbell, Pillai Riddell, Garfield, & Greenberg, 2011). A key piece to this analysis was that the impact of earlier pain scores (from within each appointment) was covaried out of the analyses to get a purer indication of what role proximal soothing played. Contrary to what we reviewed earlier with what we would expect given the infant's innate disposition to signal caregiver, parent soothing behavior had minimal impact on pain-related distress in infancy.

However, when it came to exacerbating distress, more consistent relationships to parent behavior were found. Racine, Pillai Riddell, Flora, Garfield, and Greenberg (2012) assessed the impact of verbal reassurance of infant pain-related distress at all four vaccination age groups. Findings showed that at all four ages, the use of verbal reassurance increased infant pain-related distress. At first glance, it is odd to think that verbal reassurance (i.e., statements such as, "you're ok" and "it's almost over"), which has the appearance of appearing sensitive, would increase infant pain-related distress. These findings corroborated work by several research teams (Chambers, Craig, & Bennett, 2002; Cohen, Bernard, McClelland, & MacLaren, 2005; Lisi et al., 2013; Sweet & McGrath, 1998). Moreover, some suggest that this may be due to a disconnect between what the parent is saying ("It's okay") and what the infant is experiencing (highest distress). These comments may be subversively communicating parental anxiety, and/or that too much use of verbal reassurance is enacted when parents have no other effective soothing techniques.

The Impact of Caregiver Sensitivity on Infant Pain

Findings reviewed earlier are slightly puzzling from a pain management perspective. The idea behind infant pain as a more heavily-weighted social construct is that the infant and caregiver work in a reciprocal fashion where the infant signals pain and the caregiver responds to this pain in predictable ways. However, as Lisi et al. (2013) showed, an increased amount of soothing behaviors will not necessarily lead to changes in pain response, or may have the opposite effect of increasing the pain response. What is missing in the equation of the social context of infant pain is understanding the "how" subsuming the "what." Soothing behaviors are only soothing if they are conducted in a manner that the infant finds soothing.

In fact, it may be that particular soothing strategies that parents believe to be effective are simply not what their particular infant wants or needs in the minutes following a painful stimulus. Thus, an important component of caregiver pain assessment and management, is how attuned or sensitive, the caregiver is to the infant, and what he or she needs in that immediate moment (see also Chap. 4). This is a more complex process than simply increasing the frequency of soothing behaviors.

In the vaccination context, caregiver sensitivity is defined as a caregiver following how the infant's needs change over the vaccination appointment, as opposed to simply focusing on increasing the quantity of soothing behaviors (Pillai Riddell & Chambers, 2007; Pillai Riddell & Racine, 2009). From the perspective of models such as the DIAPR model (Pillai Riddell, 2009), it is the parent who is attuned to the changing needs of the infant and is accordingly able to change their management strategies, who will be most successful in reducing infant pain-related distress (e.g., Din, Pillai Riddell, & Gordner, 2009; Pillai Riddell et al., 2011). Thus, examining sensitivity is not just about what the parent is doing, it is *how* they are doing it.

Pillai Riddell et al. (2011) used the OUCH cohort to assess whether caregivers higher in sensitivity had infants with lower pain-related distress in the vaccination context. Sensitivity was measured using the Emotional Availability Scales, 4th Edition (Biringen, 2008), which operationalizes sensitivity as a parent's ability to follow the child's lead, structure environments to optimize child interactions and refrain from hostile/intrusive behaviors. Following the OUCH cohort at 2, 4, 6, and 12 months using the same methodology described above, researchers found that caregiver sensitivity and infant pain-related distress were negatively related. This meant that the more sensitive the caregiver, the less pain-related distress displayed by the infant. As would be expected from an attachment perspective, this relationship grew stronger as the infant aged, with the strongest negative relationship seen at 12 months. From an infant mental health and child development perspective, these findings are unsurprising as the attachment relationship is becoming more reliable at 12 months (Ainsworth et al., 1978). By 12 months, the infant and parent have had more time to bond socially and emotionally, and the attunement to the infant's needs becomes easier to follow with time.

Returning to Racine et al. (2012) study on verbal reassurance, it was found that caregivers, who scored higher in sensitivity, used less verbal reassurance. Although sensitivity did not moderate the relationship between verbal reassurance and infant pain at that age, it is important to note that these parents are likely more attuned to the fact that verbal reassurance is not working, and could be reducing their use of this in turn of more optimal strategies. These studies are some of the first to demonstrate that it is not merely the quantity of soothing behaviors, but rather the quality and the fit of these behaviors with the infant's needs that is important in the infant pain context. This is not to say quantity is irrelevant as it has also been demonstrated that highly sensitive mothers typically use more soothing behaviors than extremely insensitive caregivers (Atkinson et al., 2015).

Brand new work coming out on the preschool wave of the OUCH Cohort is showing that both parent behavior and sensitivity during infant vaccinations are predicting how preschoolers approach and express pain. Racine et al. (2016) had initially hypothesized that greater pain expressed during infant vaccinations would predict greater anticipatory distress to the preschool vaccination. No relationships were found. However, one of the strongest relationships with anticipatory distress to the preschool vaccination was that caregiver sensitivity during the 12-month vaccination was predicting preschooler anticipatory distress.

Examining children's pain responses after their preschool vaccination, Campbell et al. (2017) examined the predictive ability of caregiver sensitivity and caregiver proximal soothing during the 12-month vaccination. Interestingly, both caregiver sensitivity and proximal soothing from infancy predicted the parallel caregiver variable during the preschool vaccination, demonstrating the stability within the young child's primary pain social context. However, only the pathway from proximal soothing during infant vaccination to caregiver coping promoting behavior during the preschool vaccination predicted preschooler pain regulation. Even more fascinating is that attachment theorists have noted that during the first year of life key frontal lobe and language brain structures are developing in concurrent fashion, as key cognitive pathways implicated in attachment. Campbell et al. (2017) showed that proximal soothing during the infant vaccination predicted language acquisition at preschool age and caregiver sensitivity during the infant vaccination negatively predicted executive functioning dysfunction at preschool age. By showing these significant relationships between key cognitive skills and parent behavior during infant vaccination, they demonstrate a notable example of how the infant's social context in pain (i.e., parent soothing) significantly predicts future cognitive functioning in children. Likely because it is representative of caregiver responding across other distress contexts, a caregiver's behavioral responses to infant acute pain seems to contribute to lasting social and cognitive processes for the child.

Naturalistic observation of the caregiver soothing and infant pain behavior has provided fruitful information in understanding the relationships between what parents do and how it influences their infant's pain. During infant vaccinations they have been shown to reflect the emerging attachment relationship. This observational data can also be used to generate experimental data on parental pain management strategies that can positively support child through randomized controlled trials. Several large systematic reviews have been released to assess the efficacy of parent-led, non-pharmacological pain management strategies on pain outcomes in either premature or healthy infants (Harrison et al., 2016; Johnston et al., 2014; Pillai Riddell et al., 2015; Shah, Herbozo, Aliwalas, & Shah, 2012).

Experimental Evidence of the Influence of Parental Pain Management Behaviors

In two separate Cochrane reviews regarding the efficacy of breastfeeding in reducing pain-related distress in healthy infants during heel lance or venipuncture, researchers showed that breastfeeding had a significant reduction in heart rate increase and crying (total time crying, first cry, and crying proportion), and behavioral measures of pain-related distress over control conditions, with effect sizes ranging from moderate to large (Harrison et al., 2016; Shah et al., 2012). Of note, Shah et al. examined the impact of breastmilk via syringe and while not as effective as breastfeeding, it was shown to make some mixed efficacy on pain responding.

A separate Cochrane review assessed the efficacy of skin-to-skin/kangaroo care on pain-related distress in premature infants (Johnston et al., 2014). Skin-to-skin contact allows for full tactile stimulation of the infant as a diaper-clad infant is placed directly on the mother's chest. This review found that although skin-to-skin care was found to be effective over control conditions in reducing premature and healthy infants' responses to a painful stimulus, the quality of the research, particularly during the initial reactivity, was low.

Pillai Riddell et al. (2015) meta-analyzed the efficacy of 22 separate non-pharmacological pain management strategies (excluding skin-to-skin and breast-feeding) used in the immediate pain reactivity phase (first 30 s following painful stimuli) and regulation phase (minutes following the noxious stimuli), across three infant age categories: premature (born less than 37 weeks gestation), neonate (0–1 year), and older infants (1–3 years). Of these 22 non-pharmacological strategies, the following utilized the parent: massage/touch, rocking/holding, toy distraction, parent presence, and structured parent involvement (i.e., parent coaching). The largest effect of parent-led interventions over control in minimizing pain-related distress was seen for rocking/holding in healthy infants up to 1 year of age (neonates), in the immediate regulatory period following a painful stimulus. However, it is important to note that the effect sizes observed in this review were relatively small, and these findings were based on very low, to low quality evidence.

Recently, a new randomized-controlled trial examined the impact of a 5-min parent coaching video (The ABCD's of pain management; informed by an attachment framework) on the vaccination distress of 6- and 18-month-olds (Pillai Riddell et al., 2017). These age groups were selected to be significantly before and significantly after the attachment relationship first starts consolidating to see if it affected the power of the intervention. The intervention video was based on extensive observations of the OUCH cohort and core attachment principles. The video discussed four easy strategies for parents to use to better support their infant during vaccination (i.e., assess their own Anxiety because their worry affects their child's pain, Belly breathe to help calm themselves down, bring their distressed child in for a Calm, Close Cuddle, and Distract only when the child has passed the peak distress reaction). Results confirmed an interaction effect of the coaching video, such that a reduction in pain was only seen between the treatment and control infants that were 18 months of age. These findings suggest that the influence of the parental social context on an infant's pain expression is developing and likely stronger after the attachment relationship becomes more stable.

Conclusion

Due to their unique developmental stage, infant pain is much more dependent on the social context and the social context's most powerful agent—the caregiver—than at any other stage in the life span. This chapter reviews evidence to suggest that attachment theory is an important lens in which to understand infant pain behavior because attachment theory demands a dyadic approach to understanding both pained infants and their caregivers. Looking to the vaccination context our research has linked both parent and infant pain behaviors to the classic Attachment categorizations as theorized by Bolby and operationalized by Ainsworth and colleagues. Parents who conduct more proximal soothing during infant vaccinations have children who have a higher chance of being securely attached. Moreover, we reported that at 12 months of age securely attached children respond to pain-related distress with behaviors that bring them closer to parent. Consistent with the attachment relationship strengthening over the first year of life, we also described that the relationship between parental behaviors and infant pain responding strengthen over the first year. Finally, research examining pain management strategies that capitalize on the attachment relationship (i.e., that bring the parent closer during infant pain-related distress) shows strong experimental evidence to bolster the relevance of Attachment Theory to the young child in pain.

Assessing and managing infant pain through an attachment lens also acknowledges that infants are in a critical period of development in terms of developing core schemas about pain/distress and their own ability to regulate pain-related distress. Research has shown that how a caregiver soothes their pained infant impacts outcomes that extend beyond the clinic room. Given pain has been posited as a clear context that would trigger a human's attachment system across the life span, future research should examine how Attachment Theory impacts pain responding across developmental stages. Moreover, as the field of attachment evolves, more dimensional approaches to attachment measurement may be developed that could prove more powerful to incorporate by pain researchers.

References

Ainsworth, M., Blehar, M., Waters, E., & Wall, S. (1978). *Patterns of attachment*. Hillsdale, NJ: Lawrence Erlbaum Associates.

Atkinson, N., Gennis, H., Racine, N., Pillai Riddell, R., Garfield, H., & Greenberg, S. (2015). Caregiver emotional availability, caregiver soothing behaviors, and infant pain during immunization. *Journal of Pediatric Psychology, 40*(10), 1105–1114.

Biringen, Z. (2008). *The emotional availability (EA) scales manual* (4th ed.). Retrieved from www.emotionalavailability.com

Bowlby, J. (1969/1982). *Attachment and loss: Vol. 1. Attachment*. New York, NY: Basic Books.

Campbell, L., Pillai Riddell, R., Garfield, H., & Greenberg, S. (2011). A cross-sectional examination of the relationships between caregiver proximal soothing and infant pain over the first year of life. *Pain, 154*, 813–823.

Campbell, L., Riddell, P., Cribbie, R., Garfield, H., & Greenberg, S. (2018). Preschool children's coping responses and outcomes in the vaccination context: Child and caregiver transactional and longitudinal relationships. *Pain, 159*(2), 314–330. https://doi.org/10.1097/j.pain.0000000000001092

Cassidy, J. (1994). Emotion regulation: Influences of attachment relationships. *Monographs of the Society for Research in Child Development, 59*(2–3), 228–249.

Chambers, C. T., Craig, K. D., & Bennett, S. M. (2002). The impact of maternal behavior on children's pain experiences: An experimental analysis. *Journal of Pediatric Psychology, 27*(3), 293–301.

Cohen, L. L., Bernard, R. S., McClelland, C. B., & MacLaren, J. E. (2005). Assessing medical room behavior during infants' painful procedures: The measure of adult and infant soothing and distress (MAISD). *Children's Health Care, 34*(2), 81–94.

Craig, K. D., Korol, C. T., & Pillai, R. R. (2002). Challenges of judging pain in vulnerable infants. *Clinics in Perinatology, 29*, 445–457.

Din, L., Pillai Riddell, R., & Gordner, S. (2009). Brief report: Maternal emotional availability and infant pain-related distress. *Journal of Pediatric Psychology, 34*(7), 722–726.

Harrison, D., Reszel, J., Bueno, M., Sampson, M., Shah, V. S., Taddio, A., … Turner, L. (2016). Does breastfeeding reduce vaccination pain in babies aged 1–12 months. *Cochrane Systematic Reviews, 10*, CD011248.

Hillgrove-Stuart, J., Pillai Riddell, R., Flora, D. B., Greenberg, S., & Garfield, H. (2015). Caregiver soothing behaviors after immunization and infant attachment: A longitudinal analysis. *Journal of Developmental & Behavioral Pediatrics, 36*, 682–689.

Horton, R., Pillai Riddell, R., Moran, G., & Lisi, D. (2016). Do infant behaviors following immunization predict attachment? An exploratory study. *Attachment & Human Development, 18*(1), 90–99.

Horton, R. E., Pillai Riddell, R., Flora, D. B., Moran, G., & Pederson, D. (2015). Distress regulation in infancy: Attachment and temperament in the context of acute pain. *Journal of Developmental & Behavioral Pediatrics, 36*(1), 35–44.

Johnston, C., Campbell-Yeo, M., Fernandes, A., Inglis, D., Streiner, D., & Zee, R. (2014). Skin-to-skin care for procedural pain in neonates. *Cochrane Database of Systematic Reviews, 1*, CD008435.

Kopp, C. (1982). Antecedents of self-regulation: A developmental perspective. *Developmental Psychology, 18*, 199–214.

Lisi, D., Campbell, L., Pillai Riddell, R., Garfield, H., & Greenberg, S. (2013). Naturalistic parental pain management during immunizations during the first year of life: Observational norms from the OUCH cohort. *Pain, 154*(8), 1245–1253.

Main, M., & Solomon, J. (1990). Procedures for identifying disorganized/disoriented infants during the Ainsworth Strange Situation. In M. Greenberg, D. Cicchetti, & M. Cummings (Eds.), *Attachment in the preschool years* (pp. 121–160). Chicago: University of Chicago Press.

Marvin, R., & Britner, P. (1999). Normative development: The ontogeny of attachment. In J. Cassidy & P. R. Shaver (Eds.), *Handbook of attachment: Theory, research, and clinical applications* (pp. 46–67). New York, NY: Guildford Press.

Pillai Riddell, R. (2009). Keynote award address to Canadian pain society 2009 annual meeting: Dependent yet developing: New theorizing on the unique social context of infant pain. *Pain Research and Management, 14*(2), 143.

Pillai Riddell, R., Campbell, L., Flora, D. B., Racine, N., Din Osmun, L., Garfield, H., & Greenberg, S. (2011). The relationship between caregiver sensitivity and infant pain behaviors across the first year of life. *Pain, 152*(12), 2819–2826.

Pillai Riddell, R., O'Neill, M., Campbell, L., Taddio, A., Greenberg, S., & Garfield, H. (2017). The ABCD's of pain management: A double-blind randomized controlled trial for a brief educational video for parents of young children undergoing vaccination. *Journal of Pediatric Psychology, 43*(3), 224–233. https://doi.org/10.1093/jpepsy/jsx122

Pillai Riddell, R., & Racine, N. (2009). Assessing pain in infancy: The caregiver context. *Pain Research Management, 14*, 27–32.

Pillai Riddell, R., Racine, N. M., Craig, K. D., & Campbell, L. (2013). Psychological theories and biopsychosocial models in paediatric pain. In P. J. McGrath, B. J. Stevens, S. M. Walker, & W. T. Zempsky (Eds.), Oxford textbook of paediatric pain (pp. 85–94). Oxford, England: Oxford University Press

Pillai Riddell, R. R., & Chambers, C. (2007). Parenting and pain during infancy. In K. J. Anand, B. J. Stevens, & P. J. McGrath (Eds.), *Pain in neonates and infants* (3rd ed., pp. 289–298). Amsterdam, The Netherlands: Elsevier.

Pillai Riddell, R. R., Racine, N. M., Gennis, H. G., Turcotte, K., Uman, L. S., Horton, R. E., … Lisi, D. M. (2015). Non-pharmacological management of infant and young child procedural pain. *Cochrane Database of Systematic Reviews, 12*, CD006275.

Racine, N., Pillai Riddell, R., Flora, D., Garfield, H., & Greenberg, S. (2012). A longitudinal examination of verbal reassurance during infant immunization: Occurrence and examination of emotional availability as a potential moderator. *Journal of Pediatric Psychology, 37*(8), 935–944.

Racine, N. M., Pillai Riddell, R. R., Flora, D. B., Taddio, A., Garfield, H., & Greenberg, S. (2016). Predicting preschool pain-related anticipatory distress: The relative contribution of longitudinal and concurrent factors. *Pain, 157*(9), 1918–1932.

Shah, P. S., Herbozo, C., Aliwalas, L. L., & Shah, V. S. (2012). Breastfeeding or breast milk for procedural pain in neonates. *Cochrane Database of Systematic Reviews, 12*, CD004950.

Sweet, S. D., & McGrath, P. J. (1998). Relative importance of mothers' versus medical staffs' behavior in the prediction of infant immunization pain behavior. *Journal of Pediatric Psychology, 23*, 249–256.

Williams, A. C. d. C., & Craig, K. D. (2016). Updating the definition of pain. *Pain, 157*(11), 2420–2423.

Chapter 18
An Ecological and Life Span Approach of Social Influences on Childhood Pain Experiences

Line Caes, Liesbet Goubert, and Laura Simons

Abstract Pediatric pain is a common experience that not only impacts the child but also their social environment (e.g., parents, peers, school functioning). Several models have been formulated to gain a better understanding of the social context interwoven with pediatric pain, with the Social Communications Model the most well-known and comprehensive model. More recent model development has focused on providing an explanation of specific pathways to adaptive or maladaptive pain-related functioning in children (e.g., Interpersonal Fear–Avoidance Model, Ecological Resilience–Risk Model). The purpose of the current chapter is to provide an overview of both the Interpersonal Fear–Avoidance Model and the Ecological Resilience–Risk Model, followed by a critical evaluation of their merit in furthering our understanding of pediatric chronic pain across development and within the broader social context (e.g., peers and school environment). The chapter concludes with directions for future research, model development, and clinical practice.

Keywords Pain · Child · Adolescent · Parental responses · Pain-related fear · Catastrophizing · Resilience · Peers · School environment · Developmental perspective

L. Caes (✉)
Faculty of Natural Sciences, Division of Psychology, University of Stirling, Stirling, UK
e-mail: line.caes@stir.ac.uk

L. Goubert
Department of Experimental-Clinical and Health Psychology, Ghent University,
Ghent, Belgium

L. Simons
Department of Anesthesiology, Perioperative and Pain Medicine, Stanford University School of Medicine, Stanford, Palo Alto, CA, USA

Introduction

Understanding the social consequences of pain and its reciprocal impact upon the sufferer's pain experiences are of particular importance in the pediatric pain context as children highly depend upon adults (primarily their parents) for help and care (Palermo, Valrie, & Karlson, 2014). This reciprocal relation between child pain and parental responses is well demonstrated within the influential *Social Communication Model of Pain* (Craig, 2009). Specifically, the Social Communication Model of Pain recognizes three important steps in understanding how personal pain experience within the child impacts parental behavioral responses. The first step entails the child's internal experience of pain (e.g., stinging, burning, … pain sensations), which is encoded in expressive pain behaviors (= second step, e.g., facial pain expressions, guarding behaviors, crying). These expressive pain behaviors act as cues for the parent(s), who will decode the child's expressive behavior in order to draw inferences about their child's pain experience and determine how to respond (= third step, e.g., parental pain estimation, parental emotional distress, parental protective behavior, parental distraction). Importantly, the model highlights that this parental behavioral response, may, in turn, have an impact upon the child's internal pain experience (step one) and pain expression (step two; Hadjistavropoulos et al., 2011). Considerable evidence has provided support for the assumptions of the Social Communication Model of Pain within the context of pediatric acute and chronic pain (Hadjistavropoulos et al., 2011; Palermo et al., 2014). For example, counterintuitive evidence has revealed that while parents tend to automatically engage in protective behaviors such as reassurance, these behaviors have been linked to increased child pain and disability (e.g., Lisi, Campbell, Riddell, Garfield, & Greenberg, 2013). In contrast, parental engagement in distraction, humor, or coping-promoting suggestions (e.g., suggesting their child to take a deep breath) has been associated with reduced child pain intensity and disability (Uman, Birnie, Noel, Parker, Chambers, McGrath, & Kisely 2013; Walker et al., 2006).

While the Social Communications Model is a well-known, comprehensive model of childhood pain experience, more recent model development has focused upon particular processes that may play a role in the pathway to adaptive or maladaptive pain-related functioning in children (e.g., interpersonal fear–avoidance model and the ecological resilience–risk model). Underlining the importance of the social context of the pediatric pain experience, these newer models put a strong emphasis on the role of parental interpretations and responses as well as family characteristics to fully understand childhood pain.

For example, the fear–avoidance model, originally developed for adults (Vlaeyen & Linton, 2000), has recently been adopted to the context of pediatric pain and introduced as the interpersonal fear–avoidance model (IFAM; Goubert & Simons, 2013). An important and substantial aspect of this adaptation comprised the inclusion of how parental cognitive (e.g., pain interpretation and catastrophic thinking), emotional (e.g., parental fear), and behavioral responses (e.g., parental protective behavior) and the child's catastrophic thinking, fear and avoidance behaviors influence each other in determining the child's pain-related functioning (Goubert & Simons, 2013). In a similar vein, but with a focus on protective mechanisms and resources supporting positive or effective adaptation to pediatric chronic pain, Cousins, Cohen, and Venable (2015) proposed the ecological resilience–risk model (ERRM). The ERRM emphasizes how protective factors and mechanisms within the child's social environment (i.e., family functioning, parental behavioral responses, and teacher/peer support) can enhance the child's resiliency or effective responding when faced with the adversity of chronic pain experiences (Cousins, Kalapurakkel, Cohen, & Simons, 2015).

The purpose of the current chapter is to first provide a brief overview of both the interpersonal fear–avoidance model and the ecological resilience–risk model, followed by a critical evaluation of their merit in furthering our understanding of pediatric chronic pain across development and within the broader social context (e.g., peers and school environment). To conclude, we will provide some future directions for research, model development, and clinical practice.

The Interpersonal Fear–Avoidance Model

To better understand the origins and persistence of chronic pain complaints and pain-related disability in adults (Leeuw et al., 2007) and children (Asmundson, Noel, Petter, & Parkerson, 2012), researchers have frequently relied on the fear–avoidance model (FAM). At the core of this model is the idea that catastrophic thoughts about pain (i.e., perceiving pain as a threat, ruminating about pain, and feeling helpless in coping with pain) may set the stage for pain-related fear, which, in turn, may motivate individuals to behave in ways that allow them to avoid pain (e.g., avoiding social or school-related activities that are expected to heighten pain). Yet evidence shows that persistent attempts to avoid pain often lead to maladaptive long-term consequences, such as disability and depression. Although the majority of work in this area has focused on adult pain (Crombez, Eccleston, Van Damme, Vlaeyen, & Karoly, 2012; Leeuw et al., 2007), recent evidence suggests that the very same processes may also be central to the development and maintenance of chronic pediatric pain and disability (Simons & Kaczynski, 2012; Simons, Smith, Kaczynski, & Basch, 2015). For instance, studies have shown that children with high levels of catastrophizing thoughts about pain report having more difficulty performing daily activities (Crombez et al., 2003; Guite, McCue, Sherker, Sherry, & Rose, 2011). Pain catastrophizing in children has also been shown to predict increased pain and disability 6 months later (Vervoort, Eccleston, Goubert, Buysse, & Crombez, 2010). Additionally, high levels of pain-related fear in children and adolescents have been associated with higher disability levels and more frequent physician visits (Simons, Sieberg, Carpino, Logan, & Berde, 2011).

Accumulating evidence shows that the wider social context in which the child is embedded influences their catastrophic thoughts about, as well as fear and avoidance of pain and that parents play a particularly important role in this regard. This work has led to the emergence of the *Interpersonal Fear–Avoidance Model* (IFAM) which highlights the impact that parents have on the development and maintenance of (chronic) pediatric pain (Goubert & Simons, 2013; Simons et al., 2015). In line with the social communication model of pain (Hadjistavropoulos et al., 2011), the IFAM assumes that pain takes place within a social context, with parents as the most influential agents. Specifically, a sender (in this case the child) who experiences pain may express this pain in different ways (e.g., through facial or full body pain displays and/or verbal messages), which may be observed and decoded by others (e.g., parents) (Goubert et al., 2005). As part of this decoding, parents will interpret these pain messages expressed by the child (e.g., how much does my child suffer), which may give rise to pain-related fears in the parent when pain is appraised as very threatening (i.e., catastrophic pain interpretation). These parental fears may motivate parents to engage in so-called protective behaviors, aimed at the reduction or avoidance of pain in their child. Parental attempts to protect their child from pain may however negatively impact child functioning and psychosocial development (Goubert & Simons, 2013; Simons et al., 2015; Sinclair, Meredith, Strong, & Feeney, 2016). See Fig. 18.1 for an overview.

Indeed, it has been shown that higher levels of parental catastrophizing about the child's pain are related to more child disability (Goubert, Eccleston, Vervoort, Jordan, & Crombez, 2006; Logan, Simons, & Carpino, 2012; Lynch-Jordan, Kashikar-Zuck, Szabova, & Goldschneider, 2013; Vowles, Cohen, McCracken, & Eccleston, 2010), lower school attendance (Goubert et al., 2006) and a higher tendency to restrict child activities that may augment pain (Caes, Vervoort, Eccleston,

Interpersonal Fear Avoidance Model of Pain

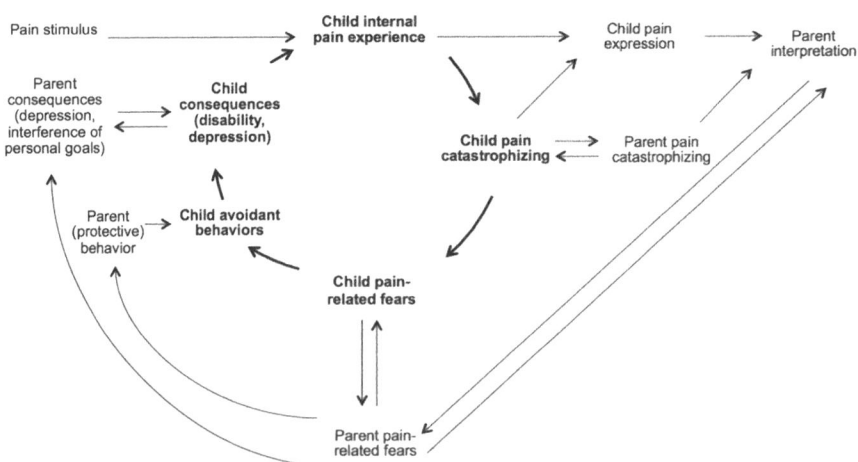

Fig. 18.1 The interpersonal fear–avoidance model (IFAM). Reproduced with permission from Goubert and Simons (2013)

Vandenhende, & Goubert, 2011). Accumulating evidence further shows that protective parenting behaviors are positively correlated with child functional disability (Claar, Simons, & Logan, 2008; Kaczynski, Claar, & Logan, 2009; Logan et al., 2012; Sieberg, Williams, & Simons, 2011; Wilson, Lewandowski, & Palermo, 2011). Preliminary prospective evidence supports this association between parental protective behaviors and child functioning. Specifically, in a cohort of 195 children and adolescents with chronic pain who presented for a multidisciplinary evaluation, it was found that baseline parental protective behavior significantly predicted child functioning at 4 months follow-up (Chow, Otis, & Simons, 2016). Of interest and supporting the assumptions of the IFAM, research has shown that parental protective behaviors mediate the relationship between parental catastrophizing and adverse child outcomes such as school functioning (Logan et al., 2012) and disability (Sieberg et al., 2011). Parental protective behaviors may fuel child avoidance behaviors, resulting in higher levels of child disability (Welkom, Hwang, & Guite, 2013).

In addition to this direct pathway by which parents may impact child outcomes through engaging in (over)protective behaviors, the IFAM also acknowledges that parents can impact children's psychosocial functioning in an indirect way, i.e., through observational learning processes (Goubert, Vlaeyen, Crombez, & Craig, 2011). When parents are highly fearful about the child's pain and perceive pain in a threatening way, fearful behaviors (such as fearful facial expressions) may be picked up by the child and fuel the child's fears and catastrophizing thoughts (Simons et al., 2015). Wilson, Moss, Palermo, and Fales (2013) for instance showed that parental catastrophizing was related to child functioning through its impact on children's catastrophizing thoughts. It has also been proposed that the way parents cope with their (own) pain may impact children's coping repertoire (Goubert et al., 2011). Although there is abundant research in adult pain on the impact of social modeling (see Craig, 1986; Helsen, Goubert, Peters, & Vlaeyen, 2011; Helsen, Goubert, & Vlaeyen, 2013; Helsen, Vlaeyen, & Goubert, 2015), the evidence in the context of pediatric pain is scarce (Goodman & McGrath, 2003; Thastum, Zachariae, Scheler, Bjerring, & Herlin, 1997).

A strength of the IFAM is the recognition of the bidirectionality between parent and child responses which not only impacts child outcomes but can also influence parental quality of life. For example, the chronification of the child's pain may fuel parents' catastrophizing and fearful thoughts, which may have as a consequence that parents become narrowly focused on alleviating their child's pain, and neglect other things they value in life (e.g., work performance or their social life). This may negatively impact parents' mood, and may eventually lead to depressive feelings in parents, which might, in turn, affect their child, leading to a vicious circle of catastrophizing/fear, avoidance, parental protection, depression, and pain (Goubert & Simons, 2013; Simons et al., 2015). Moreover, these maladaptive parent–child interactions likely result in short term and long term alterations in brain processes in the child and parent (Simons, Goubert, Vervoort, & Borsook, 2016) that manifest as alterations in physiology, behavior, and emotional state.

The Ecological Resilience–Risk Model

The *Ecological Resilience–Risk Model (ERRM)* has recently been formulated in response to the dominant focus on maladaptive coping in the context of pediatric pain. Processes and mechanisms which optimize the quality of life in families of a child experiencing chronic pain (i.e., resilience) have been largely overlooked (Cousins, Cohen, et al., 2015). Nevertheless, a substantial body of research on pediatric chronic illnesses demonstrates that many family units demonstrate substantial flexibility and resiliency in the face of ongoing interference due to chronic illness. For example, in a large-scale (N = 10,650) epidemiological study in Flemish young people (age range: 10–21 years; M_{age} = 14.33 years), 19.1% of young people reported experiencing high levels of pain accompanied by low levels of disability, thereby reflecting resilience despite being faced with chronic pain (Vervoort, Logan, Goubert, De Clercq, & Hublet, 2014). Furthermore, a recently conducted systematic review on family-level strengths or family resilience in the context of childhood cancer revealed that most families are resilient in various domains of functioning, such as family support, cohesion, positive communication, and adaptability. However, the available evidence is lacking in their usage of theoretical frameworks to guide the research question and approach. To facilitate further progression in this field, more research applying a family resilience framework is warranted (Van Schoors, Caes, Verhofstadt, Goubert, & Alderfer, 2015).

Resilience can be defined as "*a dynamic and multi-systemic progression that allows the individual to respond effectively when faced with risk or adversity (e.g., chronic pain)*" (Cousins, Cohen, et al., 2015). Importantly, the definition of resilience as well as the ERRM acknowledge that resilience originates within the individual, but can be enhanced through factors in the individual's social environment. Similar to the development of the IFAM, the ERRM for pediatric chronic pain is adapted from an adult model, namely the adult chronic pain risk–resilience model (Sturgeon & Zautra, 2013). While resilience and vulnerability were long considered as the opposites of a continuum, the chronic pain risk–resilience model introduced the idea of resilience and vulnerability being two independent but related constructs that determine the individual's pain-related trajectory. Importantly, a distinction is made between "*resilience resources*," "*resilience mechanisms*," and "*resilience outcomes*." Resilience resources are portrayed as stable characteristics (e.g., optimism and hope), while mechanisms are characterized as dynamic and modifiable processes (e.g., positive affect and positive relations) of a person and his/her social context. Resilience resources promote resilience mechanisms but minimize the impact of vulnerability factors and mechanisms, which in turn interfere with the impact of resilience resources. These resilience and vulnerability pathways determine the resilience outcomes, which consist of three distinct components: (1) sustained engagement in highly valued activities, (2) recovery from stressful experiences such as pain flares, and (3) personal growth or benefit-finding (Sturgeon & Zautra, 2013).

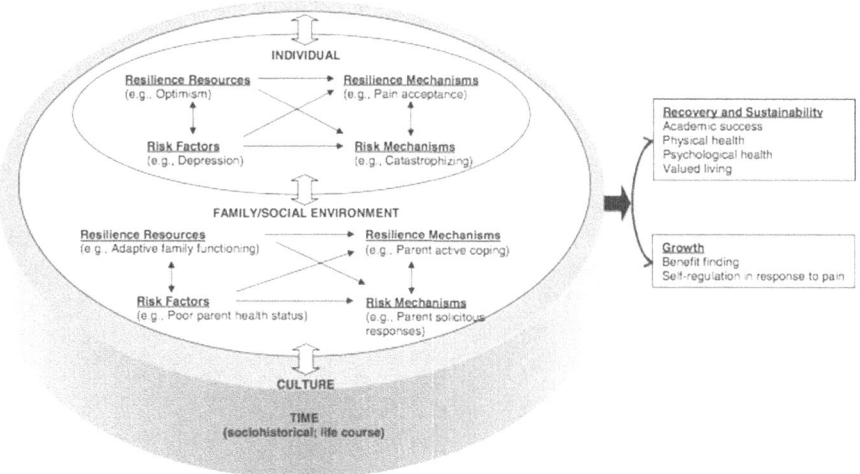

Fig. 18.2 The ecological resilience–risk model (ERRM). Reproduced with permission from Cousins, Cohen, et al. (2015)

The ERRM represents an adjustment of the adult model to account for the unique situation of childhood pain experiences. Specifically, despite the dearth of research addressing the social context as a source of resilience, the resilience resources and mechanisms available in the child's social environment play a prominent role within ERRM. The resilience and vulnerability pathways are proposed to occur within the individual itself and his/her social environment (including family, peers, school environment and culture), with a bidirectional relationship between the child's individual and social pathways determining the outcomes of the child in pain (See Fig. 18.2; Cousins, Cohen, et al., 2015).

The main goal of the ERRM is to facilitate continued research on resilience resources, mechanisms, and outcomes in pediatric chronic pain. The authors therefore highlight that further research is warranted to test and potentially refine the proposed pathways. Nevertheless, preliminary findings provide evidence for the role of resilience resources such as optimism, mindfulness, positive peer relations, teacher support, and supportive parent and family functioning in improving outcomes (e.g., increased quality of life and pain tolerance; reduced pain intensity and school absenteeism) for adolescents with chronic pain and their family (Cousins, Cohen, et al., 2015; Palermo et al., 2014; Petter, Chambers, McGrath, & Dick, 2013; Vervoort et al., 2014). With respect to identifying resilience mechanisms relevant for pediatric chronic pain, various research efforts (e.g., explorative, instrument development, and intervention studies) point to the beneficial impact of child acceptance of pain, child self-efficacy, and parental psychological flexibility on emotional and functional disability as well as improved school functioning (Carpino, Segal, Logan, Lebel, & Simons, 2014; Kalapurakkel, Carpino, Lebel, & Simons, 2015; Wallace, McCracken, Weiss, & Harbeck-Weber, 2015; Weiss et al., 2013).

Contrasting with the large body of research available on vulnerability factors when faced with pediatric chronic pain, substantial knowledge is lacking on various aspects of resiliency such as the role of positive affect, committed action, parent modeling of active coping and promotion of activity engagement, benefit finding, and self-regulation (Cousins, Cohen, et al., 2015; Cousins, Kalapurakkel, et al., 2015). Yet focusing on the role of protective factors and how they interact with vulnerability factors in the context of pediatric chronic pain is of critical importance to optimize clinical interventions. Specifically, protective factors and processes may be easier to influence and reinforce than vulnerability factors and therefore play a key role in clinical practice (Hilliard, Harris, & Weissberg-Benchell, 2012).

Critical Discussion of IFAM and ERRM

Both the IFAM and ERRM were developed in response to the need for developmentally and contextually appropriate models that reflect a child's experience of chronic pain. While both models acknowledge that developmental changes throughout childhood can influence the child's pain experience, they only provide a limited account of how exactly the proposed pathways might differ for infants, preschoolers, children and adolescents. In addition, while both models put a strong emphasis on the role of parental responses and family functioning in understanding the child's pain experience and impact on the family, the social context in childhood is broader than parental and familial influences. Particularly, in adolescence a key developmental task is gaining independence from their parents, which goes hand in hand with increased importance of and reliance on peers (Viner & Christies, 2005). Research has shown that the experience of chronic pain during childhood has the potential to impede these developing social skills (e.g., making new friends and maintaining relationships; Forgeron et al., 2010). How each of these aspects can impact the child's pain experience and how they currently are or could be incorporated within the IFAM and ERRM will be discussed below.

Developmental Perspective

The first examination of the FAM's application to pediatric pain demonstrated that there are developmental differences among children and adolescents (Simons & Kaczynski, 2012). Fear of pain had a stronger indirect role between catastrophizing and avoidant behaviors among adolescents as compared to younger children with chronic pain. This suggests that targeting fear-related pain cognitions ("I walk around in constant fear of hurting") when working with adolescents will likely yield greater gains in returning to previously avoided activities, than in younger pain patients, who are likely more responsive to a more concrete, behaviorally driven intervention.

There were also differences that emerged between younger children and adolescent patients with regard to avoidant behaviors. Adolescents reported significantly higher levels of fear–avoidance, which may be due to greater agency in choosing to avoid social or academic activities (e.g., "I cancel plans when I am in pain"), whereas younger children may have less choice in doing so (Simons & Kaczynski, 2012). This is where examining the influence of parents and even peers on this relationship is essential. It is likely that the influence of context (parents, peers) and therefore the authority for decision-making varies within childhood and thus cannot be examined as a static variable across children and adolescents. In support of this, Caes et al. (2014) revealed that parental engagement in protective behaviors prior to an invasive, painful medical procedure was related to more child non-verbal pain behavior following the procedure, but only for younger children (Caes et al., 2014). Taken together, these findings highlight the differential influence of parental behaviors depending on the child's developmental status.

The ERRM explicitly mentions the importance of an ecological framework in considering adaptation to adversity such as pain and frames the model in reference to Bronfenbrenner's ecological systems theory (Bronfenbrenner, 1979). In particular, the ERRM points to the occurrence of resilience and vulnerability pathways within time, with mutually influencing individual, familial/social, and cultural pathways. However, limited further explanation or evidence is provided on how these pathways develop across child development. A recent study examining pain catastrophizing across development does suggest the need to examine these differences (Feinstein et al., 2016). The authors found that pain catastrophizing was a significant predictor of pain interference and mobility in adolescents and young adults with chronic pain, but not for children. This is consistent with differences that emerged when testing the adult FAM in pediatric pain (Simons & Kaczynski, 2012) and reflects recent discussions that pain catastrophizing in children may simply reflect normal worry rather than a pathological process (Eccleston, Fisher, Vervoort, & Crombez, 2012). Similarly, while not explicitly accounted for in the ERRM, it is reasonable to assume that developmental states could strengthen or weaken the link between parental and child resilience resources and mechanisms. Taken together, our understanding of how vulnerability and resilience pathways within the child and their interactions with the social context (parents, peers) alter throughout development is limited and would benefit tremendously from more longitudinal research across the life span.

Role of Peers

Given the importance of peers in the psychosocial development of children and adolescents, peer support has been suggested as an important resilience mechanism (Forgeron & King, 2013; Sinclair et al., 2016). Although the IFAM (Goubert & Simons, 2013) acknowledges the role of the parental cognitive-emotional and behavioral responses in explaining the development and maintenance of children's chronic pain complaints and disability, it neglects the role of other potential social agents, such as peers. The ERRM refers to the role of social support as a resilience mechanism of adaptive child functioning in the presence of pain, but it only briefly touches on the role of peers (Cousins, Cohen, et al., 2015).

Despite not being included in the existing theoretical models, accumulating evidence suggests that disruptions to peer relationships, friendships, and social engagement are common and characterized by child avoidance of potentially fundamental social situations with friends and romantic interests (Forgeron et al., 2010). This is a major concern, especially for adolescents who develop and refine key social skills within the context of their relationships with peers. For instance, children and adolescents with chronic pain often have fewer friends than their healthy peers, they may miss opportunities for social leisure activities, and are at increased risk for victimization (for an overview, see Forgeron et al., 2010). Research also has shown that adolescents with chronic pain feel lonelier than their healthy peers (Forgeron et al., 2011), feel more distressed by negative interactions with friends, and report that friends are not always supportive because they lack insight in living with a daily condition such as chronic pain (Forgeron & McGrath, 2009). A qualitative study by Fleischman, Hains, and Davies (2011) showed that practitioners perceive a decline in adolescents' peer functioning over time, with adolescents often avoiding other peers. Practitioners attributed this avoidance of peers more to the pain than to social (in)competence. Furthermore, peers perceive adolescents with chronic pain as more withdrawn and less popular (Kashikar-Zuck et al., 2007). The latter study also showed that these adolescents had fewer reciprocated friendships (Kashikar-Zuck et al., 2007).

A study by Forgeron et al. (2011) provides preliminary understanding of the potential underlying mechanisms involved in this compromised social functioning by suggesting that social information processing may be different in adolescents with chronic pain compared to controls. It was found that adolescents with chronic pain interpreted non-supportive social situations with close friends as more distressing and expected more supportive behaviors from friends. Eccleston, Wastell, Crombez, and Jordan (2008) investigated the impact of chronic pain on social development in 110 adolescents with chronic pain. The findings showed that adolescents generally perceived themselves to be behind their peers in their psychosocial development, which could further explain the compromised social functioning in these adolescents. Of interest, strong peer relationships were associated with positive social comparisons, indicating that the presence of good peer relationships may be a resilience mechanism (Eccleston et al., 2008). This perception of being socially delayed was recently confirmed in a large cohort study of over 800 adolescents with chronic pain drawn from a community sample (Caes, Fisher, Clinch, Tobias, & Eccleston, 2015). In this large community sample of adolescents with chronic pain especially girls who experienced high levels of pain-related anxiety endorsed this feeling of being behind in their social development, thereby highlighting gender differences in how pain can impact social experiences.

Despite the fact that the majority of research focused on how pain experiences negatively impact children's engagement with peers, recently interest has been growing on how peer support can be effectively stimulated to enhance resilience and health outcomes. For example, the systematic review by Forgeron et al. (2010) also provided evidence for the power of positive friendships, which are related to improvements in pain intensity and social competence (Walker, Claar, & Garber, 2002). Furthermore, these positive friendship relations were found to counteract negative family and peer interactions (Kaminsky, Robertson, & Dewey, 2006; Walker, Garber, & Greene, 1994).

Recently, research efforts have started to focus on how to incorporate these buffering aspects of strong social support in interventions. Forgeron, Chorney, Carlson, Dick, and Plante (2015) examined, in an adolescent group who had attended a 10-week structured self-management program, whether adolescents with chronic pain wanted to befriend other adolescents suffering from chronic pain. During the course of the program, 32% became friends, 52% were interested in becoming friends with another peer suffering from chronic pain, and 15% were not interested in making friends. The most often reported peer support was emotional support, in which pain was a common topic during interactions. Kohut et al. (2016) developed an online peer mentorship intervention, the iPeer2Peer program, to enhance self-management skills of adolescents with chronic pain. In this program, young adults (18–25 years) who learned to successfully cope with their pain act as a role model and provide reinforcement to younger peers (12–18 years). Results from a feasibility trial showed that adolescents who completed the iPeer2Peer program demonstrated significant improvement in self-management skills compared to adolescents assigned to a waiting-list control group (Kohut et al., 2016). This study is one of the first to suggest that a peer mentoring intervention may be useful to help adolescents with chronic pain develop successful pain management skills.

In sum, the available evidence suggests that peer relationships may be negatively impacted by chronic pain, and that interpersonal reactions by peers, depending on their nature, can either have adverse or beneficial effects on the child's pain experience. However, research investigating the role of peer relationships and peer support in the context of pain is still in its infancy (Forgeron & King, 2013). This might be partially due to the lack of specific assessments to assess the unique impact of childhood pain experiences on social functioning and competency. More research is needed with regard to (a) the underlying mechanisms by which pain impacts friendship relations, (b) the differences with regard to the impact on female versus male friendships as well as children's versus adolescents' friendships, and (c) the impact of interventions on peer relationships and friendships (Forgeron & King, 2013).

Role of School Environment

The school environment is a paramount part of children's life, which not only focuses on learning and cognitive-emotional functioning, but is also a crucial environment for developing adequate social skills (e.g., developing social competency and a sense of self in a wider environment; Shiu, 2001). However, similar to the lack of acknowledgment of peer influences, the IFAM does not provide predictions on how the school environment could act as either a vulnerability or buffer when faced with pediatric chronic pain. The ERRM briefly highlights the role of teacher support as a potential resilience resource that can have a positive impact on the child's competence and functioning despite chronic pain experiences (Cousins, Cohen, et al., 2015). However, an in-depth account of the mechanisms explaining the protective role of the school environment is lacking.

Despite limited inclusion within the available theoretical models, the pivotal role of the school environment in a child's development has widely been acknowledged across various research efforts. The majority of the research evaluating the impact of chronic pain on the child's functioning does include the impact on school functioning. This evidence reveals that the experience of pain can have a profound negative impact on various aspects of the school experience, including children's school participation, attendance, academic achievement, peer relationships and their perceived competence in these domains (Dick & Riddell, 2010; Gorodzinsky, Hainsworth, & Weisman, 2011). The impact on school attendance has traditionally been the most widely investigated indicator of school functioning, with a substantial body of evidence pointing at elevated levels of school absences in children with chronic pain. For instance, Konijnenberg et al. (2005) found that about 51% of pediatric chronic pain patients missed 1–3 days of school per month (Konijnenberg et al., 2005). While pain intensity or duration were long assumed to be the main reason for school-related disability, Logan, Simons, Stein, and Chastain (2008) provided an interesting new perspective by highlighting the pivotal role of psychosocial factors such as pain-related depression and anxiety, as the main drivers of school impairment (Logan et al., 2008). Furthermore, Logan et al. (2008) set the stage to go beyond the sole reliance of school absenteeism as an indicator of school-related impairment. Comprehensive assessment of school functioning encompassing multiple domains including academic performance and competence, has been recommended (Logan et al., 2008).

Albeit less well understood, evidence is available for the supportive, or even buffering, role teacher support can play for children with chronic pain. For instance, having a teacher who supports child autonomy and competence has found to be associated with less school absence in children with chronic pain (Vervoort et al., 2014). The strongest influential factor explaining teachers' supportive behaviors (e.g., granting relief from responsibility and implementing accommodations for the child) seems the availability of medical evidence for the pain. However, a constructive relationship between parents and teachers was found to influence the teachers' emotional responses such as their level of sympathy (Logan, Coakley, & Scharff, 2007). These findings highlight the variety of support teachers can offer and the complexity of the underlying mechanisms explaining variety in teacher support. With respect to these underlying mechanism, the results reveal that the impact of different social agents in the child's life (e.g., parents and teachers) can interact.

Taken together, it is clear that teacher responses to chronic pain experiences by their students play an important role in understanding disability, particularly school-related disability, due to pain. While we have a good grasp on the potential detrimental impact of pediatric chronic pain on the school experience, the key aspects and underlying mechanisms of a supportive child–teacher relationship are less clear. More knowledge on the ingredients and underlying processes of a positive teacher–student relation and adequate teacher support strategies will be crucial to further our understanding of this important social influence for children with chronic pain (Sinclair et al., 2016). Taking a life span approach will be important to evaluate whether the effective aspects of a supportive teacher–student relationship and support strategies potentially differ depending on the school setting (i.e., different needs for primary, secondary, and high school students).

Future Challenges

We have come a long way in our understanding of how pediatric pain impacts the child's social functioning and how the social environment can influence a child's adjustment. However, challenges remain that will need to be overcome to substantially progress this particular aspect of childhood pain experiences. Investigation into the role of parental and family characteristics continues to be underrepresented with a recent bibliometric analysis revealing a mere 8% of pediatric pain literature dedicated to the parental and family environment (Caes et al., 2016). Even more concerning is the near absence of research involving teachers (0.29% of articles; Caes et al., 2016), which might be partially explained by the lack of theoretical guidance and availability of adequate, reliable and valid measurement tools for this particular aspect of childhood pain. While the bibliometric analyses did not specify research including peers, a similar negligence as found for teacher-involved research is to be expected. The formulation of theoretical models such as the IFAM and ERRM is of indispensable value to guide an improved understanding of the relevant factors in a child's social environment influencing adaptation to chronic pain experiences.

   It is important to note the difference between the IFAM and ERRM with respect to how they facilitate research. While the IFAM represents a theoretical model with clear and testable hypotheses, the ERRM is rather a general framework of resilience applied to the context of pediatric pain. This is useful in guiding our conceptualizations, but a theoretical model on pediatric pain resilience from which testable hypotheses can be derived may be warranted to facilitate future research efforts. As proposed within the ERRM, this theoretical model would ideally incorporate both vulnerability and resilience mechanisms to be able to reflect their connections and not just being two sides of the same coin. Consideration of vulnerability and resilience factors within a single model rather than a sole focus on either vulnerability or resilience may better explain why some children function well in the face of chronic pain. This brings the question to mind as to whether this requires drawing up a new theoretical model specifying testable resiliency pathways explaining child and parent positive adaptation, or could the ERRM stimulate an extension of the IFAM to incorporate specific resilience pathways in both child and parents as well as their interrelation with vulnerability factors. The risk associated with extending the IFAM would be to lose its current clear focus and testability of the suggested associations and pathways by creating an all-encompassing model that is too complex to evaluate. For instance, identifying different pathways of adaptation to pediatric chronic pain based on the various possible interactions between vulnerability and resilience factors brings with it its own statistical challenges. Testing these interactions would require a person-centered rather than more typical variable-centered approach to analyses. It is likely that future studies on resilient children at different stages of development (i.e., from childhood to young adulthood) are critical to shed more light on the exact mechanisms underlying resiliency to pain and their interactions with vulnerabilities. Albeit awaiting further evidence, it is reasonable to assume that the impact of parental vulnerability and resilience pathways is particularly strong in determining younger children's health-related outcomes, but gradually lessens throughout adolescence, as peers become a stronger source of resilience throughout development.

In a similar vein, it is worthwhile to consider how to either extend existing models to account for the buffering impact of supportive friendships and teacher relations or whether development of new, context-specific models is warranted. However, the research on the role of peer and teacher support is truly still in its infancy and would likely benefit from prioritizing efforts on systematic development of valid and reliable measures. Assessments of peer and teacher responses to pediatric chronic pain as well as assessments accounting for the unique challenges children with chronic pain might face with respect to social competence, friendships, and school performance are currently lacking. The availability of such measures would not only tremendously advance exploratory and treatment-related research opportunities but could also be applied in clinical practice to provide a comprehensive assessment of the challenges and improvements within the social context for children suffering from chronic pain.

A last challenge for future model development and refinement that has not yet been discussed within the context of this chapter would be the inclusion of the broader family context. The potential influence of parents is prominently featured in both the ERRM and IFAM, but the dynamic of general family functioning has not been well-articulated or studied. Broad indicators of adaptive family functioning have been identified as important and include clear communication, well-defined roles and structure, cohesion, adaptability, effective problem solving, and affect regulation (Palermo et al., 2014), but evidence for the specific mechanisms underlying their influence in pediatric chronic pain is sparse. One study published approximately a decade ago identified a subset of patients who present in a tertiary care pain clinic have moderate levels of distress and disability, but markedly low levels of family cohesion (Scharff et al., 2005). Another early study among adolescents with fibromyalgia reported higher family conflict and poor family functioning compared to healthy peers (Kashikar-Zuck et al., 2008). Most recently, among pediatric headache patients, family functioning was identified as indirectly influencing child functional disability via a child's depressive symptoms (Kaczynski, Gambhir, Caruso, & Lebel, 2016). Investigations into resilient family characteristics are largely absent from the extant literature and likely are as important in relation to child outcomes

(Cousins, Cohen, et al., 2015; Cousins, Kalapurakkel, et al., 2015). One of the key limitations of examining the relation between family characteristics and child functioning lies in inadequate measures of family functioning, which can be incredibly dynamic, particularly in response to stress. In addition, most available assessment of family functioning relies on self-report, which might be inadequate to detect the subtle dynamics of family interactions. It may be that focusing on observation of specific mechanisms that are modeled in the home, such as affect regulation, will yield more sensitive measures of the impact of family functioning than examining global measures of family functioning such as communication or cohesion.

Conclusion

While several challenges remain, the IFAM and ERRM represent the most important models currently available to understand the social context of pediatric pain experiences. Both models have stimulated further exploration and associated understanding of how child and parental multi-faceted responses to pediatric pain experiences interact in determining the child's and family adaptation to chronic pain. The main limitations associated with both models is their lack of detailed explanations on how the broader social context and developmental changes influence the child's functioning as well as the dynamic relationship between child and parental responses. With this in mind, continued efforts to provide a comprehensive insight in the social influences and consequences when faced with pediatric chronic pain utilizing an ecological (i.e., including all aspects of the child's social context) and life span (i.e., from infancy through adolescence) approach are critical.

Acknowledgments This chapter was supported by grant no. BOF15/24j/017 from the Ghent University Special Research Fund, awarded to Liesbet Goubert and Laura Simons.

References

Asmundson, G. J., Noel, M., Petter, M., & Parkerson, H. A. (2012). Pediatric fear-avoidance model of chronic pain: Foundation, application and future directions. *Pain Research and Management, 17*(6), 397–405.

Bronfenbrenner, U. (1979). *The ecology of human development: Experiments by nature and design*. Cambridge, MA: Harvard University Press.

Caes, L., Boerner, K. E., Chambers, C. T., Campbell-Yeo, M., Stinson, J., Birnie, K. A., … Schinkel, M. (2016). A comprehensive categorical and bibliometric analysis of published research articles on pediatric pain from 1975 to 2010. *Pain, 157*(2), 302–313.

Caes, L., Fisher, E., Clinch, J., Tobias, J. H., & Eccleston, C. (2015). The role of pain-related anxiety in adolescents' disability and social impairment: ALSPAC data. *European Journal of Pain, 19*(6), 842–851.

Caes, L., Vervoort, T., Devos, P., Verlooy, J., Benoit, Y., & Goubert, L. (2014). Parental distress and catastrophic thoughts about child pain: Implications for parental protective behavior in the context of child leukemia related medical procedures. *Clinical Journal of Pain, 30*(9), 787–799.

Caes, L., Vervoort, T., Eccleston, C., Vandenhende, M., & Goubert, L. (2011). Parental catastrophizing about child's pain and its relationship with activity restriction: The mediating role of parental distress. *Pain, 152*, 212–222.

Carpino, E., Segal, S., Logan, D., Lebel, A., & Simons, L. E. (2014). The interplay of pain-related self-efficacy and fear on functional outcomes among youth with headache. *The Journal of Pain, 15*, 527–534.

Chow, E. T., Otis, J. D., & Simons, L. E. (2016). The longitudinal impact of parent distress and behavior on functional outcomes among youth with chronic pain. *The Journal of Pain, 17*(6), 729–738.

Claar, R. L., Simons, L. E., & Logan, D. E. (2008). Parental response to children's pain: The moderating impact of children's emotional distress on symptoms and disability. *Pain, 138*(1), 172–179.

Cousins, L. A., Cohen, L. L., & Venable, C. (2015). Risk and resilience in pediatric chronic pain: Exploring the protective role of optimism. *Journal of Pediatric Psychology, 40*, 934–942.

Cousins, L. A., Kalapurakkel, S., Cohen, L. L., & Simons, L. E. (2015). Topical review: Resilience resources and mechanisms in pediatric chronic pain. *Journal of Pediatric Psychology, 40*(9), 840–845.

Craig, K. (1986). Social modeling influences on pain. In R. Sternbach (Ed.), *The psychology of pain* (2nd ed., pp. 67–96). New York, NY: Raven Press.

Craig, K. D. (2009). The social communication model of pain. *Canadian Psychology/Psychologie Canadienne, 50*(1), 22.

Crombez, G., Bijttebier, P., Eccleston, C., Mascagni, T., Mertens, G., Goubert, L., & Verstraeten, K. (2003). The child version of the pain catastrophizing scale (PCS-C): A preliminary validation. *Pain, 104*, 369–646.

Crombez, G., Eccleston, C., Van Damme, S., Vlaeyen, J. W., & Karoly, P. (2012). Fear-avoidance model of chronic pain: The next generation. *The Clinical Journal of Pain, 28*(6), 475–483.

Dick, B. D., & Riddell, R. P. (2010). Cognitive and school functioning in children and adolescents with chronic pain: A critical review. *Pain Research and Management, 15*(4), 238–244.

Eccleston, C., Fisher, E. A., Vervoort, T., & Crombez, G. (2012). Worry and catastrophizing about pain in youth: A reappraisal. *Pain, 153*(8), 1560–1562.

Eccleston, C., Wastell, S., Crombez, G., & Jordan, A. (2008). Adolescent social development and chronic pain. *European Journal of Pain, 12*(6), 765–774.

Feinstein, A. B., Sturgeon, J. A., Bhandari, R. P., Dunn, A., Rico, T., Kao, M. C., & Darnall, B. D. (2016). The impact of pain catastrophizing on outcomes: A developmental perspective across children, adolescents and young adults with chronic pain. *The Journal of Pain, 18*, 144–154.

Fleischman, K. M., Hains, A. A., & Davies, W. H. (2011). Practitioner perceptions of peer relationships in adolescents with chronic pain. *Journal of Child Health Care, 15*(1), 50–58.

Forgeron, P., & King, S. (2013). Pain, social relationships, and school. In P. McGrath, B. Stevens, S. Walker, & W. Zempsky (Eds.), *Oxford textbook of paediatric pain* (pp. 119–126). Oxford, England: Oxford University Press.

Forgeron, P., & McGrath, P. J. (2009). Self-identified needs of youth with chronic pain. *Journal of Pain Management, 1*, 163–172.

Forgeron, P. A., Chorney, J. M., Carlson, T. E., Dick, B. D., & Plante, E. (2015). To befriend or not: Naturally developing friendships amongst a clinical group of adolescents with chronic pain. *Pain Management Nursing, 16*(5), 721–732.

Forgeron, P. A., King, S., Stinson, J. N., McGrath, P. J., MacDonald, A. J., & Chambers, C. T. (2010). Social functioning and peer relationships in children and adolescents with chronic pain: A systematic review. *Pain Research and Management, 15*(1), 27–41.

Forgeron, P. A., McGrath, P., Stevens, B., Evans, J., Dick, B., Finley, G. A., & Carlson, T. (2011). Social information processing in adolescents with chronic pain: My friends don't really understand me. *Pain, 152*(12), 2773–2780.

Goodman, J. E., & McGrath, P. J. (2003). Mothers' modeling influences children's pain during a cold pressor task. *Pain, 104*(3), 559–565.

Gorodzinsky, A. Y., Hainsworth, K. R., & Weisman, S. J. (2011). School functioning and chronic pain: A review of methods and measures. *Journal of Pediatric Psychology, 36*(9), 991–1002.

Goubert, L., Craig, K. D., Vervoort, T., Morley, S., Sullivan, M. J. L., Williams, A. C., … Crombez, G. (2005). Facing others in pain: The effects of empathy. *Pain, 118*(3), 285–288.

Goubert, L., Eccleston, C., Vervoort, T., Jordan, A., & Crombez, G. (2006). Parental catastrophizing about their child's pain. The parent version of the Pain Catastrophizing Scale (PCS-P): A preliminary validation. *Pain, 123*(3), 254–263.

Goubert, L., & Simons, L. E. (2013). Cognitive styles and processes in paediatric pain. In P. McGrath, B. Stevens, S. Walker, & W. Zempsky (Eds.), *Oxford textbook of paediatric pain* (pp. 95–101). Oxford, England: Oxford University Press.

Goubert, L., Vlaeyen, J. W., Crombez, G., & Craig, K. D. (2011). Learning about pain from others: An observational learning account. *The Journal of Pain, 12*(2), 167–174.

Guite, J. W., McCue, R. L., Sherker, J. L., Sherry, D. D., & Rose, J. B. (2011). Relationships among pain, protective parental responses, and disability for adolescents with chronic musculoskeletal pain: The mediating role of pain catastrophizing. *The Clinical Journal of Pain, 27*(9), 775–781.

Hadjistavropoulos, T., Craig, D. C., Cano, A., Goubert, L., Jackson, P. L., Mogil, J. S., … Fitzgerald, T. D. (2011). A biopsychosocial formulation of pain communication. *Psychological Bulletin, 137*, 910–939.

Helsen, K., Goubert, L., Peters, M. L., & Vlaeyen, J. W. (2011). Observational learning and pain-related fear: An experimental study with colored cold pressor tasks. *The Journal of Pain, 12*(12), 1230–1239.

Helsen, K., Goubert, L., & Vlaeyen, J. W. (2013). Observational learning and pain-related fear: Exploring contingency learning in an experimental study using colored warm water immersions. *The Journal of Pain, 14*(7), 676–688.

Helsen, K., Vlaeyen, J. W., & Goubert, L. (2015). Indirect acquisition of pain-related fear: An experimental study of observational learning using coloured cold metal bars. *PLoS One, 10*(3), e0117236.

Hilliard, M. E., Harris, M. A., & Weissberg-Benchell, J. (2012). Diabetes resilience: A model of risk and protection in type 1 diabetes. *Current Diabetes Reports, 12*(6), 739–748.

Kaczynski, K., Gambhir, R., Caruso, A., & Lebel, A. (2016). Depression as a mediator of the relation between family functioning and functional disability in youth with chronic headaches. *Headache, 56*(3), 491–500.

Kaczynski, K. J., Claar, R. L., & Logan, D. E. (2009). Testing gender as a moderator of associations between psychosocial variables and functional disability in children and adolescents with chronic pain. *Journal of Pediatric Psychology, 34*(7), 738–748.

Kalapurakkel, S., Carpino, E. A., Lebel, A., & Simons, L. E. (2015). "Pain can't stop me": Examining pain self-efficacy and acceptance as resilience processes among youth with chronic headache. *Journal of Pediatric Psychology, 40*, 926–933.

Kaminsky, L., Robertson, M., & Dewey, D. (2006). Psychological correlates of depression in children with recurrent abdominal pain. *Journal of Pediatric Psychology, 31*(9), 956–966.

Kashikar-Zuck, S., Lynch, A. M., Graham, T. B., Swain, N. F., Mullen, S. M., & Noll, R. B. (2007). Social functioning and peer relationships of adolescents with juvenile fibromyalgia syndrome. *Arthritis Care & Research, 57*(3), 474–480.

Kashikar-Zuck, S., Lynch, A. M., Slater, S., Graham, T. B., Swain, N. F., & Noll, R. B. (2008). Family factors, emotional functioning, and functional impairment in juvenile fibromyalgia syndrome. *Arthritis Care & Research, 59*(10), 1392–1398.

Kohut, S. A., Stinson, J. N., Ruskin, D., Forgeron, P., Harris, L., van Wyk, M., … Campbell, F. (2016). iPeer2Peer program: A pilot feasibility study in adolescents with chronic pain. *Pain, 157*(5), 1146–1155.

Konijnenberg, A. Y., Uieterwaal, C. S. P. M., Kimpen, J. L. L., van der Hoeven, J., Buitetlaar, J. K., & de Graeff-Meeder, E. R. (2005). Children with unexplained chronic pain: Substantial impairment in everyday life. *Archives of Diseases in Childhood, 90*, 680–688.

Leeuw, M., Goossens, M. E. J. B., Linton, S. J., Crombez, G., Boersma, K., & Vlaeyen, J. (2007). The fear-avoidance model of musculoskeletal pain: Current state of scientific evidence. *Journal of Behavioral Medicine, 30*, 77–94.

Lisi, D., Campbell, L., Riddell, R. P., Garfield, H., & Greenberg, S. (2013). Naturalistic parental pain management during immunizations during the first year of life: Observational norms from the OUCH cohort. *Pain, 154*(8), 1245–1253.

Logan, D. E., Coakley, R. M., & Scharff, L. (2007). Teachers' perceptions of and responses to adolescents with chronic pain syndromes. *Journal of Pediatric Psychology, 32*(2), 139–149.

Logan, D. E., Simons, L. E., & Carpino, E. A. (2012). Too sick for school? Parent influences on school functioning among children with chronic pain. *Pain, 153*(2), 437–443.

Logan, D. E., Simons, L. E., Stein, M. J., & Chastain, L. (2008). School impairment in adolescents with chronic pain. *The Journal of Pain, 9*(5), 407–416.

Lynch-Jordan, A. M., Kashikar-Zuck, S., Szabova, A., & Goldschneider, K. R. (2013). The interplay of parent and adolescent catastrophizing and its impact on adolescents' pain, functioning, and pain behavior. *The Clinical Journal of Pain, 29*(8), 681.

Palermo, T. M., Valrie, C. R., & Karlson, C. W. (2014). Family and parent influences on pediatric chronic pain: A developmental perspective. *American Psychologist, 69*(2), 142.

Petter, M., Chambers, C. T., McGrath, P. J., & Dick, B. D. (2013). The role of trait mindfulness in the pain experience of adolescents. *The Journal of Pain, 14*, 1709–1718.

Scharff, L., Langan, N., Rotter, N., Scott-Sutherland, J., Schenck, C., Tayor, N., … Masek, B. (2005). Psychological, behavioral, and family characteristics of pediatric patients with chronic pain: A 1-year retrospective study and cluster analysis. *The Clinical Journal of Pain, 21*(5), 432–438.

Shiu, S. (2001). Issues in the education of students with chronic illness. *International Journal of Disability, Development and Education, 48*(3), 269–281.

Sieberg, C. B., Williams, S., & Simons, L. (2011). Do parent protective responses mediate the relation between parent distress and child functional disability among children with chronic pain? *Journal of Pediatric Psychology, 36*, 1043–1051.

Simons, L. E., Goubert, L., Vervoort, T., & Borsook, D. (2016). Circles of engagement: Childhood pain and parent brain. *Neuroscience & Biobehavioral Reviews, 68*, 537–546.

Simons, L. E., & Kaczynski, K. J. (2012). The fear avoidance model of chronic pain: Examination for pediatric application. *The Journal of Pain, 13*(9), 827–835.

Simons, L. E., Sieberg, C. B., Carpino, E., Logan, D., & Berde, C. (2011). The Fear of Pain Questionnaire (FOPQ): Assessment of pain-related fear among children and adolescents with chronic pain. *The Journal of Pain, 12*(6), 677–686.

Simons, L. E., Smith, A., Kaczynski, K., & Basch, M. (2015). Living in fear of your child's pain: The parent fear of pain questionnaire. *Pain, 156*(4), 694.

Sinclair, C. M., Meredith, P., Strong, J., & Feeney, R. (2016). Personal and contextual factors affecting the functional ability of children and adolescents with chronic pain: A systematic review. *Journal of Developmental & Behavioral Pediatrics, 37*(4), 327–342.

Sturgeon, J. A., & Zautra, A. J. (2013). Psychological resil- ience, pain catastrophizing, and positive emotions: Perspectives on comprehensive modeling of individual pain adaptation. *Current Pain and Headache Reports*, 17, 1–9.

Thastum, M., Zachariae, R., Scheler, M., Bjerring, P., & Herlin, T. (1997). Cold pressor pain: Comparing responses of juvenile arthritis patients and their parents. *Scandinavian Journal of Rheumatology, 26*(4), 272–279.

Uman, L. S., Birnie, K. A., Noel, M., Parker, J. A., Chambers, C. T., McGrath, P. J., & Kisely, S. R. (2013). Psychological interventions for needle-related procedural pain and distress in children and adolescents. *Cochrane Database of Systematic Reviews, 10*(10), CD005179. https://doi.org/10.1002/14651858.CD005179.pub3.

Van Schoors, M., Caes, L., Verhofstadt, L. L., Goubert, L., & Alderfer, M. A. (2015). Systematic review: Family resilience after pediatric cancer diagnosis. *Journal of Pediatric Psychology, 40*(9), 856–868.

Vervoort, T., Eccleston, C., Goubert, L., Buysse, A., & Crombez, G. (2010). Children's catastrophic thinking about their pain predicts pain and disability 6 months later. *European Journal of Pain, 14*(1), 90–96.

Vervoort, T., Logan, D. E., Goubert, L., De Clercq, B., & Hublet, A. (2014). Severity of pediatric pain in relation to school-related functioning and teacher support: An epidemiological study among school-aged children and adolescents. *Pain, 155*(6), 1118–1127.

Viner, R., & Christies, D. (2005). ABC of adolescence: Adolescent development. *British Medical Journal, 330*(7486), 301–304.

Vlaeyen, J. W., & Linton, S. J. (2000). Fear-avoidance and its consequences in chronic musculoskeletal pain: A state of the art. *Pain, 85*(3), 317–332.

Vowles, K. E., Cohen, L. L., McCracken, L. M., & Eccleston, C. (2010). Disentangling the complex relations among caregiver and adolescent responses to adolescent chronic pain. *Pain, 151*(3), 680–686.

Walker, L. S., Claar, R. L., & Garber, J. (2002). Social consequences of children's pain: When do they encourage symptom maintenance? *Journal of Pediatric Psychology, 27*(8), 689–698.

Walker, L. S., Garber, J., & Greene, J. W. (1994). Somatic complaints in pediatric patients: A prospective study of the role of negative life events, child social and academic competence, and parental somatic symptoms. *Journal of Consulting and Clinical Psychology, 62*(6), 1213.

Walker, L. S., Williams, S. E., Smith, C. A., Garber, J., Van Slyke, D. A., & Lipani, T. A. (2006). Parent attention versus distraction: Impact on symptom complaints by children with and without chronic functional abdominal pain. *Pain, 122*(1), 43–52.

Wallace, D. P., McCracken, L. M., Weiss, K. E., & Harbeck-Weber, C. (2015). The role of parent psychological flexibility in relation to adolescent chronic pain: Further instrument development. *The Journal of Pain, 16*, 235–246.

Weiss, K. E., Hahn, A., Wallace, D. P., Biggs, B., Bruce, B. K., & Harrison, T. E. (2013). Acceptance of pain: Associations with depression, catastrophizing, and functional disability among children and adolescents in an interdisciplinary chronic pain rehabilitation program. *Journal of Pediatric Psychology, 38*, 756–765.

Welkom, J. S., Hwang, W. T., & Guite, J. W. (2013). Adolescent pain catastrophizing mediates the relationship between protective parental responses to pain and disability over time. *Journal of Pediatric Psychology, 38*, 541–550.

Wilson, A. C., Lewandowski, A. S., & Palermo, T. M. (2011). Fear-avoidance beliefs and parental responses to pain in adolescents with chronic pain. *Pain Research and Management, 16*(3), 178–182.

Wilson, A. C., Moss, A., Palermo, T. M., & Fales, J. L. (2013). Parent pain and catastrophizing are associated with pain, somatic symptoms, and pain-related disability among early adolescents. *Journal of Pediatric Psychology, 39*(4), 418–426.

Chapter 19
Pain in Older Adults: Caregiver Challenges

Thomas Hadjistavropoulos and Natasha L. Gallant

Abstract This chapter focuses on the social context of pain in older adults with a special emphasis on caregiver–care recipient dyads. Pain is highly prevalent among older persons and, especially when it is combined with frailty and dementia, can contribute to caregiver challenges such as caregiver burden (i.e., a perception that caregiving is having a negative impact on caregiver psychological, social or spiritual functioning). Caregivers often have difficulty accurately estimating/evaluating the patient's pain (especially in instances where the care recipient presents with limited ability to communicate due to dementia) and in selecting the appropriate actions to help palliate the pain. Despite these challenges, there is a paucity of research specifically focusing on caregivers of older adults with pain. We review the studies that have been conducted in this area and conclude with practical recommendations for caregivers of older pain sufferers and with recommendations for future research.

Keywords Caregiver burden · Aging · Elderly · Dementia · Alzheimer's disease

Pain in Older Adults: Caregiver Challenges

Biopsychosocial formulations of the pain experience emphasize the social context of pain (e.g., Hadjistavropoulos et al., 2011; Prkachin & Craig, 1995). According to such formulations, the internal experience of pain is encoded in expressive behavior which, in turn, can be decoded and understood by others (including caregivers) who may then provide care and assistance. Sometimes the detection and decoding of pain signals by caregivers can present challenges. Older adults, for example, are often stoic about and reluctant to express their pain (Yong, Gibson, de Horne, & Helme, 2001). Pain that is not explicitly communicated could lead caregivers to make inaccurate judgements about the pain experience. In addition, caregivers may

T. Hadjistavropoulos (✉) · N. L. Gallant
Department of Psychology and Centre on Aging and Health, University of Regina,
Regina, SK, Canada
e-mail: Thomas.Hadjistavropoulos@uregina.ca

© Springer International Publishing AG, part of Springer Nature 2018   415
T. Vervoort et al. (eds.), *Social and Interpersonal Dynamics in Pain*,
https://doi.org/10.1007/978-3-319-78340-6_19

make inaccurate attributions about pain-related changes in patient behavior (e.g., deflated mood, reduced activity). Caregivers may incorrectly assume, for instance, that the patient is dissatisfied with the home environment which could lead to increased tensions. The focus of this chapter is on the social context of pain in older adults with an emphasis on the caregiver–care recipient dyad. Emphasis is placed on caregiver–care recipient communication and the challenges that can be experienced within the caregiving context.

Pain in Older Adults: Extent of the Problem

Our population is aging rapidly. In 2014, just over 46 million persons in the USA (15% of the population) were at least 65 years of age and this number is projected to rise to 88 million (22% of the population) by 2050 (Colby & Ortman, 2015). According to Statistics Canada (2015), 15% of the Canadian population was over 65 years in 2013 and it is projected that between 23% and 25% of Canadians will be over 65 years by 2033. Similar trends have been observed in other countries (He, Goodkind, & Kowal, 2016).

Old age is most often accompanied by loss of muscle strength, increasing bone fragility, and decreasing ability of tissues to function normally (Freemont & Hoyland, 2007). Consequently, there is an increased risk of fractures as well as other fall-related injuries in old age (Gheno, Cepparo, Rosca, & Cotten, 2012). Moreover, aging has been associated with an increased prevalence of chronic health conditions such as arthritis, cancer, and cardiovascular disease. In fact, almost 80% of older adults have at least one chronic health problem (Centers for Disease Control and Prevention & The Merck Company Foundation, 2007).

Many of the health conditions that accompany aging are associated with increased pain. As an example, pain is a central issue among older adults with cancer (Bernabei et al., 1998). Compounding the problem, when older adults are diagnosed with cancer, they are more likely to be diagnosed in the later stages of the disease (Delgado-Guay & Bruera, 2008), which involve a much higher prevalence of pain compared to earlier stages (van den Beuken-van Everdingen et al., 2007). Cancer pain also tends to remain underassessed and undertreated in this population, thus exacerbating the problem (Bernabei et al., 1998; Cleeland et al., 1994; Hofmann, Farnon, Javed, & Posner, 1998) and the associated caregiver challenges. As older patients with cancer are increasingly cared for in the home (Ferrell, Cohen, Rhiner, & Rozek, 1991), family members are tasked with taking a caregiving role.

As a result of increased injuries and chronic health conditions among older adults, pain is very prevalent in this population. Based on a systematic review examining a variety of studies, it was concluded that 46–73% of older adults living in the community suffer from pain (Takai, Yamamoto-Mitani, Okamoto, Koyama, & Honda, 2010). The prevalence estimates varied from study to study as a function of methodology (Takai et al., 2010). Prevalence estimates for people who live in long-term care facilities are as high as 80%, but these estimates may also vary substantially from study to study (Charlton, 2005; Takai et al., 2013). These estimates (Takai et al., 2010, 2013) tend to focus on pain in general and not specifically on pain that would be described as chronic.

Complicating the increased frailty and pain that may accompany older age is an increased prevalence of dementia and cognitive decline. Dementia affects 1 in 10 people over 70 years of age (Plassman et al., 2007) with one third of people over 85 years of age suffering from dementia (Alzheimer's Association, 2014). Due to the cognitive and linguistic impairments that accompany the dementing condition, an older person's ability to effectively communicate the subjective state of pain can be affected. More specifically, moderate to severe dementia interferes with ability to effectively communicate one's pain experience. In contrast to verbal communication, nonverbal pain expressions seem to remain relatively intact even in moderate to advanced dementia although those with dementia tend to react to pain with more vigor than their cognitively intact counterparts (e.g., Hadjistavropoulos, LaChapelle, MacLeod, Snider, & Craig, 2000; Kunz, Scharmann, Hemmeter, Schepelmann, & Lautenbacher, 2007).

Limitations in ability to engage in verbal communication pose special challenges for caregivers who then find themselves in a position of having to decode the more ambiguous nonverbal signals in an effort to understand what their loved one is experiencing. As such, the problem of pain undertreatment is more pronounced in people with dementia as compared to their cognitively intact counterparts (Hadjistavropoulos et al., 2009). Further compounding the problem, pain in patients with dementia frequently results in the display of aggression and other types of behavioral disturbances (Cipher, Clifford, & Roper, 2006). These types of reactions, resulting from pain, are often misattributed to a psychiatric condition rather than pain, resulting in the administration of psychotropic medications which increase the risk of death in frail elders (Ballard et al., 2009; Cipher et al., 2006).

Caregiving

There are over 2.7 million Canadian and 65.7 million American informal caregivers of ill or disabled older persons (National Alliance for Caregiving & American Association of Retired Persons, 2009). Moreover, 20–25% of these informal caregivers are older adults themselves (Alecxih, Zeruld, & Olearczyl, 2001; Cranswick & Dosman, 2008). Health policy changes as well as an increased reliance on home care and outpatient care for many older persons with significant health conditions, including pain, have resulted in an increased need for family and friends to assume caregiving responsibilities (Chappell, 1993). These responsibilities involve performing many activities (e.g., self-care, medication reminders) for the care recipient that he or she may not be able to perform. Moreover, although our population is aging, there is a trend that the available resources for families to provide care to older adults have diminished given that family size has been steadily decreasing and divorce rates have been increasing (Zarit & Heid, 2015). These shrinking caregiving resources, combined with the demands of care, can result in an exhaustive and overwhelming experience.

Caregiver burden is defined as the extent to which caregivers perceive caregiving as having a negative effect on their physical, financial, or spiritual functioning (Zarit, Todd, & Zarit, 1986). Burden is an important issue in the caregiving experience as over 50% of informal caregivers are estimated to suffer from medium or high caregiver burden (National Alliance for Caregiving & American Association of Retired Persons, 2009).

The stress associated with caregiver burden is linked to negative outcomes for the caregiver. As an example, caregiver burden is inversely related to the caregiver's self-reported physical and mental health (e.g., Abdollahpour, Nedjat, Noroozian, Salimi, & Majdzadeh, 2014; Chen, Chen, & Chu, 2015; Morimoto, Schreiner, & Asano, 2003). Burden is also associated with immunological changes for the care provider. Compared to sex-, age-, and income-matched controls, for instance, wound healing is significantly slower to repair among informal caregivers (Kiecolt-Glaser, Marucha, Malarkey, Mercado, & Glaser, 1995). Antibody responses to the influenza virus vaccine were also significantly less effective for caregivers compared to a control group (Kiecolt-Glaser, Glaser, Gravenstein, Malarkey, & Sheridan, 1996). Moreover, von Känel et al. (2008) have demonstrated that caregivers are at increased risk of coronary heart disease when compared to a control group. Consequences of experiencing caregiver burden even include a 63% increased risk of death over a period of 4 years (Schulz & Beach, 1999). Caregiving has also been associated with depression, which represents a condition that is distinct from but associated with caregiver burden (Clyburn, Stones, Hadjistavropoulos, & Tuokko, 2000; Cohen & Eisdorfer, 1988).

Demographic, psychosocial, and contextual risk factors for increased caregiver burden have been identified. In a recent review of the literature concerning caregiver burden, for instance, Adelman, Tmanova, Delgado, Dion, and Lachs (2014) reported that female caregivers (who represent the majority of caregivers; National Alliance for Caregiving and American Association of Retired Persons, 2015) and caregivers with depression, lower educational attainment, financial stress, or social isolation experienced increased caregiver burden. Characteristics of the relationship between caregivers and care recipients were also identified as playing a role in increased burden for the caregiver. That is, living with the care recipient, spending more time providing care, perceiving distress in the care recipient, and not having a choice in becoming a caregiver (e.g., being unable to afford assisted living accommodations for their loved one) tended to result in higher levels of caregiver burden (Adelman et al., 2014). Moreover, among family caregivers looking after care recipients with dementia, spousal caregivers have been shown to experience greater burden than caregivers who are adult children of the care recipient (Joling et al., 2010; Kim, Chang, Rose, & Kim, 2012). Behavioral problems have been identified as the most consistent contributor to the burden experienced by those caring for care recipients with dementia (van der Lee, Bakker, Duivenvoorden, & Dröes, 2014).

Caregiving in the Context of Pain

Although social support networks may shrink as people age (e.g., friends and family members dying, children moving away), such networks provide caregiving and are associated with greater life satisfaction in older patients suffering from chronic pain-related conditions such as osteoarthritis (Ferreira & Sherman, 2007). Moreover, older adults, like younger persons, consider social support to be important in their effort to cope with persistent pain (Martin, Schoster, Woodard, & Callahan, 2012; Molton & Terrill, 2014).

Social and material support provided by informal caregivers have a positive impact on the pain sufferers' functioning (Burckhardt, 1985; Faucett & Levine, 1991; Murphy, Creed, & Jayson, 1988; Turner & Noh, 1988), although when such support is excessive, to the point that it becomes solicitous, it can lead to increased expressions of pain and disability (Boothby, Thorn, Overduin, & Ward, 2004; Campbell, Jordan, & Dunn, 2012; McCracken, 2005; Paulsen & Altmaier, 1995; Pence, Thorn, Jensen, & Romano, 2008). Moreover, strained family relationships (e.g., marital conflict), which imply a weaker social support network, can lead to increases in reported pain severity (Burns et al., 2013; Schwartz, Slater, & Birchler, 1996).

Chronic pain can cause significant functional limitations that can impact a variety of functioning dimensions such as ability to carry out chores at home, mobility, and self-care (Covinsky, Lindquist, Dunlop, & Yelin, 2009). As a result, family members of pain patients have to carry out additional responsibilities. Related to the context of the older adult, pain tends to be undertreated in older persons (Ferrell et al., 2001; Hadjistavropoulos et al., 2007) and this undertreatment would likely increase caregiver burden. It is important to recognize, however, that caregiving roles and responsibilities evolve over time as the older pain patients' functioning needs may fluctuate. Related to this point, in many instances, older patients manage their pain with minimal assistance from caregivers (McPherson, Hadjistavropoulos, Devereaux, & Lobchuk, 2014). Irrespective of fluctuations in patient need for care, patient suffering remains a source of stress for the caregiver.

Ojeda et al. (2014) conducted a study focusing on pain patient caregivers. While the study was not exclusively focused on older adults, over one third of the sample was over 65 years of age. The researchers concluded that chronic pain significantly affected the family environment with perceptions of patient sadness, modification of leisure activities and patient sleep difficulties being among the factors that had a negative impact on the family.

In another study on pain patient caregivers, and using a qualitative descriptive approach, McPherson, Hadjistavropoulos, Lobchuk, and Kilgour (2013) reported that caregivers sometimes felt more distress about their family member's cancer pain than did the patients themselves. That is, caregivers expressed a great deal of distress, in response to seeing their loved one in pain, including a sense of hopelessness in their effort to manage pain. Caregivers were also worried about the effects of patient suffering on their own health and, consequently, there was anger expressed toward both the patient and the health professional for not adequately managing the pain. McPherson et al. (2013) also found that patients, who were not living with the caregiver, had a strong sense of wanting to remain independent and were, therefore, reluctant to seek help. Interestingly, the extent of caregiving differed across family caregivers. Some caregivers played a secondary role in helping patients self-manage their pain, whereas other caregivers played a more central role that involved assessing pain and implementing pain management strategies for their family member. When cancer pain was mild to moderate, but not when it was severe, patients and their family caregivers were more able to accept the pain in order to continue functioning in their daily lives. When patients and their family caregivers described their relationship as close, the cancer pain did not appear to elicit changes in the relationship. In fact, caregivers appreciated being able to help their family member and reported an increased closeness emanating from the experience of cancer pain, although this was only found when patients described their pain as mild to moderate.

An added challenge of caregiving for older adults with pain is that their caregivers (e.g., spouses) have an increased likelihood of being older adults themselves, given that the majority of caregivers are over 50 years of age and almost 20% are over 65 years old (National Alliance for Caregiving & American Association of Retired Persons, 2015). Older adult caregivers are more likely to suffer from pain than their younger counterparts. Jones, Hadjistavropoulos, Janzen, and Hadjistavropoulos (2011), for instance, found that level of caregiver pain predicts ability to cope with caregiving. That is, caregiver pain ratings were associated with caregiver burden including physical and emotional burden.

McPherson et al. (2014) showed that, although the caregiver–care recipient relationship was usually described as cooperative and supportive, challenges to this alliance can occur. Some patients, for example, are reluctant to relinquish roles, insisting to remain independent despite requiring assistance. This may lead patients to not disclose pain, which is not uncommon among older adults. Patients may also be concealing pain in order to avoid burdening caregivers (Dar, Beach, Barden, & Cleeland, 1992; McPherson, Wilson, & Murray, 2007). That is, a barrier to an adequate understanding of an older person's pain is that older adults tend to be more stoic about their pain and less likely to report it than younger individuals (Lyons, Langille, & Duck, 2006; Yong et al., 2001).

Caregiver perceptions of the patient could also interfere with ability to adequately decode pain. Redinbaugh, Baum, DeMoss, Fello, and Arnold (2002), for example, examined factors that were associated with the accuracy of family caregivers' estimates of pain in a sample of patients with a mean age of 64 years ($SD = 16.3$). They examined disparities in pain ratings between patients and their caregivers. The greatest disparities (i.e., caregivers assigning higher and more disparate patient pain scores) involved caregivers who perceived their loved one as experiencing very high levels of distress secondary to pain and caregivers who were themselves distressed about their loved one's pain. Related to the issue of pain communication, a persistent style of catastrophizing on the part of the patient (which tends to be associated with more intensive pain displays; Sullivan, Adams, & Sullivan, 2004; Sullivan, Martel,

Tripp, Savard, & Crombez, 2006) can also become a source of strain/burden for caregivers (Cano, 2004). In turn, negative responses on the part of the caregivers (irrespective of care-recipient age) may make it more difficult for the sufferer to cope with their pain condition (e.g., Claar, Simons, & Logan, 2008; McCracken, 2005). Underscoring the importance of the caregiver having a good understanding of a patient's pain, Mehta, Cohen, Ezer, Carnevale, and Ducharme (2011) found that caregivers of patients (average patient age was 69.8 years) who were unable to distinguish among different types of pain selected pain control approaches that were not necessarily appropriate.

Once caregivers interpret pain messages, most often, they will take actions to palliate the pain. Indeed, McPherson et al. (2013) found that, in response to behavioral reactions (e.g., asking for help, paralinguistic vocalizations) of elders with cancer pain, caregivers responded by taking actions to help alleviate the pain such as by encouraging administration of medications. Education and an interdisciplinary approach to pain management (Stanos, 2012), preferably with caregiver involvement (Ferrell, Grant, Chan, Ahn, & Ferrell, 1995), would help not only with the pain control of the older person but also with the challenges that the caregiver faces.

Caregivers of Pain Patients with Dementia

The caregiver of the dementia patient who also has pain would be challenged not only by the caregiving related to the pain condition but also by the dementia and the need to accommodate memory, linguistic, and other related patient impairments. Dementia, especially in the moderate to severe stages, can impose increased challenges in pain communication given the associated cognitive limitations. When pain cannot be communicated verbally, caregivers would need to be especially attuned to important behavioral and contextual indicators of pain.

In the context of older adults with dementia, although some signs of pain may appear obvious, caregivers often miss nonverbal indicators (Eritz & Hadjistavropoulos, 2011). Rather than drawing their conclusion largely based on pain behavior, they seem to be making inferences about patient pain based on situational/contextual information (e.g., beliefs on whether a given situation is likely to be painful). Unsurprisingly, caregivers who spend the most time with the patient are the least likely to miss pain-related nonverbal cues (Eritz & Hadjistavropoulos, 2011).

Helping caregivers focus on patient nonverbal behavior is extremely important. As indicated earlier, pain in patients with dementia tends to be associated with increased aggression and behavioral disturbance (Cipher et al., 2006). This aggression may be misattributed to causes unrelated to pain (e.g., a psychiatric disturbance or lack of appreciation for the caregiver's effort) which could result in the administration of psychotropic medications that can hasten death in frail seniors (Ballard et al., 2009; Cipher et al., 2006). Being attuned to nonverbal pain behavior (e.g., facial expressions of pain, paralinguistic vocalizations that are typically indicative of pain, rubbing or guarding the affected area) could potentially lead to effective intervention and thus reductions in behavioral disturbance.

One way of assisting caregivers to effectively attend to patient pain behavior may be through use of standardized observational checklists. In order to help address the challenges of associated with the limited communication of pain in dementia, a number of behavioral observational tools have been developed for this population (Aubin, Giguère, Hadjistavropoulos, & Verreault, 2007; Chan, Hadjistavropoulos, Williams, & Lints-Martindale, 2014; Warden, Hurley, & Volicer, 2003). These tools have been shown to be reliable and valid in the identification of pain behaviors (Hadjistavropoulos et al., 2014). Although most validation studies of such tools are based on use by health care staff, recent research has provided evidence that lay-people can also provide valid responses to the tools (Ammaturo et al., 2017), creating the possibility of informal caregivers using such tools with some instruction from a health professional. Guidance from a health professional is recommended in order to achieve adequate standardization of administration conditions, use an appropriate individualized approach to assessment as per written guidelines, and effective reporting of observational checklist results to health professionals (Hadjistavropoulos, Dever Fitzgerald, & Marchildon, 2010).

A study involving use of the Pain Assessment Checklist for Seniors with Limited Ability to Communicate (PACSLAC; Fuchs-Lacelle, Hadjistavropoulos, & Lix, 2008) demonstrated that when nursing staff assess pain in older adults on a regular basis they experience decreased burnout and less stress compared to nursing staff who do not regularly assess pain. Findings from the same study also suggested that regular pain assessment led to better pain management. If improved pain care is likely to reduce behavioral disturbance (in the case of dementia patients; Cipher et al., 2006; Fuchs-Lacelle et al., 2008) and nurse stress in professional caregiving contexts, it would be reasonable to expect that regular pain assessment and good pain care could result in improved levels of informal caregiver stress. Nonetheless, this is a speculation that should be investigated.

To optimize decoding of dementia patient communication and attempts to intervene in order to palliate pain, consideration should also be given to the issue of caregiver perceptions of patient personhood. Personhood refers to a status or standing bestowed upon an individual by other people in social contexts (Kitwood & Bredin, 1992). The construct of personhood implies trust, recognition, and respect. Recent evidence shows that many people may have the tendency to perceive people with dementia as having reduced personhood (Hunter et al., 2013). This tendency is likely related to people with dementia having reduced memory and consciousness as well as a reduced ability to think logically (Hadjistavropoulos, 2016). Hunter et al. (2013) demonstrated that the extent to which patients are perceived as having personhood may affect quality of pain care (e.g., the likelihood that analgesics will be administered). Although the Hunter et al. (2013) study involved health professionals as research participants, it is likely that its findings generalize to informal caregivers as well. Many educational and support programs (e.g., webinars, group educational and support sessions) offered through organizations such as the Alzheimer Society of Canada and other similar organizations are designed to enhance perceptions about the personhood of individuals with dementia.

Conclusions and Recommendations

The literature on caregivers of older adults with pain is quite limited. Nonetheless, we conclude with some recommendations based on research findings and/or consensus guidelines related to caregivers of older pain patients. That said, most of these recommendations would likely be equally applicable to all caregivers.

Recommendations for Future Research

We were surprised to discover that the research literature on caregiving for older patients suffering from chronic pain is very limited, compared to caregiving associated with other health conditions and populations (e.g., Javalkar et al., 2017; Stansfeld et al., 2017) with only a small number of studies conducted. There is clearly a need for more research in this area.

While there are many possible research domains that can be pursued in this area, we highlight a few here. Specifically, there is a need to evaluate more systematically the impact of a care-recipient pain condition on caregiver burden independent of other non-pain related conditions that the care recipient may be presenting with. That is, it would be important to understand the extent to which care recipient chronic pain is an independent contributor to burden. Moreover, there is a need for development and evaluation of interventions designed to educate and assist caregivers of older adults with pain in areas such as pain monitoring and management. Programs designed to help such caregivers cope with their caregiving role also need to be developed and evaluated.

General Recommendations for Caregivers

1. Caregivers can play a key role in the assessment of the chronic pain patient by offering their unique perspective and important information about the functioning of the individual with chronic pain (Hadjistavropoulos et al., 2007). It is very common for clinicians to involve family members (i.e., informal caregivers) in the assessment of the pain client.

2. Caregivers are more likely to succeed in their caregiving role if they ensure that they take good care of their own mental and physical well-being. Clinicians are advised to evaluate the extent to which the caregiving role takes a toll on the caregiver and intervene either directly or indirectly (e.g., through appropriate referral) in order to maximize caregivers' well-being.
3. Evaluation of the caregiver's level of social support provided to the patient is important. While an optimal level of social support is critical in the rehabilitation of the pain patient (Burckhardt, 1985; Faucett & Levine, 1991; Murphy et al., 1988; Turner & Noh, 1988), when this support becomes solicitous, it can be counterproductive (Boothby et al., 2004; Campbell et al., 2012; McCracken, 2005; Paulsen & Altmaier, 1995; Pence et al., 2008). Helping caregivers provide support that is attuned to the specific needs of the pain sufferer is of critical importance.
4. Marital distress can increase with chronic pain (Burns et al., 2013; Schwartz et al., 1996). It is recommended that appropriate referral for couples therapy be pursued in such cases.
5. It would be important for caregivers and care recipients to discuss their caregiving goals as some findings suggest that caregivers and care recipients may have discrepant goals (McPherson et al., 2014). That is, caregivers may have the goal of helping the patient become completely pain free, whereas patients may prioritize maximization of independence which could be negatively impacted by side effects of certain medications.
6. Although medication tends to represent a primary approach to pain management, seeking information about other treatment modalities (e.g., physiotherapy, occupational therapy) that may be helpful to the care recipient is also important.

Special Recommendations for Caregivers of Older Adults with Dementia

Given that patients with dementia, depending on the level of cognitive and linguistic impairment, may have difficulty monitoring and/or reporting their pain, it would be important for caregivers to fulfill that role. Recent research has shown that laypeople can complete, in a valid fashion, observational pain assessment tools for people with dementia (e.g., PACSLAC-II; Chan et al., 2014]; Pain Assessment in Advanced Dementia [PAINAD; Warden et al., 2003]) that were originally developed for use by nursing staff (Ammaturo et al., 2017). Health professionals can provide instructions to caregivers and help optimize the completion of administration of such observational tools.

The PACSLAC-II, which is one of the tools that has been validated for use by informal caregivers, does not use cutoff scores given that substantial individual differences in the expression of pain exist among individuals with dementia. Instead, it is recommended that an individualized approach be adopted that involves the regular administration of the tool under consistent circumstances (e.g., during personal care or over the course of an evening) and recording the scores in a diary. Deviations from one's regular pattern of scores may be indicative of changes in pain levels that would need to be discussed with a health professional. More details on the use of tools like the PACSLAC-II can be found in Hadjistavropoulos, Dever Fitzgerald, and Marchildon (2010).

Caregivers of pain patients with dementia can also be encouraged to facilitate increased involvement in pleasant activities for their loved one as a means of enhancing caregiver mood (e.g., Teri, Longsdon, Uomoto, & McCurry, 1997) and distracting themselves from pain. Moreover, identifying and modifying environmental triggers (e.g., noise, monotonous situations) of distress may be helpful.

References

Abdollahpour, I., Nedjat, S., Noroozian, M., Salimi, Y., & Majdzadeh, R. (2014). Caregiver burden: The strongest predictor of self-rated health in caregivers of patients with dementia. *Journal of Geriatric Psychiatry and Neurology, 27*, 172–180.

Adelman, R. D., Tmanova, L. L., Delgado, D., Dion, S., & Lachs, M. S. (2014). Caregiver burden: A clinical review. *Journal of the American Medical Association, 311*, 1052–1059.

Alecxih, L. M. B., Zeruld, S., & Olearczyl, B. (2001). *Characteristics of caregivers based on the survey of income and program participation. National Family Caregiver Support Program: Selected Issue Briefs.* Falls Church, VA: The Lewin Group.

Alzheimer's Association. (2014). 2014 Alzheimer's disease facts and figures. *Alzheimer's & Dementia, 10*. Retrieved from https://www.alz.org/downloads/facts_figures_2014.pdf

Ammaturo, D., Hadjistavropoulos, T. & Williams, J. (2017). Pain in dementia: Use of observational pain assessment tools by people who are not health professionals. *Pain Medicine, 18*, 1895–1907.

Aubin, M., Giguère, A., Hadjistavropoulos, T., & Verreault, R. (2007). Évaluation systématique des instruments pour mesurer la douleur chez les personnes âgées ayant des capacités réduites à communiquer. *Pain Research & Management, 12*, 195–203.

Ballard, C., Hanney, M. L., Theodoulou, M., Douglas, S., McShane, R., Kossakowski, K., … Investigators, D. A. R. T.-A. D. (2009). The dementia antipsychotic withdrawal trial (DART-AD): Long-term follow-up of a randomised placebo-controlled trial. *The Lancet Neurology, 8*, 151–157.

Bernabei, R., Gambassi, G., Lapane, K., Landi, F., Gatsonis, C., Dunlop, R., … Mor, V. (1998). Management of pain in elderly patients with cancer. *The Journal of the American Medical Association, 279*, 1877–1882.

Boothby, J. L., Thorn, B. E., Overduin, L. Y., & Ward, L. C. (2004). Catastrophizing and perceived partner responses to pain. *Pain, 109*, 500–506.

Burckhardt, C. S. (1985). The impact of arthritis on quality of life. *Nursing Research, 34*, 11–18.

Burns, J. W., Peterson, K. M., Smith, D. A., Keefe, F. J., Porter, L. S., Schuster, E., & Kinner, E. (2013). Temporal associations between spouse criticism/hostility and pain among patients with chronic pain: A within-couple daily diary study. *Pain, 154*, 2715–2721.

Campbell, P., Jordan, K. P., & Dunn, K. M. (2012). The role of relationship quality and perceived partner responses with pain and disability in those with back pain. *Pain Medicine, 13*, 204–214.

Cano, A. (2004). Pain catastrophizing and social support in married individuals with chronic pain: The moderating role of pain duration. *Pain, 110*, 656–664.

Centers for Disease Control and Prevention & The Merck Company Foundation. (2007). *The state of aging and health in America 2007*. Whitehouse Station, NJ: The Merck Company Foundation.

Chan, S., Hadjistavropoulos, T., Williams, J., & Lints-Martindale, A. (2014). Evidence-based development and initial validation of the Pain Assessment Checklist for Seniors with Limited Ability to Communicate-II (PACSLAC-II). *Clinical Journal of Pain, 30*, 816–824.

Chappell, N. L. (1993). Implications of shifting health care policy for caregiving in Canada. *Journal of Aging & Social Policy, 5*, 39–55.

Charlton, J. E. (2005). *Core curriculum for professional education in pain* (3rd ed.). Seattle, WA: IASP Press.

Chen, M.-C., Chen, K.-M., & Chu, T.-P. (2015). Caregiver burden, health status, and learned resourcefulness of older caregivers. *Western Journal of Nursing Research, 37*, 767–780.

Cipher, D. J., Clifford, P. A., & Roper, K. D. (2006). Behavioral manifestations of pain in the demented elderly. *Journal of the American Medical Directors Association, 7*(6), 355–365.

Claar, R. L., Simons, L. E., & Logan, D. E. (2008). Parental response to children's pain: The moderating impact of children's emotional distress on symptoms and disability. *Pain, 138*, 172–179.

Cleeland, C. S., Gonin, R., Hatfield, A. K., Edmonson, J. H., Blum, R. H., Stewart, J. A., & Pandya, K. J. (1994). Pain and its treatment in outpatients with metastic cancer. *The New England Journal of Medicine, 330*, 592–596.

Clyburn, L. D., Stones, M. J., Hadjistavropoulos, T., & Tuokko, H. (2000). Predicting caregiver burden and depression in Alzheimer's disease. *Journal of Gerontology, 55B*, S2–S13.

Cohen, D., & Eisdorfer, C. (1988). Depression in family members caring for a relative with Alzheimer's disease. *Journal of the American Geriatrics Society, 36*, 885–889.

Colby, S. L., & Ortman, J. M. (2015). Projections of the size and composition of the U.S. population: Population estimates and projections. In *Current population reports* (pp. 25–1143). Washington, DC: U.S. Census Bureau.

Covinsky, K. E., Lindquist, K., Dunlop, D. D., & Yelin, E. (2009). Pain, functional limitations, and aging. *Journal of the American Geriatrics Society, 57*, 1556–1561.

Cranswick, K., & Dosman, D. (2008). *Eldercare: What we know today*. Ottawa, ON: Statistics Canada.

Dar, R., Beach, C. M., Barden, P. L., & Cleeland, C. S. (1992). Cancer pain in the marital system: A study of patients and their spouses. *Journal of Pain and Symptom Management, 7*, 87–93.

Delgado-Guay, M. O., & Bruera, E. (2008). Management of pain in the older person with cancer. *Oncology, 22*, 56–61.

Eritz, H., & Hadjistavropoulos, T. (2011). Do informal caregivers consider non-verbal behavior when they assess pain in people with dementia? *Journal of Pain, 12*, 331–339.

Faucett, J. A., & Levine, J. D. (1991). The contributions of interpersonal conflict to chronic pain in the presence or absence of organic pathology. *Pain, 44*, 35–43.

Ferreira, V. M., & Sherman, A. M. (2007). The relationship of optimism, pain and social support to well-being in older adults with osteoarthritis. *Aging & Mental Health, 11*, 89–98.

Ferrell, B. R., Cohen, M., Rhiner, M., & Rozek, A. (1991). Pain as a metaphor for illness. Part II: Family caregivers' management of pain. *Oncology Nursing Forum, 18*, 1315–1321.

Ferrell, B. R., Grant, M., Chan, J., Ahn, C., & Ferrell, B. A. (1995). The impact of cancer pain education on family caregivers of elderly patients. *Oncology Nursing Forum, 22*, 1211–1218.

Ferrell, B. R., Novy, D., Sullivan, M. D., Banja, J., Dubois, M. Y., Gitlin, M. C., … Livovich, J. (2001). Ethical dilemmas in pain management. *The Journal of Pain, 2*, 171–180.

Freemont, A. J., & Hoyland, J. A. (2007). Morphology, mechanisms and pathology of musculoskeletal aging. *The Journal of Pathology, 211*, 252–259.

Fuchs-Lacelle, S., Hadjistavropoulos, T., & Lix, L. (2008). Pain assessment as intervention: A study of older adults with severe dementia. *Clinical Journal of Pain, 24*, 697–707.

Gheno, R., Cepparo, J. M., Rosca, C. E., & Cotten, A. (2012). Musculoskeletal disorders in the elderly. *Journal of Clinical Imaging Science, 2*. https://doi.org/10.4103/2156-7514.99151

Hadjistavropoulos, T. (2016). Recognizing pain in dementia. In L. Garcia-Larrea & P. Jackson (Eds.), *Pain and the conscious brain* (pp. 167–181). Philadelphia: Walters Kluwer Health.

Hadjistavropoulos, T., Craig, K. D., Duck, S., Cano, A., Goubert, L., Jackson, P. L., ... Fitzgerald, T. D. (2011). A biopsychosocial formulation of pain communication. *Psychological Bulletin, 137*, 910–939.

Hadjistavropoulos, T., Dever Fitzgerald, T., & Marchildon, G. (2010). Practice guidelines for assessing pain in older persons who reside in long-term care facilities. *Physiotherapy Canada, 62*(2), 104–113.

Hadjistavropoulos, T., Herr, K., Prkachin, K., Craig, K., Gibson, S., Lukas, L., & Smith, J. (2014). Pain assessment in elderly adults with dementia. *The Lancet Neurology, 13*(12), 1216–1227.

Hadjistavropoulos, T., Herr, K., Turk, D. C., Fine, P. G., Dworkin, R. H., Helme, R., ... Williams, J. (2007). An interdisciplinary expert consensus statement on assessment of pain in older persons. *Clinical Journal of Pain, 23*(Suppl), S1–S43.

Hadjistavropoulos, T., LaChapelle, D., MacLeod, F., Snider, B., & Craig, K. D. (2000). Measuring movement exacerbated pain in cognitively impaired frail elders. *The Clinical Journal of Pain, 16*, 54–63.

Hadjistavropoulos, T., Marchildon, G. P., Fine, P. G., Herr, K., Palley, H. A., Kaasalainen, S., & Béland, F. (2009). Transforming long-term care pain management in North America: The policy–clinical interface. *Pain Medicine, 10*, 506–520.

He, W., Goodkind, D., & Kowal, P. (2016). An aging world: 2015. In *International population reports* (pp. 1–165). Washington, DC: U.S. Census Bureau.

Hofmann, M. T., Farnon, C. U., Javed, A., & Posner, J. D. (1998). Pain in the elderly hospice patient. *American Journal of Hospice and Palliative Medicine, 15*, 259–265.

Hunter, P. V., Hadjistavropoulos, T., Smythe, W. E., Malloy, D. C., Kaasalainen, S., & Williams, J. (2013). The personhood in dementia questionnaire (PDQ): Establishing an association between beliefs about personhood and health providers' approaches to person-centred care. *Journal of Aging Studies, 27*, 276–287.

Javalkar, K., Rak, E., Phillips, A., Haberman, C., Ferris, M., & Van Tilburg, M. (2017). Predictors of caregiver burden among mothers of children with chronic conditions. *Children (Basel)*. https://doi.org/10.3390/children4050039.

Joling, K. J., van Hout, H. P. J., Schellevis, F. G., van der Horst, H. E., Scheltens, P., Knol, D. L., & van Marwijk, H. W. J. (2010). Incidence of depression and anxiety in the spouses of patients with dementia: A naturalistic cohort study of recorded morbidity with a 6-year follow-up. *The American Journal of Geriatric Psychiatry, 18*, 146–153.

Jones, S. L., Hadjistavropoulos, H. D., Janzen, J. A., & Hadjistavropoulos, T. (2011). The relation of pain and caregiver burden in informal older adult caregivers. *Pain Medicine, 12*, 51–58.

Kiecolt-Glaser, J. K., Glaser, R., Gravenstein, S., Malarkey, W. B., & Sheridan, J. (1996). Chronic stress alters the immune response to influenza virus vaccine in older adults. *Proceedings of the National Academy of Science of the United States of America, 93*, 3043–3047.

Kiecolt-Glaser, J. K., Marucha, P. T., Malarkey, W. B., Mercado, A. M., & Glaser, R. (1995). Slowing of wound healing by psychological stress. *The Lancet, 346*, 1194–1196.

Kim, H., Chang, M., Rose, K., & Kim, S. (2012). Predictors of caregiver burden in caregivers of individuals with dementia. *Journal of Advanced Nursing, 68*, 846–855.

Kitwood, T., & Bredin, K. (1992). Towards a theory of dementia care: Personhood and well-being. *Ageing and Society, 12*, 269–287.

Kunz, M., Scharmann, S., Hemmeter, U., Schepelmann, K., & Lautenbacher, S. (2007). The facial expression of pain in patients with dementia. *Pain, 15*, 22–228.

Lyons, R. F., Langille, L., & Duck, S. (2006). Difficult relationship–relationship difficulties: Relationship adaptation and chronic health problems. In D. C. Kirkpatrick, S. Duck, & M. K. Foley (Eds.), *Relating difficulty* (pp. 203–224). Mahwah, NJ: Lawrence Erlbaum.

Martin, K. R., Schoster, B., Woodard, J., & Callahan, L. F. (2012). What community resources do older community-dwelling adults use to manage their osteoarthritis? A formative examination. *Journal of Applied Gerontology, 31*, 661–684.

McCracken, L. M. (2005). Social context and acceptance of chronic pain: The role of solicitous and punishing responses. *Pain, 113*, 155–159.

McPherson, C., Wilson, K., & Murray, M. (2007). Feeling like a burden: Exploring the perspectives of patients at the end of life. *Social Science & Medicine, 64*, 417–427.

McPherson, C. J., Hadjistavropoulos, T., Devereaux, A., & Lobchuk, M. M. (2014). A qualitative investigation of the roles and perspectives of older patients with advanced cancer and their family caregivers in managing pain in the home. *BMC Palliative Care, 13*, 293–300.

McPherson, C. J., Hadjistavropoulos, T., Lobchuk, M. M., & Kilgour, K. N. (2013). Cancer-related pain in older adults receiving palliative care: Patient and family caregiver perspectives on the experience of pain. *Pain Research & Management, 18*, 293–300.

Mehta, A., Cohen, S. R., Ezer, H., Carnevale, F. A., & Ducharme, F. (2011). Striving to respond to palliative care patients' pain at home: A puzzle for family caregivers. *Oncology Nursing Forum, 38*, E37–E45.

Molton, I. R., & Terrill, A. L. (2014). Overview of persistent pain in older adults. *The American Psychologist, 69*, 197–207.

Morimoto, T., Schreiner, A. S., & Asano, H. (2003). Caregiver burden and health-related quality of life among Japanese stroke caregivers. *Age and Ageing, 32*, 218–223.

Murphy, S., Creed, F., & Jayson, M. I. (1988). Psychiatric disorder and illness behaviour in rheumatoid arthritis. *British Journal of Rheumatology, 27*, 357–363.

National Alliance for Caregiving & American Association of Retired Persons. (2009). *Caregiving in the U.S.* National Alliance for Caregiving. Washington, DC.

National Alliance for Caregiving & American Association of Retired Persons. (2015). *Caregiving in the U.S.* National Alliance for Caregiving. Washington, DC.

Ojeda, B., Salazar, A., Dueñas, M., Torres, L. M., Micó, J. A., & Failde, I. (2014). The impact of chronic pain: The perspective of patients, relatives, and caregivers. *Families, Systems, & Health, 32*, 399–407.

Paulsen, J. S., & Altmaier, E. M. (1995). The effects of perceived versus enacted social support on the discriminative cue functions of spouses for pain behavior. *Pain, 60*, 103–110.

Pence, L., Thorn, B. E., Jensen, M. P., & Romano, J. M. (2008). Examination of perceived spouse responses to patient well and pain behavior in patients with headache. *Clinical Journal of Pain, 24*, 654–661.

Plassman, B. L., Langa, K. M., Fisher, G. G., Heeringa, S. G., Weir, D. R., Ofstedal, M. B., … Wallace, R. B. (2007). Prevalence of dementia in the United States: The aging, demographics, and memory study. *Neuroepidemiology, 29*, 125–132.

Prkachin, K. M., & Craig, K. D. (1995). Expressing pain: The communication and interpretation of facial pain signals. *Journal of Nonverbal Behavior, 19*, 191–205.

Redinbaugh, E. M., Baum, A., DeMoss, C., Fello, M., & Arnold, R. (2002). Factors associated with the accuracy of family caregiver estimates of patient pain. *Journal of Pain and Symptom Management, 23*, 31–38.

Schulz, R., & Beach, S. R. (1999). Caregiving as a risk factor for mortality: The Caregiver Health Effects Study. *Journal of the American Medical Association, 282*, 2215–2219.

Schwartz, L., Slater, M. A., & Birchler, G. R. (1996). The role of pain behaviors in the modulation of marital conflict in chronic pain couples. *Pain, 65*(2–3), 227–233.

Stanos, S. (2012). Focused review of interdisciplinary pain rehabilitation programs for chronic pain. *Current Pain and Headache Reports, 16*, 147–152.

Stansfeld, J., Stoner, C.R., Wenborn, J., Vernooij-Dassen, M., Moniz-Cook, E., & Orrell, M. (2017). Positive psychology outcome measures for family caregivers of people living with dementia: A systematic review. *International Psychogeriatrics.* https://doi.org/10.1017/S1041610217000655.

Statistics Canada. (2015). Population projections for Canada, provinces and territories (91-520-X). Retrieved from http://www5.statcan.gc.ca/olc-cel/olc.action?objId=91-520-X&objType=2&lang=en&limit=0

Sullivan, M. J. L., Adams, H., & Sullivan, M. E. (2004). Communicative dimensions of pain cata-strophizing: Social cueing effects on pain behaviour and coping. *Pain, 107,* 220–226.

Sullivan, M. J. L., Martel, M. O., Tripp, D., Savard, A., & Crombez, G. (2006). The relation between catastrophizing and the communication of pain experience. *Pain, 122,* 282–288.

Takai, Y., Yamamoto-Mitani, N., Okamoto, Y., Koyama, K., & Honda, A. (2010). Literature review of pain prevalence among older residents of nursing homes. *Pain Management Nursing, 11,* 209–223.

Takai, Y., Yamamoto-Mitani, N., Suzuki, M., Furuta, Y., Sato, A., & Fujimaki, Y. (2013). Developing and validating a Japanese version of the assessment of pain in elderly people with communication impairment. *Archives of Gerontology and Geriatrics, 57,* 403–410.

Teri, L., Longsdon, R. G., Uomoto, J., & McCurry, S. M. (1997). Behavioral treatment of depression in dementia patients: A controlled clinical trial. *Journals of Gerontology Series B: Psychological Sciences and Social Sciences, 52,* P159–P166.

Turner, R. J., & Noh, S. (1988). Physical disability and depression: A longitudinal analysis. *Journal of Health and Social Behavior, 29,* 23–37.

van den Beuken-van Everdingen, M. H., de Rijke, J. M., Kessels, A. G., Schouten, H. C., van Kleef, M., & Patijn, J. (2007). Prevalence of pain in patients with cancer: A systematic review of the past 40 years. *Annals of Oncology, 18,* 1437–1449.

van der Lee, J., Bakker, T. J. E. M., Duivenvoorden, H. J., & Dröes, R.-M. (2014). Multivariate models of subjective caregiver burden in dementia: A systematic review. *Aging Research Reviews, 15,* 76–93.

von Känel, R., Mausbach, B. T., Patterson, T. L., Dimsdale, J. E., Aschbacher, K., Mills, P. J., … Grant, I. (2008). Increased Framingham coronary heart disease risk score in dementia caregivers relative to non-caregiving controls. *Gerontology, 54,* 131–137.

Warden, V., Hurley, A. C., & Volicer, L. (2003). Development and psychometric evaluation of the Pain Assessment in Advanced Dementia (PAINAD) scale. *Journal of the American Medical Directors Association, 4,* 9–15.

Yong, H.-H., Gibson, S. J., de Horne, D. J. L., & Helme, R. D. (2001). Development of a pain assessment questionnaire to assess stoicism and cautiousness for possible age differences. *Journal of Gerontology: Psychological Sciences, 56,* 279–284.

Zarit, S. H., & Heid, A. R. (2015). Assessment and treatment of family caregivers. In P. A. Lichtenberg & B. T. Mast (Eds.), *APA handbook of clinical geropsychology (Vol. 2)* (pp. 521–552). Washington, DC: APA Press.

Zarit, S. H., Todd, P. A., & Zarit, J. M. (1986). Subjective burden of husbands and wives as caregivers: A longitudinal study. *The Gerontologist, 26,* 260–266.

Part VII
Societal Context

Chapter 20
Sex and Gender as Social-Contextual Factors in Pain

Edmund Keogh

Abstract Pain does not operate in a social vacuum. The environment we are in, and the people who occupy it can influence how pain is perceived, experienced, and managed. This chapter argues that sex and gender are relevant social-contextual factors that should be considered when exploring and managing pain. It illustrates this by reviewing the evidence for sex differences in pain, before exploring why these male–female differences might exist. Central to psychosocial accounts is the notion of gender, which points to sociocultural influences, and the impact that gender-based beliefs and expectations have on pain and pain-related behavior. A range of relevant evidence for sex and gender as social context is presented, including research into dyadic interactions, pain expression, and communication. This chapter should be of interest to those studying social-contextual and interpersonal factors in pain, as well as those interested in understanding how social factors help explain why men and women vary in pain.

Keywords Pain · Sex · Gender · Masculinity · Femininity · Gender roles ·
Nonverbal behavior · Communication

Introduction

Pain does not operate in a social vacuum. The environment we are in, and the people who occupy it can influence how pain is perceived, experienced, and managed. This chapter argues that sex and gender are relevant social-contextual factors that should be considered when exploring and managing pain. It illustrates this by reviewing the evidence for sex differences in pain, before exploring why these male–female differences might exist. Central to psychosocial accounts is the notion of gender, which points to sociocultural influences, and the impact that gender-based beliefs and expectations have on pain and pain-related behavior. A range of relevant evidence

E. Keogh (✉)
Department of Psychology, University of Bath, Bath, UK
e-mail: e.m.keogh@bath.ac.uk

433

for sex and gender as social context is presented, including research into dyadic interactions, pain expression, and communication. This chapter should be of interest to those studying social-contextual and interpersonal factors in pain, as well as those interested in understanding how social factors help explain why men and women vary in pain.

Definitions: Sex and Gender

Given this chapter considers sex and gender as factors in pain, it makes sense to define both terms first. This is particularly important as sex and gender are often used interchangeably, and can create confusion (Muehlenhard & Peterson, 2011; Unger, 1979). Sex is typically used when referring to physiological differences between males and females, and includes genetics, anatomy, and hormonal and immune functioning. Sex can also be used as a more general term to refer to categorical male–female differences. Therefore, for the purposes of the current chapter, "sex" will be used when making explicit reference to physiological factors, and/or referring to dichotomous male–female comparisons.

Gender is most often used to refer to the wider psychosocial and cultural aspects of pain (Bernardes, Keogh, & Lima, 2008). It incorporates constructs such as masculinity and femininity, and what it means to be "male" and "female" within a particular context, culture and time. Gender is thought to be less fixed, in that it is open to change and reflects situational influences. The term "gender" will therefore be used when focusing on the psychosocial and cultural influences around how male and female pain behaviors are defined, develop, and manifest. Given the focus here on social contextual factors in pain, gender will clearly form an important aspect in this chapter.

Evidence for Sex Differences in Pain

In order to argue that sex and gender are relevant social-contextual factors in pain, we need to first establish that there is evidence for male–female variability in pain. Fortunately, there are extensive reviews on this topic, so this section will only briefly summarize this work (Chin, Fillingim, & Ness, 2013; Fillingim, King, Ribeiro-Dasilva, Rahim-Williams, & Riley 3rd., 2009; Keogh, 2013). It will consider evidence from laboratory and epidemiological studies, as well as clinical and treatment outcome research.

Sex Differences in Experimentally Induced Pain

One approach to investigating sex differences in pain is to look at whether men and women differ in how they experience and respond to experimentally induced pain (Fillingim et al., 2009; Mogil, 2012). The advantage of these laboratory-based approaches is that the type of pain stimulus can be standardized, so that we are sure of the precise nature and location of pain. It also allows for systematic and highly controlled investigations. What these studies show is that women typically exhibit a lower threshold and tolerance to pain when compared to men. Furthermore, this heightened female sensitivity has been shown across a range of types of induced pain, including thermal, pressure, and electrical stimulation (Riley, Robinson, Wise, Myers, & Fillingim, 1998).

There is, however, variation in these sex-based effects, and inconsistencies have also been reported (Racine et al., 2012a). For example, the strength of male–female differences can depend on the type of pain induction method used, with one meta-analysis suggesting stronger effects for pressure pain and electrical stimulation, and weaker effects for thermal methods (Riley et al., 1998). Another source of variation is thought to be age. Sex differences in pain are less often reported in children, and seem to become more apparent around puberty and into adulthood. While this has been sporadically tested in laboratory, only recently has it been possible to collate relevant information and test this empirically (Boerner, Birnie, Caes, Schinkel, & Chambers, 2014). Boerner et al. (2014) conducted a meta-analysis of sex difference effects in healthy children and adolescents responses to experimental pain. They reported that in older aged children (i.e., aged over 12 years), girls reported a higher intensity to cold pressor pain than boys, and that generally boys had a higher tolerance to thermal heat pain. Interestingly, for heat pain, younger boys also had a higher threshold than girls. This points to the possibility that there may be sex differences in younger groups, but only for some types of pain. As will become apparent later, these studies are particularly interesting in light of suggestions that early developmental factors in children influence the establishment of gender-based identity, which can impact on pain behaviors. Less is known, however, about male–female differences in pain within older age groups.

Sex Differences in Clinical Pain Prevalence

Alongside laboratory studies, there is also clinical evidence for sex differences in pain. For example, epidemiological investigations point to sex difference in the prevalence of pain, both generally, and across a range of specific painful conditions (LeResche, 1999, 2013). What these studies typically show is that women report higher levels of pain when compared to men (Fayaz, Croft, Langford, Donaldson, & Jones, 2016; Johannes, Le, Zhou, Johnston, & Dworkin, 2010; Kennedy, Roll, Schraudner, Murphy, & McPherson, 2014; Tsang et al., 2008). For example, in a

US-based study, persistent pain was reported to be 16.2% for men and 21.6% for women (Kennedy et al., 2014). In a review spanning 17 different countries, Tsang et al. (2008) reported that 44.9% of females and 31.4% of males reported chronic pain. Such reports are consistent with the general global trend that women carry a greater burden of disease compared to men, where many of the most common diseases associated with disability feature pain (DALYs & Collaborators, 2016).

Females also show greater a prevalence for a range of specific painful conditions including lower back pain, migraine and tension type headache, irritable bowel syndrome, arthritic conditions, fibromyalgia, and cancer-related and postsurgical pain (Fillingim et al., 2009; Tighe, Riley, & Fillingim, 2014). Similar to experimental pain studies, some sex differences in painful clinical conditions can vary by age (LeResche, 2013). For example, sex differences in temporomandibular disorder and some headache-related conditions peak during reproductive years, often starting around puberty. Greater prevalence of pain in females can also be seen in healthcare utilization, including access to pain services and analgesic usage (Antonov & Isacson, 1998; Hargreave et al., 2010; Sarganas et al., 2015; Weir, Browne, Tunks, Gafni, & Roberts, 1996). For example, females report consuming higher prescription and over-the-counter analgesics. While this may very well suggest that women experience more pain, this could also reflect different pain control (analgesic) strategies used to manage pain.

Sex Differences in Pain Treatment Responses

There may also be sex differences in responses to pharmacological treatments. One systematic review and meta-analysis of around 50 opioid treatment studies concluded there are sex differences in analgesic responsiveness, with greater analgesia found in adult females for morphine analgesia in both patient controlled analgesia and experimental pain (Niesters et al., 2010). There are also suggestions for sex differences in the side effects associated with some analgesics (Ciccone & Holdcroft, 1999). However, only a few studies to date have considered sex differences in placebo analgesia, which is surprising given the role that (sex- and gender-related) expectations might have in pain responses (Butcher & Carmody, 2012).

There have been fewer investigations into sex differences in other types of pain treatment, such as psychosocial and multidisciplinary interventions (Jensen, Bergstrom, Ljungquist, Bodin, & Nygren, 2001; Keogh, McCracken, & Eccleston, 2005; McGeary, Mayer, Gatchel, Anagnostis, & Proctor, 2003; Pieh et al., 2012). Although some adult male–female differences have been reported, outcomes are difficult to interpret given the limited number of studies that have directly considered sex as a factor. A recent systematic review and meta-analysis has, however, been conducted into sex differences in psychological interventions for children and adolescents with chronic pain (Boerner, Eccleston, Chambers, & Keogh, 2017). This study found that there may be pretreatment sex differences in anxiety and depression (both higher in girls), although treatment outcome effects were generally similar for boys and girls. One difference that was found, however, was that girls with chronic non-headache pain benefited from treatment on disability-related outcomes, whereas this was not found in boys. This review also revealed that of the studies included, many more girls than boys were recruited into the clinical trials.

The general reluctance to directly consider sex as a potential moderator of pain treatments remains a problem, and limits the conclusions we can make. However, there are tentative suggestions that sex may play a role in some pain treatment responses.

Explanations for Sex and Gender Differences in Pain

What the above section demonstrates is that there are potentially important male–female differences in pain and analgesia. Females are typically found to report and experience more pain across a range of conditions and situations, when compared to males. The question that naturally arises from this work is to ask why such differences should occur. Explanations are multifaceted, reflecting biological/physiological, psychological, and social factors (Fillingim, 2017; Keogh, 2013; Sorge & Totsch, 2017). The next section will examine these biopsychosocial factors, but given the interest in social-contextual influences, particular attention will be given to the role that gender has in these male–female differences.

Biological Explanations for Sex Differences in Pain

A range of physiological factors have been proposed to account for male–female differences in pain (Melchior, Poisbeau, Gaumond, & Marchand, 2016; Sorge & Totsch, 2017). These include genetic factors (Fillingim et al., 2005; Mogil et al., 2003), cortical differences (Gupta et al., 2017), endogenous inhibitory systems (Popescu, LeResche, Truelove, & Drangsholt, 2010), and, more recently, immune functioning (Rosen, Ham, & Mogil, 2017). However, most attention has been placed on the role that sex hormones may have, with estrogen being linked to an increased vulnerability to pain (Craft, Mogil, & Aloisi, 2004). Further evidence for the sex hormone hypothesis stems from observations that changes to pain sensitivity can coincide with changes in hormonal profiles, such as around puberty, across the menstrual cycle and during pregnancy (Hazes, 1991; LeResche, 2013). The effects of the menstrual cycle on pain have been reported in healthy adults in studies utilizing experimental pain methods (Riley, Robinson, Wise, & Price, 1999; Sherman & LeResche, 2006), as well as within clinical pain studies where changes in hormonal status have been related to changes in pain experience (LeResche, Mancl, Sherman, Gandara, & Dworkin, 2003). Furthermore, menstrual cycle-related effects on pain may extend to analgesia, with at least one study reporting changes in opioid analgesia across different menstrual phases (Ribeiro-Dasilva et al., 2011). However, inconsistencies have also been reported, possibly due to differences in the methods used to ascertain menstrual phase.

There are also social evolutionary approaches that might help explain why men and women experience and express pain in different ways. For example, a greater general vulnerability to painful conditions might have led to a greater sensitivity to pain sensations in women (Berkley, 1997). Similarly, different sex-specific pressures may exist around showing or hiding pain from others, as these may signal vulnerability to others. It has also been suggested that historically a greater reliance on non-kin based social networks among women existed, resulting in a greater reliance on verbal and nonverbal processes to aid interpersonal interactions and social bonding (Vigil, 2009). Such explanations would seem relevant to the communication of pain as well.

Gender-based Explanations for Male–Female Variation in Pain

What the above section starts to illustrate is that as well as understanding the physiological mechanisms for male–female variation in pain, we also need to understand the psychosocial and interpersonal factors involved. Here, emotional and cognitive processes are considered important to our understanding of male–female pain, with gender-based approaches receiving particular attention (Keogh, 2013). The starting point is the view that there are socially-determined, often stereotypical beliefs associated with being male and female, which in turn influence how we behave, view, and interact with others. A key distinction is made between socially constructed masculine and feminine behaviors: masculinity typically refers to stoic (less emotional), independent and aggressive behaviors patterns, and are most commonly associated with being male, whereas femininity, typically reflects a more emotionally responsive, socially oriented and nurturing set of behaviors, that are often associated with being female. However, masculinity is not exclusively male, nor femininity exclusively female, as these characteristics are shared behavior patterns that are socially learnt in both males and females. From a social learning perspective, our gender identity, and associated behaviors, is shaped early on in life by close family members and friends, then influenced by key social institutions such as school and education, followed by the workplace, and media and society (Bussey & Bandura, 1999). While gender can be viewed as stable, more contemporary approaches take the view that gender is a more fluid construct; less fixed and more flexible, and contextually determined.

If we apply this gender-based approach to pain, we can start to think about stereotypical beliefs about how men and women are expected to behave when they are in pain. Such expectations might also result in differences in actual pain behaviors, especially in terms of how pain is expressed, reported, and dealt with. For example, someone who strongly identifies with a masculine-type identity, may be less willing or feel able to express pain to others, and may avoid seeking help (Keogh, 2015). Similarly, gender-based expectations about pain may impact on how observers view and interpret the pain expressed by others, and even affect our responses to those in pain. A further consideration is to view social interactions around pain as being influenced by the sex and gender-context people find themselves in. For example, pain expression may not only be influenced by the sex of the person in pain, but also the sex-congruence between those involved in dyadic interactions.

The flexible nature of gender also means we can consider different levels of gender analysis, and apply this to pain (Bernardes et al., 2008). For example, we can examine stable gender-based (personality) traits, as well as more situational and contextual ways of behaving in a gendered way. Here we can draw on ideas such as "doing gender" (West & Zimmerman, 1987), which reflects the wider social context in which behaviors occur. We can also consider certain environments as being gendered, with occupations and work settings being examples where independence and nurturing may be reflected to different degrees. From this, different social environments and interpersonal interactions may also be considered gendered, with some being more or less conducive to expressing and supporting those in pain.

Sex and Gender Factors in Dyadic Social Interactions

Given the relevance of social contextual factors for pain, and that sex and gender impact on social interactions, it would seem likely that sex and gender are relevant contextual factors in pain. This section will present the evidence for this view, focusing on the sex-based dyadic interactions across a range of different interpersonal situations.

Sex of Observer Effects in the Laboratory

One way to investigate sex-based dyadic effects has been to manipulate the gender context in which experimental pain studies have been conducted, and see how this affects pain reporting (Kallai, Barke, & Voss, 2004; Levine & Desimone, 1991). For example, Levine and Desimone (1991) reported one of the first studies to do this, by varying the sex of the experimenter in a cold pressor study. They found pain reports were lower in male participants who were accompanied by female experimenters. There have been further attempts to examine these sex of experimenter effects, although mixed results are reported. For example, Kallai et al. (2004) found opposite-sex experimenter effects in both male and female participants, whereas others report opposite-sex effects may be more reliable in males than females (Aslaksen, Myrbakk, Hoifodt, & Flaten, 2007; Gijsbers & Nicholson, 2005). However, there are also failures to find sex-experimenter effects, and other inconsistent patterns (Vigil, Rowell, Alcock, & Maestes, 2014; Weisse, Foster, & Fisher, 2005).

Other types of male–female observer effects have also been examined (Edwards, Eccleston, & Keogh, 2017; Gougeon, Gaumond, Goffaux, Potvin, & Marchand,

2016; Jackson, Iezzi, Chen, Ebnet, & Eglitis, 2005; McClelland & McCubbin, 2008). Some have looked at whether the sex of a stranger-observer affects pain. For example, one study varied the sex of a virtual stranger, by presenting different audio-visual stimuli while participants engaged in a pain task (Vigil, Torres, Wolff, & Hughes, 2014). They found that pain reports were higher when male participants were presented with opposite sex stimuli—with no such effect found among females. In another study, Jackson et al. (2005) found that the type of interpersonal transactions that occurs between dyads is important, with distraction and encouragement found to be more likely to affect the pain responses of females, rather than males.

Some studies have examined different types of interpersonal relationships in dyadic interactions. For example, in an experimental pain study on healthy adults, McClelland and McCubbin (2008) found that female participants reported more pain when accompanied by a same-sex friend. In a series of experiments, Edwards et al. (2017) systematically considered the effect that same and opposite sex friends had on participant's cold pressor pain reports. They found that males were less likely to report pain (higher tolerance) when accompanied by a same-sex friend. Interestingly, no observer sex difference effect was found when participants were accompanied by an opposite-sex friend or a romantic partner.

Together these studies suggest that not only is the sex congruence of the dyad relevant to how experimental pain is reported, but that the nature (social context) of the relationship between those involved in a painful event may be relevant as well.

Parent–Child Interactions

The nature of the relationship among those involved in interpersonal interactions has also been examined within families, and in particular within parent–child dyads. Here it is possible to look at whether parents view their child's pain in a sex-specific way (Goodenough et al., 1999; Heden, von Essen, & Ljungman, 2016; Moon et al., 2008). For example, Moon et al. (2008) found that mothers rated the cold pressor pain responses of sons and daughters in a similar way, whereas fathers rated their sons as being in more pain than their daughters. However, in a study looking at needle pain, Goodenough et al. (1999) found that the concordance between child and parental ratings was high, and did not differ by sex of child. Interestingly, this study did find a general sex effect in that the difference between unpleasantness and pain intensity scores was greater in girls than boys.

As well as estimating a child's pain, there have been investigations into whether the sex of parents affects how they behave towards a child in pain (Goubert, Vervoort, De Ruddere, & Crombez, 2012; Vervoort, Huguet, Verhoeven, & Goubert, 2011). Vervoort et al. (2011) found that parental behaviors around pain were related to children's pain outcomes in a sex-specific way. For fathers, the degree of solicitous pain behavior was found to be related to child pain catastrophizing, whereas in mothers, it was parental discouragement that was related. In addition, the link between a child's level of catastrophizing and their pain-related disability depended on the level of solicitous behavior in fathers. In another study, Goubert et al. (2012) used a vignette approach where they asked mothers and fathers to imagine their child in pain, and what they would do in response. Similar levels of solicitousness were reported by mothers and fathers, but fathers reported that they were more likely to engage in discouraging responses. There was also a suggestion that among fathers, their levels of catastrophizing were related to such responses. Others have shown that both the mother's and father's levels of pain catastrophizing may be related to their child's pain, but in different ways (Hechler et al., 2011).

Given these parent-related findings, a question that arises is why such attitudes and behaviors affect a child's pain. One line of research has been to investigate the effect of parents as models for pain behaviors, and whether this differentially affects boys and girls (Boerner, Chambers, McGrath, LoLordo, & Uher, 2017; Goodman & McGrath, 2003; Tsao et al., 2006). In one of the only studies to consider *both*, the sex of the parent *and* sex of the child to examine social modelling effects has on pain behaviors, Boerner, Chambers, et al. (2017) recruited children aged between 6 and 8 years into a cold pressor task. They asked parents to either exaggerate or mini-mize their pain responses, while their child watched. Interestingly, when the child completed the cold pressor task, girls were found to report higher pain intensity levels than boys when they had seen their parent exaggerate their pain response. This study suggest that social modelling around pain may indeed have sex-specific effects, with girls being more sensitive (or more willing) to respond to others exag-gerated pain responses.

What the above section indicates is that, although there certainly seem to be sex-related influences that affect both parental and child pain behaviors, there are also inconsistencies in what is found. This means that it is difficult to draw any specific conclusions about the precise direction of sex-related effects in parent–child inter-actions at present.

Dyadic Interactions between Spouses

Another way of examining family-based interactions has been to focus on spousal social support around pain (Cano, Barterian, & Heller, 2008; Cano, Johansen, & Franz, 2005; Romano et al., 1995). Some studies have looked at the behavioral pat-terns that spouses exhibit when interacting with patients in pain, with some also considering this in a sex-specific way (Fillingim, Doleys, Edwards, & Lowery, 2003; Leong, Cano, & Johansent, 2011; Newton-John & Williams, 2006; Romano, Turner, & Clancy, 1989; Smith, Keefe, Caldwell, Romano, & Baucom, 2004). For example, Fillingim et al. (2003) found that solicitous behaviors in spouses were related to pain outcomes in male and female patients, but in different ways. Higher levels of spousal solicitous behavior were related to more self-reported pain and disability in men, whereas it was more closely related to lower tolerance, interfer-ence and high opioid medication usage in women. In another study, Newton-John and Williams (2006) found that male spouses were more likely to report engaging in solicitous behaviors. Others have looked at behavioral activity levels. For example, Smith et al. (2004) asked 50 chronic pain patients to engage in various household tasks, and observed the spousal support behaviors, and found wives were more likely to engage in facilitative behaviors than husbands.

The perceived nature of the relationship a patient has with their spouse has also been considered. For example, Romano et al. (1989) found that among women there was a stronger relationship between their emotional (negative) well-being and perceived level of dysfunction in the spouse. However, in the Newton-John and Williams (2006) study reported above, they did not find any differences in overall relationship satisfaction. Others have look at different interpersonal factors, including empathy and anger, to see what role these experiences might play in pain (Burns, Johnson, Mahoney, Devine, & Pawl, 1996; Gougeon et al., 2016). For example, Gougeon et al. (2016) asked males and females to watch a video of either themselves or a spouse in pain, while also engaging in a pain induction task. They found that pain inhibition was related to higher levels of empathy in women when compared to men.

Together, these investigations not only suggests that spousal interactions are relevant but that how patients perceived the support provided by their partners, as well as how patients perceived their spouse's well-being, can play a role in pain and pain-related disability.

Dyadic Interactions between Healthcare Professional and Patients

Good patient–doctor interactions are important for healthcare, and both the type and amount of communication can vary by sex of physician (Jefferson, Bloor, Birks, Hewitt, & Bland, 2013; Roter & Hall, 2004; Sandhu, Adams, Singleton, Clark-Carter, & Kidd, 2009). For example, some have found female physicians take a more patient-focused approach, spending longer communicating with patients, and especially within same-sex dyadic interactions. Sex-related differences in dyadic patient–doctor interactions have also been considered within the specific context of pain (Chen et al., 2008; Deepmala, Franz, Aponte, Agrawal, & Jiang, 2013; Raftery, Smithcoggins, & Ghen, 1995; Safdar et al., 2009; Vigil & Alcock, 2014; Weisse, Sorum, & Dominguez, 2003). For example, Vigil and Alcock (2014) looked at patient records and found that when pain intensity was reported to be high, both male and female patients reported higher levels of pain to female health practitioners.

Others have looked at whether there are physician sex differences in treatment choices around pain. For example, Raftery et al. (1995) found that female patients receive more medications, including stronger analgesics. Female physicians have also been found to prescribe more pharmacological treatments (Veldhuijzen et al., 2013). However, results are mixed, in that some report a same-sex bias in both female and male practitioners (Safdar et al., 2009), whereas others fail to find differences (Uri, Elias, Behrbalk, & Halpern, 2015). In an attempt to collate this work, Deepmala et al. (2013) conducted a systematic review, and concluded that sex-related factors do play a role in prescription trends. For example, female providers were found to be more conservative in the prescription of opioids, although other fairly complex results were found. These authors speculated that a greater awareness of female vulnerability to pain, especially by female physicians, may play a role in these prescription differences.

Analogue studies allow for the careful control of patient information, and an opportunity to consider how patient's sex influences how observers rate another person's pain (Bernardes, Costa, & Carvalho, 2013; Hirsh, Alqudah, Stutts, & Robinson, 2008; Hirsh, Hollingshead, Matthias, Bair, & Kroenke, 2014; Robinson & Wise, 2003; Schafer, Prkachin, Kaseweter, & Williams, 2016; Torres et al., 2013; Wandner et al., 2013). For example, Bernardes et al. (2013) conducted a vignette study with general practitioners and found males placed greater emphasis on evidence of pathology when making treatment referrals for psychological treatments. Some have used virtual patients, looking at whether the sex of the patient affects healthcare decisions, despite presenting identical information about pain. Hirsh et al. (2008) found that irrespective of the judge's sex, virtual female patients were judged to be in more pain and worse at coping with pain. When Schafer et al. (2016) asked medical students to view virtual male and female patients presenting with identical nonverbal pain signals and contextual information, female patients were judged to have less pain, and more likely to exaggerate it, especially if also perceived to be low in trustworthiness. Male patients were more likely to be "prescribed" analgesics, whereas females were more likely to be considered for psychological interventions.

Like the previous section on sex-related effects in parent–child interactions, it is also difficult to draw specific conclusions around the role sex has on the interpersonal interactions between patients and healthcare providers. One effect that does seem to be emerging, however, is the tendency for the pain of female patients to be rated in a more negative manner than that of male patients by healthcare professionals, even when the information presented is essentially the same. Better understanding about these sex-related biases, and the potential effects they have on treatment is warranted.

The Sex and Gender Context of Pain: Psychosocial Mechanisms

Given sex and gender are likely interpersonal and contextual factors that influence the experience of pain, a key question to ask is why this might happen and what the core mechanisms for such an effect might be. This section will consider two interrelated areas. The first focuses on gender-based beliefs and expectations about pain, whereas the second considers how sex and gender impacts on how individuals express and communicate pain.

Gender-based Beliefs about Pain

Research into gender identity and gender-based beliefs helps provide a better understanding as to why sex and gender impact on pain. As outlined above, a person's gender identity not only influences the beliefs and expectations we have about our own pain and how it is expressed, but also how we view the pain of others. Such beliefs, in turn, are thought to impact on how we behave when we are in pain, and how we behave in the pain-related interactions we have with other people.

Investigations into gender-based beliefs confirm that there are some pain-related behaviors which are more closely associated with being male or female (Bernardes, Silva, Carvalho, Costa, & Pereira, 2014; Robinson et al., 2001). Men are perceived to be stoic when they are in pain, less likely to ask for help, and generally take an avoidant approach, whereas women are viewed as more emotionally expressive and willing to seek help around health issues. Certain types of pain and pain coping behaviors are also thought to be more typical of men and women (Bernardes et al., 2014; Keogh & Denford, 2009). Bernardes et al. (2014) found that when adults were asked to freely associate around sex-typical pain, musculoskeletal pain was associated with men, whereas a wider range of pains were associated with women e.g., headache, abdominal/back pain, and pain related to reproductive systems. Similarly, stereotypical beliefs about the type of pain coping strategies that men and women employ exist. For example, Keogh and Denford (2009) found that men were viewed as being more likely to engage in distraction, whereas women more likely to catastrophize. There are also gender-related judgments that people placed on those who express pain, with pain behaviors being rated as more acceptable when displayed by women than men (Hobara, 2005).

Given the existence of stereotypical gender-based beliefs about pain and pain behaviors, a related question to ask is whether gender traits affect actual pain experiences (Alabas, Tashani, Tabasam, & Johnson, 2012; Racine et al., 2012b). A systematic review by Alabas et al. (2012) concluded that individuals who report higher levels of masculinity, or indicate they are less sensitive to pain when compared to the typical man, were found to show reduced sensitivity to experimental pain, i.e., higher pain threshold and tolerance.

As well as one's own pain experiences, gender-based beliefs also seem to affect how we view others when they are in pain. For example, gender-role expectations about pain endurance have been found to predict how observers viewed another person's pain (Robinson & Wise, 2003). Others have looked at the flexibility of gender, viewing it as a more fluid construct that changes (Bernardes et al., 2008; Keogh, 2015; West & Zimmerman, 1987). For example, experimental instructions around gender-role expectations have been found to moderate observable sex differences in pain (Fowler, Rasinski, Geers, Helfer, & France, 2011; Robinson, Gagnon, Riley, & Price, 2003). One recent study used a manipulation to threaten gender roles, and found this increased men's experimental pain tolerance levels (Berke, Reidy, Miller, & Zeichner, 2017).

The reciprocal relationship between pain and gender has also been considered, and in particular whether pain can affect gender identity (Keogh, 2015). Here it has been reported that males with chronic pain conditions can report a loss of gender identity, which some have taken to suggest that pain may have a "demasculinizing" effect (Ahlsen, Bondevik, Mengshoel, & Solbraekke, 2014; Paulson, Danielson, & Norberg, 1999). Interestingly, it also seems that prior knowledge of a pain state can affect how observers perceived the gender identity of another person (Bernardes & Lima, 2010, 2011).

Clearly, gender roles, beliefs and expectations play an important role in helping to understand and explain how and why social factors have an impact on the variation that can be found between men and women in the perception and experience of pain.

Nonverbal Pain Communication

A second approach that could help us better understand social factors in male–female variation in pain is to focus on how men and women communicate pain. As we have already seen there may be sex-related biases in how pain is interpreted and responded to, which may stem from differences in how pain signals are encoded and/or decoded (Keogh, 2015). Much of the work described in the previous sections of this chapter has relied on verbal descriptors of pain. However, pain is communicated through a combination of both verbal and nonverbal processes (Craig, 2009; Hadjistavropoulos et al., 2011), and so nonverbal signals are also relevant. There are a range of nonverbal signals that people can use to communicate pain to others, include facial expressions (grimaces), vocalizations (groaning), and bodily posture/movements (guarding). However, most studies focus on facial expressions.

A question to ask is whether there are sex and gender differences in the way in which facial expression of pain expressions are transmitted or encoded. For example, are there differences in the basic signals that are used to communicate pain between men and women? There certainly seem to be unique facial codes that are specific to pain, and that contextual factors can impact on its encoding (Craig & Patrick, 1985; Prkachin, 1992a, 1992b, 2005; Vlaeyen et al., 2009). We also know that there may be general sex differences in the encoding of emotional expressions (Hall, 2006; Keogh, 2014). Females are typically more expressive, or willing to display, a range of emotional expressions when compared to men. A good example, is smiling, where females are more likely to smile compared to men (LaFrance, Hecht, & Levy Paluck, 2003), and that social context plays a moderating role. However, when it comes to the cues associated with the encoding of pain-related expressions, few studies are directly designed to consider sex differences. Of those studies conducted, most do not find male–female differences, and in the few that do, inconsistent effects are reported (Craig, Hyde, & Patrick, 1991; Kunz, Gruber, & Lautenbacher, 2006; Prkachin & Solomon, 2009; Simon, Craig, Gosselin, Belin, & Rainville, 2008). This is somewhat surprising given the cognate evidence from emotional expression research, where we might expect a sex difference in pain encoding to emerge. Therefore, the best that we can currently say is that there is a lack of consistent evidence for sex differences in the encoding of pain through facial expression cues.

Although there are inconsistent effects associated with pain encoding, they may of course be differences in how facial expressions of pain are detected or recognized by others. This is particularly important in the context of interpersonal interactions such as caregiving, where it is important to be able to appropriately recognize and act on another personal pain. Like encoding studies, there is a large body of evidence that has considered sex differences in the decoding of non-pain expressions. Again, the general pattern that emerges is that females show a general recognition advantage for emotional expressions (Hall & Matsumoto, 2004; McClure, 2000). In terms of pain expression recognition, there are again somewhat mixed results. However, there are some studies where sex differences have been found (Hirsh et al., 2008; Moon et al., 2008; Prkachin, 2005; Riva, Sacchi, Montali, & Frigerio, 2011; Simon et al., 2008; Vervoort, Goubert, & Crombez, 2009). For example, Prkachin et al. (2004) reports a study in which women were found to be more sensitive to facial pain cues. In a second study, Hirsh et al. (2008) presented virtual patients expressing pain, who varied in terms of their sex. Female faces were rated as having greater levels of pain by both male and female observers. However, there are also examples of studies where sex differences have not been found, and few studies have considered gender-related factors in nonverbal pain communication.

Even so, a nonverbal communication approach to pain would certainly seem to provide a useful framework from which to consider how men and women may differ in pain (Keogh, 2014). There are also well-developed methods that could translate to novel investigations of sex differences, including the role of other channels of nonverbal communication, such as vocalizations and body movements (Walsh, Eccleston, & Keogh, 2014).

Summary and Conclusions

This chapter considers the roles that sex and gender have as social contextual factors in pain. Both factors can affect the way in which an individual behaves when in pain, as well as how observers interact with someone in pain. This has particular relevance when we consider the many social interactions that patients have, including friends, family, coworkers, and healthcare professionals.

A central theme within this chapter has been the notion of gender, and how beliefs and expectations around masculinity and femininity impact on pain, and play a role in interpersonal interactions. This approach also highlights that gender-based beliefs and attitudes are potentially malleable and context dependent, which means they provide an opportunity for intervention. This is particularly relevant when considering the way in which gender beliefs might affect how carers judge and respond to someone in pain. This approach also enables us to think about pain in new and novel ways.

An interesting, yet largely unexplored avenue of work could be to consider whether interpersonal interactions and contexts around pain are themselves "gendered." For example, men are less well represented in self-management support interventions for long-term conditions, and it may be that this could be improved by designing interventions in a gender-relevant way (Flurey et al., 2017; Galdas et al., 2014). The "men's shed" approach is a good example of where this approach has been successfully used, and it would be interesting to see if this could be used within the context of pain also.

In conclusion, a sex and gender approach to pain is not only relevant to those with interests in social factors, but also informs those investigating the role of sex and gender as to the relevance of social contextual and interpersonal factors to better understand male–female variation in pain and analgesia.

References

Ahlsen, B., Bondevik, H., Mengshoel, A. M., & Solbraekke, K. N. (2014). (Un)doing gender in a rehabilitation context: A narrative analysis of gender and self in stories of chronic muscle pain. *Disability and Rehabilitation, 36*(5), 359–366.

Alabas, O. A., Tashani, O. A., Tabasam, G., & Johnson, M. I. (2012). Gender role affects experimental pain responses: A systematic review with meta-analysis. *European Journal of Pain, 16*(9), 1211–1223.

Antonov, K. I., & Isacson, D. G. (1998). Prescription and nonprescription analgesic use in Sweden. *Annals of Pharmacotherapy, 32*(4), 485–494.

Aslaksen, P. M., Myrbakk, I. N., Hoifodt, R. S., & Flaten, M. A. (2007). The effect of experimenter gender on autonomic and subjective responses to pain stimuli. *Pain, 129*(3), 260–268.

Berke, D. S., Reidy, D. E., Miller, J. D., & Zeichner, A. (2017). Take it like a man: Gender-rhreatened men's experience of gender role discrepancy, emotion activation, and pain tolerance. *Psychology of Men & Masculinity, 18*(1), 62–69.

Berkley, K. J. (1997). Sex differences in pain. *Behavioral & Brain Sciences, 20*(3), 371–380.

Bernardes, S. F., Costa, M., & Carvalho, H. (2013). Engendering pain management practices: The role of physician sex on chronic low-back pain assessment and treatment prescriptions. *The Journal of Pain, 14*(9), 931–940.

Bernardes, S. F., Keogh, E., & Lima, M. L. (2008). Bridging the gap between pain and gender research: A selective literature review. *European Journal of Pain, 12*(4), 427–440.

Bernardes, S. F., & Lima, M. L. (2010). Being less of a man or less of a woman: Perceptions of chronic pain patients' gender identities. *European Journal of Pain, 14*(2), 194–199.

Bernardes, S. F., & Lima, M. L. (2011). On the contextual nature of sex-related biases in pain judgments: The effects of pain duration, patient's distress and judge's sex. *European Journal of Pain, 15*(9), 950–957.

Bernardes, S. F., Silva, S. A., Carvalho, H., Costa, M., & Pereira, S. (2014). Is it a (fe) male pain? Portuguese nurses' and laypeople's gendered representations of common pains. *European Journal of Pain, 18*(4), 530–539.

Boerner, K. E., Birnie, K. A., Caes, L., Schinkel, M., & Chambers, C. T. (2014). Sex differences in experimental pain among healthy children: A systematic review and meta-analysis. *Pain, 155*(5), 983–993.

Boerner, K. E., Chambers, C. T., McGrath, P. J., LoLordo, V., & Uher, R. (2017). The impact of parental modeling on child pain responses: The role of parent and child sex. *The Journal of Pain, 18*(6), 702–715.

Boerner, K. E., Eccleston, C., Chambers, C. T., & Keogh, E. (2017). Sex differences in the efficacy of psychological therapies for the management of chronic and recurrent pain in children and adolescents: A systematic review and meta-analysis. *Pain, 158*(4), 569–582.

Burns, J. W., Johnson, B. J., Mahoney, N., Devine, J., & Pawl, R. (1996). Anger management style, hostility and spouse responses: Gender differences in predictors of adjustment among chronic pain patients. *Pain, 64*(3), 445–453.

Bussey, K., & Bandura, A. (1999). Social cognitive theory of gender development and differentiation. *Psychological Review, 106*(4), 676–713.

Butcher, B. E., & Carmody, J. J. (2012). Sex differences in analgesic response to ibuprofen are influenced by expectancy: A randomized, crossover, balanced placebo-designed study. *European Journal of Pain, 16*(7), 1005–1013.

Cano, A., Barterian, J. A., & Heller, J. B. (2008). Empathic and nonempathic interaction in chronic pain couples. *Clinical Journal of Pain, 24*(8), 678–684.

Cano, A., Johansen, A. B., & Franz, A. (2005). Multilevel analysis of couple congruence on pain, interference, and disability. *Pain, 118*(3), 369–379.

Chen, E. H., Shofer, F. S., Dean, A. J., Hollander, J. E., Baxt, W. G., Robey, J. L., et al. (2008). Gender disparity in analgesic treatment of emergency department patients with acute abdominal pain. *Academic Emergency Medicine, 15*(5), 414–418.

Chin, M. L., Fillingim, R. B., & Ness, T. J. (Eds.). (2013). *Pain in women.* Oxford: Oxford University Press.

Ciccone, G. K., & Holdcroft, A. (1999). Drugs and sex differences: A review of drugs relating to anaesthesia. *British Journal of Anaesthesia, 82*(2), 255–265.

Craft, R. M., Mogil, J. S., & Aloisi, A. M. (2004). Sex differences in pain and analgesia: The role of gonadal hormones. *European Journal of Pain, 8*(5), 397–411.

Craig, K. D. (2009). The social communication model of pain. *Canadian Psychology, 50*(1), 22–32.

Craig, K. D., Hyde, S. A., & Patrick, C. J. (1991). Genuine, suppressed and faked facial behavior during exacerbation of chronic low back pain. *Pain, 46*(2), 161–171.

Craig, K. D., & Patrick, C. J. (1985). Facial expression during induced pain. *Journal of Personality and Social Psychology, 48*(4), 1080–1091.

DALYs, G. B. D., & Collaborators, H. (2016). Global, regional, and national disability-adjusted life-years (DALYs) for 315 diseases and injuries and healthy life expectancy (HALE), 1990–2015: A systematic analysis for the Global Burden of Disease Study 2015. *Lancet, 388*(10053), 1603–1658.

Deepmala, D., Franz, L., Aponte, C., Agrawal, M., & Jiang, W. (2013). Identification of provider characteristics influencing prescription of analgesics: A systematic literature review. *Pain Practice, 13*(6), 504–513.

Edwards, R., Eccleston, C., & Keogh, E. (2017). Observer influences on pain: An experimental series examining same-sex and opposite-sex friends, strangers, and romantic partners. *Pain, 158*(5), 846–855.

Fayaz, A., Croft, P., Langford, R. M., Donaldson, L. J., & Jones, G. T. (2016). Prevalence of chronic pain in the UK: A systematic review and meta-analysis of population studies. *BMJ Open, 6*(6), e010364.

Fillingim, R. B. (2017). Individual differences in pain: Understanding the mosaic that makes pain personal. *Pain, 158*(Suppl 1), S11–S18.

Fillingim, R. B., Doleys, D. M., Edwards, R. R., & Lowery, D. (2003). Spousal responses are differentially associated with clinical variables in women and men with chronic pain. *Clinical Journal of Pain, 19*(4), 217–224.

Fillingim, R. B., Kaplan, L., Staud, R., Ness, T. J., Glover, T. L., Campbell, C. M., et al. (2005). The A118G single nucleotide polymorphism of the mu-opioid receptor gene (OPRM1) is associated with pressure pain sensitivity in humans. *The Journal of Pain, 6*(3), 159–167.

Fillingim, R. B., King, C. D., Ribeiro-Dasilva, M. C., Rahim-Williams, B., & Riley, J. L., 3rd. (2009). Sex, gender, and pain: A review of recent clinical and experimental findings. *The Journal of Pain, 10*(5), 447–485.

Flurey, C. A., Hewlett, S., Rodham, K., White, A., Noddings, R., & Kirwan, J. R. (2017). "You obviously just have to put on a brave face": A qualitative study of the experiences and coping styles of men with rheumatoid arthritis. *Arthritis Care & Research, 69*(3), 330–337.

Fowler, S. L., Rasinski, H. M., Geers, A. L., Helfer, S. G., & France, C. R. (2011). Concept priming and pain: An experimental approach to understanding gender roles in sex-related pain differences. *Journal of Behavioral Medicine, 34*(2), 139–147.

Galdas, P., Darwin, Z., Kidd, L., Blickem, C., McPherson, K., Hunt, K., ... Richardson, G. (2014). The accessibility and acceptability of self-management support interventions for men with long term conditions: A systematic review and meta-synthesis of qualitative studies. *BMC Public Health, 14*, 1230.

Gijsbers, K., & Nicholson, F. (2005). Experimental pain thresholds influenced by sex of experimenter. *Perceptual and Motor Skills, 101*(3), 803–807.

Goodenough, B., Thomas, W., Champion, G. D., Perrott, D., Taplin, J. E., von Baeyer, C. L., et al. (1999). Unravelling age effects and sex differences in needle pain: Ratings of sensory intensity and unpleasantness of venipuncture pain by children and their parents. *Pain, 80*(1–2), 179–190.

Goodman, J. E., & McGrath, P. J. (2003). Mothers' modeling influences children's pain during a cold pressor task. *Pain, 104*(3), 559–565.

Goubert, L., Vervoort, T., De Ruddere, L., & Crombez, G. (2012). The impact of parental gender, catastrophizing and situational threat upon parental behaviour to child pain: A vignette study. *European Journal of Pain, 16*(8), 1176–1184.

Gougeon, V., Gaumond, I., Goffaux, P., Potvin, S., & Marchand, S. (2016). Triggering descending pain inhibition by observing ourselves or a loved-one in pain. *Clinical Journal of Pain, 32*(3), 238–245.

Gupta, A., Mayer, E. A., Fling, C., Labus, J. S., Naliboff, B. D., Hong, J. Y., et al. (2017). Sex-based differences in brain alterations across chronic pain conditions. *Journal of Neuroscience Research, 95*(1–2), 604–616.

Hadjistavropoulos, T., Craig, K. D., Duck, S., Cano, A., Goubert, L., Jackson, P. L., et al. (2011). A biopsychosocial formulation of pain communication. *Psychological Bulletin, 137*(6), 910–939.

Hall, J. A. (2006). Women's and men's nonverbal communication: Similarities, differences, stereotypes, and origins. In V. Manusov & M. L. Patterson (Eds.), *The SAGE handbook of nonverbal communication* (pp. 208–218). London: Sage Publishers.

Hall, J. A., & Matsumoto, D. (2004). Gender differences in judgments of multiple emotions from facial expressions. *Emotion, 4*(2), 201–206.

Hargreave, M., Andersen, T. V., Nielsen, A., Munk, C., Liaw, K. L., & Kjaer, S. K. (2010). Factors associated with a continuous regular analgesic use-a population-based study of more than 45,000 Danish women and men 18–45 years of age. *Pharmacoepidemiology and Drug Safety, 19*(1), 65–74.

Hazes, J. M. (1991). Pregnancy and its effect on the risk of developing rheumatoid arthritis. *Annals of the Rheumatic Diseases, 50*(2), 71–72.

Hechler, T., Vervoort, T., Hamann, M., Tietze, A. L., Vocks, S., Goubert, L., Hermann, C., Wager, J., Blankenburg, M., Schroeder, S., & Zernikow, B. (2011). Parental catastrophizing about their child's chronic pain: Are mothers and fathers different? *European Journal of Pain, 15*(5), e1–e9.

Heden, L., von Essen, L., & Ljungman, G. (2016). The relationship between fear and pain levels during needle procedures in children from the parents' perspective. *European Journal of Pain, 20*(2), 223–230.

Hirsh, A. T., Alqudah, A. F., Stutts, L. A., & Robinson, M. E. (2008). Virtual human technology: Capturing sex, race, and age influences in individual pain decision policies. *Pain, 140*(1), 231–238.

Hirsh, A. T., Hollingshead, N. A., Matthias, M. S., Bair, M. J., & Kroenke, K. (2014). The influence of patient sex, provider sex, and sexist attitudes on pain treatment decisions. *The Journal of Pain, 15*(5), 551–559.

Hobara, M. (2005). Beliefs about appropriate pain behavior: Cross-cultural and sex differences between Japanese and Euro-Americans. *European Journal of Pain, 9*(4), 389–393.

Jackson, T., Iezzi, T., Chen, H., Ebnet, S., & Eglitis, K. (2005). Gender, interpersonal transactions, and the perception of pain: An experimental analysis. *The Journal of Pain, 6*(4), 228–236.

Jefferson, L., Bloor, K., Birks, Y., Hewitt, C., & Bland, M. (2013). Effect of physicians' gender on communication and consultation length: A systematic review and meta-analysis. *Journal of Health Services Research & Policy, 18*(4), 242–248.

Jensen, I. B., Bergstrom, G., Ljungquist, T., Bodin, L., & Nygren, A. L. (2001). A randomized controlled component analysis of a behavioral medicine rehabilitation program for chronic spinal pain: Are the effects dependent on gender? *Pain, 91*(1–2), 65–78.

Johannes, C. B., Le, T. K., Zhou, X. L., Johnston, J. A., & Dworkin, R. H. (2010). The prevalence of chronic pain in United States adults: Results of an internet-based survey. *The Journal of Pain, 11*(11), 1230–1239.

Kallai, I., Barke, A., & Voss, U. (2004). The effects of experimenter characteristics on pain reports in women and men. *Pain, 112*(1–2), 142–147.

Kennedy, J., Roll, J. M., Schraudner, T., Murphy, S., & McPherson, S. (2014). Prevalence of persistent pain in the US adult population: New data from the 2010 National Health Interview Survey. *The Journal of Pain, 15*(10), 979–984.

Keogh, E. (2013). Role of psychosocial factors and psychological interventions. In M. L. Chin, R. B. Fillingim, & T. J. Ness (Eds.), *Pain in women* (pp. 94–105). Oxford: Oxford University Press.

Keogh, E. (2014). Gender differences in the nonverbal communication of pain: A new direction for sex, gender, and pain research? *Pain, 155*(10), 1927–1931.

Keogh, E. (2015). Men, masculinity, and pain. *Pain, 156*(12), 2408–2412.

Keogh, E., & Denford, S. (2009). Sex differences in perceptions of pain coping strategy usage. *European Journal of Pain, 13*(6), 629–634.

Keogh, E., McCracken, L. M., & Eccleston, C. (2005). Do men and women differ in their response to interdisciplinary chronic pain management? *Pain, 114*(1–2), 37–46.

Kunz, M., Gruber, A., & Lautenbacher, S. (2006). Sex differences in facial encoding of pain. *The Journal of Pain, 7*(12), 915–928.

LaFrance, M., Hecht, M. A., & Levy Paluck, E. (2003). The contingent smile: A meta-analysis of sex differences in smiling. *Psychological Bulletin, 129*(2), 305–334.

Leong, L. E. M., Cano, A., & Johansent, A. B. (2011). Sequential and base rate analysis of emotional validation and invalidation in chronic pain couples: Patient gender matters. *The Journal of Pain, 12*(11), 1140–1148.

LeResche, L. (1999). Gender considerations in the epidemiology of chronic pain. In I. K. Crombie, P. R. Croft, S. J. Linton, L. LeResche, & M. Von Korff (Eds.), *Epidemiology of pain* (pp. 43–52). Seattle: IASP Press.

LeResche, L. (2013). Epidemiology of pain conditions with higher prevalence in women. In C. Chin, R. B. Fillingim, & T. J. Ness (Eds.), *Pain in women* (pp. 3–15). Oxford: Oxford University Press.

LeResche, L., Mancl, L., Sherman, J. J., Gandara, B., & Dworkin, S. F. (2003). Changes in temporomandibular pain and other symptoms across the menstrual cycle. *Pain, 106*(3), 253–261.

Levine, F. M., & Desimone, L. L. (1991). The effects of experimenter gender on pain report in male and female subjects. *Pain, 44*(1), 69–72.

McClelland, L. E., & McCubbin, J. A. (2008). Social influence and pain response in women and men. *Journal of Behavioral Medicine, 31*(5), 413–420.

McClure, E. B. (2000). A meta-analytic review of sex differences in facial expression processing and their development in infants, children, and adolescents. *Psychological Bulletin, 126*(3), 424–453.

McGeary, D. D., Mayer, T. G., Gatchel, R. J., Anagnostis, C., & Proctor, T. J. (2003). Gender-related differences in treatment outcomes for patients with musculoskeletal disorders. *The Spine Journal, 3*(3), 197–203.

Melchior, M., Poisbeau, P., Gaumond, I., & Marchand, S. (2016). Insights into the mechanisms and the emergence of sex-differences in pain. *Neuroscience, 338*, 63–80.

Mogil, J. S. (2012). Sex differences in pain and pain inhibition: Multiple explanations of a controversial phenomenon. *Nature Reviews Neuroscience, 13*(12), 859–866.

Mogil, J. S., Wilson, S. G., Chesler, E. J., Rankin, A. L., Nemmani, K. V., Lariviere, W. R., et al. (2003). The melanocortin-1 receptor gene mediates female-specific mechanisms of analgesia in mice and humans. *Proceedings of the National Academy of Sciences of the United States of America, 100*(8), 4867–4872.

Moon, E. C., Chambers, C. T., Larochette, A. C., Hayton, K., Craig, K. D., & McGrath, P. J. (2008). Sex differences in parent and child pain ratings during an experimental child pain task. *Pain Research & Management, 13*(3), 225–230.

Muehlenhard, C. L., & Peterson, Z. D. (2011). Distinguishing between sex and gender: History, urrent conceptualizations, and implications. *Sex Roles, 64*(11–12), 791–803.

Newton-John, T. R., & Williams, A. C. (2006). Chronic pain couples: Perceived marital interactions and pain behaviours. *Pain, 123*(1–2), 53–63.

Niesters, M., Dahan, A., Kest, B., Zacny, J., Stijnen, T., Aarts, L., et al. (2010). Do sex differences exist in opioid analgesia? A systematic review and meta-analysis of human experimental and clinical studies. *Pain, 15*(1), 61–68.

Paulson, M., Danielson, E., & Norberg, A. (1999). Nurses' and physicians' narratives about long-term non-malignant pain among men. *Journal of Advanced Nursing, 30*(5), 1097–1105.

Pieh, C., Altmeppen, J., Neumeier, S., Loew, T., Angerer, M., & Lahmann, C. (2012). Gender differences in outcomes of a multimodal pain management program. *Pain, 153*(1), 197–202.

Popescu, A., LeResche, L., Truelove, E. L., & Drangsholt, M. T. (2010). Gender differences in pain modulation by diffuse noxious inhibitory controls: A systematic review. *Pain, 150*(2), 309–318.

Prkachin, K. M. (1992a). The consistency of facial expressions of pain: A comparison across modalities. *Pain, 51*(3), 297–306.

Prkachin, K. M. (1992b). Dissociating spontaneous and deliberate expressions of pain: Signal detection analyses. *Pain, 51*(1), 57–65.

Prkachin, K. M. (2005). Effects of deliberate control on verbal and facial expressions of pain. *Pain, 114*(3), 328–338.

Prkachin, K. M., Mass, H., & Mercer, S. R. (2004). Effects of exposure on perception of pain expression. *Pain, 111*(1–2), 8–12.

Prkachin, K. M., & Solomon, P. E. (2009). The structure, reliability and validity of pain expression: Evidence from patients with shoulder pain. *Pain, 139*(2), 267–274.

Racine, M., Tousignant-Laflamme, Y., Kloda, L. A., Dion, D., Dupuis, G., & Choiniere, M. (2012a). A systematic literature review of 10 years of research on sex/gender and experimental pain perception—Part 1: Are there really differences between women and men? *Pain, 153*(3), 602–618.

Racine, M., Tousignant-Laflamme, Y., Kloda, L. A., Dion, D., Dupuis, G., & Choiniere, M. (2012b). A systematic literature review of 10 years of research on sex/gender and pain perception—Part 2: Do biopsychosocial factors alter pain sensitivity differently in women and men? *Pain, 153*(3), 619–635.

Raftery, K. A., Smithcoggins, R., & Ghen, A. H. (1995). Gender-associated differences in emergency department pain management. *Annals of Emergency Medicine, 26*(4), 414–421.

Ribeiro-Dasilva, M. C., Shinal, R. M., Glover, T., Williams, R. S., Staud, R., Riley, J. L., 3rd, et al. (2011). Evaluation of menstrual cycle effects on morphine and pentazocine analgesia. *Pain, 152*(3), 614–622.

Riley, J. L., Robinson, M. E., Wise, E. A., Myers, C. D., & Fillingim, R. B. (1998). Sex differences in the perception of noxious experimental stimuli: A meta-analysis. *Pain, 74*(2–3), 181–187.

Riley, J. L., Robinson, M. E., Wise, E. A., & Price, D. D. (1999). A meta-analytic review of pain perception across the menstrual cycle. *Pain, 81*(3), 225–235.

Riva, P., Sacchi, S., Montali, L., & Frigerio, A. (2011). Gender effects in pain detection: Speed and accuracy in decoding female and male pain expressions. *European Journal of Pain, 15*(9), 985.e1–985.e11.

Robinson, M. E., Gagnon, C. M., Riley, J. L., & Price, D. D. (2003). Altering gender role expectations: Effects on pain tolerance, pain threshold, and pain ratings. *The Journal of Pain, 4*(5), 284–288.

Robinson, M. E., Riley, J. L., Myers, C. D., Papas, R. K., Wise, E. A., Waxenberg, L. B., et al. (2001). Gender role expectations of pain: Relationship to sex differences in pain. *The Journal of Pain, 2*(5), 251–257.

Robinson, M. E., & Wise, E. A. (2003). Gender bias in the observation of experimental pain. *Pain, 104*(1–2), 259–264.

Romano, J. M., Turner, J. A., & Clancy, S. L. (1989). Sex differences in the relationship of pain patient dysfunction to spouse adjustment. *Pain, 39*(3), 289–295.

Romano, J. M., Turner, J. A., Jensen, M. P., Friedman, L. S., Bulcroft, R. A., Hops, H., et al. (1995). Chronic pain patient-spouse behavioral interactions predict patient disability. *Pain, 63*(3), 353–360.

Rosen, S., Ham, B., & Mogil, J. S. (2017). Sex differences in neuroimmunity and pain. *Journal of Neuroscience Research, 95*(1–2), 500–508.

Roter, D. L., & Hall, J. A. (2004). Physician gender and patient-centered communication: A critical review of empirical research. *Annual Review of Public Health, 25*, 497–519.

Safdar, B., Heins, A., Homel, P., Miner, J., Neighbor, M., DeSandre, P., et al. (2009). Impact of physician and patient gender on pain management in the emergency department: A multicenter study. *Pain Medicine, 10*(2), 364–372.

Sandhu, H., Adams, A., Singleton, L., Clark-Carter, D., & Kidd, J. (2009). The impact of gender dyads on doctor-patient communication: A systematic review. *Patient Education and Counseling, 76*(3), 348–355.

Sarganas, G., Buttery, A. K., Zhuang, W., Wolf, I. K., Grams, D., Rosario, A. S., et al. (2015). Prevalence, trends, patterns and associations of analgesic use in Germany. *BMC Pharmacology & Toxicology, 16*, 28.

Schafer, G., Prkachin, K. M., Kaseweter, K. A., & Williams, A. C. D. (2016). Health care providers' judgments in chronic pain: The influence of gender and trustworthiness. *Pain, 157*(8), 1618–1625.

Sherman, J. J., & LeResche, L. (2006). Does experimental pain response vary across the menstrual cycle? A methodological review. *American Journal of Physiology: Regulatory, Integrative and Comparative Physiology, 291*(2), R245–R256.

Simon, D., Craig, K. D., Gosselin, F., Belin, P., & Rainville, P. (2008). Recognition and discrimination of prototypical dynamic expressions of pain and emotions. *Pain, 135*(1–2), 55–64.

Smith, S. J., Keefe, F. J., Caldwell, D. S., Romano, J., & Baucom, D. (2004). Gender differences in patient-spouse interactions: A sequential analysis of behavioral interactions in patients having osteoarthritic knee pain. *Pain, 112*(1–2), 183–187.

Sorge, R. E., & Totsch, S. K. (2017). Sex differences in pain. *Journal of Neuroscience Research, 95*(6), 1271–1281.

Tighe, P. J., Riley, J. L., & Fillingim, R. B. (2014). Sex differences in the incidence of severe pain events following surgery: A review of 333,000 pain scores. *Pain Medicine, 15*(8), 1390–1404.

Torres, C. A., Bartley, E. J., Wandner, L. D., Alqudah, A. F., Hirsh, A. T., & Robinson, M. E. (2013). The influence of sex, race, and age on pain assessment and treatment decisions using virtual human technology: A cross-national comparison. *Journal of Pain Research, 6*, 577–588.

Tsang, A., Von Korff, M., Lee, S., Alonso, J., Karam, E., Angermeyer, M. C., et al. (2008). Common chronic pain conditions in developed and developing countries: Gender and age differences and comorbidity with depression-anxiety disorders. *The Journal of Pain, 9*(10), 883–891.

Tsao, J. C. I., Lu, Q., Myers, C. D., Kim, S. C., Turk, N., & Zeltzer, L. K. (2006). Parent and child anxiety sensitivity: Relationship to children's experimental pain responsivity. *The Journal of Pain, 7*(5), 319–326.

Unger, R. K. (1979). Toward a redefinition of sex and gender. *American Psychologist, 34*(11), 1085–1094.

Uri, O., Elias, S., Behrbalk, E., & Halpern, P. (2015). No gender-related bias in acute musculo-skeletal pain management in the emergency department. *Emergency Medicine Journal, 32*(2), 149–152.

Veldhuijzen, D. S., Karhof, S., Leenders, M. E., Karsch, A. M., & van Wijck, A. J. (2013). Impact of physicians' sex on treatment choices for low back pain. *Pain Practice, 13*(6), 451–458.

Vervoort, T., Goubert, L., & Crombez, G. (2009). The relationship between high catastrophizing children's facial display of pain and parental judgment of their child's pain. *Pain, 142*(1–2), 142–148.

Vervoort, T., Huguet, A., Verhoeven, K., & Goubert, L. (2011). Mothers' and fathers' responses to their child's pain moderate the relationship between the child's pain catastrophizing and dis-ability. *Pain, 152*(4), 786–793.

Vigil, J. M. (2009). A socio-relational framework of sex differences in the expression of emotion. *Behavioral & Brain Sciences, 32*(5), 375–390.

Vigil, J. M., & Alcock, J. (2014). Tough guys or sensitive guys? Disentangling the role of examiner sex on patient pain reports. *Pain Research & Management, 19*(1), E9–E12.

Vigil, J. M., Rowell, L. N., Alcock, J., & Maestes, R. (2014). Laboratory personnel gender and cold pressor apparatus affect subjective pain reports. *Pain Research & Management, 19*(1), E13–E18.

Vigil, J. M., Torres, D., Wolff, A., & Hughes, K. (2014). Exposure to virtual social stimuli modu-lates subjective pain reports. *Pain Research & Management, 19*(4), E103–E108.

Vlaeyen, J. W., Hanssen, M., Goubert, L., Vervoort, T., Peters, M., van Breukelen, G., et al. (2009). Threat of pain influences social context effects on verbal pain report and facial expression. *Behaviour Research and Therapy, 47*(9), 774–782.

Walsh, J., Eccleston, C., & Keogh, E. (2014). Pain communication through body posture: The development and validation of a stimulus set. *Pain, 155*(11), 2282–2290.

Wandner, L. D., George, S. Z., Lok, B. C., Torres, C. A., Chuah, J. H., & Robinson, M. E. (2013). Pain assessment and treatment decisions for virtual human patients. *Cyberpsychology Behavior and Social Networking, 16*(12), 904–909.

Weir, R., Browne, G., Tunks, E., Gafni, A., & Roberts, J. (1996). Gender differences in psychoso-cial adjustment to chronic pain and expenditures for health care services used. *Clinical Journal of Pain, 12*(4), 277–290.

Weisse, C. S., Foster, K. K., & Fisher, E. A. (2005). The influence of experimenter gender and race on pain reporting: Does racial or gender concordance matter? *Pain Medicine, 6*(1), 80–87.

Weisse, C. S., Sorum, P. C., & Dominguez, R. E. (2003). The influence of gender and race on physicians' pain management decisions. *The Journal of Pain, 4*(9), 505–510.

West, C., & Zimmerman, D. H. (1987). Doing gender. *Gender & Society, 1*(2), 125–151.

Chapter 21
Race and Pain: A Dual Injustice

Brian Blake Drwecki

Abstract The evidence presented in this chapter highlights the existence of a dual injustice—members of nondominant racial groups are more than likely to experience pain, while these same individuals are also more than likely to have their pain discounted by and undertreated by healthcare professionals. Evidence is presented from numerous national, racial, and ethnic contexts, and this chapter utilizes evidence that crosses historical, social, psychological, biological, and medical research. The antecedents, consequences, causes, and potential solutions to this dual injustice are examined and discussed with the recognition that the literal pain and suffering of people of color is at stake.

Keywords Race · Pain · Psychology · Medical decision-making · Racial injustice · Racial oppression · Racism · Empathy · Genetics · Culture

Pain and race have many attributes in common. They are difficult to define and somewhat subjective, but the experiences of both are real, tangible, and sometimes life changing. Both can impact one's life in ways that individuals without these experiences find difficult to fathom and understand. In its most noble pursuit, science attempts to unravel truths in an effort to improve humanity. When the relationship between race and pain are examined scientifically, it becomes clear that these two elusive concepts weave a tangled web that impacts the lives of numerous individuals across the globe and highlights how the concept of race is inextricably linked to the experience of pain.

An examination of societies across the globe indicates marked privileges for racial and ethnic groups considered, for the most part, White, while people of color and members of historically marginalized racial groups live lives where oppression is omnipresent. Research across numerous fields, nations, and interracial contexts unpacks the pervasiveness of these privileges and disadvantages, not only in an America but also in numerous global contexts. For example, membership in a

B. B. Drwecki (✉)
Regis University, Denver, CO, USA
e-mail: bdrwecki@regis.edu

marginalized racial group is associated with (1) mortality disparities in ethnic minorities in Estonia (Baburin, Lai, & Leinsalu, 2011), Maori in New Zealand (Bramley, Hebert, Jackson, & Chassin, 2004), Indigenous people of Australia (Bramley et al., 2004), American Indians in America's pacific northwest (Dankovchik, Hoopes, Warren-Mears, & Knaster, 2015), Native Alaskans in Alaska (Dankovchik et al., 2015), South African Black populations (Jinabhai, Coovadia, & Abdool-Karim, 1986), Black populations in America (Kochanek, Arias, & Anderson, 2013), Roma in Slovakia (Rosicova et al., 2015), and ethnic minorities in Mongolia (Surenjav et al., 2016); (2) disparities in infant mortality for South African Black populations (Bachmann, London, & Barron, 1996), First nations and Inuit populations in Quebec (Chen et al., 2015), indigenous populations in Western Australia (Freemantle et al., 2006), indigenous people in Siberia (Leonard, Keenleyside, & Ivakine, 1997), Black populations in America (Matthews, MacDorman, & Thoma, 2015), African and South Asian populations in the Netherlands (Ravelli et al., 2013); (3) marked economic disadvantages such as access to and cost of economic capital for ethnic minorities in the Netherlands (Aalbers, 2007), Black individuals in America (Blanchflower, Levine, & Zimmerman, 2003), Latinx individuals in America (Bocian, Ernst, & Li, 2008), and non-White individuals in the UK (Deku, Kara, & Molyneux, 2016); marked discrimination in obtaining employment in entry-level positions for Indigenous, Italian, Chinese, and Middle Eastern individuals in Australia (Booth, Leigh, & Varganova, 2012), Black populations in South Africa (Kingdon & Knight, 2004) and America (Pager, 2003); and marked income and wealth gaps that disadvantage Black and Latinx racial groups in the USA (Proctor, Semega, & Kollar, 2015) with additional evidence suggesting general racial economic advantage for dominant racial groups in Belize, Brazil, Canada, India, Israel, Japan, Malaysia, New Zealand, South Africa, and Trinidad and Tobago (Darity & Nembhard, 2000); (4) marked educational disadvantages and segregation for Black individuals in South Africa (Christopher, 2015), numerous racial and ethnic groups across, Belgium, Britain, France, the Netherlands, and Sweden (Heath, Rothon, & Kilpi, 2008), Black and South Asian individuals in England (Johnston, Burgess, Wilson, & Harris, 2006), numerous non-White groups in the Netherlands (Karsten et al., 2006), and Roma across numerous European nations (O'Nions, 2010); (4) marked inequalities in all aspects of the criminal justice system for Black and Latinx individuals in the USA (Alexander, 2012), Black and First Nations groups in Canada (Trevethan & Rastin, 2007), ethnic minorities in the Netherlands (Komen & Schooten, 2009), Black individuals in the UK (Sharp & Atherton, 2007), and for numerous racial groups across the globe (Sudbury, 2014); and (5) of particular interest to this investigation, substantial global racial disparities in health (Beck et al., 2010; Casas-Zamora & Ibrahim, 2004; Smedley, Stith, & Nelson, 2003), including well-documented racial disparities in pain experience and pain treatment that will be reviewed in this chapter. This is by no means a comprehensive review; however, it illustrates that racial injustice is a global phenomenon with tremendous and abhorrent impact on one's life. Being a person of color in this world is associated with numerous disadvantages, unfair treatment, death, pain, and inequality, and this global context must remain at the forefront of discussions of racial disparities in any field, particularly pain.

In terms of pain specifically, the evidence indicates what I am calling a dual injustice, where individuals of oppressed racial groups both experience more pain and are more than likely to have their pain undertreated in clinical context. Nonetheless, in order to understand why this dual injustice exists, it is important to briefly examine the history of race as a concept and construct. As the next section will attest, race has not always existed and is a relatively recent social invention.

Race: A Historical and Sociological Primer

It is possible that some readers of this chapter have never contemplated the origins and history of race, likely assuming that humans have always categorized and dehumanized each other based on skin and hair phenotypes, that this racial categorization is hardwired in humans, and that humans are wary of those who look different from themselves. Evidence does not support this narrative. In fact, evidence from various fields generally highlights that race is a recent social invention with racial conflict developing in modern times (American Anthropological Association, 1998; American Association of Physical Anthropologists, 1996; Lopez, 1994; Smedley, 1998; Smedley & Smedley, 2005; Snowden, 1983). The anthropological evidence is so strong that it is conceived of as a fact similar to how climate scientists view global warming as an undeniable scientific fact (American Anthropological Association, 1998; American Association of Physical Anthropologists, 1996). While a complete review of this topic is beyond the scope of this chapter, some of the evidence is worth presentation. For example, modern population trends suggests racial segregation is commonplace (Bolt, Phillips, & Kempen, 2010), but this appears to be a modern development. Undoubtedly, geographic isolation in different physical environments led to the development of what we now consider racial phenotypes; however, when technology, luck, or further migratory patterns put humans into contact, the result, more often than not, is the sharing of genes (Jorde & Wooding, 2004). This is additionally seen in the historical facts that Alexander the Great officially encouraged the men in his armies to marry the women of newly acquired provinces who undoubtedly possessed diverse racial phenotypes, and the soldiers were happy to oblige (Godolphin, 1942; Smedley, 1998); art from the Roman and Greek empires depicts individuals of various racial phenotypes interacting in everyday life (Snowden, 1983); when individuals of different racial phenotypes were incorporated into these empires, they were endowed with not only equal privileges of a citizen but often earned positions of power and prestige (Smedley & Smedley, 2005); and race was not a barrier to trade (Smedley, 1998). Furthermore, in one of the earliest written acknowledgements of racial phenotype, the great historian Herodotus proclaimed that racial phenotypes "certainly amount to but little" (Godolphin, 1942). People saw what we call race, but it held very little meaning. The usage of the word "race" provides greater evidence that race is a modern social construct as the word "race" has drastically changed in both meaning and usage from the early 1500s where it was a rarely used word synonymous with the words "like," "type," "kind," and "sort" to the late 1700s where it was widely used almost exclusively to hierarchically arrange groups of people interacting in the Americas (Allen, 1994; Smedley & Smedley, 2005). Even the application of race has changed over the years as evinced by the fact that numerous groups considered White today were not considered White in the near distant past (Brodkin, 1998; McDermott & Samson, 2005). Clearly, societies were not always separated by race, and race was not always used as a tool of social oppression, but what led to the invention of race?

Inventions invariably serve a purpose, so we must ask ourselves what was the purpose of race during the colonial period in which it was invented? It is no coincidence that race was invented during the period during which European nations were colonizing the American Continents and Africa; enslaving, displacing, and murdering Africans en masse with the establishment of the trans-Atlantic slave trade and committing numerous acts of genocide against indigenous people (Zinn, 2010). Nonetheless, this was ironically the period of history during which the enlightenment beliefs of democracy, equality, civil rights, justice, and freedom were becoming the dominant political philosophy of Europe (Smedley & Smedley, 2005). How could European peoples simultaneously enslave and murder entire groups of people while believing in these cherished enlightenment ideals? The answer is that people with different skin and hair phenotypes were considered distinct, hierarchically arranged groups with Europeans being the most civilized and advanced. This scheme was invented to suggest that only Europeans were truly human, and thus, oppressing non-European groups was natural and part of the natural order of the world (Jefferson, 1787). Modern psychological evidence suggests that these hierarchical beliefs and abhorrent beliefs about the human essence persist, albeit in nonconscious memory stores (Goff, Eberhardt, Williams, & Jackson, 2008).

For the purposes of this chapter, I adopt the stance that race is a modern invention, a social construct and not a biological reality or an inescapable truth of human life (see Smedley & Smedley, 2005; Yudell, Roberts, DeSalle, & Tishkoff, 2016 for reviews). Race was originally invented to develop a hierarchy of human social groups and justify abhorrent acts of oppression committed by European nations and their peoples. Over time, this construct became embedded in our societies, evolved, and exists in our minds as stereotypes and prejudice. For example, psychologically, race is associated, in our minds, with a seemingly never ending list of stereotypes where people of color are erroneously perceived to be less intelligent (Amodio & Devine, 2006), less moral (Alter, Stern, Granot, & Balcetis, 2016), less inclined to be successful at business and leadership (Rosette, Leonardelli, & Phillips, 2008), more criminal (Eberhardt, Goff, Purdie, & Davies, 2004), more violent (Devine, 1989), more promiscuous (Rosenthal & Lobel, 2016), worse parents (Rosenthal & Lobel, 2016), highly rhythmic (Devine & Elliot, 1995), athletic (Devine & Elliot, 1995), and even perceived to have a greater pain tolerance (Trawalter, Hoffman, & Waytz, 2012). Considering the aforementioned evidence that race impacts one's quality of life globally, the idea that race impacts the experience of pain makes logical sense as racial oppression is not a pleasant experience. In fact, the chronic and widespread experience of racial oppression may have a chronic impact on both the psychological experience of pain and biological processes that form the foundation of the physiological pain response.

Race and Pain: A Dual Injustice

Research indicates that individuals from traditionally oppressed and marginalized racial groups are experiencing, for the most part, more pain. Throughout this paper, I marshal evidence that these racial pain disparities are indicative of a complex relationship between the social construct of race, interpersonal cognitive and emotional processes, and the biological pain response. In particular, this paper focuses on what I am calling a dual injustice: the apparent fact that individuals of marginalized groups experience more pain and are also more than likely to have this pain undertreated. Interestingly, evidence suggests that the experience of more pain is observable in both clinical and presumably healthy nonclinical populations.

Experimental Pain Disparities and Pain in Nonclinical Populations

Before a complete discussion of racial disparities in clinical pain, it is prudent to examine racial pain disparities in nonclinical, presumably healthy, individuals. Experimental investigations of pain, where painful stimuli are presented under highly controlled laboratory circumstances and the pain response of participants is carefully monitored, show racial pain disparities. One of the first demonstrations of racial disparities in experimental pain came from the early work of Chapman demonstrating that Black Americans living in the South exhibited a lower pain threshold and tolerance than White Americans living in the North (Chapman & Jones, 1944). Since 1944, scientists have amassed a substantial body of work examining racial disparities in experimental pain between nonclinical Black and White Americans. Two recent meta-analyses have examined these racial disparities in experimental pain (Kim et al., 2017; Rahim-Williams, Riley, Williams, & Fillingim, 2012), with both analyses indicating that nonclinical African American participants exhibit lower pain tolerances with effect sizes in the moderate to large range across numerous experimental pain modalities, and both analyses provide evidence of higher pain ratings with effect sizes in the moderate range. Additionally, Kim et al. (2017) found no evidence of racial disparities in pain thresholds with Rahim-Williams et al. (2012) reporting that African Americans have lower pain thresholds with effect sizes in the small to moderate range. Considering that the results of these meta-analyses summarize numerous studies of racial disparities in experimental pain across Black and White American populations, a relatively clear picture emerges: presumably healthy, nonclinical Black Americans are more responsive to pain stimuli than Healthy, nonclinical White Americans.

Both of the aforementioned meta-analyses examined experimental pain disparities in numerous racial groups. Rahim-Williams et al. (2012) specifically combined all the pain scores of these non-White and non-Black individuals and found evidence of disparities in experimental pain where this conglomerate "minority" group showed somewhat similar, but weaker and less consistent, experimental pain disparities as Black individuals. However, by analyzing numerous racial groups together, important differences between groups could be lost. Kim et al. (2017) took a different approach and did not group all non-Black people of color together into one large non-White group. Kim et al. (2017) specifically found that individuals of Asian heritage and background show heightened pain intensity in comparison to White individuals, but do not differ in terms of pain tolerance or threshold. Similarly, Latinx individuals exhibit a lower pain tolerance and lower pain intensity than White individuals. Overall, this evidence suggests that numerous non-White racial groups exhibit greater pain and greater pain sensitivity in comparison to White racial groups. Furthermore, race is utilized in numerous national contexts, and racial oppression is hardly an exclusively American phenomenon. While evidence examining racial experimental pain disparities from a non-American context is rare, two European studies indicate similar patterns. Particularly, South Asian individuals in Britain generally showed heightened pain sensitivity in comparison to British White individuals (Watson, Latif, & Rowbotham, 2005) and South Indian individuals in Denmark showed heightened pain sensitivity in comparison to Danish White individuals (Gazerani & Arendt-Nielsen, 2005). As mentioned earlier, the boundaries of Whiteness have changed over time, and research suggests that socially disadvantaged groups of "ethnic Whites" in America also exhibited greater pain sensitivity than privileged White groups considered, at the time, to be "native Whites" (Zborowski, 1952). Interestingly, some studies do not find evidence of the same pattern for all racial groups. For example, Native American people demonstrate a greater pain tolerance in comparison to European groups (Palit et al., 2013). Nonetheless, while more research examining racial disparities in experimental pain across racial contexts is needed, in general, research suggests that nonclinical members of racially oppressed groups exhibit some evidence of greater pain responsivity than White individuals. This enhanced pain responsivity does not extend to all measures of pain, but the overall pattern of results and numerous meta-analyses suggest aspects of the pain response are altered by race.

Mechanisms

Why would racial disparities in experimental pain show, for the most part, a consistent pattern across numerous racial and national contexts? Current research does not provide a definitive answer to the mechanism(s) underlying these findings. However, three mechanisms deserve greater attention: Experienced Injustice and Social Exclusion, Genetics, and Cultural differences in pain coping strategies.

Experienced Injustice and Social Exclusion and Pain

Pain is a complex physiological and emotional response, and recent research has suggested that pain is, in part, social. That is, various forms of social rejection and exclusion literally hurt (Eisenberger & Lieberman, 2004; MacDonald & Leary, 2005; Panksepp, 1998). While "social pain" was originally conceived as a meta-phor, it has been argued that the neurobiological pain response was adapted to respond to social exclusion in an effort to promote survival and success through maintaining social inclusion and group membership (Eisenberger & Lieberman, 2004; MacDonald & Leary, 2005; Nelson & Panksepp, 1998). In line with this con-ception of pain, the experience of social exclusion in humans, is consequently asso-ciated with an affective experience consistent with physical pain (Chen, Williams, Fitness, & Newton, 2008; Riva, Wirth, & Williams, 2011; Zisook, Devaul, & Click, 1982), and individual differences in physical pain sensitivity are positively corre-lated with individual differences in sensitivity to the pain of social exclusion (Eisenberger, Jarcho, Lieberman, & Naliboff, 2006). However, the most convincing evidence comes from research using brain imaging techniques where many of the same neurobiological structures activated during the experience of physical pain are activated during the experience of social exclusion. For example, experiencing social exclusion in a computer simulated ball tossing game leads to not only greater feelings of pain distress but also greater activation of anterior cingulate cortex (ACC) (Eisenberger, Lieberman, & Williams, 2003), a brain area associated with greater feelings of pain distress for physically induced pain (Rainville, Duncan, Price, Carrier, & Bushnell, 1997; Sawamoto et al., 2000). Likewise, prefrontal cor-tex (PFC) activation downregulates the physiological ACC response during the experience of socially induced pain distress (Eisenberger et al., 2003) similar to how the PFC downregulates ACC response during the experience of physically induced pain distress (Bantick et al., 2002; Brooks, Nurmikko, Bimson, Singh, & Roberts, 2002; Eisenberger et al., 2003; Longe et al., 2001; Petrovic, Petersson, Ghatan, Stone-Elander, & Ingvar, 2000). Additionally, exposure to the picture of a former partner following an unwanted breakup leads to activation in brain regions associated with the first person experience of pain (Kross, Berman, Mischel, Smith, & Wager, 2011). Together, this evidence suggests that pain is, in part, a sociometer that provides feedback about social status and social relationships. This is a particu-larly important revelation for this discussion, as members of historically marginal-ized racial groups experience an extreme, pervasive, and chronic form of social exclusion that cannot be practically or ethically replicated in a traditional laboratory setting.

Race is used to exclude and disadvantage individuals from society (Delgado & Stefancic, 2012). This is witnessed in global patterns of residential segregation, where people of color live in the most impoverished (Bolt et al., 2010), polluted neighborhoods (Adeola, 2000; Brulle & Pellow, 2006; Laurian, 2008) with access to the worst education (Chadderton & Edmonds, 2015; Christopher, 2015; Heath et al., 2008; Jenkins, Micklewright, & Schnepf, 2008; Johnston et al., 2006; Karsten et al., 2006; O'Nions, 2010; Szulkin & Jonsson, 2007). Furthermore, people of color in varied cultural contexts are often told, explicitly, to leave the country or to "go back" to a perceived place of origin (Bacallao & Smokowski, 2007; Hein, 2000). Exclusion from society is also a literal reality for many people of color in nations across the globe where racist policing and justice practices are commonplace (Alexander, 2012; Komen & Schooten, 2009; Miller, 2010; Sharp & Atherton, 2007; Sudbury, 2014; Trevethan & Rastin, 2007). Furthermore, in the USA, individuals with the strongest Black phenotypes are more than likely to be permanently excluded from society with a death sentence (Eberhardt et al., 2004). This evidence suggests that people of color experience a chronic and institutionalized form of social exclusion. Considering that minor and fleeting laboratory manipulations of social exclusion have observable effects on the pain response, it is logical to hypothesize that the impact of such chronic and pervasive social exclusion is leading to the observed racial disparities in experimental pain described above.

Some additional evidence supports this hypothesis. For example, healthy African Americans who perceive the greatest amount of racial discrimination in their lives also report the lowest heat pain tolerances in controlled laboratory experiments. Likewise, older African Americans seeking treatment from the Veterans Administration show a similar correlation, where experiences of racial discrimination in American society leads to greater global reports of body pain (Burgess et al., 2009). Furthermore, in a study examining the relationship between perceived discrimination and the experience of everyday back pain, it was found that the perception of lifetime discrimination was the strongest individual predictor of back pain for Black participants (Edwards, 2008). Furthermore, the specific measures of discrimination utilized by these studies highlight the relationships between social exclusion and racism. For example, Edwards (2008) utilized a scale constructed by Mays and Cochran (2001) which asks participants to indicate if their identity was associated with many outcomes including social exclusion: "not hired for a job," "fired from a job," "discouraged by teacher from continuing education," "prevented from renting or buying a home," and "forced out from neighborhood by neighbors." Burgess et al. (2009) utilized the Experience of Discrimination scale (Krieger, Smith, Naishadham, Hartman, & Barbeau, 2005) which asks participants to indicate if their race has ever affected various exclusionary behaviors like "getting hired or getting a job," "getting housing," "getting medical care," "getting services in a store or restaurant." Thus, the measures of perceived racial discrimination utilized in these investigations define racial discrimination, in part, as exclusion. Furthermore, experiences of racial social exclusion are directly associated with an intensified pain response. For example, having a strong ethnic identity is associated with greater experimental pain sensitivity for Latinx and African American participants (F. B. Rahim-Williams et al., 2007). Thus, individuals who most strongly associate with their racial groups would most likely exhibit increased pain sensitivity. Considering that individuals with the strongest ethnic identities are also more than likely to perceive racial discrimination (Sellers & Nicole, 2003), it is likely that these individuals would most likely perceive and experience the social exclusion of racism. The hypothesis that the social exclusion of racism is altering the pain response of nondominant racial groups is bolstered by the evidence above.

Nonetheless, pain additionally is associated with changes in biological processes, and if the social exclusion of racism has a chronic impact on pain systems, one would expect these basic biological processes associated with pain to be modulated by race. Research examining race and these biological responses is limited; however, research examining African Americans supports this claim. Specifically, African Americans show a more sensitive nociceptive flexion reflex than White participants (Campbell et al., 2008b), a reduced diffuse noxious inhibitory controls (a tendency for one painful stimulus to inhibit pain from a second noxious stimulus), indicating differences in endogenous pain inhibition where African Americans are less effective at pain inhibition than White participants (Campbell et al., 2008a). Similarly, research indicates that the biological factors of blood pressure, allopregnanolone immunoreactivity, hypothalamic–pituitary–adrenal axis activation that theoretically affect the intensity of pain experience and perception in European Americans, have little predictive validity for Black individuals (Mechlin, Maixner, Light, Fisher, & Girdler, 2005; Mechlin, Morrow, Maixner, & Girdler, 2007). Finally, evidence indicates that African Americans have lower concentrations of plasma levels of oxytocin (Grewen, Light, Mechlin, & Girdler, 2008), a hormone associated with social affiliation (Feldman, 2012; Feldman, Weller, Zagoory-Sharon, & Levine, 2007), and these differential levels, in part, mediate racial disparities in experimental pain response (Grewen et al., 2008). Despite the suggestion of this evidence, a direct connection between experiencing long-terms forms of the social exclusion that is racism and the modulation of the biological processes associated with pain, frankly, does not exist. This will be a difficult, potentially unethical, question to examine, but it appears possible that chronic exposure to the social exclusion that is racism may alter biological processes that, in turn, alter the experience of pain. Considering that cross-race differences in the biological aspects of the pain response exist, examining and ruling out potential genetic influence is warranted.

Genetics

The aforementioned biological differences warrant an investigation of genetic influence. Nonetheless, genetic investigations into racial disparities in experimental pain do not provide compelling evidence of genetic influence. To my knowledge, only one study examines the genetic mechanisms underlying racial differences in experimental pain (Hastie et al., 2012). This investigation focused exclusively on the Mu-opioid receptor (OPRM1) A118G. African Americans have a lower proportion of the G allele than European American or Latinx individuals, and previous research in mainly European American samples links variants in this gene to alteration in pain sensitivity (Hastie et al., 2012). The results of this investigation replicated previous findings of racial experimental pain disparities, but the genetic analyses did not directly connect population differences in allelic variation to variation in pain. Interestingly, the results showed that White individuals with one or two copies of the G allele showed a markedly decreased pain sensitivity, while African American and Latinx participants with this genetic composition exhibited a nonsignificant increase in pain sensitivity. The authors suggest the possibility that other, unexamined, genes may be driving this race by gene interaction; however, I must caution against such hypotheses as genetics are extremely unlikely to explain racial differences in health and behavior and likely represent a historical pattern of thinking where unsupported racialized science has biased the scientific process (Goodman, 2000; Yudell et al., 2016). Current genetic data examining this question does not provide compelling evidence that racial experimental pain disparities are driven by genetics, and genetic data, in general, indicates that cross-race genetic variation is not only minimal, but often when genetic variation is observed, it is likely due to the history of how these social constructs were formed and defined (Morning, 2014). Individuals interested in examining the genetic underpinnings of race should be extremely cautious and specific. Racial variations developed as a result of specific environments and geographical realities and lead to specific changes in a few heritable genes, but these genes are not present in all people of a specific race, as the geographic ancestry of people of the same race is not identical (Jorde & Wooding, 2004). It is not only problematic, but also potentially unscientific, to utilize race as a shorthand for geographic isolation and subsequent genetic variation when the geographic ancestry is not the same for all people of an apparent, socially constructed race. Furthermore, considering that genes and social environment interact and including measures of social environment has proven useful in understanding the impact of genes on behavior (Caspi & Moffitt, 2006), it is important to begin to include direct measures of social environment in addition to direct measures of genetic composition when examining racial pain disparities because, as evinced above, the social and political environment experienced by marginalized racial groups is drastically different than the social and political environment experienced by privileged racial groups. By incorporating this reality into our scientific hypotheses, we may rediscover what many scientists already know, race is a much more robust social construct than a genetic construct (Smedley & Smedley, 2005; Yudell et al., 2016).

Cultural Differences in Pain Coping Strategies

Racial groups not only differ in sensitivity to experimental pain, but also differ in coping strategies. For example, African Americans, in comparison to European Americans, are more than likely to engage in catastrophizing when exposed to painful stimuli in a laboratory (Forsythe, Thorn, Day, & Shelby, 2011; Meints & Hirsh, 2015; Meints, Stout, Abplanalp, & Hirsh, 2017) and utilize prayer in response to real-world pain and laboratory-controlled pain stimuli (Cano, Mayo, & Ventimiglia, 2006; Edwards, Moric, Husfeldt, Buvanendran, & Ivankovich, 2005; Jordan, Lumley, & Leisen, 1998; Meints & Hirsh, 2015; Meints et al., 2017). Experimental evidence further indicates that cross-racial differences in experimental pain sensitivity are partially mediated by cross-racial differences in coping strategies (Forsythe et al., 2011; Meints & Hirsh, 2015; Meints et al., 2017). Interestingly, prayer and spirituality assist individuals in coping with a racially oppressive system (Lyris & Constantine, 2006) and prove beneficial in other health contexts (Cooper, Thayer, & Waldstein, 2014). Likewise, an important aspect of catastrophizing, feeling as if pain is not under one's direct control, may also be an effective coping mechanism for racial oppression, as attributing negative life outcomes to the specific external and uncontrollable factor of racism fosters maintenance of self-esteem (Crocker & Major, 1989; Major, Spencer, Schmader, Wolfe, & Crocker, 1998). Thus, while direct coping strategies clearly play a role in racial disparities in experimental pain, the social and political context in which these strategies have developed is important to understanding and responding to these disparities, especially considering that these coping strategies prove beneficial in managing other forms of racism.

Summary

A body of research has emerged documenting racial differences in experimental pain experience with healthy, nonclinical populations of Black and Latinx Americans exhibiting greater sensitization to pain than White Americans in controlled laboratory settings. Some evidence likewise suggests that other racially marginalized groups from various cultural and national contexts exhibit similar patterns of enhanced pain sensitivity. Furthermore, neurobiological evidence, while far from being conclusive, indicates that the biological processes associated with pain show modulation by race and provide some evidence of a biological component of these observed experimental pain disparities. However, the limited research examining the genetic underpinnings of these biological modulations falls very short in accounting for observed biological and psychological differences. Nonetheless, evidence examining the effect of perceived and experienced discrimination on experimental pain sensitivity indicates that experiencing racism, oppression, and discrimination in one's daily life leads to enhanced pain in controlled laboratory investigations. Considering that (1) research not examining race or racism shows a clear relationship between social exclusion, heightened pain sensitivity, and heightened activation of pain relevant neurobiological structures, and (2) racism is essentially an extreme form of social exclusion, it is logical to hypothesize that the chronic social exclusion of living in a racially oppressive society alters biological processes associated with the experience of pain. Nonetheless, no research has directly examined this hypothesis, and conducting such research may prove difficult and potentially unethical. Additionally, cross-racial differences in pain coping strategies do partially mediate cross-racial differences in experimental pain experience; however, these cross-racial strategical differences are also likely affected by the experience of racism omnipresent in the lives of racially marginalized group members. Racial disparities in the pain experience of nonclinical individuals are alarming as they suggest that living as a member of an oppressed racial group literally hurts. Much more research is needed to fully understand the causes and mechanisms of these pain disparities, but it appears highly likely that experiencing racial injustice, marginalization, and oppression drastically alters the pain system of healthy, nonclinical individuals.

Clinical Pain Disparities

In addition to racial disparities in experimental pain, some research highlights another disturbing fact: racially marginalized groups experience greater pain in numerous clinical settings. For example, African Americans experience more pain after operations in general (Faucett, Gordon, & Levine, 1994), when fighting numerous forms of cancer (Green, Montague, & Hart-Johnson, 2009), when living with chronic pain (Chen et al., 2005; Riley III et al., 2002), and even when living with arthritis (Creamer, Lethbridge-Cejku, & Hochberg, 1999). These disparities extend to patients receiving specialized pain treatment at a state-of-the-art pain clinic (Edwards, Doleys, Fillingim, & Lowery, 2001). While a majority of this research specifically focuses on racial disparities between White and Black Americans, research indicates similar disparities for other racial groups in America and for other nations (Nicholl et al., 2015; Peres, Iser, Peres, Malta, & Antunes, 2012; van der Hammen, de Roos, Sabelis, & Janssen, 2010).

There are many potential reasons for these disparities in clinical contexts. First, considering the previous discussion, it is possible that racial disparities in experimental pain may impact racial disparities in clinical pain. Likewise, socioeconomic status plays a considerable role in racial health disparities (Williams, 1999) and pain specifically (Green & Hart-Johnson, 2012); however, racial disparities in pain experience, while lessened, remain substantial after controlling for economic factors (Green & Hart-Johnson, 2012). Furthermore, racial segregation can also lead to racial pain disparities as healthcare facilities serving racially marginalized groups often provide objectively worse care (Bach, Pham, Schrag, Tate, & Hargraves, 2004; Epstein, 2004; Haider et al., 2012) and facilities like pharmacies that serve racially marginalized groups are less likely to carry pain medicines needed to ameliorate pain (Green, Ndao-Brumblay, West, & Washington, 2005).

Nonetheless, a majority of research examining the causes of racial pain disparities focuses on racial bias in pain treatment decisions, with healthcare professionals' treatment decisions showing strong evidence of systematic racial bias. This statement is supported by a meta-analysis summarizing 20 years of research, the analysis found such marked pain treatment disparities that the authors proclaimed: "These findings unequivocally point to the evidence that race and ethnicity matters in clinical pain treatment outcomes and the size of the difference is sufficiently large to warrant clinical safety and quality concerns" (Meghani, Byun, & Gallagher, 2012). Evidence of racial bias in pain treatment decisions has also been found in other national contexts and across numerous racial groups (Beck & Falkson, 2001; Kurita, Sjøgren, Juel, Højsted, & Ekholm, 2012).

Taken together, these findings suggest a dual injustice. Members of marginalized racial groups are more responsive and sensitive to pain, but also more than likely to receive lower quality pain treatment. In order to understand pain treatment disparities, an examination of the cognitive and emotional processes that may drive these effects is warranted.

Cognitive Biases

In-Group Emotion Recognition Advantage

Is it possible that the pain of marginalized racial group members is not being perceived by members of advantaged racial groups? Psychological evidence suggests that this may in fact be a cause of these disparities. In a comprehensive meta-analysis examining recognition of emotional expressions across numerous racial, national, ethnic, and social groups, evidence indicates a marked advantage for in-group emotion recognition (Elfenbein & Ambady, 2002). Furthermore, this analysis found cultural groups that comprised the numerical minority were better at identifying emotional expressions of the numerical majority than the numerical majority was at identifying the emotional expressions of the numerical minority. Furthermore, this analysis shows that groups with the highest levels of interpersonal contact were the least likely to show the in-group emotional recognition advantage. In terms of pain treatment, it is possible that the pain of racial groups who are underrepresented in medicine is simply not being recognized. Some evidence supports this possibility. For example, physicians are more than likely to underestimate the pain of Black patients relative to White patients (Staton et al., 2007); however, while the sample of physicians was predominately White (66%), it was also highly diverse considering that 6% were African American and 28% of physicians were from other racial groups. Thus, while this finding does not rule out an in-group pain perception bias, the fact that a large portion of the sample was not White suggests that factors other than one's in-group may also drive these responses. The experimental investigations of Trawalter, Hoffman, and colleagues (Hoffman, Trawalter, Axt, & Oliver, 2016; Trawalter & Hoffman, 2015; Trawalter et al., 2012) consistently find that in vignette studies where individuals are asked to imagine how individuals of different races feel, participants consistently rate the pain of African Americans to be less than the pain of European Americans. Considering that these studies do not simply examine the recognition of pain intensity from an objective expression of pain, and instead rely on imagination of how a painful event (i.e., a paper cut or a broken bone) affects pain, it is possible that factors other than basic emotional recognition and perception are driving these effects. The impressive work of Adam Hirsh utilizes virtual human technology (i.e., the presentation of human-like avatars where variables like pain expression, race, and gender are easily manipulated) finds mixed evidence with some investigations finding evidence that race impacts perceptions of pain and pain treatment of lay people and medical professionals alike with African American avatars being perceived as experiencing higher levels of pain (Hirsh, George, & Robinson, 2009; Stutts, Hirsh, George, & Robinson, 2010) or does not find evidence of racial disparities in pain perception (Alqudah, Hirsh, Stutts, Scipio, & Robinson,

2010; Hirsh, Alqudah, Stutts, & Robinson, 2008; Torres et al., 2013). While this work is impressive, it is difficult to interpret, not only for the fact that the observed racial treatment disparities are in the opposite direction from those found in clinical settings, but also for the fact that it is unclear if the specific avatars utilized by this research activate different psychological processes than non-virtual human targets. Nonetheless, no published research that I am aware of examines if the in-group pain recognition advantage extends to expressions of pain from non-virtual human targets. Thus cross-racial disparities in pan perception may drive pain treatment disparities; however, more research is needed to provide greater clarity.

Stereotypes and Prejudice

As eloquently pointed out in a recent review paper by Sophie Trawalter and Kelly Hoffman (Trawalter & Hoffman, 2015), racial pain stereotypes have historically been utilized since the early days of colonialism and slavery to justify both the oppression of Black people and the social structures responsible for this oppression. Furthermore, the work of Trawalter, Hoffman, and numerous colleagues indicates that these stereotypes are not only present, but they affect perceptions of experienced pain. In the most eye-opening investigation of this phenomenon, Hoffman and colleagues (Hoffman et al., 2016) found that nearly 73% of laypersons and 50% of medical students at a prestigious medical school endorsed at least one false and racist biological belief about African Americans: "Black's nerve endings are less sensitive than whites," "Blacks' skin is thicker than whites'," and "Blacks have stronger immune systems than whites." Furthermore, endorsing these beliefs was associated with more inaccurate treatment decisions for Black patients vs White patients and perceiving Black pain to be less severe than White pain. Interestingly, the aforementioned work of Trawalter and colleagues shows that racial bias in pain perception is mediated by perceived privilege. That is, when participants viewed an individual as having a difficult life, full of adversity or as being in a low status economic position relative to the participant, they also viewed the target as being less affected by pain (Trawalter et al., 2012). It appears that complex cognitive structures exist that have the primary purpose of convincing individuals that systematically disadvantaged peoples feel less pain, a cognitive response that not only results in inadequate pain treatment but also likely ameliorates feelings of guilt and compunction that come with privilege (Jost, Banaji, & Nosek, 2004).

As noted elsewhere (Trawalter & Hoffman, 2015), research examining racial prejudice, defined as antipathy or negative affect towards a specific group, is not associated with pain treatment biases. This extends to both explicit and implicit measures of racial prejudice. Nonetheless, overall basic cognitions and complicated stereotypes appear to play some role in precipitating racial pain treatment biases, and honing one's basic ability to recognize cross-racial pain while simultaneously unlearning these racist pain stereotypes appears one potential answer to reducing racial pain treatment biases.

Empathy

In terms of emotional responses, research indicates that empathy may play a particularly important role in pain treatment biases. In studies investigating the empathetic response, research indicates that simply learning of one's negative life circumstance (Batson, Lishner, & Stocks, 2015) or viewing a pain face elicits psychological and neural processes indicative of empathy (Botvinick et al., 2005; Saarela & Finnäs, 2014). Decades of research finds that empathy, in turn, leads to prosocial motivations and helping responses (Batson et al., 2015). Thus, under normal circumstances, pain is communicated to others who, in turn, feel empathy, and, as a result, provide help.

Interestingly, research indicates that humans do not always respond to pain with empathy or helping. This is particularly true when pain and suffering is expressed by racial out-group members. For example, the pain of an envied out-group member can elicit joy, Schadenfreude, and other positive emotions (Cikara, Botvinick, & Fiske, 2011). Likewise, research indicates an empathy gap, where individuals experience more empathy for racial in-group members (Gutsell & Inzlicht, 2012) which likely precipitates the racial helping gap (Saucier, Miller, & Doucet, 2005; Stürmer, Snyder, Kropp, & Siem, 2006) where African Americans receive less help in emergency situations when need is the highest (Saucier et al., 2005). Evidence also indicates a corresponding empathy bias. For example, when White Italians and African Immigrants living in Italy view the pain of a racial in-group, they exhibit a physiological response similar to the first-person experience of pain; however, this response is not present when observing racial out-group members experience pain. Interestingly, a study by Contreras-Huerta, Baker, Reynolds, Batalha, and Cunnington (2013) replicated these effects using racial groups, but the effects did not extend to the minimal group paradigm where random groups are created and then utilized to examine psychological effects. This fact indicates that the findings are not driven by the presence of any opposing social group, but appear to be specific to racial groups. Thus, one may begin to hypothesize that the pain of racially marginalized out-group members will not elicit the same empathetic and emotional responses as the pain of in-group members. This fact is particularly important considering that people of color, particularly Black Americans, Latinx individuals, and Native Americans are extremely underrepresented in the medical field (Merchant & Omary, 2010; Sullivan, 2004), and thus members of these racial groups are unlikely to receive care from a person with their same racial background. Considering the aforementioned research documenting in-group cognitive and emotional advantages in pain recognition, and pain response, underrepresentation in medicine is not simply unfair, it may contribute to racial pain treatment disparities. In terms of pain treatment, evidence suggests that empathy is associated with pain treatment disparities in American and Canadian contexts (Drwecki, Moore, Ward, & Prkachin, 2011; Kaseweter, Drwecki, & Prkachin, 2012). Specifically, these studies indicate that experiencing racial disparities in empathy are strongly correlated with providing racial disparities in pain treatment. Furthermore, empathy-inducing perspective taking interventions have reduced racial biases in pain treatment decisions (Drwecki et al., 2011; Wandner, Torres, Bartley, George, & Robinson, 2015), showing that empathy is not only a cause of racial disparities in pain treatment but also an effective intervention. Additional experiments suggest that these empathy biases are implicit and potentially, nonconscious (Mathur, Richeson, Paice, Muzyka, & Chiao, 2014). Together, this evidence highlights that while many factors likely precipitate racial disparities in clinical pain experience, one important factor is the cognitive and emotional processes of healthcare professionals and the decision made by these healthcare professionals as a result.

Conclusions

The evidence presented in this chapter highlights the existence of a dual injustice—members of nondominant racial groups are more than likely to experience pain, while these same individuals are also more likely to have their pain discounted by and undertreated by healthcare professionals. While a majority of evidence examining the relationship between race and pain comes from an American context, it is important to point out that many citations utilized in this short review are from non-American racial contexts. Some are likely perplexed by the consistency of these findings across racial, ethnic, and national lines. The fact of the matter is that race is a social, not a biological, construct that has been used to oppress people of color across the globe since the time period when colonization began to take shape. This oppression includes institutionalized forms of social exclusion where individuals are both discriminated against and excluded from many aspects in numerous abhorrent ways as documented at the beginning of this chapter. Considering that research provides a strong link between social exclusion and pain, it is not illogical to hypothesize that the chronic social exclusion that members of marginalized racial groups face is altering basic pain responses. Nonetheless, while no research directly connects experiencing chronic racism to pain responsivity, research examining self-reports of perceived discrimination highlights a relationship to experimental pain responsivity. Furthermore, genetic evidence examining these disparities is limited at best and does not provide strong evidence of a genetic predisposition driving experimental pain disparities. Nonetheless, pain, like all psychological phenomenon, is, in part, driven by biological processes, and evidence suggests that neurobiological pain responses are also different in individuals from marginalized racial groups. However, this is not evidence of a genetic predisposition, as all psychological experiences, not just pain, are instantiated in a biological brain that produces biological changes in response to environmental events. Additionally, it is important to recognize that cultural differences in pain coping strategies undeniably play a role in constructing experimental disparities; however, these coping strategies, may themselves, be responses to living in an oppressive social structure.

Furthermore, marginalized racial group members experience pain disparities in clinical settings, and while many potential causes of these disparities exist, it is clear that the behavior and decisions of healthcare professionals are biased against individuals from marginalized racial groups. These biases are likely driven by numerous psychological processes, and evidence indicates that racial empathy biases and the maintenance of racist social beliefs are two factors that undoubtedly play a role.

An important question is what can be done by healthcare professionals to reduce the pain and suffering that members of marginalized racial groups are experiencing. My own research (Drwecki et al., 2011) shows that racial disparities in pain treatment can be reduced via an empathy inducing, perspective taking intervention where healthcare professionals simple "imagine how your patient feels about his or her pain and how this pain is affecting his or her life" directly prior to making the final pain treatment decisions. This is an admittedly simple solution that effectively targets one small part of the larger problem. However, results suggesting that medical students, and presumably medical professionals, hold beliefs that are frankly dehumanizing and racist like the beliefs that African Americans "have less sensitive nerve endings," points out that racialized science continues to impact the minds, thoughts, beliefs, and treatment decisions of individuals. As scientists and medical professionals it is important to conduct research into the history of the social construction of race. It is also important to examine the often unexamined notion that race is a biological construct, and finally it is dually important to be wary of racial explanations of phenomenon. Take sickle cell disease as an example. The existence of higher sickle cell prevalence in African communities can likely lead to thoughts that race is biologically real and finite. Nonetheless, this disease has nothing to do with biological race; it is simply passed on to individuals whose ancestors lived in areas where malaria was common (i.e., Africa, the Mediterranean, and South America). Nearly 8% of African Americans are susceptible to this disorder, because nearly 8% of African American have ancestors from areas where malaria resistance was an evolutionary adaptation. Furthermore, Latinx individuals and White individuals from the Mediterranean are also susceptible to this disorder because they too had ancestors from areas where malaria resistance was an evolutionary adaptation. Thus, race is being used as a proxy for geographical ancestry. Using geographical ancestry is a much more prudent approach in understanding who is more than likely to have the genetic predisposition for sickle cell. Unfortunately, most Black American descendants of slaves do not know their geographical origins because a system of global oppression has led to the massive loss of one's ancestral history. So, in America today, it may be prudent to examine African American populations for the presence of the sickle cell trait, but this is the result of racism, not evidence for the existence of race.

Overall, the evidence presented in this chapter highlights the existence of a dual injustice whereby members of marginalized racial groups are not only more responsive to pain but this pain is more than likely to be undertreated by healthcare professionals. This evidence suggests that numerous societies have constructed racial privileges and disadvantages that may, in turn, chronically alter pain responsivity while simultaneously shaping the biases and behaviors of the very healthcare professionals who are charged with ameliorating this pain. That is, our societies, nations, communities, healthcare professionals, laypersons, and even ourselves participate in a system of oppression that both causes pain for racially marginalized individuals and simultaneously discounts it. Some research presented in this review suggests that the individual level biases can be reduced; however, we must not be Pollyannaish. Eradicating this dual injustice will require more than changing the behavior of a few individuals, it will also require dismantling a system of relative White skin privilege that permeates many social structures across the globe.

References

Aalbers, M. B. (2007). Place-based and race-based exclusion from mortgage loans: Evidence from three cities in the Netherlands. *Journal of Urban Affairs, 29*(1), 1–29. https://doi.org/10.1111/j.1467-9906.2007.00320.x

Adeola, F. O. (2000). Cross-National Environmental Injustice and human rights issues: A review of evidence in the developing world. *American Behavioral Scientist, 43*(4), 686–706. https://doi.org/10.1177/00027640021955496

Alexander, M. (2012). *The new Jim crow: Mass incarceration in the age of colorblindness*. The New Press.

Allen, T. W. (1994). *The invention of the white race: The origin of racial oppression in Anglo-America*. Verso.

Alqudah, A. F., Hirsh, A. T., Stutts, L. A., Scipio, C. D., & Robinson, M. E. (2010). Sex and race differences in rating others' pain, pain-related negative mood, pain coping, and recommending medical help. *Journal of Cyber Therapy and Rehabilitation, 3*(1), 63–70.

Alter, A. L., Stern, C., Granot, Y., & Balcetis, E. (2016). The "bad is black" effect: Why people believe evildoers have darker skin than do-Gooders. *Personality and Social Psychology Bulletin, 42*(12), 1653–1665. https://doi.org/10.1177/0146167216669123

American Anthropological Association. (1998). *American Anthropological Association Statement on "Race."* Retrieved from http://www.aaanet.org/stmts/racepp.htm

American Association of Physical Anthropologists. (1996). AAPA statement on biological aspects of race. *American Journal of Physical Anthropology, 101*(4), 569–570. https://doi.org/10.1002/ajpa.1331010408

Amodio, D. M., & Devine, P. G. (2006). Stereotyping and evaluation in implicit race Bias: Evidence for independent constructs and unique effects on behavior. *Journal of Personality and Social Psychology, 91*(4), 652–661. https://doi.org/10.1037/0022-3514.91.4.652

Baburin, A., Lai, T., & Leinsalu, M. (2011). Avoidable mortality in Estonia: Exploring the differences in life expectancy between Estonians and non-Estonians in 2005-2007. *Public Health, 125*(11), 754-762. https://doi.org/10.1016/j.puhe.2011.09.005

Bacallao, M. L., & Smokowski, P. R. (2007). The costs of getting ahead: Mexican family system changes after immigration. *Family Relations, 56*(1), 52–66. https://doi.org/10.1111/j.1741-3729.2007.00439.x

Bach, P. B., Pham, H. H., Schrag, D., Tate, R. C., & Hargraves, J. L. (2004). Primary care physicians who treat blacks and whites. *The New England Journal of Medicine, 351*(6), 575–584. https://doi.org/10.1056/NEJMsa040609

Bachmann, M., London, L., & Barron, P. (1996). Infant mortality rate inequalities in the western Cape Province of South Africa. *International Journal of Epidemiology, 25*(5), 966–972.

Bantick, S. J., Wise, R. G., Ploghaus, A., Clare, S., Smith, S. M., & Tracey, I. (2002). Imaging how attention modulates pain in humans using functional MRI. *Brain: A Journal of Neurology, 125*(Pt 2), 310–319.

Batson, C. D., Lishner, D. A., & Stocks, E. L. (2015). The empathy—Altruism hypothesis. In D. A. Schroeder, W. G. Graziano, D. A. Schroeder (Ed), & W. G. Graziano (Ed) (Eds.), *The Oxford handbook of prosocial behavior.* (pp. 259–281). New York, NY, US: Oxford University Press.

Beck, S., Wojdyla, D., Say, L., Betran, A. P., Merialdi, M., Requejo, J. H., … Look, P. F. V. (2010). The worldwide incidence of preterm birth: A systematic review of maternal mortality and morbidity. *Bulletin of the World Health Organization, 88*(1), 31–38. https://doi.org/10.1590/S0042-96862010000100012

Beck, S. L., & Falkson, G. (2001). Prevalence and Management of Cancer Pain in South Africa. *Pain, 94*(1), 75–84. https://doi.org/10.1016/S0304-3959(01)00343-8

Blanchflower, D. G., Levine, P. B., & Zimmerman, D. J. (2003). Discrimination in the small-business credit market. *Review of Economics and Statistics, 85*(4), 930–943. https://doi.org/10.1162/003465303772815835

Bocian, D. G., Ernst, K. S., & Li, W. (2008). Race, ethnicity and subprime home loan pricing. *Journal of Economics and Business, 60*(1–2), 110–124. https://doi.org/10.1016/j.jeconbus.2007.10.001

Bolt, G., Phillips, D., & Kempen, R. V. (2010). Housing policy, (De)segregation and social mixing: An international perspective. *Housing Studies, 25*(2), 129–135. https://doi.org/10.1080/02673030903564838

Booth, A. L., Leigh, A., & Varganova, E. (2012). Does ethnic discrimination vary across minority groups? Evidence from a field experiment*. *Oxford Bulletin of Economics and Statistics, 74*(4), 547–573. https://doi.org/10.1111/j.1468-0084.2011.00664.x

Botvinick, M., Jha, A. P., Bylsma, L. M., Fabian, S. A., Solomon, P. E., & Prkachin, K. M. (2005). Viewing facial expressions of pain engages cortical areas involved in the direct experience of pain. *NeuroImage, 25*(1), 312–319. https://doi.org/10.1016/j.neuroimage.2004.11.043

Bramley, D., Hebert, P., Jackson, R., & Chassin, M. (2004). Indigenous disparities in disease-specific mortality, a cross-country comparison: New Zealand, Australia, Canada, and the United States. *The New Zealand Medical Journal, 117*(1207), U1215.

Brodkin, K. (1998). *How Jews became white folks and what that says about race in America.* Rutgers University Press.

Brooks, J. C. W., Nurmikko, T. J., Bimson, W. E., Singh, K. D., & Roberts, N. (2002). fMRI of thermal pain: Effects of stimulus laterality and attention. *NeuroImage, 15*(2), 293–301. https://doi.org/10.1006/nimg.2001.0974

Brulle, R. J., & Pellow, D. N. (2006). Environmental justice: Human health and environmental inequalities. *Annual Review of Public Health, 27*(1), 103–124. https://doi.org/10.1146/annurev.publhealth.27.021405.102124

Burgess, D. J., Grill, J., Noorbaloochi, S., Griffin, J. M., Ricards, J., van Ryn, M., & Partin, M. R. (2009). The effect of perceived racial discrimination on bodily pain among older African American men. *Pain Medicine (Malden, Mass.), 10*(8), 1341–1352. https://doi.org/10.1111/j.1526-4637.2009.00742.x

Campbell, C. M., France, C. R., Robinson, M. E., Logan, H. L., Geffken, G. R., & Fillingim, R. B. (2008a). Ethnic differences in diffuse noxious inhibitory controls (DNIC). *The Journal of Pain, 9*(8), 759–766. https://doi.org/10.1016/j.jpain.2008.03.010

Campbell, C. M., France, C. R., Robinson, M. E., Logan, H. L., Geffken, G. R., & Fillingim, R. B. (2008b). Ethnic differences in the nociceptive flexion reflex (NFR). *Pain, 134*(1–2), 91–96. https://doi.org/10.1016/j.pain.2007.03.035

Cano, A., Mayo, A., & Ventimiglia, M. (2006). Coping, pain severity, interference, and disability: The potential mediating and moderating roles of race and education. *Journal of Pain, 7*(7), 459–468. https://doi.org/10.1016/j.jpain.2006.01.445

Casas-Zamora, J. A., & Ibrahim, S. A. (2004). Confronting health inequity: The global dimension. *American Journal of Public Health, 94*(12), 2055–2058.

Caspi, A., & Moffitt, T. E. (2006). Gene–environment interactions in psychiatry: Joining forces with neuroscience. *Nature Reviews Neuroscience, 7*(7), 583–590. https://doi.org/10.1038/nrn1925

Chadderton, C., & Edmonds, C. (2015). Refugees and access to vocational education and training across Europe: A case of protection of white privilege? *Journal of Vocational Education and Training, 67*(2), 136–152.

Chapman, W. P., & Jones, C. M. (1944). Variations in cutaneous and visceral pain sensitivity in normal subjects 1. *Journal of Clinical Investigation, 23*(1), 81–91.

Chen, I., Kurz, J., Pasanen, M., Faselis, C., Panda, M., Staton, L. J., … Cykert, S. (2005). Racial differences in opioid use for chronic nonmalignant pain. *Journal of General Internal Medicine, 20*(7), 593–598. https://doi.org/10.1111/j.1525-1497.2005.0106.x

Chen, L., Xiao, L., Auger, N., Torrie, J., McHugh, N. G.-L., Zoungrana, H., & Luo, Z.-C. (2015). Disparities and trends in birth outcomes, perinatal and infant mortality in aboriginal vs. non-aboriginal populations: A population-based study in Quebec, Canada 1996-2010. *PLoS One, 10*(9), e0138562. https://doi.org/10.1371/journal.pone.0138562

Chen, Z., Williams, K. D., Fitness, J., & Newton, N. C. (2008). When hurt will not heal: Exploring the capacity to relive social and physical pain. *Psychological Science, 19*(8), 789–795. https://doi.org/10.1111/j.1467-9280.2008.02158.x

Christopher, A. J. (2015). Educational attainment in South Africa: A view from the census 1865-2011. *History of Education, 44*(4), 503–522.

Cikara, M., Botvinick, M. M., & Fiske, S. T. (2011). Us versus them: Social identity shapes neural responses to intergroup competition and harm. *Psychological Science, 22*(3), 306–313. https://doi.org/10.1177/0956797610397667

Contreras-Huerta, L. S., Baker, K. S., Reynolds, K. J., Batalha, L., & Cunnington, R. (2013). Racial Bias in neural empathic responses to pain. *PLoS One, 8*(12), e84001. https://doi.org/10.1371/journal.pone.0084001

Cooper, D. C., Thayer, J. F., & Waldstein, S. R. (2014). Coping with racism: The impact of prayer on cardiovascular reactivity and post-stress recovery in African American women. *Annals of Behavioral Medicine, 47*(2), 218–230. https://doi.org/10.1007/s12160-013-9540-4

Creamer, P., Lethbridge-Cejku, M., & Hochberg, M. C. (1999). Determinants of pain severity in knee osteoarthritis: Effect of demographic and psychosocial variables using 3 pain measures. *The Journal of Rheumatology, 26*(8), 1785–1792.

Crocker, J., & Major, B. (1989). Social stigma and self-esteem: The self-protective properties of stigma. *Psychological Review, 96*(4), 608–630. https://doi.org/10.1037/0033-295X.96.4.608

Dankovchik, J., Hoopes, M. J., Warren-Mears, V., & Knaster, E. (2015). Disparities in life expectancy of Pacific Northwest American Indians and Alaska natives: Analysis of linkage-corrected life tables. *Public Health Reports (Washington, DC: 1974), 130*(1), 71–80.

Darity, W., & Nembhard, J. G. (2000). Racial and ethnic economic inequality: The international record. *The American Economic Review, 90*(2), 308–311.

Deku, S. Y., Kara, A., & Molyneux, P. (2016). Access to Consumer Credit in the UK. *The European Journal of Finance, 22*(10), 941–964. https://doi.org/10.1080/1351847X.2015.1019641

Delgado, R., & Stefancic, J. (2012). *Critical race theory: An introduction*. NYU Press.

Devine, P. G. (1989). Stereotypes and prejudice: Their automatic and controlled components. *Journal of Personality and Social Psychology, 56*(1), 5–18. https://doi.org/10.1037/0022-3514.56.1.5

Devine, P. G., & Elliot, A. J. (1995). Are racial stereotypes really fading? The Princeton trilogy revisited. *Personality and Social Psychology Bulletin, 21*(11), 1139–1150. https://doi.org/10.1177/01461672952111002

Drwecki, B. B., Moore, C. F., Ward, S. E., & Prkachin, K. M. (2011). Reducing racial disparities in pain treatment: The role of empathy and perspective-taking. *Pain, 152*(5), 1001–1006. https://doi.org/10.1016/j.pain.2010.12.005

Eberhardt, J. L., Goff, P. A., Purdie, V. J., & Davies, P. G. (2004). Seeing black: Race, crime, and visual processing. *Journal of Personality and Social Psychology, 87*(6), 876–893. https://doi.org/10.1037/0022-3514.87.6.876

Edwards, R. R. (2008). The Association of Perceived Discrimination with low back pain. *Journal of Behavioral Medicine, 31*(5), 379–389. https://doi.org/10.1007/s10865-008-9160-9

Edwards, R. R., Doleys, D. M., Fillingim, R. B., & Lowery, D. (2001). Ethnic differences in pain tolerance: Clinical implications in a chronic pain population. *Psychosomatic Medicine, 63*(2), 316–323. https://doi.org/10.1097/00006842-200103000-00018

Edwards, R. R., Moric, M., Husfeldt, B., Buvanendran, A., & Ivankovich, O. (2005). Ethnic similarities and differences in the chronic pain experience: A comparison of African American, hispanic, and white patients. *Pain Medicine (Malden, Mass.), 6*(1), 88–98. https://doi.org/10.1111/j.1526-4637.2005.05007.x

Eisenberger, N. I., Jarcho, J. M., Lieberman, M. D., & Naliboff, B. D. (2006). An experimental study of shared sensitivity to physical pain and social rejection. *Pain, 126*(1–3), 132–138. https://doi.org/10.1016/j.pain.2006.06.024

Eisenberger, N. I., & Lieberman, M. D. (2004). Why rejection hurts: A common neural alarm system for physical and social pain. *Trends in Cognitive Sciences, 8*(7), 294–300. https://doi.org/10.1016/j.tics.2004.05.010

Eisenberger, N. I., Lieberman, M. D., & Williams, K. D. (2003). Does rejection hurt? An fMRI study of social exclusion. *Science, 302*(5643), 290–292. https://doi.org/10.1126/science.1089134

Elfenbein, H. A., & Ambady, N. (2002). Is there an in-group advantage in emotion recognition? *Psychological Bulletin, 128*(2), 243–249. https://doi.org/10.1037/0033-2909.128.2.243

Epstein, A. M. (2004). Health Care in America — Still too separate, not yet equal. *New England Journal of Medicine, 351*(6), 603–605. https://doi.org/10.1056/NEJMe048181

Faucett, J., Gordon, N., & Levine, J. (1994). Differences in postoperative pain severity among four ethnic groups. *Journal of Pain and Symptom Management, 9*(6), 383–389. https://doi.org/10.1016/0885-3924(94)90175-9

Feldman, R. (2012). Oxytocin and social affiliation in humans. *Hormones and Behavior, 61*(3), 380–391. https://doi.org/10.1016/j.yhbeh.2012.01.008

Feldman, R., Weller, A., Zagoory-Sharon, O., & Levine, A. (2007). Evidence for a Neuroendocrinological Foundation of Human Affiliation: Plasma oxytocin levels across pregnancy and the postpartum period predict mother-infant bonding. *Psychological Science, 18*(11), 965–970. https://doi.org/10.1111/j.1467-9280.2007.02010.x

Forsythe, L. P., Thorn, B., Day, M., & Shelby, G. (2011). Race and sex differences in primary appraisals, catastrophizing, and experimental pain outcomes. *The Journal of Pain, 12*(5), 563–572. https://doi.org/10.1016/j.jpain.2010.11.003

Freemantle, C. J., Read, A. W., de Klerk, N. H., McAullay, D., Anderson, I. P., & Stanley, F. J. (2006). Patterns, trends, and increasing disparities in mortality for aboriginal and non-aboriginal infants born in Western Australia, 1980-2001: Population database study. *Lancet, 367*(9524), 1758–1766. https://doi.org/10.1016/S0140-6736(06)68771-0

Gazerani, P., & Arendt-Nielsen, L. (2005). The impact of ethnic differences in response to capsaicin-induced trigeminal sensitization. *Pain, 117*(1–2), 223–229. https://doi.org/10.1016/j.pain.2005.06.010

Godolphin, F. R. B. (1942). *The Greek historians: The complete and unabridged works of Herodotus, Thucydides, Xenophon.* Arrian: Random House.

Goff, P. A., Eberhardt, J. L., Williams, M. J., & Jackson, M. C. (2008). Not yet human: Implicit knowledge, historical dehumanization, and contemporary consequences. *Journal of Personality and Social Psychology, 94*(2), 292–306. https://doi.org/10.1037/0022-3514.94.2.292

Goodman, A. H. (2000). Why genes Don't count (for racial differences in health). *American Journal of Public Health, 90*(11), 1699–1702.

Green, C. R., & Hart-Johnson, T. (2012). The association between race and neighborhood socioeconomic status in younger black and white adults with chronic pain. *The Journal of Pain, 13*(2), 176–186. https://doi.org/10.1016/j.jpain.2011.10.008

Green, C. R., Montague, L., & Hart-Johnson, T. A. (2009). Consistent and breakthrough pain in diverse advanced Cancer patients: A longitudinal examination. *Journal of Pain and Symptom Management, 37*(5), 831–847. https://doi.org/10.1016/j.jpainsymman.2008.05.011

Green, C. R., Ndao-Brumblay, S. K., West, B., & Washington, T. (2005). Differences in prescription opioid analgesic availability: Comparing minority and white pharmacies across Michigan. *The Journal of Pain, 6*(10), 689–699. https://doi.org/10.1016/j.jpain.2005.06.002

Grewen, K. M., Light, K. C., Mechlin, B., & Girdler, S. S. (2008). Ethnicity is associated with alterations in oxytocin relationships to pain sensitivity in women. *Ethnicity & Health, 13*(3), 219–241. https://doi.org/10.1080/13557850701837310

Gutsell, J. N., & Inzlicht, M. (2012). Intergroup differences in the sharing of emotive states: Neural evidence of an empathy gap. *Social Cognitive and Affective Neuroscience, 7*(5), 596–603. https://doi.org/10.1093/scan/nsr035

Haider, A. H., Ong'uti, S., Efron, D. T., Oyetunji, T. A., Crandall, M. L., Scott, V. K., … Cornwell, E. E. (2012). Association between hospitals caring for a disproportionately high percentage of minority trauma patients and increased mortality: A Nationwide analysis of 434 hospitals. *Archives of Surgery, 147*(1), 63–70. https://doi.org/10.1001/archsurg.2011.254

Hastie, B. A., Riley, J. L., Kaplan, L., Herrera, D. G., Campbell, C. M., Virtusio, K., … Fillingim, R. B. (2012). Ethnicity interacts with the OPRM1 gene in experimental pain sensitivity. *Pain, 153*(8), 1610–1619. https://doi.org/10.1016/j.pain.2012.03.022

Heath, A. F., Rothon, C., & Kilpi, E. (2008). The second generation in Western Europe: Education, unemployment, and occupational attainment. *Annual Review of Sociology, 34*(1), 211–235. https://doi.org/10.1146/annurev.soc.34.040507.134728

Hein, J. (2000). Interpersonal discrimination against Hmong Americans: Parallels and variation in microlevel racial inequality. *Sociological Quarterly, 41*(3), 413–429. https://doi.org/10.1111/j.1533-8525.2000.tb00085.x

Hirsh, A. T., Alqudah, A. F., Stutts, L. A., & Robinson, M. E. (2008). Virtual human technology: Capturing sex, race, and age influences in individual pain decision policies. *Pain, 140*(1), 231–238. https://doi.org/10.1016/j.pain.2008.09.010

Hirsh, A. T., George, S. Z., & Robinson, M. E. (2009). Pain assessment and treatment disparities: A virtual human technology investigation. *Pain, 143*(1–2), 106–113. https://doi.org/10.1016/j.pain.2009.02.005

Hoffman, K. M., Trawalter, S., Axt, J. R., & Oliver, M. N. (2016). Racial Bias in pain assessment and treatment recommendations, and false beliefs about biological differences between blacks and whites. *Proceedings of the National Academy of Sciences, 113*(16), 4296–4301. https://doi.org/10.1073/pnas.1516047113

Jefferson, T. (1787). *Notes on the state of Virginia.*

Jenkins, S. P., Micklewright, J., & Schnepf, S. V. (2008). Social segregation in secondary schools: How does England compare with other countries? *Oxford Review of Education, 34*(1), 21–37.

Jinabhai, C. C., Coovadia, H. M., & Abdool-Karim, S. S. (1986). Socio-medical indicators of health in South Africa. *International Journal of Health Services: Planning, Administration, Evaluation, 16*(1), 163–176.

Johnston, R., Burgess, S., Wilson, D., & Harris, R. (2006). School and residential ethnic segregation: An analysis of variations across England's local education authorities. *Regional Studies, 40*(9), 973–990. https://doi.org/10.1080/00343400601047390

Jordan, M. S., Lumley, M. A., & Leisen, J. C. (1998). The relationships of cognitive coping and pain control beliefs to pain and adjustment among African-American and Caucasian women with rheumatoid arthritis. *Arthritis Care and Research, 11*(2), 80–88.

Jorde, L. B., & Wooding, S. P. (2004). Genetic variation, classification and "race". *Nature Genetics, 36*, S28–S33. https://doi.org/10.1038/ng1435

Jost, J. T., Banaji, M. R., & Nosek, B. A. (2004). A decade of system justification theory: Accumulated evidence of conscious and unconscious bolstering of the status quo. *Political Psychology, 25*(6), 881–919. https://doi.org/10.1111/j.1467-9221.2004.00402.x

Karsten, S., Felix, C., Ledoux, G., Meijnen, W., Roeleveld, J., & Van Schooten, E. (2006). Choosing segregation or integration? The extent and effects of ethnic segregation in Dutch cities. *Education and Urban Society, 38*(2), 228–247.

Kaseweter, K. A., Drwecki, B. B., & Prkachin, K. M. (2012). Racial differences in pain treatment and empathy in a Canadian sample. *Pain Research & Management, 17*(6), 381–384.

Kim, H. J., Yang, G. S., Greenspan, J. D., Downton, K. D., Griffith, K. A., Renn, C. L., … Dorsey, S. G. (2017). Racial and ethnic differences in experimental pain sensitivity: Systematic review and meta-analysis. *Pain, 158*(2), 194–211. https://doi.org/10.1097/j.pain.0000000000000731

Kingdon, G. G., & Knight, J. (2004). Race and the incidence of unemployment in South Africa. *Review of Development Economics, 8*(2), 198–222. https://doi.org/10.1111/j.1467-9361.2004.00228.x

Kochanek, K. D., Arias, E., & Anderson, R. N. (2013). How did cause of death contribute to racial differences in life expectancy in the United States in 2010? *NCHS Data Brief, 125*, 1–8.

Komen, M., & Schooten, E. V. (2009). Ethnic disparities in Dutch juvenile justice. *Journal of Ethnicity in Criminal Justice, 7*(2), 85–106. https://doi.org/10.1080/15377930902929182

Krieger, N., Smith, K., Naishadham, D., Hartman, C., & Barbeau, E. M. (2005). Experiences of discrimination: Validity and reliability of a self-report measure for population health research on racism and health. *Social Science & Medicine (1982), 61*(7), 1576–1596. https://doi.org/10.1016/j.socscimed.2005.03.006

Kross, E., Berman, M. G., Mischel, W., Smith, E. E., & Wager, T. D. (2011). Social rejection shares somatosensory representations with physical pain. *Proceedings of the National Academy of Sciences, 108*(15), 6270–6275. https://doi.org/10.1073/pnas.1102693108

Kurita, G. P., Sjøgren, P., Juel, K., Højsted, J., & Ekholm, O. (2012). The burden of chronic pain: A cross-sectional survey focusing on diseases, immigration, and opioid use. *Pain, 153*(12), 2332–2338. https://doi.org/10.1016/j.pain.2012.07.023

Laurian, L. (2008). Environmental injustice in France. *Journal of Environmental Planning and Management, 51*(1), 55–79. https://doi.org/10.1080/09640560701712267

Leonard, W. R., Keenleyside, A., & Ivakine, E. (1997). Recent fertility and mortality trends among aboriginal and nonaboriginal populations of Central Siberia. *Human Biology, 69*(3), 403–417.

Longe, S. E., Wise, R., Bantick, S., Lloyd, D., Johansen-Berg, H., McGlone, F., & Tracey, I. (2001). Counter-stimulatory effects on pain perception and processing are significantly altered by attention: An fMRI study. *Neuroreport, 12*(9), 2021–2025.

Lopez, I. F. H. (1994). The social construction of race: Some observations on illusion, fabrication, and choice. *Harvard Civil Rights-Civil Liberties Law Review, 29*, 1.

Lyris, E., & Constantine, M. G. (2006). Racism-related stress, Africultural coping, and religious problem-solving among African Americans. *Cultural Diversity and Ethnic Minority Psychology, 12*(3), 433–443. https://doi.org/10.1037/1099-9809.12.3.433

MacDonald, G., & Leary, M. R. (2005). Why does social exclusion hurt? The relationship between social and physical pain. *Psychological Bulletin, 131*(2), 202–223. https://doi.org/10.1037/0033-2909.131.2.202

Major, B., Spencer, S., Schmader, T., Wolfe, C., & Crocker, J. (1998). Coping with negative stereotypes about intellectual performance: The role of psychological disengagement. *Personality and Social Psychology Bulletin, 24*(1), 34–50. https://doi.org/10.1177/0146167298241003

Mathur, V. A., Richeson, J. A., Paice, J. A., Muzyka, M., & Chiao, J. Y. (2014). Racial Bias in pain perception and response: Experimental examination of automatic and deliberate processes. *The Journal of Pain, 15*(5), 476–484. https://doi.org/10.1016/j.jpain.2014.01.488

Matthews, T. J., MacDorman, M. F., & Thoma, M. E. (2015). Infant mortality statistics from the 2013 period linked birth/infant death data set. *National Vital Statistics Reports: From the Centers for Disease Control and Prevention, National Center for Health Statistics, National Vital Statistics System, 64*(9), 1–30.

Mays, V. M., & Cochran, S. D. (2001). Mental Health Correlates of Perceived Discrimination Among Lesbian, Gay, and Bisexual Adults in the United States. *American Journal of Public Health, 91*(11), 1869–1876.

McDermott, M., & Samson, F. L. (2005). White racial and ethnic identity in the United States. *Annual Review of Sociology, 31*, 245–261.

Mechlin, B., Maixner, W., Light, K. C., Fisher, J. M., & Girdler, S. S. (2005). African Americans show alterations in endogenous pain regulatory mechanisms and reduced pain tolerance to experimental pain procedures. *Psychosomatic Medicine, 67*(6), 948–956. https://doi.org/10.1097/01.psy.0000188466.14546.68

Mechlin, B., Morrow, A. L., Maixner, W., & Girdler, S. S. (2007). The relationship of Allopregnanolone immunoreactivity and HPA-Axis measures to experimental pain sensitivity. Pain, 131(1–2), 142–152. https://doi.org/10.1016/j.pain.2006.12.027

Meghani, S. H., Byun, E., & Gallagher, R. M. (2012). Time to take stock: A meta-analysis and systematic review of analgesic treatment disparities for pain in the United States. *Pain Medicine, 13*(2), 150–174. https://doi.org/10.1111/j.1526-4637.2011.01310.x

Meints, S. M., & Hirsh, A. T. (2015). In vivo praying and catastrophizing mediate the race differences in experimental pain sensitivity. *The Journal of Pain, 16*(5), 491–497. https://doi.org/10.1016/j.jpain.2015.02.005

Meints, S. M., Stout, M., Abplanalp, S., & Hirsh, A. T. (2017). Pain-related rumination, but not magnification or helplessness, mediates race and sex differences in experimental pain. *The Journal of Pain, 18*, 332. https://doi.org/10.1016/j.jpain.2016.11.005

Merchant, J. L., & Omary, M. B. (2010). Underrepresentation of underrepresented minorities in academic medicine: The need to enhance the pipeline and the pipe. *Gastroenterology, 138*(1), 19–26.e3. https://doi.org/10.1053/j.gastro.2009.11.017

Miller, J. (2010). Stop and search in England: A reformed tactic or business as usual? *British Journal of Criminology, 50*(5), 954–974. https://doi.org/10.1093/bjc/azq021

Morning, A. (2014). Does genomics challenge the social construction of race? *Sociological Theory, 32*(3), 189–207. https://doi.org/10.1177/0735275114550881

Nelson, E. E., & Panksepp, J. (1998). Brain substrates of infant–mother attachment: Contributions of opioids, oxytocin, and norepinephrine. *Neuroscience & Biobehavioral Reviews, 22*(3), 437–452. https://doi.org/10.1016/S0149-7634(97)00052-3

Nicholl, B. I., Smith, D. J., Cullen, B., Mackay, D., Evans, J., Anderson, J., … Mair, F. S. (2015). Ethnic differences in the association between depression and chronic pain: Cross sectional Results from UK biobank. *BMC Family Practice, 16*(128), 128. https://doi.org/10.1186/s12875-015-0343-5

O'Nions, H. (2010). Different and unequal: The educational segregation of Roma pupils in Europe. *Intercultural Education, 21*(1), 1–13. https://doi.org/10.1080/14675980903491833

Pager, D. (2003). The mark of a criminal record. *American Journal of Sociology, 108*(5), 937–975. https://doi.org/10.1086/ajs.2003.108.issue-5

Palit, S., Kerr, K. L., Kuhn, B. L., Terry, E. L., Delventura, J. L., Bartley, E. J., … Rhudy, J. L. (2013). Exploring pain processing differences in native Americans. *Health Psychology, 32*(11), 1127–1136. https://doi.org/10.1037/a0031057

Panksepp, J. (1998). *Affective neuroscience: The foundations of human and animal emotions.* New York: Oxford University Press.

Peres, M. A., Iser, B. P. M., Peres, K. G., Malta, D. C., & Antunes, J. L. F. (2012). Contextual and individual inequalities in dental pain prevalence among Brazilian adults and elders. *Cadernos De Saude Publica, 28*(Suppl), s114–s123.

Petrovic, P., Petersson, K. M., Ghatan, P. H., Stone-Elander, S., & Ingvar, M. (2000). Pain-related cerebral activation is altered by a distracting cognitive task. *Pain, 85*(1–2), 19–30.

Proctor, B. D., Semega, J. L., & Kollar, M. A. (2015). Income and Poverty in the United States: 2015. Retrieved from http://www.census.gov/library/publications/2016/demo/p60-256.html

Rahim-Williams, B., Riley, J. L., Williams, A. K. K., & Fillingim, R. B. (2012). A quantitative review of ethnic group differences in experimental pain response: Do biology, psychology, and culture matter? *Pain Medicine, 13*(4), 522–540. https://doi.org/10.1111/j.1526-4637.2012.01336.x

Rahim-Williams, F. B., Riley, J. L., Herrera, D., Campbell, C., Hastie, B. A., & Fillingim, R. B. (2007). Ethnic identity predicts experimental pain sensitivity in African Americans and Hispanics. *Pain, 129*(1–2), 177–184. https://doi.org/10.1016/j.pain.2006.12.016

Rainville, P., Duncan, G. H., Price, D. D., Carrier, B., & Bushnell, M. C. (1997). Pain affect encoded in human anterior cingulate but not somatosensory cortex. *Science, 277*(5328), 968–971. https://doi.org/10.1126/science.277.5328.968

Ravelli, A. C. J., Schaaf, J. M., Eskes, M., Abu-Hanna, A., de Miranda, E., & Mol, B. W. J. (2013). Ethnic disparities in perinatal mortality at 40 and 41 weeks of gestation. *Journal of Perinatal Medicine, 41*(4), 381–388. https://doi.org/10.1515/jpm-2012-0228

Riley, J. L., III, Wade, J. B., Myers, C. D., Sheffield, D., Papas, R. K., & Price, D. D. (2002). Racial/ethnic differences in the experience of chronic pain. *Pain, 100*(3), 291–298. https://doi.org/10.1016/S0304-3959(02)00306-8

Riva, P., Wirth, J. H., & Williams, K. D. (2011). The consequences of pain: The social and physical pain overlap on psychological responses. *European Journal of Social Psychology, 41*(6), 681–687. https://doi.org/10.1002/ejsp.837

Rosenthal, L., & Lobel, M. (2016). Stereotypes of black American women related to sexuality and motherhood. *Psychology of Women Quarterly, 40*(3), 414–427. https://doi.org/10.1177/0361684315627459

Rosette, A. S., Leonardelli, G. J., & Phillips, K. W. (2008). The white standard: Racial Bias in leader categorization. *Journal of Applied Psychology, 93*(4), 758–777. https://doi.org/10.1037/0021-9010.93.4.758

Rosicova, K., Reijneveld, S. A., Madarasova Geckova, A., Stewart, R. E., Rosic, M., Groothoff, J. W., & van Dijk, J. P. (2015). Inequalities in mortality by socioeconomic factors and Roma ethnicity in the two biggest cities in Slovakia: A multilevel analysis. *International Journal for Equity in Health, 14*(123), 123. https://doi.org/10.1186/s12939-015-0262-z

Saarela, J., & Finnäs, F. (2014). Infant mortality and ethnicity in an indigenous European population: Novel evidence from the Finnish population register. *Scientific Reports, 4*(4214). https://doi.org/10.1038/srep04214

Saucier, D. A., Miller, C. T., & Doucet, N. (2005). Differences in helping whites and blacks: A meta-analysis. *Personality and Social Psychology Review, 9*(1), 2–16. https://doi.org/10.1207/s15327957pspr0901_1

Sawamoto, N., Honda, M., Okada, T., Hanakawa, T., Kanda, M., Fukuyama, H., … Shibasaki, H. (2000). Expectation of pain enhances responses to nonpainful somatosensory stimulation in the anterior cingulate cortex and parietal operculum/posterior insula: An event-related functional magnetic resonance imaging study. *Journal of Neuroscience, 20*(19), 7438–7445.

Sellers, R. M., & Nicole, J. (2003). The role of racial identity in perceived racial discrimination. *Journal of Personality and Social Psychology, 84*(5), 1079–1092. https://doi.org/10.1037/0022-3514.84.5.1079

Sharp, D., & Atherton, S. (2007). To serve and protect? The experiences of policing in the Community of Young People from black and other ethnic minority groups. *The British Journal of Criminology, 47*(5), 746–763. https://doi.org/10.1093/bjc/azm024

Smedley, A. (1998). "Race" and the construction of human identity. *American Anthropologist, 100*(3), 690–702. https://doi.org/10.1525/aa.1998.100.3.690

Smedley, A., & Smedley, B. D. (2005). Race as biology is fiction, racism as a social problem is real: Anthropological and historical perspectives on the social construction of race. *American Psychologist, 60*(1), 16–26. https://doi.org/10.1037/0003-066X.60.1.16

Smedley, B. D., Stith, A. Y., & Nelson, A. R. (2003). *Unequal treatment: Confronting racial and ethnic disparities in health care.* (B. D. Smedley, A. Y. Stith, & A. R. Nelson, Eds.). Washington, DC: National Academies Press.

Snowden, F. M. (1983). *Before color prejudice: The ancient view of blacks.* Harvard University Press.

Staton, L. J., Panda, M., Chen, I., Genao, I., Kurz, J., Pasanen, M., … Cykert, S. (2007). When race matters: Disagreement in pain perception between patients and their physicians in primary care. *Journal of the National Medical Association, 99*(5), 532–538.

Stürmer, S., Snyder, M., Kropp, A., & Siem, B. (2006). Empathy-motivated helping: The moderating role of group membership. *Personality and Social Psychology Bulletin, 32*(7), 943–956. https://doi.org/10.1177/0146167206287363

Stutts, L. A., Hirsh, A. T., George, S. Z., & Robinson, M. E. (2010). Investigating patient characteristics on pain assessment using virtual human technology. *European Journal of Pain, 14*(10), 1040–1045. https://doi.org/10.1016/j.ejpain.2010.04.003

Sudbury, J. (2014). *Global lockdown: Race, gender, and the prison-industrial complex*. Routledge.

Sullivan, L. W. (2004, September). Missing Persons: Minorities in the Health Professions, A Report of the Sullivan Commission on Diversity in the Healthcare Workforce [Report Document or Other Monograph]. Retrieved January 6, 2017, from http://www.aacn.nche.edu/Media/pdf/SullivanReport.pdf

Surenjav, E., Sovd, T., Yoshida, Y., Yamamoto, E., Reyer, J. A., & Hamajima, N. (2016). Trends in amenable mortality rate in the Mongolian population, 2007-2014. *Nagoya Journal of Medical Science, 78*(1), 55–68.

Szulkin, R., & Jonsson, J. O. (2007). Ethnic segregation and educational outcomes in Swedish comprehensive schools. Stockholm University Linnaeus Center. Retrieved from http://www.diva-portal.org/smash/record.jsf?pid=diva2:176854

Torres, C. A., Bartley, E. J., Wandner, L. D., Alqudah, A. F., Hirsh, A. T., & Robinson, M. E. (2013). The influence of sex, race, and age on pain assessment and treatment decisions using virtual human technology: A cross-National Comparison. *Journal of Pain Research, 6*, 577–588. https://doi.org/10.2147/JPR.S46295

Trawalter, S., & Hoffman, K. M. (2015). Got pain? Racial Bias in perceptions of pain. *Social and Personality Psychology Compass, 9*(3), 146–157. https://doi.org/10.1111/spc3.12161

Trawalter, S., Hoffman, K. M., & Waytz, A. (2012). Racial Bias in perceptions of others' pain. *PLoS One, 7*(11), e48546. https://doi.org/10.1371/journal.pone.0048546

Trevethan, S., & Rastin, C. J. (2007). *A profile of visible minority offenders in the federal Canadian correctional system*. Retrieved January 4, 2017, from http://www.csc-scc.gc.ca/research/r144-eng.shtml

van der Hammen, T., de Roos, A. M., Sabelis, M. W., & Janssen, A. (2010). Order of invasion affects the spatial distribution of a reciprocal Intraguild predator. *Oecologia, 163*(1), 79–89. https://doi.org/10.1007/s00442-010-1575-7

Wandner, L. D., Torres, C. A., Bartley, E. J., George, S. Z., & Robinson, M. E. (2015). Effect of a perspective-taking intervention on the consideration of pain assessment and treatment decisions. *Journal of Pain Research, 8*, 809–818. https://doi.org/10.2147/JPR.S88033

Watson, P. J., Latif, R. K., & Rowbotham, D. J. (2005). Ethnic differences in thermal pain responses: A comparison of south Asian and white British healthy males. *Pain, 118*(1–2), 194–200. https://doi.org/10.1016/j.pain.2005.08.010

Williams, D. R. (1999). Race, socioeconomic status, and health the added effects of racism and discrimination. *Annals of the New York Academy of Sciences, 896*(1), 173–188. https://doi.org/10.1111/j.1749-6632.1999.tb08114.x

Yudell, M., Roberts, D., DeSalle, R., & Tishkoff, S. (2016). Taking race out of human genetics. *Science, 351*(6273), 564–565. https://doi.org/10.1126/science.aac4951

Zborowski, M. (1952). Cultural components in responses to Pain1. *Journal of Social Issues, 8*(4), 16–30. https://doi.org/10.1111/j.1540-4560.1952.tb01860.x

Zinn, H. (2010). *A People's history of the United States*. Harper Collins.

Zisook, S., Devaul, R. A., & Click, M. A. (1982). Measuring symptoms of grief and bereavement. *The American Journal of Psychiatry, 139*(12), 1590–1593. https://doi.org/10.1176/ajp.139.12.1590

Part VIII
Towards Change: Targets and Methods for Intervention

Chapter 22
Toward Change: Targeting Individual and Interpersonal Processes in Therapeutic Interventions for Chronic Pain

Rocio de la Vega, Emma Fisher, and Tonya M. Palermo

Abstract Pain demands attention of the individual experiencing it, but also involves a dynamic process between the individual in pain and relevant observers. Observers may include healthcare providers, employers, friends, romantic partners, and family members, among others. Observers can play an important role in understanding of pain diagnosis and treatment, in helping patients feel motivated to participate in treatments and engage in self-care behaviors, and in the individual's long-term coping with chronic pain. Interpersonal processes that underlie communication about pain are dynamic and may change over time due to learned responses from the individual or observer. For example, the characteristics of the individual in pain may influence the observer's likelihood of offering assistance or providing empathic support versus their likelihood of criticizing and invalidating the individual in pain. In turn, the observer's reaction may influence the individual in pain such as leading to positive or negative expectations for pain treatment or leading to feelings of empathic understanding versus feelings of being stigmatized. In this chapter, we summarize individual and interpersonal processes from the perspective of the individual in pain versus the observer. Next, we highlight examples of interventions that aim to modify these individual or interpersonal processes to move toward

R. de la Vega
Department of Rehabilitation Medicine, University of Washington, Seattle, WA, USA

Center for Child Health, Behavior, and Development, Seattle Children's Research Institute, Seattle, WA, USA

E. Fisher
Center for Child Health, Behavior, and Development, Seattle Children's Research Institute, Seattle, WA, USA

T. M. Palermo (✉)
Center for Child Health, Behavior, and Development, Seattle Children's Research Institute, Seattle, WA, USA

Department of Anesthesiology and Pain Medicine, University of Washington, Seattle, WA, USA
e-mail: tonya.palermo@seattlechildrens.org

© Springer International Publishing AG, part of Springer Nature 2018
T. Vervoort et al. (eds.), *Social and Interpersonal Dynamics in Pain*,
https://doi.org/10.1007/978-3-319-78340-6_22

change in the pain experience. Last, we present ideas for future research to develop novel treatments targeted toward change in individual or interpersonal processes that underlie pain communication.

Keywords Pain · Interpersonal processes · Communication · Interventions · Observer · Expectations · Empathy · Stigma

Individual Processes

Individual processes influence the experience of pain. For example, the individual in pain has their own core beliefs about pain and how pain should be treated that may influence interactions with healthcare professionals and motivation and preferences toward specific pain interventions. In this section, we explore expectations, stigma, and validation as three potentially modifiable factors that are central to observers' responses and that may influence the individual's experience of chronic pain and its treatment.

Expectations

Expectations can determine the healthcare that people pursue, as well as their receptivity to and adherence to recommended treatments. Expectations may be influenced by past experiences of pain or by medical knowledge about pain and pain treatment. A substantial body of research in adults with chronic pain has identified treatment expectations as a robust predictor of treatment outcomes. For example, in an observational cohort study of 2272 patients receiving multidisciplinary pain treatment, higher expectations of treatment success were associated with greater change in pain-related outcomes (pain intensity, catastrophizing, depression, pain interference, and satisfaction) (Cormier, Lavigne, Choinière, & Rainville, 2016). Related, greater adherence to cognitive behavioral treatments has also been associated with greater improvements in symptoms of pain, disability and depression (Nicholas et al., 2012). Cormier et al. (2016) suggest that patients with greater expectancies are more likely to be optimistic and adherent to treatments, and higher expectations can reduce anxiety.

fMRI studies have provided neurobiological evidence of the role of treatment expectations in the pain experience. In one study investigating acupuncture versus sham therapy, those with high expectations across both treatments reported lower pain intensity compared to those with lower expectations (Kong et al., 2009). Further supporting these findings, fMRI activity showed decreased activity in brain regions associated with processing pain signals (e.g., anterior cingulate cortex, medial pre frontal cortex) in the group with high expectations, demonstrating the modulating analgesic effect of positive expectations. Other studies have likewise found that when pain is induced experimentally and treatment expectancies are assessed, providing expectations for analgesia leads to lower pain ratings and specific expected neural changes in brain regions associated with pain processing (Schenk, Sprenger, Geuter, & Buchel, 2014).

A systematic review of back pain patients concluded that there was a gap between patient expectations and services offered by healthcare professionals. In a summary of 12 qualitative and eight quantitative studies, findings demonstrated that patients had four primary expectations when visiting a healthcare professional with back pain. Patients wanted: (1) a diagnosis of their pain problem, (2) instructions or advice on pain management, (3) effective relief for their pain condition, and (4) sickness certification (Verbeek, Sengers, Riemens, & Haafkens, 2004). In a more recent study of expectations for pain clinic visits, patients similarly expected from the visit to receive pain relief, education on the cause of pain, and a definitive diagnosis (Calpin, Imran, & Harmon, 2017); pain physicians, on the other hand, expected to formulate a management plan, conduct a patient assessment for the cause of pain, and educate patients on the cause of pain. Although research has not specifically examined the impact of whether patient treatment expectations are met in their healthcare encounters, a mismatch in expectations would be anticipated to reduce adherence to treatment.

Very limited research has been conducted on children's expectations for pain treatment to understand whether similar patterns to adults are observed. Because parents are primarily responsible for bringing their child for evaluation and treatment, parents' expectations likely play an important role. There are several studies demonstrating that children and parents expect physiotherapy, psychotherapy, medical intervention and complementary and alternative medicine (i.e., hypnosis, massage, acupuncture) to be most helpful for the child's chronic pain (Guite et al., 2014; Tsao et al., 2005). Further, holding positive expectations regarding the beneficial effects of psychological treatment and biofeedback treatment were related to subsequent adherence to psychological interventions offered to children in a pain clinic (Simons, Logan, Chastain, & Cerullo, 2010). However, there has been no investigation of the relationship between children's treatment expectations and outcomes. It is unclear if there are developmental differences in the effect of expectations on the pain experience or whether parent expectations would have a stronger relationship to treatment outcomes; further research in pediatric pain populations is needed.

Stigma

As outlined within Chap. 12, studies indicate that a large number of people with chronic pain feel stigmatized by others (e.g., Waugh, Byrne, & Nicholas, 2014). Stigma can be internalized, meaning those with chronic pain develop their own thoughts that are negative and stigmatizing about having pain, or the stigma may be experienced from the attitudes or behaviors from others toward the individual in pain. Chronic pain can be invisible to the observer, without physical signs, and because pain is assessed subjectively, it can be difficult to describe and convey to others. For these reasons, observers of people with pain can become suspicious, not trusting that pain is as severe or disabling as patients report.

People with chronic pain can feel stigmatized by observers including friends, family, healthcare providers, and the wider society (De Ruddere & Craig, 2016). Within the workplace, people with chronic pain have felt hostility from colleagues and managers and describe injustice of chronic pain (McParland, Eccleston, Osborn, & Hezseltine, 2011). For children with chronic pain, social stigma may be experienced through negative interactions with teachers and the school system as well as through isolation and the loss of social interactions and perceiving themselves as 'different' from peers (Eccleston, Wastell, Crombez, & Jordan, 2008; Forgeron, Evans, McGrath, Stevens, & Finley, 2013).

Higher stigma is associated with reduced hope, lower self-esteem and empowerment, and increased symptom severity in people with mental illnesses (Livingston & Boyd, 2010). However, less research has investigated the effects of stigma on physical and emotional health in patients with chronic pain. In the few studies in this area, patient perception of others discounting or not understanding their pain condition is related to poorer physical and mental health (Kool, van Middendorp, Lumley, Bijlsma, & Geenen, 2013). Further, patients perceiving higher levels of stigma report lower self-efficacy and self-esteem, even when depressive symptoms are accounted for (Waugh et al., 2014).

Validation

Contrary to stigma, validation by an observer provides legitimacy to an individual who has chronic pain (see also Chap. 13). It conveys that an observer believes the symptom reporting of the individual with chronic pain. People with chronic pain have reported that they feel others think their pain is imagined or exaggerated and when diagnostic tests do reveal an underlying pathology for their pain, patients often describe feeling relieved (Rhodes, McPhillips-Tangum, Markham, & Klenk, 1999). However, patients that did not agree with their diagnosis also reported higher pain, disability, and more maladaptive coping strategies (Geisser & Roth, 1998). This is congruent with cultural expectations within modern Western medical culture that when individuals experience pain they seek a biomedical explanation for illness (Eccleston, 2013).

Other groups, including parents and spouses also search for validation of their child's or partner's condition. Parents describe searching for a medical diagnosis for their child's pain, and that they struggle to convince others of the severity of the child's pain problem (Jordan, Eccleston, & Osborn, 2007), confronting societal disbelief and even accusations of harming their child (e.g., Munchausen syndrome)

(Jordan et al., 2007). In another qualitative study, Noel, Beals-Erickson, Law, Alberts, and Palermo (2016), characterized parents' narratives about their child's pain into those signifying distress versus resilience. Distress narratives were characterized by having unresolved diagnoses of the child's pain, pessimism, and negative affect. Resilience narratives, on the other hand, were typically more positive, had a resolved diagnosis of the child's pain, and were more optimistic, highlighting the importance of having the child's diagnosis confirmed or validated. Similarly, validation between individuals with chronic pain and their spouses is also important. In couples in which a spouse expresses more validation and empathy for their partner's pain, better marital satisfaction has been found (Cano, Barterian, & Heller, 2008).

Communication with healthcare professionals is a primary context for patients to communicate and receive validation for their pain. In a systematic review by Verbeek et al. (2004), patients reported that they wanted healthcare professionals to communicate with them with confidence, and to listen to their pain problem with understanding and respect. The diagnosis given for the patient's pain problem was perceived as part of this validation. Diagnoses that change over time, or are perceived as inadequate can be associated with mistrust and decreased patient satisfaction.

In summary, individual processes including expectations, stigma, and validation are three potentially modifiable factors that may influence and be influenced by interactions with an observer. In the next section, we take the reverse perspective from the standpoint of the observer focusing on observer processes that may influence the individual's experience of chronic pain and its treatment.

Observer Processes

Adequate management of pain ultimately relies upon the understanding abilities of an observer (Craig, 2009). There are several characteristics that may influence the way people perceive and react to others' pain, and we focus on two of them that are potentially modifiable: attitude implicit bias and empathy.

Attitude Implicit Bias

This term refers to "relatively unconscious and relatively automatic features of prejudiced judgment and social behavior" (Brownstein, 2016). A number of studies show that perceptions of people with pain are usually more negative than of healthy people, in that people with pain are judged as less competent and more depressed (Ashton-James, Richardson, Williams, Bianchi-Berthouze, & Dekker, 2014). These biases may have a significant impact on the individual with pain, leading to differences in the treatment options offered (Hollingshead, Matthias, Bair, & Hirsh, 2015). As highlighted in a recent systematic review, biases are particularly pronounced for females and racial minorities (Hampton, Cavalier, & Langford, 2015). The experience of bias may also lead to feelings of stigma or victimization as reviewed earlier. Perceptions of others' pain are subjective and change as a function of the implicit biases held toward personal characteristics of the one in pain (e.g., diagnosis, race, and sex) and vary by observer relationship role (Torres et al., 2013; Hirsh, Hollingshead, Ashburn-Nardo, & Kroenke, 2015; Wandner et al., 2014).

Clarity of a medical diagnosis is a determining factor in bias in other's perception (see also Chap. 12). In this regard, it is noteworthy that studies including several groups of observers (e.g., general population, nurses, physicians, and physiotherapists) show that observers tend to rate other's pain as lower if it is chronic or has an unclear diagnosis (i.e., there is no medical evidence to justify it) (De Ruddere & Craig, 2016; Samolsky Dekel et al., 2016).

In children, observers' biases have also been found when medical evidence is not available for the child's pain condition. For example, in a study using a vignette methodology, teachers were more likely to endorse physical causes for pain, perceive the pain as more severe and impairing if medical evidence was supplied (Logan, Catanese, Coakley, & Scharff, 2007; Logan, Coakley, & Scharff, 2006). In addition, teachers were also more likely to provide relief and make accommodations for the student if medical information concerning the pain condition was provided.

Race is another source of bias regarding pain judgments (Hall et al., 2015). Several studies conclude that Black people are usually judged as being less sensitive to pain (Trawalter, Hoffman, & Waytz, 2012). This is despite data from studies testing experimental pain sensitivity (Morris et al., 2015; Riley et al., 2014) finding that Black individuals are more (rather than less) sensitive to pain. Racial bias toward others' pain occurs both in adults and children; individuals develop this racial bias between 7 and 10 years of age (Dore, Hoffman, Lillard, & Trawalter, 2014).

Women are usually viewed as more sensitive to pain than men, although in experimental studies, sex differences do not consistently emerge for sensitivity to different pain stimuli (Racine et al., 2012). In a recent study, healthcare professionals were asked to rate pain intensity of video-recorded patients and to recommend a treatment for them; women were estimated to have less pain than men. Moreover, women who were deemed untrustworthy (but not men) were judged to exaggerate their pain more and have less pain. Consequently, providers were more likely to recommend psychological treatment for women's chronic pain in contrast to men who were more likely to be recommended analgesics for their pain (Schäfer, Prkachin, Kaseweter, & Williams, 2016).

Depending on the role of the observer (i.e., the relationship with the one in pain), the accuracy of the judgments of pain in others varies. For example, nurses and physicians tend to underestimate patient's pain (e.g., pain in the elderly, burn pain, or cancer pain). These effects are moderated by a central tendency in pain judgments (i.e., overrating low pain and underrating high pain levels) and years of experience (Solomon, 2001). In a study of couples with one member having chronic pain, it was found that men perceived a higher number of pain-related interactions and that they had a tendency to respond to them in a more solicitous way than women (Newton-John & de C Williams, 2006). When the one in pain is a child it has been well established that the judgments by a proxy are not accurate (Kamper, Dissing, & Hestbaek, 2016; Zhou, Roberts, & Horgan, 2008). However, nurses were found to be more accurate in judging facial expressions of pain (that could be neutral, faked, or genuine) than parents (Boerner, Chambers, Craig, Pillai Riddell, & Parker, 2013), and fathers were more accurate judging their children's pain than mothers (Moon et al., 2008).

Empathy

Empathy can be defined as "the action of understanding, being aware of, being sensitive to, and vicariously experiencing the feelings, thoughts, and experience of another without having the feelings, thoughts, and experience fully communicated in an objectively explicit manner" (Medical Definition of Empathy, n.d.). Being empathic toward others' pain and the resulting behavior (Goubert et al., 2005) may help those in pain to feel validated. Recent studies have been conducted to understand the neurological correlates of pain empathy in adults (e.g., Bucchioni et al., 2016; Fabi & Leuthold, 2016; Majdandžić, Amashaufer, Hummer, Windischberger, & Lamm, 2016; Mischkowski, Crocker, & Way, 2016), concluding that the prefrontal areas play a determinant role. Moreover, the personal characteristics of the one in pain moderate the effect of empathy of the observer; empathy is higher when the individual in pain is perceived as similar to the observer (Majdandžić et al., 2016).

Empathy toward pain starts to develop at an early age, being present in children as young as 18 months (Bandstra, Chambers, McGrath, & Moore, 2011). However, in comparison to empathy toward other emotional states (i.e., sadness) pain empathy is not as robust. Fewer prosocial behaviors are shown toward those in pain compared to those displaying sadness (Bandstra et al., 2011).

Empathy from a significant other may influence the experience of the one in pain. A recent controlled study, conducted in a laboratory setting, found that the touch from a significant other (a romantic partner touching their partner's skin, in this case) had a higher analgesic effect than touch from non-empathic partners or strangers (Goldstein, Shamay-Tsoory, Yellinek, & Weissman-Fogel, 2016), illustrating the potential beneficial effects for modifying pain perception.

Empathy toward the thoughts or feelings of the one in pain is also moderated by the characteristics (e.g., anxiety) of both the observer and the one in pain. For example, in a study with couples, partners' level of catastrophizing about their partners' pain was associated with empathy toward thoughts (e.g., knowing that the one in pain is thinking that the other is not understanding the situation), whilst pain severity of the one in pain was associated with empathy toward feelings (e.g., knowing that the one in pain is feeling frustrated) (Leonard, Issner, Cano, & Williams, 2013). Similarly, parents with high catastrophizing toward their children's pain paid more attention to their child's pain behavior (Vervoort et al., 2011). In another study, parents with distress narratives (negative affect and an unresolved orientation toward the child's diagnosis) had higher catastrophizing than parents with resilience narratives (Noel et al., 2016).

In summary, attitude implicit bias and empathy are two potentially modifiable observer processes that may influence interactions with the individual in pain, and differ by characteristics of the observer and the one in pain.

Interventions

Several interventions have been developed to modify individual and interpersonal processes within the context of pain and other chronic illnesses. In this section, we describe interventions targeted at (1) modifying expectations, (2) improving communication, and (3) improving attitudes, empathy, and validation. Interventions have been delivered to patients with chronic pain and to observers of a patient in pain (e.g., healthcare professional, spouse, parent, teacher, peer).

Expectations Interventions

Adapting expectations for treatment could be an important target of intervention given the treatment moderation effects found where individuals with higher expectations benefit the most from pain treatments. Interventions to enhance personal expectations are relevant to any treatment (e.g., medication, psychological intervention, physical therapy), and thus have broad applicability. Such interventions might also be applicable to any age group, although there are limited data in younger and older populations. Children and adolescents have been excluded from the systematic reviews and meta-analyses on the topic; however, there are several relevant studies in the procedural pain literature with children. For example, in one study conducted with children 6–12 years old, a picture book explaining a blood draw procedure was successfully used to set positive expectations about the procedure and subsequently led to reduced pain intensity (Zieger, Praskova, Busse, & Barth, 2013). Although, to the best of our knowledge, no research has been conducted specifically in the elderly regarding expectation interventions, it has been recommended as a treatment target (Reid, 2016). In addition, we are not aware of any interventions targeting observer expectations, although this is a potentially fruitful avenue for future intervention development, which could influence the behaviors, support, and care offered by providers, parents, and other observers for the patient. Here we discuss two of the most studied interventions to alter personal expectations in patients: verbal suggestions and mental imagery.

Verbal suggestion interventions involving making explicit favorable statements about a treatment (either an active treatment or a placebo) have successfully increased patients' outcome expectancies and reduced pain. The verbal suggestion itself may include a statement to induce positive expectancies, such as "The treatment you have just been given is known to powerfully reduce pain in some patients." This has been the most studied intervention, and findings from a meta-analysis show that it has a medium to large effect on pain relief in samples of adults with various types of chronic pain (e.g., migraines, back pain, and irritable bowel syndrome) (Peerdeman et al., 2016).

Mental imagery consists of inviting the patient to imagine an ideal future or outcome, like creating a mental image of him or herself healing or experiencing the benefits of the treatment. This specific manner of using mental imagery is intended to increase expectations of treatment success. In some applications of mental imagery, relaxation and positive statements are taught to the patient as well. There is moderate support for mental imagery from six studies included in the Peerdeman review (Peerdeman et al., 2016) in patients undergoing colonoscopy, cancer pain, abortion, coronary angiography, head and neck surgery, and IV therapy. All of the studies include samples with acute pain (e.g., surgery) with the exception of one study with patients with cancer-related pain. The effects on pain relief are shown to be small.

Communication Interventions

Communication between the observer and the one in pain is a key element that may be used to ease the pain experience. In this regard, there are a number of interventions that specifically target communication which we describe below. These interventions aim to improve both the communication from clinicians to patients and from patients to clinicians, and also communication among patients and couples/family members.

From Clinicians to Patients One study has delivered an intervention to nurses directed at communicating pain to hospitalized patients with a variety of medical-surgical diagnoses (Alaloul, Williams, Myers, Jones, & Logsdon, 2015). The researchers found that providing the nurses with guidelines about communication strategies led to improved communication and also improved patient satisfaction with pain treatment. Strategies to improve communication included using whiteboards to write down information, implementing script-based communication, and conducting hourly rounds.

Established strategies for improving pain communication are scarce; however, there are established strategies in other chronic health conditions such as cancer. We review these here as they may also be applicable to chronic pain. A Cochrane review examining the effectiveness of communication skills training for healthcare professionals (e.g., teaching skills for building rapport, structuring the interviews, initiating the session, gathering information, giving explanations, planning interventions, and closing the session) found beneficial effects for improving information gathering and supportive skills with cancer patients. For example, after receiving communication interventions, healthcare professionals were more likely to use open questions and to show empathy toward patients (Moore, Rivera Mercado, Grez Artigues, & Lawrie, 2013).

From Patients to Clinicians To our knowledge, there have not been any pain communication interventions applied to patients to enhance their communication to their healthcare provider. There is an existing literature in other clinical encounters. Two systematic reviews may be relevant, including a review of patient knowledge translation strategies for clinical encounters in general (Gagliardi et al., 2015) and a review of interventions seeking to improve communication between pediatric patients or their parents and medical providers (Kodjebacheva, Sabo, & Xiong, 2016).

Gagliardi et al.'s review (Gagliardi et al., 2015) includes 16 studies investigating varied strategies such as providing printed materials or access to websites in samples of patients with cancer ($n = 11$) and arthritis ($n = 5$) with the goal of providing them with information about how to enhance communication with a healthcare provider and to activate their proactive behavior in this respect. Results of this review demonstrated that providing guidance and prompts to facilitate communication with healthcare professionals had positive effects on increasing patient self-efficacy, readiness to ask questions, and the amount of patient–provider communication.

The review centered on pediatric patients (Kodjebacheva et al., 2016) highlights a number of interventions delivered to clinicians, parents, or children. Interventions targeted at clinicians in 15 studies were delivered via educational seminars, lectures, and printed materials on effective communication. A further 13 studies consisted of simulation sessions and role-play with fictitious patients (medical visits or counseling session with standardized patients and a feedback session). These interventions were shown to enhance the clinician's patient-centered interviewing skills. Five studies delivered interventions to parents; they comprised role-playing to encourage questions, providing written information booklets, and a video to promote communication. Studies generally found that parent satisfaction and communication were improved. Finally, one study with children watching a role-modeling video of children communicating with a physician was included; researchers found that viewing the video helped children to build better rapport with physicians and to recall their recommendations about the treatment.

Communication Among Patients and Family Members Several published interventions in osteoarthritis patients and their partners have aimed to specifically improve communication between these dyads (Martire, Schulz, Keefe, Rudy, & Starz, 2008). For example, in one study, 103 couples participated in an intervention based on the Arthritis Self-Management Program and either participated in patient-only groups or couples groups. The six week group intervention for patients included information about the etiology and treatment of arthritis, self-management strategies, communication skills, and coping with negative emotion. The intervention for couples was similar in format and content with the addition of couples' examples when possible such as explaining effective and ineffective strategies for requesting spousal assistance (e.g., pain expressions or asking for help). When comparing the couple interventions with patient-centered ones, a greater decrease in the spouses' punishing responses (like anger or irritation) was found at post-treatment as well as higher perceived spouse support at a six-month follow-up.

Additional research has been conducted with participants with other health problems. In a meta-analysis regarding interventions for couples with chronic illnesses (Martire, Schulz, Helgeson, Small, & Saghafi, 2010), 33 studies were reviewed, including a subset with chronic pain (n = 4) and arthritis (n = 7). In general, these studies including couple interventions demonstrated greater effects on reducing depression, improving marital functioning, and decreasing pain than patient-only interventions. The authors conclude that targeting spouse communication may be important to enhance the benefit of chronic illness interventions.

While most of the pediatric chronic pain intervention studies with parents have focused on changing parent behavior, several studies have provided multifaceted interventions to parents including interventions to improve parent–child communication. For example, Palermo et al. (2016) conducted a randomized controlled multicenter trial of a Web-based intervention for adolescents with mixed types of chronic pain and their parents. In this study, 138 families were allocated to an Internet-delivered cognitive-behavioral intervention and 135 to Internet-delivered education intervention. The program consisted of 9 h of intervention (4 h for adolescents, 4 h for parents, and 1 h of coaching). Parents learned a range of strategies including operant strategies, modeling, supporting independence, and enhancing communication about pain with their child. As a result of the intervention, among other benefits to youth, parental responses to pain behaviors significantly improved: the intervention group experienced small to medium effects on reducing maladaptive behaviors (i.e., significantly greater reduction in protective behaviors) compared to the attention control group.

Stigma, Empathy, and Validation Interventions

Few interventions have been conducted in observers of patients with chronic pain, including healthy bystanders, healthcare professionals, or parents/spouses to reduce stigma, or increase empathy and validation.

Interventions that target stigma and knowledge are predominantly educational. De Ruddere and Craig (2016, see also Chap. 12) suggest that interventions to address stigma should be threefold: intrapersonal, interpersonal, and structural. Further, pain education to healthcare professionals has been recommended to increase understanding of the causes and consequences of chronic pain within a biopsychosocial model (De Ruddere & Craig, 2016). Interventions that have been targeted at changing attitudes regarding pain management include education interventions for healthcare professionals. These educational interventions aim to change behavior (i.e., assessing pain scores, reconciling differences between patients' and nurses' pain scores) through didactic presentations on pain management for patients with acute pain and cancer pain. Although positive effects on provider behavior are seen immediately after intervention, they are not maintained over time (Gustafsson & Borglin, 2013; Schreiber et al., 2014). However, interventions altering thoughts and behaviors of healthcare providers, spouses, and families of those with chronic pain have not yet been developed or evaluated.

There is also a literature on interventions delivered to the public, students, healthcare professionals, or people with mental health problems that aim to reduce stigma. Interventions delivered to observers are predominantly educational consisting of mental health education, education about stigma, history of mental illness, and education about self-harm or other specific mental health conditions. These interventions have found positive effects for reducing stigma about mental health problems (Clement et al., 2013; Mehta et al., 2015). Specifically, positive benefits of intervention were found on reductions of attitude biases regarding mental health. Interventions delivered to people with mental health conditions are psychoeducational or cognitive-behavioral including skills to increase self-esteem, and develop adaptive coping skills to deal with stigma when it is encountered.

Perspective-taking is a treatment approach that has been used to increase empathy of observers toward people in pain. Within experimental paradigms, observers are asked to imagine the thoughts, feelings, or emotions of those experiencing pain. For example, in an experiment where a group of undergraduates and registered nurses were asked to take the perspective of Black and White patients, those in the perspective-taking group showed less racial treatment bias compared to those in a control group. Being reminded to take perspectives of others could be a powerful influencer on how providers make treatment recommendations for patients with chronic pain (Drwecki, Moore, Ward, & Prkachin, 2011; see also Chap. 3). Similar findings have been demonstrated in romantic couples undergoing a laboratory pain stimulus. In one study, the perspective-taking group was told to imagine how their partner (who was putting their hand in a cold bath) felt and what emotions they might be feeling. In this perspective-taking group, compared to a control group (that received only a description of the task), partners expressed more empathy, and participants reported less pain and perceived greater validation from their partner (Leong, Cano, Wurm, Lumley, & Corley, 2015).

Future Research Agenda

In this chapter, we explore a number of individual and interpersonal processes that can influence interactions about pain and the subsequent pain experience. Expectations, stigma, and validation are three potentially modifiable individual processes that may influence and be influenced by interactions with an observer. In turn, empathy and attitude implicit bias are observer processes that may influence the individual's experience of chronic pain and its treatment. At present, there have been very few interventions to address these individual or interpersonal processes for individuals with chronic pain. However, relevant studies of communication and expectancy interventions have been conducted in acute pain, general medical, and other chronic conditions.

Here we outline several key recommendations that will extend future intervention research in this area:

A Developmental Approach Is Needed to Address Individual and Interpersonal Processes that Influence Pain

Both social communication skills and the influence and impact of social experiences change over the life span. As one example, during adolescence and young adulthood, peer and romantic relationships increase in importance. Developmentally informed opportunities exist to intervene that are tailored to particular social communication needs across the life span. A recent pilot study to develop and test the feasibility, acceptability, and impact of a tailored peer mentorship program for young adults with chronic pain (Ahola Kohut et al., 2016; Stinson et al., 2016) is illustrative. This program provided modeling and reinforcement by peers (trained young adults with chronic pain who have learned to successfully manage their pain) to enhance independence around self-management of chronic pain in adolescents and young adults. Similarly, couple interventions may meet important developmental needs in middle or older adulthood. Future research is needed to capitalize on knowledge of developmental changes and social needs across the life span.

Research is Needed to Link Theories of Social Communication in Pain to Specific Intervention Targets

We reviewed several potentially modifiable targets (expectations, stigma, validation, attitude implicit bias, and empathy); however, with the exception of expectancy interventions, other intervention strategies delivered to date have not been tightly linked to these targets. Often interventions address broad goals of education, knowledge, and communication, which might not be specific enough to lead to change in these targeted individual and interpersonal processes. In a similar vein, outcome measures that reflect these individual and interpersonal processes in addition to other pain-related outcomes also need to be included in intervention studies to understand specific treatment effects. We encourage research that is linked to theories of social communication in the development of interventions and measurement of outcomes to address individual and interpersonal processes.

Promising Interventions Tested in Other Medical Populations May be Applied to Chronic Pain

As reviewed, there have been promising interventions intended to address provider communication and stigma in general medical and mental health populations that could be adapted and applied to chronic pain. Particularly drawing from the research base in mental health and cancer, it will be important for researchers to understand similarities and differences in the needs of individuals with chronic pain and relevant observers to these other populations in order to tailor interventions.

Studies of Basic Communication Patterns Between Providers and Patients are Needed to Guide Interventions

There is a gap in understanding of basic patterns of communication that are associated with optimal outcomes for patients with chronic pain. Ideally, such studies can capture both the content and patterns of communication between providers and patients during medical visits for chronic pain. Following patients longitudinally will provide novel insight into the impact of communication patterns on patient response and adherence to pain treatment. This research is expected to guide interventions with increased specificity for targeting communication patterns that maximize patient response.

In conclusion, there are many opportunities available for developing and implementing therapeutic interventions that could lead to change in individual and interpersonal processes in the chronic pain experience. The field is ripe for research on basic social communication processes to guide interventions as well as for translation of interventions from other fields to chronic pain.

References

Ahola Kohut, S., Stinson, J. N., Ruskin, D., Forgeron, P., Harris, L., van Wyk, M., … Campbell, F. (2016). iPeer2Peer program. *Pain, 157*(5), 1146–1155. https://doi.org/10.1097/j.pain.0000000000000496

Alaloul, F., Williams, K., Myers, J., Jones, K. D., & Logsdon, M. C. (2015). Impact of a script-based communication intervention on patient satisfaction with pain management. *Pain Management Nursing, 16*(3), 321–327. https://doi.org/10.1016/j.pmn.2014.08.008

Ashton-James, C. E., Richardson, D. C., Williams, A. C., Bianchi-Berthouze, N., & Dekker, P. H. (2014). Impact of pain behaviors on evaluations of warmth and competence. *Pain, 155*(12), 2656–2661. https://doi.org/10.1016/j.pain.2014.09.031

Bandstra, N. F., Chambers, C. T., McGrath, P. J., & Moore, C. (2011). The behavioural expression of empathy to others' pain versus others' sadness in young children. *Pain, 152*(5), 1074–1082. https://doi.org/10.1016/j.pain.2011.01.024

Torres, C. A., Bartley, E. J., Wandner, L. D., Alqudah, A. F., Hirsh, A. T., & Robinson, M. E. (2013). The influence of sex, race, and age on pain assessment and treatment decisions using virtual human technology: A cross-national comparison. *Journal of Pain Research, 6,* 577. https://doi.org/10.2147/JPR.S46295

Boerner, K. E., Chambers, C. T., Craig, K. D., Pillai Riddell, R. R., & Parker, J. A. (2013). Caregiver accuracy in detecting deception in facial expressions of pain in children. *Pain, 154*(4), 525–533. https://doi.org/10.1016/j.pain.2012.12.015

Brownstein, M. (2016). *Implicit bias.* Retrieved September 27, 2016, from http://plato.stanford.edu/archives/spr2016/entries/implicit-bias/

Bucchioni, G., Fossataro, C., Cavallo, A., Mouras, H., Neppi-Modona, M., & Garbarini, F. (2016). Empathy or ownership? Evidence from corticospinal excitability during pain observation. *Journal of Cognitive Neuroscience, 28,* 1–12. https://doi.org/10.1162/jocn_a_01003

Calpin, P., Imran, A., & Harmon, D. (2017). A comparison of expectations of physicians and patients with chronic pain for pain clinic visits. *Pain Practice, 17*(3), 305–311. https://doi.org/10.1111/papr.12428

Cano, A., Barterian, J. A., & Heller, J. B. (2008). Empathic and nonempathic interaction in chronic pain couples. *The Clinical Journal of Pain, 24*(8), 678–684. https://doi.org/10.1097/AJP.0b013e31816753d8

Clement, S., Lassman, F., Barley, E., Evans-Lacko, S., Williams, P., Yamaguchi, S., Slade, M., Rusch, N., & Thornicroft, G. (2013). Mass media interventions for reducing mental health-related stigma. *Cochrane Database Syst Rev,* (7), Cd009453.https://doi.org/10.1002/14651858.CD009453.pub2

Cormier, S., Lavigne, G. L., Choinière, M., & Rainville, P. (2016). Expectations predict chronic pain treatment outcomes. *Pain, 157*(2), 329–338. https://doi.org/10.1097/j.pain.0000000000000379

Craig, K. D. (2009). The social communication model of pain. *Canadian Psychology, 50*(1), 22–32. https://doi.org/10.1037/a0014772

De Ruddere, L., & Craig, K. D. (2016). Understanding stigma and chronic pain. Pain, 157(8), 1607–1610. https://doi.org/10.1097/j.pain.0000000000000512

Dore, R. A., Hoffman, K. M., Lillard, A. S., & Trawalter, S. (2014). Children's racial bias in perceptions of others' pain. *British Journal of Developmental Psychology, 32*(2), 218–231. https://doi.org/10.1111/bjdp.12038

Drwecki, B. B., Moore, C. F., Ward, S. E., & Prkachin, K. M. (2011). Reducing racial disparities in pain treatment: The role of empathy and perspective-taking. *Pain, 152*(5), 1001–1006. https://doi.org/10.1016/j.pain.2010.12.005

Eccleston, C. (2013). A normal psychology of everyday pain. *International Journal of Clinical Practice. Supplement, 178,* 47–50. https://doi.org/10.1111/ijcp.12051

Eccleston, C., Wastell, S., Crombez, G., & Jordan, A. L. (2008). Adolescent social development and chronic pain. *European Journal of Pain, 12*(6), 765–774.

Fabi, S., & Leuthold, H. (2016). Empathy for pain influences perceptual and motor processing: Evidence from response force, ERPs, and EEG oscillations. *Social Neuroscience, 12*(6), 701–716. 10.1080/17470919.2016.1238009

Forgeron, P. A., Evans, J., McGrath, P. J., Stevens, B., & Finley, G. A. (2013). Living with difference: Exploring the social self of adolescents with chronic pain. *Pain Research & Management, 18*(6), e115–e123.

Gagliardi, A. R., Légaré, F., Brouwers, M. C., Webster, F., Badley, E., & Straus, S. (2015). Patient-mediated knowledge translation (PKT) interventions for clinical encounters: A systematic review. *Implementation Science, 11*(1), 26. https://doi.org/10.1186/s13012-016-0389-3

Geisser, M. E., & Roth, R. S. (1998). Knowledge of and agreement with chronic pain diagnosis: Relation to affective distress, pain beliefs and coping, pain intensity, and disability. *Journal of Occupational Rehabilitation, 8*(1), 73–88. https://doi.org/10.1023/a:1023060616201

Goldstein, P., Shamay-Tsoory, S. G., Yellinek, S., & Weissman-Fogel, I. (2016). Empathy predicts an experimental pain reduction during touch. *The Journal of Pain., 17,* 1049. https://doi.org/10.1016/j.jpain.2016.06.007

Goubert, L., Craig, K. D., Vervoort, T., Morley, S., Sullivan, M. J. L., de C Williams AC, Cano, A., & Crombez, G. (2005). Facing others in pain: the effects of empathy. *Pain, 118*(3), 285–288. 10.1016/j.pain.2005.10.025

Guite, J. W., Kim, S., Chen, C.-P., Sherker, J. L., Sherry, D. D., Rose, J. B., & Hwang, W.-T. (2014). Treatment expectations among adolescents with chronic musculoskeletal pain and their parents before an initial pain clinic evaluation. *The Clinical Journal of Pain, 30*(1), https://doi.org/10.1097/AJP.0b013e3182851735

Gustafsson, M., & Borglin, G. (2013). Can a theory-based educational intervention change nurses' knowledge and attitudes concerning cancer pain management? A quasi-experimental design. *BMC Health Services Research, 13*(328). https://doi.org/10.1186/1472-6963-13-328

Hall, W. J., Chapman, M. V., Lee, K. M., Merino, Y. M., Thomas, T. W., Payne, B. K., … Coyne-Beasley, T. (2015). Implicit racial/ethnic Bias among health care professionals and its influence on health care outcomes: A systematic review. *American Journal of Public Health, 105*(12), e60–e76. https://doi.org/10.2105/AJPH.2015.302903

Hampton, S. B., Cavalier, J., & Langford, R. (2015). The influence of race and gender on pain management: A systematic literature review. *Pain Management Nursing, 16*(6), 968–977. https://doi.org/10.1016/j.pmn.2015.06.009

Hirsh, A. T., Hollingshead, N. A., Ashburn-Nardo, L., & Kroenke, K. (2015). The interaction of patient race, provider Bias, and clinical ambiguity on pain management decisions. *The Journal of Pain, 16*(6), 558–568. https://doi.org/10.1016/j.jpain.2015.03.003

Hollingshead, N. A., Matthias, M. S., Bair, M. J., & Hirsh, A. T. (2015). Impact of race and sex on pain management by medical trainees: A mixed methods pilot study of decision making and awareness of influence. *Pain Medicine, 16*(2), 280–290. https://doi.org/10.1111/pme.12506

Jordan, A. L., Eccleston, C., & Osborn, M. (2007). Being a parent of the adolescent with complex chronic pain: An interpretative phenomenological analysis. *European Journal of Pain, 11*(1), 49.

Kamper, S. J., Dissing, K. B., & Hestbaek, L. (2016). Whose pain is it anyway? Comparability of pain reports from children and their parents. *Chiropractic & Manual Therapies, 24*(1), 24. https://doi.org/10.1186/s12998-016-0104-0

Kodjebacheva, G. D., Sabo, T., & Xiong, J. (2016). Interventions to improve child-parent-medical provider communication: A systematic review. *Social Science & Medicine, 166*, 120–127. https://doi.org/10.1016/j.socscimed.2016.08.003

Kong, J., Kaptachuk, T. J., Polich, G., Kirsch, I. V., Vangel, M., Zyloney, C., … Gollub, R. (2009). An fMRI study on the interaction and dissociation between expectation of pain relief and acupuncture treatment. *NeuroImage, 47*(3), 1066–1076. https://doi.org/10.1016/j.neuroimage.2009.05.087

Kool, M. B., van Middendorp, H., Lumley, M. A., Bijlsma, J. W. J., & Geenen, R. (2013). Social support and invalidation by others contribute uniquely to the understanding of physical and mental health of patients with rheumatic diseases. *Journal of Health Psychology, 18*(1), 86–95. https://doi.org/10.1177/1359105312436438

Leonard, M. T., Issner, J. H., Cano, A., & Williams, A. M. (2013). Correlates of spousal empathic accuracy for pain-related thoughts and feelings. *The Clinical Journal of Pain, 29*(4), 324–333. https://doi.org/10.1097/AJP.0b013e3182527bfd

Leong, L. E. M., Cano, A., Wurm, L. H., Lumley, M. A., & Corley, A. M. (2015). A perspective-taking manipulation leads to greater empathy and less pain during the cold pressor task. *The Journal of Pain, 16*(11), 1176–1185. https://doi.org/10.1016/j.jpain.2015.08.006

Livingston, J. D., & Boyd, J. E. (2010). Correlates and consequences of internalized stigma for people living with mental illness: A systematic review and meta-analysis. *Social Science & Medicine, 71*(12), 2150–2161.

Logan, D. E., Catanese, S. P., Coakley, R. M., & Scharff, L. (2007). Chronic pain in the classroom: Teachers? Attributions about the causes of chronic pain. *Journal of School Health, 77*(5), 248–256. https://doi.org/10.1111/j.1746-1561.2007.00200.x

Logan, D. E., Coakley, R. M., & Scharff, L. (2006). Teachers' perceptions of and responses to adolescents with chronic pain syndromes. *Journal of Pediatric Psychology, 32*(2), 139–149. https://doi.org/10.1093/jpepsy/jsj110

Majdandžić, J., Amashaufer, S., Hummer, A., Windischberger, C., & Lamm, C. (2016). The selfless mind: How prefrontal involvement in mentalizing with similar and dissimilar others shapes empathy and prosocial behavior. *Cognition, 157*, 24–38. https://doi.org/10.1016/j.cognition.2016.08.003

Martire, L. M., Schulz, R., Helgeson, V. S., Small, B. J., & Saghafi, E. M. (2010). Review and meta-analysis of couple-oriented interventions for chronic illness. *Annals of Behavioral Medicine, 40*(3), 325–342. https://doi.org/10.1007/s12160-010-9216-2

Martire, L. M., Schulz, R., Keefe, F. J., Rudy, T. E., & Starz, T. W. (2008). Couple-oriented education and support intervention for osteoarthritis: Effects on spouses' support and responses to patient pain. *Families, Systems, & Health, 26*(2), 185–195. https://doi.org/10.1037/1091-7527.26.2.185

McParland, J. L., Eccleston, C., Osborn, M., & Hezseltine, L. (2011). It's not fair: An interpretative phenomenological analysis of discourses of justice and fairness in chronic pain. *Health, 15*(5), 459–474. https://doi.org/10.1177/1363459310383593

Medical Definition of Empathy. (n.d.). Retrieved September 27, 2016, from http://www.merriam-webster.com/dictionary/empathy

Mehta, N., Clement, S., Marcus, E., Stona, A.-C., Bezborodovs, N., Evans-Lacko, S., … Thornicroft, G. (2015). Evidence for effective interventions to reduce mental health-related stigma and discrimination in the medium and long term: Systematic review. *The British Journal of Psychiatry, 207*(5), 377–384. https://doi.org/10.1192/bjp.bp.114.151944

Mischkowski, D., Crocker, J., & Way, B. M. (2016). From painkiller to empathy killer: Acetaminophen (paracetamol) reduces empathy for pain. *Social Cognitive and Affective Neuroscience, 11*(9), 1345–1353. https://doi.org/10.1093/scan/nsw057

Moon, E. C., Chambers, C. T., Larochette, A.-C., Hayton, K., Craig, K. D., & McGrath, P. J. (2008). Sex differences in parent and child pain ratings during an experimental child pain task. *Pain Research & Management, 13*(3), 225–230.

Moore, P. M., Rivera Mercado, S., Grez Artigues, M., & Lawrie, T. A. (2013). Communication skills training for healthcare professionals working with people who have cancer. In P. M. Moore (Ed.), *Cochrane database of systematic reviews*. Chichester, UK: Wiley. https://doi.org/10.1002/14651858.CD003751.pub3

Morris, M. C., Walker, L., Bruehl, S., Hellman, N., Sherman, A. L., & Rao, U. (2015). Race effects on temporal summation to heat pain in youth. *Pain, 156*(5), 917–922. https://doi.org/10.1097/j.pain.0000000000000129

Newton-John, T. R., & de C Williams, A. C. (2006). Chronic pain couples: Perceived marital interactions and pain behaviours. *Pain, 123*(1), 53–63. 10.1016/j.pain.2006.02.009

Nicholas, M. K., Asghari, A., Corbett, M., Smeets, R. J. E. M., Wood, B. M., Overton, S., … Beeston, L. (2012). Is adherence to pain self-management strategies associated with improved pain, depression and disability in those with disabling chronic pain? *European Journal of Pain, 16*(1), 93–104. https://doi.org/10.1016/j.ejpain.2011.06.005

Noel, M., Beals-Erickson, S. E., Law, E. F., Alberts, N., & Palermo, T. M. (2016). Characterizing the pain narratives of parents of youth with chronic pain. *The Clinical Journal of Pain, 32*, 849. https://doi.org/10.1097/AJP.0000000000000346

Palermo, T. M., Law, E. F., Fales, J., Bromberg, M. H., Jessen-Fiddick, T., & Tai, G. (2016). Internet-delivered cognitive-behavioral treatment for adolescents with chronic pain and their parents. *Pain, 157*(1), 174–185. https://doi.org/10.1097/j.pain.0000000000000348

Peerdeman, K. J., van Laarhoven, A. I. M., Keij, S. M., Vase, L., Rovers, M. M., Peters, M. L., & Evers, A. W. M. (2016). Relieving patients' pain with expectation interventions. *Pain, 157*(6), 1179–1191. https://doi.org/10.1097/j.pain.0000000000000540

Racine, M., Tousignant-Laflamme, Y., Kloda, L. A., Dion, D., Dupuis, G., & Choinière, M. (2012). A systematic literature review of 10 years of research on sex/gender and experimental pain perception – Part 1: Are there really differences between women and men? *Pain, 153*(3), 602–618. https://doi.org/10.1016/j.pain.2011.11.025

Reid, M. C. (2016). Expanding targets for intervention in later life pain. *Clinics in Geriatric Medicine, 32*(4), 797–805. https://doi.org/10.1016/j.cger.2016.06.009

Rhodes, L. A., McPhillips-Tangum, C. A., Markham, C., & Klenk, R. (1999). The power of the visible: The meaning of diagnostic tests in chronic back pain. *Social Science & Medicine, 48*(9), 1189–1203.

Riley, J. L., Cruz-Almeida, Y., Glover, T. L., King, C. D., Goodin, B. R., Sibille, K. T., … Fillingim, R. B. (2014). Age and race effects on pain sensitivity and modulation among middle-aged and older adults. *The Journal of Pain, 15*(3), 272–282. https://doi.org/10.1016/j.jpain.2013.10.015

Samolsky Dekel, B. G., Gori, A., Vasarri, A., Sorella, M. C., Di Nino, G., & Melotti, R. M. (2016). Medical evidence influence on inpatients and nurses pain ratings agreement. *Pain Research and Management, 2016*, 1–11. https://doi.org/10.1155/2016/9267536

Schäfer, G., Prkachin, K. M., Kaseweter, K. A., & Williams, A. C. de C. (2016). Health care providers' judgments in chronic. *Pain, 157*(8), 1618–1625. 10.1097/j.pain.0000000000000536

Schenk, L. A., Sprenger, C., Geuter, S., & Buchel, C. (2014). Expectation requires treatment to boost pain relief: An fMRI study. *Pain, 155*(1), 150–157. https://doi.org/10.1016/j.pain.2013.09.024

Schreiber, J. A., Cantrell, D., Moe, K. A., Hench, J., McKinney, E., Preston Lewis, C., Weir, A., & Brockopp, D. (2014). Improving knowledge, assessment, and attitudes related to pain management: Evaluation of an intervention. *Pain Management Nursing, 15*(2), 474–481. 10.1016/j.pmn.2012.12.006

Simons, L. E., Logan, D. E., Chastain, L., & Cerullo, M. (2010). Engagement in multidisciplinary interventions for pediatric chronic pain: Parental expectations, barriers, and child outcomes. *The Clinical Journal of Pain, 26*(4), 291–299. https://doi.org/10.1097/AJP.0b013e3181cf59fb

Solomon, P. (2001). Congruence between health professionals' and patients' pain ratings: A review of the literature. *Scandinavian Journal of Caring Sciences, 15*(2), 174–180. https://doi.org/10.1046/j.1471-6712.2001.00027.x

Stinson, J., Ahola Kohut, S., Forgeron, P., Amaria, K., Bell, M., Kaufman, M., … Spiegel, L. (2016). The iPeer2Peer program: A pilot randomized controlled trial in adolescents with juvenile idiopathic arthritis. *Pediatric Rheumatology, 14*(1), 48. https://doi.org/10.1186/s12969-016-0108-2

Trawalter, S., Hoffman, K. M., & Waytz, A. (2012). Racial bias in perceptions of others' pain. *PLoS One, 7*(11), e48546. https://doi.org/10.1371/journal.pone.0048546

Tsao, J. C. I., Meldrum, M., Bursch, B., Jacob, M. C., Kim, S. C., & Zeltzer, L. K. (2005). Treatment expectations for CAM interventions in pediatric chronic pain patients and their parents. *Evidence-based Complementary and Alternative Medicine, 2*(4), 521–527. https://doi.org/10.1093/ecam/neh132

Verbeek, J., Sengers, M. J., Riemens, L., & Haafkens, J. (2004). Patient expectations of treatment for back pain: A systematic review of qualitative and quantitative studies. *Spine (Phila Pa 1976), 29*(20), 2309–2318.

Vervoort, T., Caes, L., Crombez, G., Koster, E., Van Damme, S., Dewitte, M., & Goubert, L. (2011). Parental catastrophizing about children's pain and selective attention to varying levels of facial expression of pain in children: A dot-probe study. Pain, 152(8), 1751–1757. https://doi.org/10.1016/j.pain.2011.03.015

Wandner, L. D., Heft, M. W., Lok, B. C., Hirsh, A. T., George, S. Z., Horgas, A. L., … Robinson, M. E. (2014). The impact of patients' gender, race, and age on health care professionals' pain management decisions: An online survey using virtual human technology. *International Journal of Nursing Studies, 51*(5), 726–733. https://doi.org/10.1016/j.ijnurstu.2013.09.011

Waugh, O. C., Byrne, D. G., & Nicholas, M. K. (2014). Internalized stigma in people living with chronic pain. The Journal of Pain, 15(5), 550.e1–550550.e10. doi:https://doi.org/10.1016/j.jpain.2014.02.001

Zhou, H., Roberts, P., & Horgan, L. (2008). Association between self-report pain ratings of child and parent, child and nurse and parent and nurse dyads: Meta-analysis. *Journal of Advanced Nursing, 63*(4), 334–342. https://doi.org/10.1111/j.1365-2648.2008.04694.x

Zieger, B., Praskova, M., Busse, E., & Barth, M. (2013). A prospective randomised control study: Reduction of Children's pain expectation using a picture book during blood withdrawal. *Klinische Pädiatrie, 225*(3), 110–114. https://doi.org/10.1055/s-0033-1343481

Part IX
Conclusion

Chapter 23
Where We've Been, Where We're at, Where Do We Go from Here?

Kenneth M. Prkachin, Kai Karos, Tine Vervoort, and Zina Trost

Abstract The goal of this volume has been to bring together "state-of-the-science" narrative reviews of major directions in the study of social and interpersonal dimensions of pain. This final chapter takes a broad overview of the field, placing the individual contributions in context. It begins with a historical overview, situating the field of social/interpersonal influences on pain within the evolution of ideas about the psychology of pain. Key conceptual and empirical contributions arising from the individual chapters are identified. In the final section, important gaps in our knowledge are identified and directions for future research that we think have the potential to be very fruitful are given. Particular emphasis is placed on the value of expanding the domain of inquiry to incorporate social influences at a macro level.

Keywords Pain · Social influence · Interpersonal influence · History · Research directions

A recent general interest article for the magazine *Psychology Today* introduced the work of pain psychologists, observing that application of the concepts of psychology to the problems of pain might be seen as a surprising area of focus for

K. M. Prkachin (✉)
Department of Psychology, University of Northern British Columbia,
Prince George, BC, Canada
e-mail: Ken.Prkachin@unbc.ca

K. Karos
Research Group on Health Psychology, KU Leuven, Leuven, Belgium
e-mail: Kai.Karos@kuleuven.be

T. Vervoort
Department of Experimental-Clinical and Health Psychology, Ghent University,
Ghent, Belgium
e-mail: Tine.Vervoort@ugent.be

Z. Trost
Department of Psychology, University of Alabama at Birmingham, Birmingham, AL, USA
e-mail: Ztrost1@uab.edu

psychology. What should be surprising is the idea that application of the concepts and methods of psychology and related fields in the social, behavioral, and biological sciences would surprise anyone at this time in the development of pain science and care. Observations highlighting the influence of variables regarded as the subject matter of psychology—for example, the situational contexts in which pain occurs (Beecher, 1959)—can be found distributed across the scientific literature for more than a century, albeit sporadically. The Gate Control Theory (Melzack & Wall, 1965), which was a revolutionary advance in large part because of its recognition of the crucial importance of "higher" central nervous system processes—i.e., motivation, affect, and cognition, is more than 50 years old. Methods of treatment for pain that target behavioral, affective, and cognitive changes and which arise from psychological conceptualization are almost as venerable (Fordyce, Fowler, Lehman, & DeLateur, 1968; Turk, Meichenbaum, & Genest, 1983). There is consensus that access to cognitive-behavioral treatments should be considered a best practice for many clinical settings of pain. Perusal of any issue of the journal *Pain* since its inception should be enough to establish that psychological approaches are common and a core feature of the field.

From its historical origins, the field of pain psychology has matured to a point at which sub-specialties have become recognizable. The present volume is the first to comprehensively survey the existing literature on the psychology of pain as viewed through a social-interpersonal lens, which has evolved to be recognized as a foundational dimension to pain scholarship and care. In this final chapter we take a long view of the field, placing it within a historical context, highlighting key empirical and conceptual contributions to emerge from this literature, and pointing to what we consider to be fruitful future directions under the headings, "Where we've been," "Where we're at," and "Where do we go from here?"

Where We've Been

Origins: Early behavioral approaches to pain. Psychological inquiry has historically skewed to the intrapersonal—toward characterizing the fundamental dimensions of individuals' pain experiences, such as their intensity, unpleasantness, endurability, and associated personal fear or anxiety, and explaining their determinants and variability in terms of intrapersonal processes (mental or physiological) or as the residue of experience navigating the physical and social environment. As psychological concepts began to be applied to the understanding of pain it was therefore natural that a similar approach predominated. Thus, early inquiry saw the emergence of basic process studies, such as Melzack and Scott's (1957) early work showing that early experiential deprivation diminished the pain response in dogs. Studies of basic perceptual processes in humans addressed issues such as the properties of the stimulus–response relationship for nociceptive stimulation, relative to that for other sensory modalities (Sternbach & Tursky, 1964; Stevens, 1961), the distinction between sensory and affective components of the pain experience

(Gracely, McGrath, & Dubner, 1978a) and their relative responsiveness to different interventions (Gracely, McGrath, & Dubner, 1978b; Gracely, Dubner, & McGrath, 1979). Experimental studies in humans documented the plasticity of pain responses to numerous influences such as suggestion (Clark & Goodman, 1974), placebo (Clark, 1969), personality traits (Dougher, 1979), affective states (Zelman, Howland, Nichols, & Cleeland, 1991), cognitive influences such as distraction and pain-related attention (McCaul & Haugtvedt, 1982), and so on.

The 1960s and 1970s witnessed the first significant application of mainstream psychological concepts to the problem of clinical pain, first with the emergence of the operant model (Fordyce, 1976; Fordyce et al., 1968). Based in a variant of Skinnerian behaviorism, the operant model had both an interpretive and an intervention component. It began with the now obvious but, for its time profound observation that we can only infer the existence and properties of pain by observing the behavior of the sufferer. If that is true, then it follows that behaviors that form the basis of our inferences about pain in others could, in principle, be responsive to any variable known to influence behavior. The behavioral theory prominent at the time, influenced by the powerful impact of operant conditioning, emphasized that behaviors can be controlled by their antecedents and their consequences. Applying this lens, the interpretive component of the behavioral model emphasized that, in certain circumstances, "pain behaviors" can come under the control of their consequences. The theory sensitized theorists and clinicians to the idea that pain behaviors could be strengthened by certain consequences that naturally follow when a person displays them, including positive reinforcement by social attention and reward, and negative reinforcement by the avoidance of further pain or other aversive consequences.

The interpretive component also provided a lens for framing interventions. If certain pain behaviors are increased by positive reinforcement, then disrupting the behavior-positive reinforcement contingency should diminish pain behaviors. If pain behaviors are being maintained by negative reinforcement, then interventions that diminish the effects of negative reinforcement should also diminish the behaviors. The conceptual clarity of the model and its apparent implications for clinical intervention, coupled with enthusiasm arising from the successes and growth of the behavior modification movement, led to its widespread adoption and application. This was abetted further by increasing awareness of the public health crisis posed by widespread chronic pain, prompting an accelerated development of the field of clinical pain psychology. The 1970s and 1980s also witnessed the rapid growth of cognitive-behavioral theory and its application to pain theory and intervention (Turk et al., 1983). Related to the behavioral model, cognitive-behavioral approaches introduced an expanded set of concepts, such as cognitive mediation of experience, catastrophic thinking, self-management, and self-efficacy to both pain science and treatment.

Both behavioral and cognitive-behavioral approaches have provided valuable insights into the determinants and effects of pain and have served as bases for intervention. However, their roots in classical intrapsychic and experiential models have not effectively facilitated (and may have in fact impeded) a comprehensive understanding of pain from a biopsychosocial perspective. For example, while the behavioral approach performed a service by drawing attention to the fact that observable changes in behavior are the universal basis for inferences about pain, it also (likely because of its epistemological roots in concepts of the arbitrariness of the operant and the equipotentiality of behavior) invoked a monolithic construct of "pain behavior." This was the idea that any pain behavior had a limited number of determinants, as reflected in the subordinate concepts of "respondent pain" (pain behaviors caused by injury) and "operant pain" (pain behaviors controlled by their consequences). Although some of the consequences posited to have a regulatory role included social responses to pain behaviors (such as expressions of sympathy or solicitousness on the part of those who witnessed pain) and thereby highlighted the importance of the proximate social environment, there was little to no recognition of the idea that different kinds of pain behaviors had markedly different functions or were differentially susceptible to similar determinants.

Empirical inquiry has increasingly demonstrated that, pain behavior is not a unitary construct: different pain behaviors have different functions (Martel & Sullivan, this volume, Chap. 5) pointing rather to an interplay of individual, motivational, temporal, and contextual factors. Further, more recent evidence (e.g., Clark, Leonard, Cano, & Pester; Vervoort & Trost, this volume, Chaps. 4 and 13) shows that there is great heterogeneity in the impact of observer responses. Indeed, observer responses have no universal a priori effect but depend on various other factors, such as sufferer characteristics and motivational factors (e.g., the current goals and needs of the observer or the sufferer. For example, people feel supported or validated by different type of responses, some responses are more helpful for some than others and these mediating perceptions can affect the outcomes of certain consequences to the expression of pain (Clark, Leonard, Cano, & Pester, this volume, Chap. 13). Moreover, there is not only heterogeneity across individuals but also across time. Just as needs and goals dynamically change across time, so does the impact of observer responses to pain.

Arguably, these early cognitive and behavioral perspectives may have had their greatest impact in drawing attention to the public elements of pain and raising curiosity about their structure, determinants and function. Why do people and other animals engage in several different kinds of behavior during or in relation to pain? Why do people respond to others in pain as they do, and what are the effects of those responses? What are the relationships among different types of pain-related behaviors? Systematic inquiry regarding these considerations set the stage for contemporary biopsychosocial conceptualizations of pain.

Emergence of a broader biopsychosocial perspective. Even before the rise of the aforementioned models, there had been conceptual approaches and individual observations highlighting the public aspects of pain and their social nature. In *The Expression of the Emotions in Man and Animals*, Darwin (1955/1872) described changes in behavior occasioned by the occurrence of pain, embedded within a broader discussion of phylogenetic continuities among emotional and motivational states. Largely ignored, Darwin's ideas relevant to the social dimension of pain were rediscovered during the emergence of the field of affective science in the latter part of the twentieth century. Although Darwin's descriptions are at variance with what empirical research has subsequently shown about how people behave when they are in pain, his inclusion of pain in one of the first scientific treatments of affective states and his emphasis of phylogenetic continuity across those states laid the foundation for more recent incorporation of evolutionary thinking into explanations of the social and interpersonal functions of pain (Williams & Kappesser, this volume, Chap. 1). Darwin's early application likewise highlights the continued relevance of comparative approaches to pain inquiry.

Elsewhere, there were isolated examples of empirical research that made use of specific publicly observable behaviors in the service of addressing basic scientific questions. For example, in a series of studies conducted in the 1930s and 1940s investigators such as Chapman and Jones (1944) made use of a behavior they termed the "pain reaction threshold" (defined as the point at which a potentially nociceptive stimulus would produce a narrowing of the outer canthus of the eyes) to evaluate pain sensitivity. Chapman and Jones used the pain reaction threshold as an endpoint because of what they believed to be its superior reliability relative to alternative ways of gauging pain sensitivity. Certain issues that have become the focus of contemporary pain research are already evident in that work. For example, Chapman and Jones argued that the pain reaction threshold was insensitive to conscious efforts on the part of the sufferer to suppress it—an issue that continues to receive attention (e.g., Craig, Hyde, & Patrick, 1991). Leventhal and Sharpe (1965) examined pain during childbirth, making use of a system for observing public behavior developed on a rational basis, and reporting that parity, reflecting experience with childbirth pain, was associated with a diminished behavioral response. Using more conventional methods for studying pain, such as measurement of experimental pain thresholds, others documented differences between ethnic groups (Sternbach, 1965; Wolff & Langley, 1968). Using ethnographic approaches social scientists such as Zborowski (1969) addressed the influence of broad cultural factors.

The direct impact of social and interpersonal contexts on aspects of pain was demonstrated in a program of studies by Craig and collaborators. Numerous experimental studies demonstrated that, when people experienced pain in the presence of another, their reactivity to that pain, as assessed by conventional evaluation methods such as measurements of pain threshold, tolerance, and subjective reports, came to resemble the other person's (Craig, 1986). These findings were significant in at least two specific ways. First, they drew attention to the malleability of reactions to pain, highlighting a social, interpersonal mechanism for their transmission. Second, they raised questions about the nature of social influence—were the effects of social modeling simply a kind of acquiescence to the social pressures of the situation—an artifact of the dependence of the methodology on measures known to be highly responsive to self-control and demand characteristics? Evidence began to suggest that such effects were broad in scope, extending to "hard" psychophysical indicators such as magnitude estimates and stimulus discriminability (Craig, Best, & Ward, 1975; Craig & Coren, 1975) and physiological reactions (Craig & Prkachin, 1978), thus running counter to the argument that the changes were superficial and reflected little of the fundamentals of pain.

Emphasis on the overt behavioral features of pain arising from the behavioral approach raised the question whether social influences could be demonstrated on actual overt pain-related behavior. Initial approaches to this question made use of judgment study methodology and focused on an overt behavior that is ubiquitous and captured relatively easily in natural or laboratory settings—facial expression. Recordings of people subjected to social influences were shown to judges who were asked to indicate, purely by observing facial expressions, how much pain the person was in. Results demonstrated that differences in pain intensity could be measured sensitively by relying on facial expression. These findings supported the conclusion that social influences on pain extended to this type of overt pain behavior. Basing measurement of the pain reaction on the perceptions of observers reinforced the idea that pain occurs in a social, interpersonal context, turning attention to the other component of the dyad—the observer of suffering (Prkachin & Craig, 1985; Prkachin, Currie, & Craig, 1983).

Influence of emotion theory. Broader trends in psychological science also began to influence the psychology of pain. In the late 1960s and 1970s, as psychology became more open to a range of concepts, the study of emotions experienced a renaissance. This renaissance was abetted by the rediscovery of Darwin's work on emotion with its emphasis on the adaptive properties of motivational and emotional states and their phylogenetic continuity. In developing his views on emotions, Darwin had emphasized the manner in which they are expressed across species. Extending his arguments to account for human emotions, this also led to a focus on facial expression. An evolutionary account views emotions and motivated states as adaptations to life conditions common to humans, leading to the expectation that their expressions would be consistent in form across cultures. This was a testable prediction which was taken up by Paul Ekman and colleagues in a series of studies examining judgments of facial expressions across cultures (Ekman, Sorenson, & Friesen, 1969; Ekman & Friesen, 1978). Although the conclusions continue to generate controversy (Gendron, Roberson, van der Vyer, & Barrett, 2014), results of these studies were seen as supporting the universality hypothesis and the broader evolutionary framework on emotion. More generally, these early studies, with their emphasis on facial expression as a vehicle for studying internal processes ordinarily considered as subjective states, contributed in a significant way to the emergence of theoretical perspectives in which facial expressions, their regulation, and social effects occupied a central position. Ekman's (2006) neurocultural model of emotion, for example, posits the existence of a limited number of "basic" emotions (happiness, surprise, sadness, anger, disgust, and fear), recognizable universally by their distinct facial appearance. They are subject to partial control by virtue of their regulation by voluntary and involuntary neural systems. This mixture of control systems provides a basis by which social and cultural processes, operating largely through interpersonal influences can modulate the expression of emotions through "display rules." This mechanism allows for circumstances in which people may suppress, exaggerate, modulate, or indeed, dissimulate affective states. This perspective came to have considerable influence as pain psychologists became interested in facial expression. Its impact continues to the present time as researchers persistently return to the relationship between pain expression and deception (Craig & Badali, 2004; Craig et al., 1991; Littlewort, Bartlett, & Lee, 2009; Prkachin, 1992a, 2005).

Emotion theory had even more profound influence on methodology. Although facial expressions have the advantage of being observable, they are complex, dynamic, and imbued with idiosyncratic meaning by observers, thus leading to substantial problems from the perspective of assessment and measurement. Emotion research struggled with this problem, which impeded progress. It was addressed by the development of a largely objective system for describing the facial actions contributing to emotion, the Facial Action Coding System (FACS; Ekman & Friesen, 1978; Ekman, Friesen, & Hager, 2002). The FACS permits observers to describe any visible action on the face in terms of the underlying muscular groups that produce it; 44 separate actions are identifiable.

The FACS was published and made broadly available around the same time that interest in facial expression and social influence was emerging among pain psychologists. It provided a way of addressing a question of fundamental importance: is there a distinct facial "signal" for pain and what does it look like? It was first applied to pain by LeResche (1982) who used it to characterize the facial expressions of candid photographs of people who had suffered grievous injuries. A series of studies in the 1980s and 1990s applied the FACS while assessing facial responses to various kinds of pain, both clinical and experimental (Craig & Patrick, 1985; Patrick, Craig, & Prkachin, 1986; Prkachin & Mercer, 1989; Prkachin, 1992b). Although there was some variation from study to study, a general pattern of consistency began to emerge, suggesting that pain experienced in several modalities produced a distinct expression characterized by a subset of facial actions. The chapter by Kunz, Karos, and Vervoort (this volume, Chap. 6) provides a detailed review and summary of findings in this area.

Contemporaneously, a similar model and logic began to be applied to the problem of pain in children. This work was driven by practical concerns. Young children in particular lack the verbal communication repertoire of most adults, including the ability to communicate sensitively and consistently about qualitative and intensive features of pain. Very young children cannot communicate verbally about pain at all. This places extra importance on alternative forms of evidence about pain experience, particularly in clinical contexts. A barrier that needed to be addressed in application of a system such as FACS is that, owing to their neuroanatomical immaturity and youthful skin, a system based on identification of changes to facial landmarks in adults cannot be transliterated to them directly. Variations on the FACS, based on its anatomical and non-inferential features and logic, such as BabyFACS (Oster, 2010) and the Neonatal Facial Coding System (NFCS: Grunau & Craig, 1987) were developed and validated for use with neonates and very young children and the Child Facial Coding System (CFCS; Gilbert et al., 1999) for use with older children. This work has been transformative in several respects, not least in showing the exquisite sensitivity of very young children to the effects of medical procedures; in the process contributing to the retreat of a view commonly held at the time that, because of the immaturity of their nervous systems, very young children did not experience pain in the same way as older children and adults. Relatedly, this work has contributed to improved attentiveness to the problems of pain control for children in clinical settings and has been extended to address similar concerns among other populations in which verbal communication about pain can be impaired (see Hadjistavropoulos & Gallant, Kunz et al., this volume, Chaps. 6 and 21).

A focus on how pain is expressed publicly inherently draws attention to its social nature. The behavioral model, with its focus on the regulation of pain behavior by its consequences placed further emphasis on the idea that pain often takes place in the context of dyadic and group social interaction. Evolutionary theory, too, draws attention to the reproductive fitness implications for the individual, kin, and social group of being able to control the behavior of others and of being susceptible to the influence of others by displaying a signal of suffering. Altogether, these concepts underscore the necessity of a comprehensive account that recognizes the existence of a biopsychosocial *pain communication system*. There have been several attempts to do so in the form of frameworks that identify key processes involved as pain is experienced by the individual, transformed and rendered into a behavioral expression which is registered, perceived, interpreted, and responded to by others. The first conceived of a system of beginning with an episode in which pain is experienced by an individual (Prkachin & Craig, 1995). That experience becomes encoded into a signal which is then broadcast into the social surround where it is registered and decoded by others present. Hadjistavropoulos and Craig (2002, 2004) later expanded on this framework, expanding the range of behaviors that could be understood within a communication framework. Hadjistavropoulos et al. (2011) have provided the most comprehensive iteration of a formal communication framework to date. The thrust of all these frameworks is that they take the kind of broad, "from the neuron of the sufferer to the structure of social relationships" sweep that characterizes the vast domain to which this volume is addressed.

Where We're at

This volume provides "state of the science" surveys of particular topical areas that have emerged written by recognized leaders in the field. In this section, we comment briefly on the core concepts or take-home messages that have emerged.

In her seminal 2002 paper, Amanda Williams was the first to formally apply the lens of evolutionary psychology to the social and interpersonal dimensions of pain, focusing on facial expression. That paper primarily reviewed the extant literature in terms of how it lined up against expectations arising out of evolutionary psychology such as evidence for the universality, distinctiveness, and consistency across time, stimuli, and cultures, controllability, and detectability by observers. Concluding that the evidence was encouraging, if often incomplete, Williams advocated more widespread application of contemporary evolutionary psychology concepts and offered an agenda for such research. Over the decade and a half since its publication, much of that agenda has been advanced, as attested by several of the reviews in this volume. In the present work, Williams and Kappesser (Chap. 1) go beyond the promissory note offered in the 2002 paper, highlighting the evidence for phylogenetic continuity in pain expression that has recently given rise to the development of novel approaches for assessing pain in other mammals, as also reviewed by Acland et al. (Chap. 10). Evolutionary psychology models can often be criticized for their post hoc nature—their ability to account for patterns of behavior after the fact by invoking scenarios of adaptiveness. A major contribution of the chapter by Williams and Kappesser is its description of the application of an "in silico" methodology, evaluating behavioral strategies involving injury, pain expression and agents interacting over simulated evolutionary time. This work provides a basis for understanding the circumstances under which pain may be expressed freely or be subject to one of several alternative self-modulation strategies.

For all the reasons outlined in the first section of this chapter, much of the research reported in this book has focused in one way or another on facial expression. Indeed, arguably, the study of facial expression in relation to pain is the best developed area within this field. Chap. 6, by Kunz et al., comprehensively reviews this work, focusing on some of the more recent developments showing how features of the social environment, social learning, and central control systems each affect the complexity with which pain is displayed. Additionally, this chapter reviews some of the limited information about how pain is communicated by other means and in other modalities and draws our attention to the need to better incorporate such behaviors into our thinking about the social and interpersonal nature of pain.

The complexity of pain-related behavior has been a factor limiting both scientific development and clinical application of knowledge in this field, just as the complexity of affective behavior has historically limited progress in the related field of emotion. The evolution of signals that allow others to infer pain is one adaptive answer to the challenge of managing its personal and interpersonal consequences. For humans, this is, in part, a problem of visual pattern recognition. Studies of pain expression have enabled us to learn something about what components of people's behavior are involved in communicating pain. At the same time, computer vision has made great strides in advancing understanding of visual pattern recognition (Cohn & De La Torre, 2015), leading to the question of whether we can advance understanding of and model pain communication with contemporary computer vision techniques. Chap. 7, by Hammall and Cohn, reviews the considerable progress that has been made in this field. As that chapter shows, the availability of rich data sets of recorded behavior, accompanied by precise behavioral measurement has made it clear that it is possible for computer vision systems to model the performance of trained human observers in detecting pain related behavior, at least in the face, and at least under ideal conditions. This development holds some promise of enabling more rapid growth of empirical research in the field and, indeed, of enabling studies that have heretofore been beyond the practical capabilities of human observers; for example, work on the temporal dynamics of pain behavior. Further, there are already several groups working on transforming this technology to develop systems for clinical pain assessment.

The availability of rich data sets, with recordings of pain-related behavior has also abetted the rapid growth of social neuroscience investigations, as reviewed in

Chap. 8 by Tremblay et al. As they point out, neuroimaging studies, many of which have made use of recording archives, have shown a striking correspondence between the patterns of cerebral activation observed when people experience pain first-hand and when they observe others in pain. Similar patterns of correspondence when people experience conditions of social exclusion and other distressing events have led, more recently, to conceptions of a more general sort under the rubric of "social pain," as reviewed by Karos (this volume, Chap. 9). The correspondences, though striking, are not without controversy. In particular, as both articles point out, there is a need for great caution when interpreting the psychological and social meanings imputed to them.

Similar caution is warranted when bridging the gap between animal models and humans, as proposed by Acland, Lidhar, and Martin (this volume, Chap. 10). There seems to be a striking similarity between humans and nonhuman animals (e.g., primates) in reactions to others' pain, including empathic responding, and as pointed out in Chap. 1 by Williams and Kappesser, in pain behavior and expression as well. Despite the challenges, this line of research highlights the importance of incorporating multidisciplinary methodology to unravel the dynamic interplay between pain experience, expression, and interpersonal context. Social psychology, evolutionary psychology, and neuroscience (among others) show great promise in enriching our understanding of the mechanisms underlying social modulation of pain.

Tremblay et al. (Chap. 8) point out further that much of the neuroimaging work on responses to others in pain is situated within the concept of empathy; yet empathy is not the inevitable response to witnessing suffering—a point also emphasized in a different way by Prkachin et al. (Chap. 11)—nor is pain the only affective state relevant to empathy. Their chapter ends with a nuanced overview of the numerous intrapersonal and contextual variables that have been shown to modify and modulate cerebral systems involved when we observe others in pain.

This complexity is also picked up at the behavioral level in the chapters by Martel and Sullivan (Chap. 5), De Ruddere and Tait (Chap. 6), Prkachin et al. (Chap. 11), Keogh (Chap. 20), and Drwecki (Chap. 21). Each of these treatments reviews lines of work based largely on studies of perceptual and decision-making processes of witnesses to pain. In documenting the numerous variables that have been shown to modify how people perceive the same behavioral evidence of pain—from the observer's prior exposure to suffering to the color of the sufferer's skin—this work underscores the stark fact underlying the subtitle to this book—we don't suffer alone—and foreshadows implications, both salubrious and potentially damaging, arising from the consequences of such perceptual differences.

Where Do We Go from Here?

The social dimension of pain has only recently received more widespread attention and the present book is another stepping stone in the maturation of this field. There is a wealth of opportunity for future research. The past years have seen exciting new research lines and conceptualizations which are just beginning to gather empirical support and help us to better understand the ways in which interpersonal context and the experience and communication of pain interact. We conclude this book with some suggested directions—both specific and general—that we think would be fruitful in advancing knowledge—both fundamental and applied—in this field.

A first step could be to integrate social context into existing influential models of acute and chronic pain that are already highly regarded in the field. For instance, current models emphasizing the social nature of pain such as the social communication model of pain (Craig, 2009, 2015), or the communal coping model (M. J.L. Sullivan, Martel, Tripp, Savard, & Crombez, 2006) should be updated to reflect recent developments in the field. Moreover, there is an increasing focus on motivational context in recent models of chronic pain, such as in current fear-avoidance models (Claes, Karos, Meulders, Crombez, & Vlaeyen, 2014; Crombez, Eccleston, Van Damme, Vlaeyen, & Karoly, 2012; Van Damme, Legrain, Vogt, & Crombez, 2010; Wiech & Tracey, 2013). Clearly, interpersonal needs and goals form an integral part of the motivational context and should, as highlighted by Vervoort and Trost (this volume, Chap. 4) be explicitly recognized as well. The realization that various goals, both of the person in pain and the observer, matter, has been the subject of recent conceptual proposals (see for example Vervoort & Trost, 2017; Wiech & Tracey, 2013). These proposals also call for an integration of several existing research lines in the field of pain, such as emotional, motivational, and interpersonal dimensions. A recent proposal to formally recognize the interpersonal dimension in the very definition of pain, alongside cognitive, affective, and sensory dimensions echoes the same goal (Williams & Craig, 2016).

Along similar lines, research into the interpersonal dimension of pain should not only be integrated into already existing research lines within the field, but other disciplines such as social psychology, social neuroscience, developmental psychology, or evolutionary psychology (to name just a few) should be further integrated into the field of pain research. Social psychology already puts a natural emphasis on the importance of social networks and interpersonal connection and boasts a long history of methodological and empirical findings that we now find to be more and more relevant to the experience and communication of pain. Some phenomena such as stereotyping, social exclusion and support, ostracism, stigmatization, perceptions of injustice, or validation have long been a topic of study in social psychology and are now increasingly a focus in pain research (Baumeister & Leary, 1995; De Ruddere, Bosmans, Crombez, & Goubert, 2016; De Ruddere & Craig, 2016; Miller, 2001a; Vervoort & Trost, 2016; Williams, 2016a, 2016b, 2007). In pursuing this line of inquiry, it will be important to recognize that an interpersonal focus should not be limited to the interaction of two individuals. Rather, investigation of social networks at different levels of analysis, ranging from the micro-level (e.g., dyads, small groups, family units) to the macro-level (e.g., countries, societies, cultures) will be necessary in order to develop a comprehensive framework of social influence. For instance, on a global cultural level, pain and injury can be conceptualized as violating a central tenet of social psychology and modern culture—belief in a just world (Lerner & Miller, 1978; McParland & Eccleston, 2013); the relevance of the justice motive is reflected in an exponentially growing literature supporting the deleterious impact of elevated injustice appraisals in response to pain and injury (Monden, Trost, Scott, Bogart, & Driver, 2016; Michael J L Sullivan, Scott, & Trost, 2012). Findings in this area have come to show that, in relation to non-minority counterparts, pain-related injustice appraisals are elevated among those who identify with traditionally marginalized minority racial/ethnic groups, and among individuals with fewer socioeconomic resources (Trost et al., 2015; Trost et al., under review). These findings suggest that injustice appraisals are filtered through a lens of chronic social inequity. In short, with a predominant focus on the individual, and some investigation at the micro-level, there is little research conceptualizing pain on a macro-level. We know surprisingly little about how larger systems (e.g., the healthcare system), society and culture affect the experience and communication of pain, and—as exemplified by research on ethnic/racial disparities in pain experience (Drwecki, this volume, Chap. 19; Green et al., 2003; Anderson, Green, & Payne, 2009) yet we have ample reason to believe that they do (De Ruddere & Craig, 2016; Hadjistavropoulos et al., 2011; Keogh, 2014). With (chronic) pain being a worldwide and almost universal burden, it is time to approach understanding its social dimensions on a commensurate scale.

Similarly, recent advances in social neuroscience raise interesting questions about underlying mechanisms of pain modulation by (social) context (Eisenberger, 2012, 2015). Moreover, there is a growing body of research aiming to find a representative neurological "signature" of pain (Davis, Racine, & Collett, 2012; Kucyi & Davis, 2016; Rogachov, Cheng, Erpelding, Hemington, & Crawley, 2016; Wager et al., 2013). Clearly such a signature, should it exist, will have to account for the complex modulation of pain experience by context in general, and interpersonal context in particular (Iannetti, Salomons, Moayedi, Mouraux, & Davis, 2013). In a similar vein, evolutionary psychology raises interesting questions about functionality and universality of the human pain experience. For instance, future research should focus on actively integrating concepts arising from research on humans and animals; domains which have thus far mainly coexisted in parallel. Research into communication of pain and pain behavior in general, especially in a social context, demonstrates a fascinating overlap between humans and nonhuman species such as mice (Mogil, 2015; Williams, 2002, 2016a). It also raises questions about universality within species (i.e., similarities and differences in pain communication across cultures) but also between species (i.e., what are the similarities and differences in pain behavior between humans and apes?). Evolutionary psychology provides an especially fruitful framework to facilitate translation of empirical findings between different disciplines about different cultures and species (Williams, 2016a, 2016b).

In this context, it is worth pointing out that, despite the comparatively large number of studies that have been conducted to characterize the behaviors (primarily facial) that communicate information about pain, there has yet to be a single investigation that realistically addresses one of the most fundamental questions in the field—a question arising from evolutionary psychology that has been central to much of the field of emotion, namely, "Are there human universals in the ways in which pain is communicated and perceived?" We also do not have adequate answers to the obverse question—"What are the cultural differences in how pain is expressed and perceived?" Admittedly, it is increasingly difficult to address such questions easily in an increasingly globalized world and in a climate of political and cultural sensitivity around such issues. Yet similar questions continue to be addressed in other areas (Gendron et al., 2014; Tracy & Robins, 2008), with both negative and positive results.

The social-interpersonal dimension of pain is brought into focus especially when one considers the ways in which the witness to suffering perceives and responds to the evidence of suffering in the other and many of the chapters in this volume focus specifically on this latter, "decoding" phase of social communication models. These models, and the research emanating from them, have been largely influenced by a framing of scenarios in terms of empathy, caretaking and support-seeking. Several chapters in this volume have pointed out that prosocial tendencies, feelings, and behaviors are not the inevitable response when an observer is confronted with someone in pain. Certain scenarios in which the natural response to a sufferer may be neutral or even decidedly antisocial also occur. Yet we know almost nothing directly about the factors predicting or determining those kinds of reactions. Vervoort and Trost (this volume, Chap. 4) provide some direction toward an accounting for such variability in terms of observers' goals in the context of pain-related transactions. What we do know is that antisocial and invalidating reactions to others pain can have several detrimental consequences for the person in pain such as social exclusion and stigmatization (Cohen, Quintner, Buchanan, Nielsen, & Guy, 2011; De Ruddere et al., 2016; Williams, 2016a, 2016b), pain underestimation (Kappesser & de C Williams, 2008), anger and aggression (Karos, Meulders, Goubert, & Vlaeyen, 2017; Miller, 2001b), ultimately affecting pain and recovery itself (Piotrowski, 2014; Michael J L Sullivan et al., 2009).There is a pressing need for research that explores these issues directly—research that could have profound implications for human development, personnel selection, and public policy.

Several of the chapters in this volume surveyed literature demonstrating personological and contextual influences on how evidence of pain in others is perceived. Much of that literature demonstrates that how evidence of pain is perceived is highly plastic and subject to numerous biasing influences. Indeed, one of the most widely studied phenomena is the so-called underestimation bias in which observers tend to perceive the sufferer to be in less pain than the sufferer herself. The many findings of the malleability of perceptions of others' pain are important to know about, and raise concerns about their implications for future behavior on the part of the witness, the quality of the interaction between sufferer and witness, and the outcome of the transaction. Yet most of our knowledge stops at the level of the perception of the observer. Few studies have explored the next level of interaction—the actual behavior of the observer—and even fewer have addressed what is perhaps the bigger question: "What is the outcome?" (Prkachin, Kaseweter, & Browne, 2015). (Exceptions include the work described by Constantin, Moline, and McMurtry (this volume, Chap. 14) on the observer's own nonverbal reactions to the sufferer and emerging research on responses to communications of pain (Cano & Goubert, 2017)), which has begun to document some of the positive consequences of validation.) Studies investigating the actual behaviors associated with perceptions of others' pain and of the distal consequences with which they are associated, such as health-care outcomes and quality of life, though difficult to design and conduct, are desperately needed in order to complete the picture.

Lastly, developmental psychology puts a similar emphasis on the bigger picture: The experience and communication of pain does not only differ as a function of the individual, or the context, but also across time. Pain is inherently dynamic and so is its context. A large body of research demonstrates (see for example Heathcote, Vervoort, & Noel; Caes, Goubert, & Simons; and Gennis & Pillai-Ridell, this volume, Chaps. 15, 16, and 17) that pain in children and adolescents is very different from, and yet incredibly influential for, pain in adulthood or older age. Childhood is a particularly sensitive time. Children are highly dependent upon care from others, whose responses, in turn, contribute to defining how a child expresses and experiences pain.

In general, then, our goal has to be expansion and integration. We need to expand our understanding of what pain is, how it is modulated, and how it is expressed. We need to expand the different levels of analysis, with a focus beyond an individual in pain but also incorporating its context, be it social, motivational, societal, or cultural. Along the same lines, there is a great need for the study of different populations (e.g., species, culture, age, gender). Similarly, we need to realize that a focus on a singular dimension (i.e., affective, cognitive, sensory, or social) will per definition be shortsighted and not lead to a full account of what pain actually is. While such a focus might be fruitful in the context of empirical endeavors, there is a desperate need to integrate these numerous levels of analyses into a bigger picture. To this end it is crucial to actively integrate different lines within pain research but also welcome differing disciplines outside the field of pain research. In this sense, the current book can be understood as a passionate plea for a true embrace of the biopsychosocial model of pain and its implications.

References

Anderson, K. O., Green, C. R., & Payne, R. (2009). Racial and ethnic disparities in pain: Causes and consequences of unequal care. *The Journal of Pain, 10*(12), 1187–1204. https://doi.org/10.1016/j.jpain.2009.10.002

Baumeister, R. F., & Leary, M. R. (1995). The need to belong: Desire for interpersonal attachments as a fundamental human motivation. *Psychological Bulletin, 117*(3), 497–529. https://doi.org/10.1037/0033-2909.117.3.497

Beecher, H. K. (1959). *Measurement of subjective responses: Quantitative effects of drugs.* New York: Oxford University Press.

Cano, A.-M., & Goubert, L. (2017). What's in a name: The case of emotional disclosure of pain-related distress. *Journal of Pain, 18*, 881–888.

Chapman, W. P., & Jones, C. (1944). Variations in cutaneous and visceral pain sensitivity in normal subjects. *Journal of Clinical Investigation, 23*, 81–91.

Claes, N., Karos, K., Meulders, A., Crombez, G., & Vlaeyen, J. W. S. (2014). Competing goals attenuate avoidance behavior in the context of pain. *The Journal of Pain : Official Journal of the American Pain Society, 15*, 1–10. https://doi.org/10.1016/j.jpain.2014.08.003

Clark, W. C. (1969). Sensory-decision theory analysis of the placebo effect on the criterion for pain and thermal sensitivity (d'). *Journal of Abnormal Psychology, 74*, 363–371.

Clark, W. C., & Goodman, J. S. (1974). Effects of suggestion on d' and C(x) for pain detection and pain tolerance. *Journal of Abnormal Psychology, 83*, 364–372.

Cohen, M., Quintner, J., Buchanan, D., Nielsen, M., & Guy, L. (2011). Stigmatization of patients with chronic pain: The extinction of empathy. *Pain Medicine, 12*(11), 1637–1643. https://doi.org/10.1111/j.1526-4637.2011.01264.x

Cohn, J. F., & De la Torre, F. (2015). Automated face analysis for affective computing. In R. A. Calvo, S. K. D'Mello, J. Gratch, & A. Kappas (Eds.), *Handbook of affective computing* (pp. 131–150). New York, NY: Oxford.

Craig, K. D. (1986). Social modeling influences: Pain in context. In R. A. Sternbach (Ed.), *The psychology of pain* (2nd ed., pp. 67–96). New York: Raven Press.

Craig, K. D. (2009). The social communication model of pain. *Canadian Psychology/Psychologie Canadienne, 50*(1), 22–32. https://doi.org/10.1037/a0014772

Craig, K. D. (2015). Social communication model of pain. *Pain, 156*(7), 1198–1199. https://doi.org/10.1097/j.pain.0000000000000185

Craig, K. D., & Badali, M. A. (2004). Introduction to the special series on the detection of pain deception and malingering. *Clinical Journal of Pain, 20*, 377–382.

Craig, K. D., Best, H., & Ward, L. M. (1975). Social modeling influences on psycho-physical judgments of electrical stimulation. *Journal of Abnormal Psychology, 84*, 366–373.

Craig, K. D., & Coren, S. (1975). Signal detection analyses of social modeling influences on pain expressions. *Journal of Psychosomatic Research, 19*, 105–112.

Craig, K. D., Hyde, S. A., & Patrick, C. J. (1991). Genuine, suppressed and faked facial behavior during exacerbation of chronic low back pain. *Pain, 46*, 161–172.

Craig, K. D., & Patrick, C. J. (1985). Facial expression during induced pain. *Journal of Personality and Social Psychology, 44*, 1080–1091.

Craig, K. D., & Prkachin, K. M. (1978). Social modeling influences on sensory decision theory and psychophysiological indexes of pain. *Journal of Personality and Social Psychology, 36*(8), 805–815.

Crombez, G., Eccleston, C., Van Damme, S., Vlaeyen, J. W. S., & Karoly, P. (2012). Fear-avoidance model of chronic pain: The next generation. *The Clinical Journal of Pain, 28*(6), 475–483. https://doi.org/10.1097/AJP.0b013e3182385392

Darwin, C. (1955; originally published 1872). *The expression of the emotions in man and animals*. New York: Philosophical Library.

Davis, K. D., Racine, E., & Collett, B. (2012). Neuroethical issues related to the use of brain imaging: Can we and should we use brain imaging as a biomarker to diagnose chronic pain? *Pain, 153*(8), 1555–1559. https://doi.org/10.1016/j.pain.2012.02.037

De Ruddere, L., Bosmans, M., Crombez, G., & Goubert, L. (2016). Patients are socially excluded when their pain has no medical explanation. *The Journal of Pain, 17*(9), 1028–1035. https://doi.org/10.1016/j.jpain.2016.06.005

De Ruddere, L., & Craig, K. D. (2016). Understanding stigma and chronic pain. *Pain, 157*(8), 1. https://doi.org/10.1097/j.pain.0000000000000512

Dougher, M. J. (1979). Sensory decision theory analysis of the effects of anxiety and experimental instructions on pain. *Journal of Abnormal Psychology, 88*, 137–144.

Eisenberger, N. I. (2012). The pain of social disconnection: Examining the shared neural underpinnings of physical and social pain. *Nature Reviews. Neuroscience, 13*(6), 421–434. https://doi.org/10.1038/nrn3231

Eisenberger, N. I. (2015). Social pain and the brain: Controversies, questions, and where to go from Here. *Annual Review of Psychology, 66*(1), 601–629. https://doi.org/10.1146/annurev-psych-010213-115146

Ekman, P. (2006). Cross-cultural studies of facial expression. In P. Ekman (Ed.), *Darwin and facial expression: A century of research in review* (pp. 169–222). Malor: Los Altos, CA.

Ekman, P., & Friesen, W. V. (1978). *Manual for the facial action coding system*. Palo Alto, CA: Consulting Psychologists Press.

Ekman, P., Friesen, W. V., & Hager, J. C. (2002). *Facial action coding system: Manual and investigator's guide*. Salt Lake City, UT: Research Nexus.

Ekman, P., Sorenson, E. R., & Friesen, W. V. (1969). Pan-cultural elements in facial displays of emotion. *Science, 164*, 86–88.

Fordyce, W. E. (1976). *Behavioral methods for chronic pain and illness*. St. Louis: Mosby.

Fordyce, W. E., Fowler, R. S., Lehman, J. F., & DeLateur, B. J. (1968). Some implications of learning in problems of chronic pain. *Journal of Chronic Diseases, 21*, 171–190.

Gendron, M., Roberson, D., van der Vyer, J. M., & Barrett, L. F. (2014). Perceptions of emotion from facial expression are not culturally universal: Evidence from a remote culture. *Emotion, 14*, 251–262.

Gilbert, C. A., Lilley, C. M., Craig, K. D., McGrath, P. J., Court, C. A., Bennett, S. M., & Montgomery, C. J. (1999). Postoperative pain expression in preschool children: Validation of the child facial coding system. *Clinical Journal of Pain, 15*, 192–200.

Gracely, R. H., Dubner, R., & McGrath, P. A. (1979). Narcotic analgesia: Fentanyl reduces the intensity but not the unpleasantness of painful tooth-pulp stimulation. *Science, 203*, 1261–1263.

Gracely, R. H., McGrath, P., & Dubner, R. (1978a). Ratio scales of sensory and affective verbal pain descriptors. *Pain, 5*, 5–18.

Gracely, R. H., McGrath, P., & Dubner, R. (1978b). Validity and sensitivity of ratio scales of sensory and affective verbal pain descriptors: Manipulation of affect by diazepam. *Pain, 5*, 19–29.

Green, C. R., Anderson, K. O., Baker, T. A., Campbell, L. C., Decker, S., Fillingim, R. B., … Vallerand, A. H. (2003). The unequal burden of pain: Confronting racial and ethnic disparities in pain. *Pain Medicine, 4*(3), 277–294. https://doi.org/10.1046/j.1526-4637.2003.03034.x

Grunau, R. V. E., & Craig, K. D. (1987). Pain expression in neonates: Facial action and cry. *Pain, 28*, 395–410.

Hadjistavropoulos, T., & Craig, K. D. (2002). A theoretical framework for understanding self-report and observational measures of pain: A communications model. *Behaviour Research and Therapy., 40*, 551–570.

Hadjistavropoulos, T., & Craig, K. D. (2004). Social influences and the communication of pain. In T. Hadjistavropoulos & K. D. Craig (Eds.), *Pain: Psychological perspectives* (pp. 87–112). New York, NY: Lawrence Erlbaum.

Hadjistavropoulos, T., Craig, K. D., Duck, S., Cano, A., Goubert, L., Jackson, P. L., … Fitzgerald, T. D. (2011). A biopsychosocial formulation of pain communication. *Psychological Bulletin, 137*(6), 910–939. https://doi.org/10.1037/a0023876

Iannetti, G. D., Salomons, T. V., Moayedi, M., Mouraux, A., & Davis, K. D. (2013). Beyond metaphor: Contrasting mechanisms of social and physical pain. *Trends in Cognitive Sciences, 17*(8), 371–378. https://doi.org/10.1016/j.tics.2013.06.002

Kappesser, J., & de C Williams, A. C. (2008). Pain judgements of patients' relatives: Examining the use of social contract theory as theoretical framework. *Journal of Behavioral Medicine, 31*(4), 309–317. https://doi.org/10.1007/s10865-008-9157-4

Karos, K., Meulders, A., Goubert, L., & Vlaeyen, J. W. S. (2017). The influence of social threat on pain, aggression, and empathy in women. *Journal of Pain, 19*(3), 291–300. https://doi.org/10.1016/j.jpain.2017.11.003

Keogh, E. (2014). Gender differences in the nonverbal communication of pain: A new direction for sex, gender, and pain research? *Pain, 155*(10), 1927–1931. https://doi.org/10.1016/j.pain.2014.06.024

Kucyi, A., & Davis, K. D. (2016). The neural code for pain: From single-cell electrophysiology to the dynamic pain connectome. *The Neuroscientist, 23*, 397. https://doi.org/10.1177/1073858416667716

LeResche, L. (1982). Facial expression in pain: A study of candid photographs. *Journal of Nonverbal Behavior, 7*, 46–56.

Lerner, M. J., & Miller, D. T. (1978). Just World Research and the Attribution Process: Looking Back and Ahead. *Psychological Bulletin, 85*, 1030–1051.

Leventhal, H., & Sharpe, E. (1965). Facial expressions as indicators of distress. In S. S. Tomkins & C. E. Izard (Eds.), *Affect, cognition, and personality* (pp. 296–318). New York: Springer.

Littlewort, G. C., Bartlett, M. S., & Lee, K. (2009). Automatic detection of facial expressions displayed during posed and genuine pain. *Image and Vision Computing, 27*, 1797–1803.

McCaul, K. D., & Haugtvedt, C. (1982). Attention, distraction, and cold-pressor pain. *Journal of Personality and Social Psychology, 43*, 154–162.

McParland, J. L., & Eccleston, C. (2013). "It's not fair": Social justice appraisals in the context of chronic pain. *Current Directions in Psychological Science, 22*(6), 484–489. https://doi.org/10.1177/0963721413496811

Melzack, R., & Scott, T. H. (1957). The effects of early experience on the response to pain. *Journal of Comparative and Physiological Psychology, 50*, 155–161.

Melzack, R., & Wall, P. D. (1965). Pain mechanisms: A new theory. *Science, 150*, 971–979.

Miller, D. T. (2001a). Disrespect and the experience of injustice. *Annual Review of Psychology, 52*, 527–553.

Miller, D. T. (2001b). Disrespect and the experience of injustice. *Annual Review of Psychology, 52*(1), 527–553. https://doi.org/10.1146/annurev.psych.52.1.527

Mogil, J. S. (2015). Social modulation of and by pain in humans and rodents. *Pain, 156*(4), S33–S41. https://doi.org/10.1097/01.j.pain.0000460341.62094.77

Monden, K. R., Trost, Z., Scott, W., Bogart, K. R., & Driver, S. (2016). The unfairness of it all: Exploring the role of injustice appraisals in rehabilitation outcomes. *Rehabilitation Psychology, 61*(1), 44–53. https://doi.org/10.1037/rep0000075

Oster, H. (2010). *Baby FACS: Facial action coding system for infants and young children.* New York: New York University Press.

Patrick, C. J., Craig, K. D., & Prkachin, K. M. (1986). Observer judgements of acute pain: Facial action determinants. *Journal of Personality and Social Psychology, 50*, 1291–1298.

Piotrowski, C. (2014). Chronic pain patients and loneliness: A systematic review of the literature. In *Loneliness in life: Education, business, society.* New York: McGraw Hill.

Prkachin, K. M. (1992a). Dissociating deliberate and spontaneous expressions of pain. *Pain, 51*, 57–65.

Prkachin, K. M. (1992b). The consistency of facial expressions of pain: A comparison across modalities. *Pain, 51*, 297–306.

Prkachin, K. M. (2005). Effects of deliberate control on verbal and facial expressions of pain. *Pain, 114*, 328–338.

Prkachin, K. M., & Craig, K. D. (1985). Influencing nonverbal expressions of pain: Signal detection analyses. *Pain, 21*, 399–409.

Prkachin, K. M., & Craig, K. D. (1995). Expressing pain: The communication and interpretation of facial pain signals. *Journal of Nonverbal Behavior, 19*, 191–205.

Prkachin, K. M., Currie, N. A., & Craig, K. D. (1983). Judging nonverbal expressions of pain. *Canadian Journal of Behavioral Science, 15*, 409–421.

Prkachin, K. M., Kaseweter, K. A., & Browne, M. E. (2015). Understanding the suffering of others: The sources and consequences of third-person pain. In G. Pickering & S. Gibson (Eds.), *Pain, emotion and cognition: A complex nexus* (pp. 53–72). New York: Springer.

Prkachin, K. M., & Mercer, S. (1989). Pain expression in patients with shoulder pathology: Validity, coding properties and relation to sickness impact. *Pain, 39*, 257–265.

Rogachov, A., Cheng, J. C., Erpelding, N., Hemington, K. S., & Crawley, A. P. (2016). Regional brain signal variability: a novel indicator of pain sensitivity and coping. *Pain., 157*(11), 2483–2492.

Sternbach, R. A., & Tursky, B. (1965). Ethnic differences among housewives in psychophysical and skin potential responses to electric shock. *Psychophysiology, 1*, 241–246.

Sternbach, R. A., & Tursky, B. (1964). On the psychophysical power function in electric shock. *Psychonomic Science, 1*, 217–218.

Stevens, S. S. (1961). To honor Fechner and to repeal his law. *Science, 133*, 80–86.

Sullivan, M. J. L., Martel, M. O., Tripp, D., Savard, A., & Crombez, G. (2006). The relation between catastrophizing and the communication of pain experience. *Pain, 122*(3), 282–288. https://doi.org/10.1016/j.pain.2006.02.001

Sullivan, M. J. L., Scott, W., & Trost, Z. (2012). Perceived injustice: A risk factor for problematic pain outcomes. *The Clinical Journal of Pain, 28*(6), 484–488. https://doi.org/10.1097/AJP.0b013e3182527d13

Sullivan, M. J. L., Thibault, P., Simmonds, M. J., Milioto, M., Cantin, A.-P., & Velly, A. M. (2009). Pain, perceived injustice and the persistence of post-traumatic stress symptoms during the course of rehabilitation for whiplash injuries. *Pain, 145*(3), 325–331. https://doi.org/10.1016/j.pain.2009.06.031

Tracy, J. L., & Robins, R. W. (2008). The nonverbal expression of pride: Evidence for cross-cultural recognition. *Journal of Personality and Social Psychology, 94*, 516–530.

Trost, Z., Agtarap, S., Scott, W., Driver, S., Guck, A., Reynolds, M., … Warren, A. M. (2015). Perceived injustice after traumatic injury: Associations with pain, psychological distress, and quality of life outcomes 12 months after injury. *Rehabilitation Psychology, 60*(3), 213–221. https://doi.org/10.1037/rep0000043

Turk, D. C., Meichenbaum, D. E., & Genest, M. (1983). *Pain and behavioral medicine: A cognitive behavioral perspective*. New York: Guilford Press.

Van Damme, S., Legrain, V., Vogt, J., & Crombez, G. (2010). Keeping pain in mind: A motivational account of attention to pain. *Neuroscience and Biobehavioral Reviews, 34*(2), 204–213. https://doi.org/10.1016/j.neubiorev.2009.01.005

Vervoort, T., & Trost, Z. (2016). The interpersonal function of pain. *Pain, 157*(4), 773–774. https://doi.org/10.1097/j.pain.0000000000000438

Vervoort, T., & Trost, Z. (2017). Examining affective-motivational dynamics and behavioral implications within the interpersonal context of pain. *Journal of Pain, 18*(10), 1174–1183. https://doi.org/10.1016/j.jpain.2017.03.010

Wager, T. D., Atlas, L. Y., Lindquist, M. a., Roy, M., Woo, C.-W., & Kross, E. (2013). An fMRI-based neurologic signature of physical pain. *New England Journal of Medicine, 368*(15), 1388–1397. https://doi.org/10.1056/NEJMoa1204471

Wiech, K., & Tracey, I. (2013). Pain, decisions, and actions: A motivational perspective. *Frontiers in Neuroscience, 7*(April), 1–12. https://doi.org/10.3389/fnins.2013.00046

Williams, A. C. (2002). Facial expression of pain: An evolutionary account. *The Behavioral and Brain Sciences, 25*(4), 439–88. Retrieved from http://www.ncbi.nlm.nih.gov/pubmed/12879700

Williams, A. C. (2016a). What can evolutionary theory tell us about chronic pain? *Pain, 157*(4), 788–790. https://doi.org/10.1097/j.pain.0000000000000464

Williams, A. C. (2016b). Defeating the stigma of chronic pain. *Pain, 157*(8), 1. https://doi.org/10.1097/j.pain.0000000000000530

Williams, A. C., & Craig, K. D. (2016). Updating the definition of pain. *Pain, 157*(11), 2420–2423. https://doi.org/10.1097/j.pain.0000000000000613

Williams, K. D. (2007). Ostracism. *Annual Review of Psychology, 58*, 425–452. https://doi.org/10.1146/annurev.psych.58.110405.085641

Wolff, B. B., & Langley, S. (1968). Cultural factors and the response to pain: A review. *American Anthropologist, 70*, 494–501.

Zborowski, M. (1969). *People in pain*. San Francisco: Jossey-Bass.

Zelman, D. C., Howland, E. W., Nichols, S. N., & Cleeland, C. S. (1991). The effects of induced mood on laboratory pain. *Pain, 46*, 105–111.

Index

Printed by Printforce, the Netherlands